publication for public health nurses. It later became the **Public Health Nursing Quarterly.**

1909 Mary E. Mahoney, the first professional black nurse, addressed the first conference of the National Association of Colored Graduate Nurses.

1910 Teachers College, Columbia University, New York City, established the first courses in a university for graduate nurses preparing for work in public health nursing.

"The public health movement did not create the public health nurse, it found her at work in her district, nursing the sick, watching over families and the neighborhood, and teaching in the homes those sanitary practices, those measures of personal and home hygiene which do much to prevent disease and promote health." (Adelaide Nutting, Professor and Chairman, Teacher's College, Columbia University)

1912 The National Organization of Public Health Nursing was established. Lillian D. Wald was the first president.

1914–1916 NOPHN worked closely with public health organizations: American Public Health Association, American Social Hygiene Association, American Association for Organizing Societies for Charity. The cooperation of public health oriented agencies was supported by both nurses and non-nurses.

1919 The National Health Council was reorganized after WWI to promote public health among blacks in the south. NOPHN participated in conferences and made its consultation services available to black schools of nursing. NOPHN also provided assistance in organizing a course in public health nursing at Howard University.

1920 C.E.H. Winslow, Harry S. Mustard, and Mary Breckinridge directed rural health demonstration projects in Cattaraugus County, New York;

Rutherford County, Tennessee; and the Frontier Nursing Service, Kentucky, respectively. Urban health projects, the counterparts of the rural health project, were started in New York City. Both rural and urban projects involved public health nurses who received consultation from NOPHN.

1921 By this time fifteen colleges and universities offered courses in public health nursing.

1921–1929 The Sheppard Towner Act required that states use federal and matched funds "in promoting the welfare and hygiene of maternity and infancy." Public health nurses were employed with the funds available, and maternity and infancy nursing was included in generalized public health nursing. The American Medical Association lobbied for the discontinuation of the S-T Act, and it was *not* renewed.

1922 Annie M. Brainards's *The Evolution of Public Health Nursing* was published.

1923 The Goldmark Report, sponsored and funded by the Rockefeller Foundation, was published. It was a landmark in nursing similar to the Flexner report in medicine. Goldmark stated "From our field study of the nurse in public health nursing, in private duty, and as instructor and supervisor in hospitals it is clear that there is need of a basic undergraduate training for all nurses alike, which should lead to a nursing diploma."

1924 The Yale School of Nursing was the first in the world to be established as a separate university department with an independent budget and its own dean. The 28-month course led to a Bachelor of Nursing degree and included public health, community work, and hospital service.

1926 NOPHN developed the **"Public Health Nursing Manual"** which was utilized in most public health nursing activities.

(continued on inside back cover)

Family-Centered Nursing in the Community

FAMILY-CENTERED NURSING IN THE COMMUNITY

Barbara Bryan Logan, R.N., Ph.D., F.A.A.N.
Cecilia E. Dawkins, R.N., Ph.D.

 Addison-Wesley Publishing Company
Health Sciences Division, Menlo Park, California

Reading, Massachusetts • Don Mills, Ontario • Wokingham, UK
Amsterdam • Sydney • Singapore • Tokyo • Mexico City
Bogota • Santiago • San Juan

Sponsoring editor: Thomas Eoyang

Production: Mary Forkner, Publication Alternatives; Judith Johnstone

Book design: Wendy Calmenson

Cover design: Michael Rogondino

Manuscript editor: Jonas Weisel

Illustrations: Reese Thornton, Deborah Thornton

Library of Congress
Cataloging-in-Publication Data

Logan, Barbara Bryan
    Family-centered nursing in the community.

Includes bibliographies and index.
1. Community health nursing.   2. Family medicine.
I. Dawkins, Cecilia E. II. Title.
[DNLM: 1. Community Health Nursing.
2. Family—nurses' instruction.   WY 106 L831f]
RT98.L64   1986   610.73'43   85-30623

ISBN 0-201-12684-2

The authors and publishers have exerted every effort to ensure that drug selections and dosages set forth in this text are in accord with current recommendations and practice at the time of publication. However, in view of ongoing research, changes in government regulations, and the constant flow of information relating to drug therapy and drug reactions, the reader is urged to check the package insert for each drug for any change in indications of dosage and for added warnings and precautions. This is particularly important where the recommended agent is a new and/or infrequently employed drug.

BCDEFGHIJK-HA-89876

Addison-Wesley Publishing Company, Inc.
2725 Sand Hill Road
Menlo Park, California 94025

Dedicated to our children
Nneka Jamil Logan and Keith Chester Veal
and our husbands
Arthur R. Logan and Chester L. Veal

Preface

Contemporary Community Health Nursing Practice

We live in a climate of social, political, and cultural change. Nowhere in the health care delivery system do these changes have more immediate impact than on the nursing profession in general and community health nursing in particular. An awareness of these changes is essential to community health nurses in fulfilling their mission of health promotion and maintenance.

To maximize their effectiveness with clients—individuals, families, and communities—community health nurses must remain attuned to the social/economic climate in which they practice and to society-wide changes and issues that affect their clients as well as their practice. Client issues include the changing structure and composition of families such as the decline in nuclear family structures, the increase in unmarried couples living together with and without children, and the increase in single-headed and female-headed households. The increased number of cultural and ethnic groups inhabiting inner cities in less-than-desirable situations, the women's movement with increased awareness of career choices and life-styles, and an economy that leaves more and more families to cope with the consequences of unemployment and lower living standards all affect the practice of community health nursing.

In the health field other changes continue to influence how nursing care is given in the community. One change is the maldistribution of health care professionals such that some metropolitan and suburban areas are oversupplied with health care personnel while many rural and inner city areas have few or no health professionals or facilities. Variations in third-party payer reimbursement for services, the prospective payment system, and innovative developments in medical technology and modes of health care delivery have created challenges as well as opportunities for nurses practicing in community settings. Community health nurses must devise marketing strategies and innovative ways to provide health care services in a competitive marketplace while at the same time maintaining their long-standing commitment to provide health care to the indigent and other underserved populations.

Family-Centered Nursing in the Community addresses the issues in contemporary society that affect community health nursing, and it offers recommendations and strategies for meeting the challenges of contemporary practice.

Family-Centered Nursing Practice

Community health nursing has traditionally been the specialty of nurses charged with planning and delivering community health services to aggregates, primarily those groups at risk for health problems. It is individuals in families and smaller groups, however, who are the ultimate consumers of these services. Therefore, nurses and nursing students learning about community health nursing must maintain a dual perspective. On one hand, they must understand the principles and practices of health care delivery to aggregates and, on the other, they must attend to the impact of health care on the individuals and smaller groups within the community.

Community health nurses have long understood the primary importance of the health promotion and maintenance of families. We have long recognized the capacity of the family to buffer its members from stress and anxiety, to serve as a source of strength and comfort, to promote and sustain the health of its members as well as to care for them in illness. We have come to emphasize the family as the unit of care throughout our practice and have focused health care measures on the entire family even if an individual family member initiates the nurse-family contact.

The purpose of *Family-Centered Nursing in the Community* is to integrate the areas of family and community health into a family-focused community health nursing text. The book reflects contemporary trends and changes in the family, communities, and health policies, and it demonstrates the impact of these changes on community health nursing. The underlying themes of the book are:

1. An orientation toward health promotion and prevention of illness, rather than the management of disease.
2. A thorough and forward-looking application of the nursing process to community health nursing.
3. Experiences of cultural and ethnic groups who are disproportionately overrepresented in populations at risk to health problems.

These themes are developed in the following ways:

1. Prevention is the major focus of all the chapters dealing with community health nursing in specific settings or for specific problems. Most of the chapters in Parts 3 and 4 contain discussions of primary, secondary, and tertiary prevention strategies.
2. The nursing process is discussed as it specifically applies to families and communities. Assessment, nursing diagnosis, planning, implementation strategies, and evaluation are given thorough and current treatment in Part 2.
3. In addition to offering a full chapter on culture and ethnicity, the text integrates content on cultural and ethnic issues whenever appropriate.

Audience

Family-Centered Nursing in the Community is a community health nursing text intended for undergraduate and graduate nursing students, nurse educators, and nurses practicing in the community. While fully presenting the necessary theory base underlying community health nursing, the text has been written at a level appropriate for students in baccalaureate programs.

Organization and Content

The book is divided into four parts:

1. Concepts of Community Health Nursing
2. The Community Health Nursing Process
3. Family-Centered Community Health Nursing Practice
4. Contemporary Issues and Problems in Community Health Nursing

Part 1, the first six chapters, presents the theories and concepts relevant to the community, the family, and community and family health. Chapters on culture and ethnicity and on epidemiology are also presented. This part lays the theoretical foundation for the remainder of the book.

The nine chapters in Part 2 present community health nursing as an application of the nursing process. This part accurately reflects both the current status and the future directions of the community health nursing process—and, in particular, of community and family nursing diagnosis. Three strategies basic to community health nursing practice are discussed as modes of implementation.

Part 3 covers community health nursing as it affects the family in various groups and settings across the life span.

Part 4 addresses legal and ethical issues as well as four specific health problems of pressing importance to many communities: substance abuse, chronic mental illness, adolescent pregnancy, and family violence. This part ends with a discussion of health policies and how the community health nurse can affect positive change for families and communities by political action.

Pedagogy

This text is intended to be a complete learning tool. The following aids are designed to enhance student learning:

- **Chapter Outline**
- **Learning Objectives**
- **Case Examples with Marginal Commentary**
  These examples show the concrete application of theories, concepts, and principles, and they model the relevant analysis for the student.
- **Topics for Nursing Research** These topics are not restricted to the researchable problems suggested by the chapter content, but they also include more delimited activities—segments of the nursing research process—that students can reasonably pursue. These topics are intended to extend the student's grasp of the content and to promote nursing research as a clinical and professional *value*.
- **Study Questions** These multiple-choice questions focus on a review of the chapter content.

Answers are provided in the back of the book and are keyed by page number to the chapter content needed to answer the question.

Acknowledgements

We are deeply indebted to many individuals, each of whom contributed substantially to the formulation and preparation of this book. Although it would be impossible to thank all who have given their help and encouragement, we would be remiss if we did not acknowledge some of the invaluable assistance we received.

We are particularly grateful to the contributors for their commitment to this endeavor and enthusiastic willingness to share their expertise with the reader.

We acknowledge Helen K. Grace, R.N., Ph.D., for her wise counsel, especially at the crucial beginning of this endeavor as well as throughout the project.

We are grateful to Addison-Wesley for their tremendous support of this project. We are indebted to Nancy Evans for her contributions at the critically important planning stages and for introducing us to Thomas Eoyang, our sponsoring editor. Thomas Eoyang is a devoted friend of nursing. He provided us with continual encouragement, resources, and the benefit of his excellent professional journalistic skills. He was always there when we needed him.

We would also like to thank Mary Forkner, of Publication Alternatives, and Judith Johnstone, of Addison-Wesley, for their patience and acumen in the production of this book. Their skill and judgment were instrumental in making this a timely and attractive publication.

We are grateful to the many individuals who provided secretarial support throughout the project.

We acknowledge the numerous community health nurses who informally shared their ideas with us in the development of the book and we appreciate their encouragement.

We wish to thank the following nurse educators, who reviewed the manuscript of this text at various stages and offered many helpful criticisms and suggestions:

Cheryl Anderson, Hurst, Texas

Joan Arnold, Adelphi University, Garden City, New York

Anne Benson, Northern Arizona University, Flagstaff

Sister Lucy Callaghan, University of Kansas, Kansas City

Anita Chesney, University of North Carolina, Greensboro

Maureen Cushing, Attorney-at-Law, Boston

Glenna Davenport-Cook, University of North Carolina, Charlotte

Barbara Fowler, Northern Kentucky University, Highland Heights

Evelyn R. Hayes, University of Delaware, Newark

Lee Ann Hoff, Northeastern University, Boston

Maureen Hull, Southeastern Massachusetts University, North Dartmouth

Judith Igoe, University of Colorado, Denver

Pearl Juris, Oregon Institute of Technology, Klamath Falls

Eleanor Lundeen, City College of New York

Patricia A. McAtee, University of Colorado, Denver

Alma Miles, Rush University, Chicago

Joan Mulligan, University of Wisconsin, Madison

Linda J. Perlich, University of Arizona, Tucson

Dorothy Petrowski, University of Wisconsin, Milwaukee

Linda Phillips, University of Arizona, Tucson

Susan Proctor, California State University, Sacramento

Phyllis Schubert, California State University, Fresno

Mary Schulze, University of Hartford, Connecticut

Ruth Stephenson, University of North Carolina, Charlotte

Marshelle Thobaben, Humboldt State University, Arcata, California

Joan Uhl, Seattle University

Mary Walker, University of Texas, Austin

Diann L. Zajac, Northern Kentucky University, Highland Heights

Finally, our gratitude is expressed to our families, particularly our husbands, Arthur R. Logan and Chester L. Veal, for their confidence, encouragement, and wise counsel throughout the period of this endeavor. They are truly our kindest critics and constant supporters.

Barbara Bryan Logan
Cecelia E. Dawkins

Contributors

Editors

Barbara Bryan Logan, R.N., Ph.D., F.A.A.N.
Associate Professor, Psychiatric Nursing
College of Nursing
University of Illinois at Chicago
Chicago, Illinois

Cecilia E. Dawkins, R.N., Ph.D.
Assistant Professor and Assistant Research
 Scientist, Community Health Nursing
School of Nursing
University of Michigan
Ann Arbor, Michigan

Contributors

Wealtha Yoder Alex, R.N., M.S.N.
Assistant Professor
Department of Nursing
Rockford College
Rockford, Illinois

Violet H. Barkauskas, R.N., Ph.D.
Associate Professor and Chairperson,
 Community Health Nursing
School of Nursing
University of Michigan
Ann Arbor, Michigan

Linda Bernhard, R.N., M.S.N.
Doctoral Candidate
College of Nursing
University of Illinois at Chicago
Chicago, Illinois

Nancy J. Brent, R.N., M.S., J.D.
Nurse—Attorney in solo law practice and
 Associate Professor of Nursing
St. Xavier College
Chicago, Illinois

Judith M. Cattron, R.N., M.S.
Assistant Professor, Public Health Nursing
College of Nursing
University of Illinois
Peoria, Illinois

Linda Chafetz, R.N., D.N.Sc.
Associate Professor, Mental Health and
 Community Nursing
School of Nursing
University of California, San Francisco
San Francisco, California

Shu-Pi Chen, R.N., Dr.PH.
Professor, Public Health Nursing
College of Nursing
University of Illinois at Chicago
Chicago, Illinois

Julia Cowell, R.N., Ph.D.
Assistant Professor, Public Health Nursing
College of Nursing
University of Illinois at Chicago
Chicago, Illinois

June Crayton, R.N., M.S.N.
Director, Nursing Services
Evangelical Health Systems
Bethany Hospital
Doctoral Candidate, University of Chicago
Chicago, Illinois

Alice Dan, Ph.D.
Associate Professor, Medical/Surgical Nursing
College of Nursing
University of Illinois at Chicago
Chicago, Illinois

Barbara Dancy, R.N., Ph.D.
Inpatient Clinical Psychologist
Malcolm Bliss Hospital Mental Health Center
St. Louis, Missouri

Linda Lee Daniel, R.N., M.N.
Associate Professor, Community Health Nursing
School of Nursing
University of Michigan
Ann Arbor, Michigan

Lucille Davis, R.N., Ph.D.
Associate Director, Graduate Programs in
    Nursing
Center for Nursing
Northwestern University
Chicago, Illinois

Nancy Dolphin, R.N., D.N.Sc.
Practitioner, Public Health Nursing
Durango, Colorado

Linda Edwards, R.N., Dr.P.H.
School Health Coordinator
Illinois Department of Public Health
Chicago, Illinois

Naomi E. Ervin, R.N., Ph.D.
Assistant Professor, Public Health Nursing
College of Nursing
University of Illinois at Chicago
Chicago, Illinois

Carol A. Frazier, R.N., Ph.D.
Chair, Department of Nursing
Simmons College
Boston, Massachusetts

Jean Gala, R.N., M.S.N.
Assistant Professor, Public Health Nursing
College of Nursing
University of Illinois
Peoria, Illinois

Beatrice Gilmore, R.N., M.S.N.
Chairman, Department of Nursing
Chicago State University
Chicago, Illinois

Helen Grace, R.N., Ph.D., F.A.A.N.
Program Director
W. K. Kellogg Foundation
Battle Creek, Michigan

Mary R. Haack, R.N., Ph.D.
Assistant Professor, Psychiatric Nursing
College of Nursing
University of Illinois at Chicago
Chicago, Illinois

Gertrude Hess, R.N., M.P.H.
Formerly Associate Professor, Public Health
    Nursing
College of Nursing
University of Illinois at Chicago
Chicago, Illinois

Robah Kellogg, R.N., M.P.H.
Associate Professor, Public Health Nursing
College of Nursing
University of Illinois
Peoria, Illinois

Carol Gorman Klint, R.N., M.S.
Administrator
Boon County Health Department
Belvidere, Illinois

Kathleen Knafl, Ph.D.
Professor, Psychiatric Nursing
College of Nursing
University of Illinois at Chicago
Chicago, Illinois

Rojean Madsen, Ph.D.
Assistant Professor
School of Urban Planning and Policy
University of Illinois at Chicago
Chicago, Illinois

Rose Odum, R.N., D.N.Sc., A.A.M.S.T.
Assistant Professor
School of Nursing
University of California, Los Angeles
Los Angeles, California

Nola J. Pender, R.N., Ph.D., F.A.A.N.
Professor of Community Health Nursing
Director, Health Promotion Research Program
School of Nursing
Northern Illinois University
DeKalb, Illinois

Dixie W. Ray, M.P.A.
Assistant Professor, Community Health Nursing
Indiana University School of Nursing
Indianapolis, Indiana

Clovis Semmes, Ph.D.
Assistant Professor, Black Studies Program
University of Illinois at Chicago
Chicago, Illinois

Iris Shannon, R.N., M.A.
Doctoral Candidate
School of Urban Planning and Policy
University of Illinois at Chicago
Chicago, Illinois

Denise Webster, R.N., Ph.D.
Assistant Professor, Psychiatric Nursing
College of Nursing
University of Illinois at Chicago
Chicago, Illinois

Contents

Part 2 The Community Health Nursing Process 153

Part 3   Family-Centered Community Health Nursing Practice   373

Chapter 20   Occupational Health 487

Chapter 21   Rural Health 515

Chapter 22   Women's Health 545

Chapter 23   Health of Older Adults 577

Part 4   Contemporary Issues and Problems in Community Health Nursing   609

Chapter 24   Legal and Ethical Issues in Family and Community Health Nursing 611

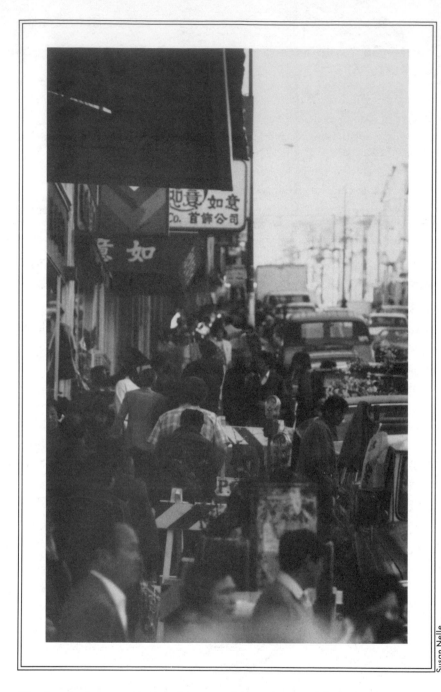

Susan Nelle

"By developing associations between the nursing model (person, environment, health, and nursing) and public health concepts, the specialty of community health nursing will be strengthened and a sound base for expanded practice roles can be established." (McKay R, Segall M: Methods and models for the aggregate. Nursing Outlook *(Nov/Dec) 1983; 31(6): 334.)*

Concepts of Community Health Nursing

Chapter 1

Community Health Nursing

Violet H. Barkauskas

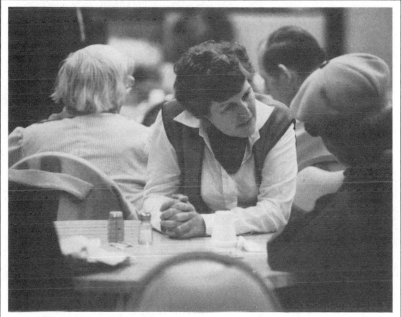

Community health nursing allows for intensive involvement with clients and their immediate environment, offering unique opportunities for meaningful interaction and participation in positive change.

Chapter Outline

Chapter Objectives

After completing this chapter, the reader will be able to:

- Differentiate community health nursing from the other specialty areas within nursing
- Describe community health nursing practice, using references from extant professional organization statements
- Explain the four predominant client groups of community health nurses
- Explain how the nursing process can be applied to the four predominant client groups of community health nurses
- Describe five different types of community health nursing roles
- Discuss three major issues in community health nursing practice

Community health nursing is an especially challenging and interesting specialty within nursing because its practice entails working with individuals, families, groups, and communities to solve health problems and meet needs basic to achieving optimal health. The work allows for intensive engagement over time, and that kind of substantive involvement offers unique opportunity for meaningful interaction and participation in positive client change and development.

Community health nursing is based on a synthesis of skills and knowledge from all the nursing specialties and from the public health sciences, which is then applied to clinical situations. In return, community health nursing provides its practitioners challenges to apply multiple skills in especially creative and independent ways. For example, community health nurses work with clients to maintain health and promote wellness in the clients' natural environments; in community agencies where they can collaborate with other professionals, community health nurses help promote and maintain the health of the whole community.

Distinguishing Characteristics of Community Health Nursing

Community health nurses functioning in various roles encounter their clients in a variety of settings. Their practice differs from others—especially nursing in acute care, institutional settings—in several ways:

- Nurses in acute care settings do not select their clients: patients are typically admitted to the institution by other health care professionals. Community health nurses have discretion in selecting clients for services and in determining the services those clients will receive. Thus, community health nursing practice is characterized by a high degree of autonomy and independence. The epidemiologic process serves as a basis to determine the groups who are at risk to health problems; community health nurses select clients from these target populations.
- Community health nurses' involvement with many clients extends over relatively long periods of time, affording frequent opportunity for continuity of care.
- The primary goals of community health nursing practice are health promotion and disease prevention. Although all nurses have these goals for clients, most nurses in acute care settings expend the major portion of efforts towards the management of human responses to pathophysiologic problems.
- Community health nursing practice requires not only assessment of clients and interventions directed to them, but also assessments of and interventions directed to clients' environments, including social, emotional, and physical environments. Further comparisons between nursing in the hospital and nursing in the community are presented in Table 1-1.

The Basic Unit of Service

The basic unit of service for community health nurses is the family. The family is important for several reasons. First, most individuals spend a large portion of their lives residing in family units. These units have potent influence on the habits and attitudes assumed by family members, such as food preferences, meal patterns, and methods of coping with stress and conflict. Thus, life-style change,

Table 1-1 Comparison of Hospital Nursing and Community Health Nursing

Hospital Nursing	Community Health Nursing
Focuses on the hospitalized patient	Focuses on families, community, and groups therein
Provides episodic nursing care	Provides distributive nursing care
Works with patients on specialty units of a hospital	Works with entire spectrum of health and illness conditions in many kinds of settings
Deals with one hospital or institution	Deals with all institutions, and community and world agencies
Coordinates care within the institution and with community nursing agency upon discharge of patient	Coordinates services provided by a variety of community agency personnel, both medical and nonmedical
Receives direction for medical therapeutics from prescriptions of physician	Receives limited direction for nursing services; medical authority distant and indirect unless in home health care category
Plans and provides individualized nursing care	Plans and provides family-centered nursing care
Limits patient autonomy within the hospital environment	Encourages family autonomy and control, except in cases of certain communicable diseases
Allows limited opportunities to observe family relationships or other indicators of health	Observes multiple factors in home environment that may change direction of health at any time
Restricts observation of typical family relationships since hospital is an artificial environment and patient is stripped of clothes and privacy	Facilitates observation of intimate relationships because usual behavior is not restricted
Limits relationships to other hospital personnel	Facilitates professional relationships with people in various disciplines other than medical; role is coordination of health care with a variety of professionals

SOURCE:
Adapted from Helvie et al, 1968 and Helvie, 1981 by JM Cattron, J Gala, and R Kellogg.

the area of most interest to community health nurses, often requires change for the family as a whole. Second, the family is a very important resource in the care of its members; for example, the parents are important caretakers of infants and children, and adult children are important resources in the care of elderly parents. Because the family is such an important and central client of community health nurses, a primary focus of this book is community health nursing practice with families. Practice with individuals, groups within communities, and communities will also be discussed because such care supports and complements care directed to families.

In this chapter and in this book the term *community health nurse* will be used as the designation for nurses in community-based practice, although the term is often used interchangeably with the term *public health nurse*. The two titles, community health nurse and public health nurse, are not always clearly differentiated and have been used to describe nurses in similar practices. Traditionally, the public health nurse title has been more closely related to nursing practice involving societal health concerns and the health of the total community or population groups at risk to health problems, especially when the services are rendered under the auspices of a governmental unit such as a local or state health department. The more recent title, community health nurse, has focussed on the health of the community as a whole, whether or not services are administered under the auspices of governmental bodies, as well as on personal health needs of individuals in communities. It has also become the more popular title. The controversy that has arisen over the use of the two terms will be discussed later in this chapter.

This chapter describes community health nursing as a subspecialty within the field of nursing. This description includes the history of the specialty, the current definition of the specialty, the conceptual bases for practice in the specialty, an overview of contemporary community health nursing roles and practice models, and a discussion of some of the issues that affect the practice.

Origins of Community Health Nursing

The past influences the present and provides valuable lessons for the future. Thus understanding the history of community health nursing is a prerequisite for fully understanding its current practice. The first section of this chapter contains a discussion of the origins of community health nursing. (For a more detailed discussion of the origins of community health nursing, the reader is referred to Kalisch and Kalisch, 1978, pp. 225–258, 365–408.)

Prior to 1900

Community health nursing has a rich history reflecting responsiveness to changing societal needs within the structure of organized health programs. Although the practice of providing care to the sick had long been an activity of religious groups, the first nonreligious organization to care for the sick was not founded until 1859. This original association was a visiting nurse service established by philanthropist William Rathbone in Liverpool, England. Mr. Rathbone's wife had received home care from a nurse during a terminal illness. Rathbone was so impressed by the care and comfort given his wife that he established a visiting nurse service for the sick poor. Mary Robinson, the first visiting nurse in Liverpool, not only cared for her sick patients, but also instructed their families in home care and general hygiene. From this program there evolved a district nurse concept in which a nurse was assigned to each of eighteen specific geographic districts within Liverpool.

In order to supply qualified nurses for district nursing, Rathbone, with the assistance of Florence Nightingale, established a training school in Liverpool. The graduates of this school, electing careers in district nursing, were called health nurses. These nurses were prepared both to care for the sick and also to provide environmental and preventive health care. An excerpt from Nightingale's *Notes on Nursing* (1859) describes an approach to health care that was unusual for its time and is still a challenge for current practice:

Minute inquiries into conditions enable us to know that in such a district, nay, in such a street, or even on one side of that street, in such a particular house, or even on one floor of that particular house will be an excess of mortality, that is, the person will die who ought not to have died before old age. . . . It is well known that the same names will be on workhouse books for generations, that is, the persons were born and brought up, and will be born and brought up, generation after generation in the conditions which make paupers. Death and disease are like the workhouse. They take from the same family, the same house, or in other words the same conditions. Why will we not observe what they are? (pp. 69–70)

Frances Root, an early graduate of the Bellevue Hospital School of Nursing in New York, initiated home care in New York City in 1817 in conjunction with the New York City Mission, a voluntary organization. Subsequent to this demonstration, visiting nurse associations were established in Buffalo in 1885 and in Boston and Philadelphia in the following year. Although the primary role of the early visiting nurses was the care of the sick in their homes, instruction to the families of the sick and to mothers and children was also a responsibility. The early visiting nurse associations relied on donations and patient fees to support services. Most associations brought in consumers as members of governing boards that directed the agencies and supervised the activities of nurses.

As the profession of nursing developed, the value of district nursing was recognized more broadly. In 1893 Lillian Wald formed a district nursing service in New York City administratively affiliated with the health department and supervised by nurses. Los Angeles was the first health department to directly employ nurses in 1898.

1900 to 1960

As nurses became more involved with individuals and families within communities, pressure grew for governments to become more accountable for the health of its citizens. By 1910 federal legislation mandated public health programs in all states. Specialized programs were developed in response to health needs and problems in such areas as infant welfare, school health, tuberculosis control, venereal disease control, and occupational health.

The first school health nurse was employed by the New York City Board of Education in 1902, and the specialty of school nursing grew rapidly.

Occupational health nursing was initiated in 1895, and communicable disease nursing followed in 1909. Maternal and child health was formalized as a nursing specialty in 1912.

A very important development occurred in 1909. Lillian Wald was instrumental in persuading the Metropolitan Life Insurance Company to reimburse home nursing services provided to its policyholders. Subsequently, other insurance companies also provided this benefit to policyholders. This early form of third-party reimbursement provided a solid financial basis for community nursing programs. Also, because this benefit was available to and utilized by families from all socioeconomic levels, visiting nurse services were no longer perceived as being only for the poor.

Prior to 1910 nurses were being prepared for community work through various formal and informal mechanisms. In 1910, faculty at Teacher's College, Columbia University developed the first academic program to prepare community health nurses. Yale University School of Nursing was the first to include community health nursing preparation for all baccalaureate students in 1923. However, it was not until after World War II that the National League for Nursing required community health nursing as a component of all accredited baccalaureate nursing curricula.

During the early days of community health nursing in the United States, nurses tended to work in specialized programs, particularly in public health departments, and the practice grew in parallel with program development within the public health departments. With the closer affiliation of nurses with health departments, the common descriptor for the field was public health nursing.

As the number of specialty service programs increased, nurses noted duplication of services as various nurses visited with multiple problems for different purposes. Subsequently, the notion of the family as the unit of service developed, and the trend from specialized to generalized services began.

During the early 1900s public health nurses had become a relatively influential group. In 1912 these nurses joined forces to become the National Organization for Public Health Nursing (NOPHN) with

Lillian Wald as the first president. This organization continued to be a strong voice for the specialty until 1952, when its membership voted for its dissolution and subsequent integration into the National League of Nursing. In 1975 a nurse historian (Fitzpatrick, 1975, p. 209) provided this summary of NOPHN's accomplishments: "It was perhaps the most progressive and socially aware group within organized nursing and was responsible for many of the innovations which helped to advance nursing towards professionalism. On a broader plane, it served to promote nursing as a major practice field within the framework of public health and contributed to many advances within that arena."

In 1918 the Rockefeller Foundation supported a research group called the Committee for the Study of Nursing Education. Their report, *Nursing and Nursing Education in the United States*, was published in 1923. Among other recommendations the report affirmed the need for the public health nursing services of teaching personal hygiene in the home, postgraduate (i.e., postdiploma) preparation for public health nursing, and collegiate education for nurses.

1960 to the Present

In the decades after World War II, baccalaureate educational programs increased and, consequently, so did the number of graduates qualified to work in public health nursing. Public health nursing became institutionalized in state, county, and city health departments, visiting nurse associations, and many other community-based health programs.

Several events during the 1960s had substantial impact on current public health nursing practice. First, preparation for public health nursing was required for baccalaureate educational program accreditation. Specialist preparation was no longer considered appropriate within post-RN or post-baccalaureate, certificate educational programs, but rather became a part of graduate degree programs. Second, a trend toward integrating public health nursing content into introductory courses for other specialty practices blurred the uniqueness of public

health nursing, particularly the community focus of care. Third, any nursing activity performed outside of an inpatient unit was considered by many to be public health nursing. The positive aspects of this latter development included increased awareness on the part of all nurses regarding the influences of family and community on health and wellness, and an increased accountability for discharge planning by hospital-based nurses. The unfortunate consequences included slowed development of the community-focused activities of the public health nurses, and a decreased prominence of the leadership in health-related social action as previously demonstrated by the early public health nurses.

During the mid-1960s to the mid-1970s, many new types of community-based workers were prepared for participation in programs developed in response to social problems in urban areas. The quality of urban life had deteriorated, and diffuse community development programs, including health programs, were proposed and implemented as solutions to those problems. Public health nurses were often participants in these programs. However, multidisciplinary programs were the norm. Therefore, it was difficult to differentiate nursing contributions from those of the total team. Although the multidisciplinary approach probably contributed to improved care, many of the contributions of public health nursing were not specifically documented.

As community-based practice became more common in nursing, the label "community health nursing" became more popular than "public health nursing." This occurred for several reasons. First, community-based health programs were being developed for a broad range of clients and from an expanded base of types of agencies. Whereas most health promotion and disease prevention programs had been provided through public health departments and directed to high-risk, low income families, newer programs were developed in many types of agencies for all types of persons. Because the nurses working in agencies other than public health nursing agencies were not technically public health nurses, and because some of them wanted to avoid the association with the poor, the label "community health nurse" became popular. Second, many public health nurses were concerned that the community and population focus of their role was becoming less prominent as many new types of health workers established roles in communities. Thus, even the nurses in public health departments often described themselves as community health nurses (Williams, 1976). The use of two labels for the same, as well as for sometimes different, practices has been a source of confusion in the specialty. The next section of this chapter includes a detailed discussion of this issue.

In 1965, an experiment was initiated that would eventually have a tremendous impact on nursing. Loretta C. Ford and Henry K. Silver initiated the first pediatric nurse practitioner program at the University of Colorado (Ford & Silver, 1967). The postbaccalaureate educational program was designed to assist public health nurses to augment their clinical skills in the care of children. After the first successful experiment, such nurse practitioner programs flourished. The scope of responsibility extended to virtually all types of ambulatory care clients. The nurse practitioner movement complemented the general nursing movement toward community-based care and multidisciplinary collaboration within health care programs, and it helped fulfill national priorities for comprehensive community health services.

The nurse practitioner movement was not and is not without its opponents. The predominant fear was that nurses would assume medical tasks and neglect the nursing care components of patient care—that is, they would be only physician substitutes.

Although graduate education in nursing had been in existence for over twenty years, the number of graduate programs in public health increased in the 1970s largely because of the interest in nurse practitioner programs and the thrust as well as federal support to prepare nurse practitioners at the graduate level. The majority of public health nursing graduate programs had one or the other of two thrusts, nurse practitioner preparation (usually family nurse practitioner preparation) or community nurse specialist preparation (Anderson et al, 1977).

The current status of community health nursing is characterized by some crisis and a significant amount of opportunity. The crisis originates from the changing role of health departments, the major employer of community health nurses. Changes are being necessitated by fiscal constraints and major budget decreases. Public health nursing positions in many traditional programs are being eliminated.

However, simultaneously, there exists a resurgence of interest in ambulatory and community-based practice. The cost of care in institutions, both acute care as well as long term care, is a major health care delivery problem. Therefore, health maintenance care, the prevention of institutionalization, and early discharge are major goals toward which community health nurses can make major contributions.

Definitions of Community Health Nursing Practice

Two recent definitional statements have been published by separate organizations in attempts to clarify the community-based, clinical nursing specialty. These statements are presented here. In addition, the definitions of public health and primary care will be presented because community health nursing practice overlaps both of those general fields.

A Conceptual Model of Community Health Nursing

In 1980 the American Nurses' Association (ANA) published *A Conceptual Model of Community Health Nursing* to define the dimensions and give direction to preparation, practice, and research in community health nursing. According to this statement:

Community health nursing is a synthesis of nursing practice and public health practice applied to promoting and preserving the health of populations. The practice is general and comprehensive. It is not limited to a particular age group or diagnosis, and is continuing, not episodic. The dominant responsibility is to the population as a whole; nursing directed to individuals, families, or groups contributes to the health of the total population. Health promotion, health maintenance, health education and management, coordination, and continuity of care are utilized in a holistic approach to the management of the health care of individuals, families, and groups in a community (American Nurses' Association, 1980, p. 2).

The definitional statement also indicates that community health nursing can provide services directly or indirectly to clients. The importance of consumer participation is stressed throughout the document.

This definition and other portions of the discussion in the full text of the *Conceptual Model* emphasize several conceptual notions, which are discussed here in some detail because they are fundamental to community health nursing practice. The first conceptual notion is that community health nursing is a synthesis of nursing practice and public health practice. As an introduction to a discussion of the implications of synthesis, nursing practice and public health practice are described separately first.

The Nursing Component of Community Health Nursing The American Nurses' Association's (1980) document *Nursing: A Social Policy Statement* proposes the following definition of nursing: "Nursing is the diagnosis and treatment of human responses to actual or potential health problems" (American Nurses' Association, 1980, p. 9). The health problems of interest to community health nurses are both potential and actual. Community-based nurses utilize strategies designed to prevent common problems (e.g., childhood accidents), to promote health in general (e.g., the teaching of stress management techniques), and to treat actual health problems (e.g., venereal disease).

Nursing practice is primarily oriented toward the care of individuals. Most of basic nursing education and a substantial portion of nursing practice is concerned with the sciences that support the understanding of the human and with the nursing care of individual patients and clients.

Archer and Fleshman (1979) identified the goal of community health nursing as the promotion of the client's optimal level of functioning, expressed as the acronym OLOF. One can argue that the objective of all nursing specialties is to assist clients to achieve OLOF. However, in acute care settings, serious physiologic problems and responses to such problems often take precedence in nursing care. The current trend toward increasingly shorter hospitalization of patients in acute care settings and the crisis nature of most hospitalizations preclude much long term health care planning or interventions directed to health promotion and potential health problems. Therefore, much of the work towards achieving OLOF must be done outside institutions and in homes, worksites, schools, and communities.

When compared, the goals of nursing as identified in the *Social Policy Statement* and the goals of community health nursing are consistent and complementary. The Archer and Fleshman statement assists in differentiating community health nursing as a specialty area within nursing, organized to assist clients to attain a level of function that is appropriate and optimal for them.

The Public Health Component of Community Health Nursing The classic definition of public health proposed by Winslow (1952) is still commonly utilized:

Public health is the science and art of preventing disease, prolonging life, and promoting physical and mental health and efficiency through organized community efforts toward a sanitary environment; the control of community infections; the education of the individual in principles of personal hygiene; the organization of medical and nursing service for the early diagnosis and treatment of disease; and the development of social machinery which will ensure to every individual in the community a standard of living adequate for the maintenance of health (p. 30).

Clearly the goals of public health are very similar to those of community health nursing. Nurses constitute the largest group of professionals in the field of public health. In large part it is through nursing efforts that many of the goals of public health are achieved.

The notion of synthesis is important to understanding community health nursing. Archer (1982) calls this synthesis the ability "to combine two or more areas of content (i.e., public health sciences and general nursing sciences) to create an outcome greater than and different from its parts (e.g., community health nursing)" (p. 442). If such a synthesis has occurred, then community health nursing should look different from both general nursing and public health practice, but should demonstrate the essence of each (Archer, 1982). The material in this chapter has already described how community health nursing is different from other nursing specialties. But what differentiates community health nursing from other public health professionals? Community health nurses have the unique ability to link and to apply programs to individuals and families and to maintain those linkages—in other words, to translate community problems and needs into services impacting on individuals and families through program planning and implementation.

The Definition and Role of Public Health Nursing in the Delivery of Health Care

In 1980 the Public Health Nursing Section of the American Public Health Association recommended the following definition for public health nursing:

Public health nursing synthesizes the body of knowledge from the public health sciences and professional nursing theories for the purpose of improving the health of the entire community. This goal lies at the heart of primary prevention and health promotion and is the foundation for public health nursing practice. To accomplish this goal, public health nurses work with groups, families, and individuals as well as in multidisciplinary teams and programs. Identifying subgroups (aggregates) within the population which are at high risk of illness, disability, or premature death and directing resources toward these groups is the most effective approach for accomplishing the goal of public health nursing. Success in reducing the risks and in improving the health of the community depends on the involvement of consumers, especially groups experiencing health risks, and others in the community, in health planning, and in self-help activities (Public Health, 1980, p. 4).

This definition is very similar to the one published by the American Nurses' Association. Both statements indicate that practice is based on both nursing as well as public health concepts, that the recipients of services include individuals, families, and communities, that consumer involvement is essential, and that the goals of services are health promotion and disease prevention. However the *Definition* emphasizes the community intervention aspects of community health nursing practice, the notion of high-risk aggregates, and primary prevention strategies.

Primary Care

As an approach to health care primary care is characteristic of the practice of some community health nurses. Primary care is, however, different from primary nursing. The term *primary nursing* indicates a nursing staffing system in which professional staff nurses who work in institutions are assigned specified caseloads of patients, each of whom has a designated nurse as the ongoing, continuous provider and/or coordinator of nursing care.

Primary care, on the other hand, is related to expanded nursing roles, and is described as having two dimensions: "(a) a person's first contact in any given episode of illness with the health care system that leads to a decision of what must be done to help resolve his problem; and (b) the responsibility for the continuum of care, i.e., maintenance of health, evaluation and management of symptoms, and appropriate referrals" (Extending the Scope, 1971, p. 2349). In their report, entitled "Extending the Scope of Nursing Practice," the members of the Secretary's Committee to Study Extended Roles for Nurses observed that public health nurses had frequently functioned as primary care providers, but that such functions were not institutionalized as a component of their role. The Committee recommended increased preparation and utilization of nurses in expanded roles because a shortage of primary care providers was identified as a major public health problem during the 1960s.

Approximately six years prior to the publication of "Extending the Scope of Nursing Practice," the evolution of a new role, nurse practitioner, had begun. The nurse practitioner was a registered nurse

who has successfully completed a formal program of study designed to prepare registered nurses to perform in an expanded role in the delivery of primary health care including the ability to:

a. Assess the health status of individuals and families through health and medical history taking, physical examination, and defining of health and developmental problems;

b. Institute and provide continuity of health care to clients (patients), work with the client to insure understanding of and compliance with the therapeutic regimen within established protocols, and recognize when to refer the client to a physician or other health care provider;

c. Provide instruction and counseling to individuals, families and groups in the areas of health promotion and maintenance, including involving such persons in planning for their health care; and

d. Work in collaboration with other health care providers and agencies to provide and, where appropriate, coordinate services to individuals and families (*Federal Register*, 1977, p. 60886).

The title "nurse practitioner" for this new role was somewhat confusing because every nurse who practices nursing is a nurse practitioner. The use of the term almost connoted that the expanded role practitioner was the "real" practitioner of nursing. Subsequent to the publication of "Extending the Scope of Nursing Practice," the nurse practitioner movement accelerated rapidly.

In 1978 members of an International Conference on Primary Health Care sponsored by the World Health Organization (WHO) and the United Nations Children's Fund described primary health care in the broad context of community health. Primary care is:

essential health care based on practical, scientifically sound and socially acceptable methods and technology made universally accessible to individuals and families in the community through their full participation and at a cost that the community and country can afford to maintain at every stage of their development in the spirit of self-reliance and self-determination. . . . It is the first level of contact of individuals, the family and community with the national health systems bringing health care as close as possible to where people live and work, and constitutes the first element of a continuing health care process (*Primary Health Care*, 1978, pp. 3–4).

This definition has been used by some to describe the core of community health nursing practice. At the community level the community health nurse assesses the health and health-related resources available to meet the basic health needs of the residents. If basic services are not available or if various portions of the community have unmet health needs or unusual health risk, the nurse works with consumers and others to obtain appropriate resources and make them available to suitable clients. The community health nurse is uniquely qualified to provide primary health care according to the WHO definition. However, other health professionals and health workers also participate in the organization and provision of primary health care.

Summary of Descriptions

Before proceeding to discussion of the practice of community health nurses, it may be useful to compare and contrast the definitions already presented to determine their similarities and differences. Several key concepts will be borrowed from Dickoff, James, and Weidenbach (1968) and Ste-

Table 1-2   Analysis of Key Concepts within Definitional Statements Pertaining to Community and Public Health Nursing and Primary Care

	STATEMENTS		
Key Concepts	ANA Conceptual Model	Definition and Role of PHN	Primary Health Care
Health Care Provider	Community health nurse	Public health nurse	Various health workers
Client Group Emphasized	Individuals Families Groups A population	A community Groups Families Individuals	A community Individuals Families
Health	Optimum self-care	State of physical, mental, and social well-being and ability to function	State of complete physical, mental and social well-being
Health Interventions (Procedures)	Health promotion Health maintenance Health education Management, coordination, and continuity of care	Primary prevention Health promotion Identify at-risk aggregates Health planning Involvement with consumers in self-help activities	Promotive, preventive curative and rehabilitative services Rehabilitative Education referral Health planning
Goals	Promote and preserve the health of populations	Improve the health of the entire community Reduce health risks	Ensure essential care

SOURCES:

American Nurses' Association Division on Community Health Nursing: *A Conceptual Model of Community Health Nursing.* Kansas City, Mo.: Author, 1980.

Public Health Nursing Section, American Public Health Association: *The Definition and Role of Public Health Nursing in the Delivery of Health Care.* Washington, DC: Author, 1980.

Primary Health Care. Geneva: World Health Organization, 1978.

vens (1984) to assist in this comparison, which is presented in Table 1-2.

The key concepts of health care provider, client, health, health intervention or procedures, and goals were selected for comparison. The health care provider in the *Primary Health Care* statement is broad and includes providers other than nurses. The notion of client across statements is similar, but the types of patients are prioritized differently with individuals having precedence in the ANA *Conceptual Model* and a community being the priority in the other statements. The concept of health is viewed very broadly and similarly in the *Definition* and *Primary Health Care.* In both cases the definition of health is more philosophical than operational. Self-care is a major theme in the *Conceptual Model.* The procedures, or interventions, of health promotion, health planning, and health education occur across statements. The identification of at-risk groups is unique in the *Definition* and curative services are a major component of *Primary Health Care*. In the area of goals, the *Conceptual Model* and the *Definition* are similar. The *Primary Health Care* statement is most broad because of the inclusion of curative services.

Although differences exist across statements, the similarities are strong. For example, the conceptual bases of community health nursing are reflected in all of them. These conceptual bases are a synthesis of the public health sciences—specifically, epidemiology and biostatistics—and of nursing practice and the sciences upon which nursing is built—specifically physiology, psychology, and sociology. The foundations for community health nursing are built on the integration and application of these sciences and practices. These conceptual bases are necessary because various groups and communities will have various needs and problems, and a broad range of knowledges and skills is necessary to maintain dynamic and effective approaches to services for diverse and complex community groups.

Conceptual Bases for Community Health Nursing Practice

The profession of nursing is developing conceptual and theoretical bases for its practice. Although a number of theorists, e.g., King (1981), Levine (1967), Orem (1980), and Rogers (1970), have proposed theories for nursing, members of the profession are not in agreement about the logic or the applicability of these theories. However, it is important to continue work in theory building, because eventually theories will be developed that are not only descriptive, as is the case with current theories, but also prescriptive and proscriptive as well. Then interventions can be guided by the theories.

This section of the chapter includes a discussion of various concepts important to community health nursing practice.

Health Promotion and Disease Prevention

Chapter 13 addresses the concept of health promotion in depth. The concept is briefly introduced here as part of the conceptual base for community health nursing. Pender (1982) indicates that health promotion "refers to activities directed toward the resources of clients that maintain or enhance well being." An example of a health promotion activity is parenting education designed to enhance the quality of expectant and actual parenthood. And Pender says prevention "refers to activities that seek to protect clients from potential or actual health threats and their harmful consequences" (p. 2). An example of prevention is immunization against childhood disease.

In public health literature prevention is described in levels—i.e., primary prevention, secondary prevention, and tertiary prevention (see Figure 1-1). The notion of levels of prevention was introduced by Leavell and Clark (1965). A recent discussion by Shamansky and Clausen (1980) clarifies the Leavell and Clark concepts in a nursing context:

Primary prevention is prevention in the true sense of the word. It precedes disease or dysfunction and is applied to a generally healthy population. . . . Primary prevention includes generalized health promotion as well as specific protection against disease.

Secondary prevention emphasizes early diagnosis and prompt intervention to halt the pathological process, thereby shortening its duration and severity. . . . Screening procedures of any type . . . are by definition secondary prevention.

Tertiary prevention comes into play when a defect of disability is fixed, stabilized, or irreversible. Rehabilitation, the goal of tertiary prevention, is more than halting the disease process itself; it is restoring the individual to an optimum level of functioning within the constraints of the disability (p. 106).

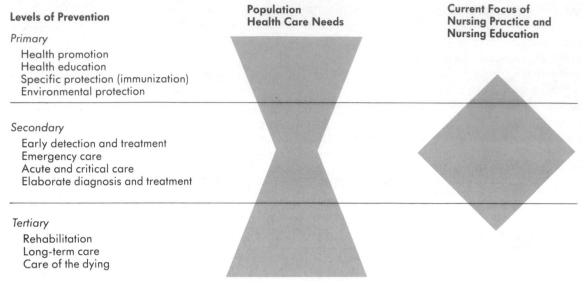

| Levels of Prevention | Population Health Care Needs | Current Focus of Nursing Practice and Nursing Education |

Levels of Prevention

Primary
   Health promotion
   Health education
   Specific protection (immunization)
   Environmental protection

Secondary
   Early detection and treatment
   Emergency care
   Acute and critical care
   Elaborate diagnosis and treatment

Tertiary
   Rehabilitation
   Long-term care
   Care of the dying

Figure 1-1 Health care levels, needs, and current nursing focus. (Adapted from a model developed by the Nursing Practice Branch, DN, BHM, HRA, DHEW, January 1979.)

Health

Health is the ultimate goal of all health care. Much practical and philosophical effort has been expended in its definition and measurement. Smith (1981) reviewed the various notions of health relevant to community health nursing practice and proposed that health can be viewed from four models: (1) eudaimonistic, (2) adaptive, (3) role-performance, and (4) clinical. In the *eudaimonistic model* health is considered the ideal state in which a person can achieve self-actualization, or fulfillment and complete development of potential. Health in the *adaptive model* is the "condition of the organism in which it can engage in effective interaction with its physical and social environment" (p. 45). This model characterizes a person's ability to adjust to a changing environment. In the *role-performance model* health represents a person's ability to perform social roles effectively. Lastly, health in the *clinical model* is the "absence of signs or symptoms of disease or disability as identified by medical science" (p. 46). Smith suggests that the various models of health constitute a continuum of views about health, with the clinical model being the narrowest view and the eudaimonistic being the most holistic. Concepts of health are further discussed in Chapter 4.

Community health nursing practice generally has goals beyond the clinical model of health; however, the actual health goal or model selected depends on many factors, including agency goals and resources. It is important that the community health nurse establish a concept of health that is congruent with self, the employing agency, and client goals and capabilities. Setting too high a health goal can produce frustration and failure. Setting too low a health goal can be wasteful of resources.

Client

The term *client* denotes a person who is not only a recipient of services but also an active negotiator

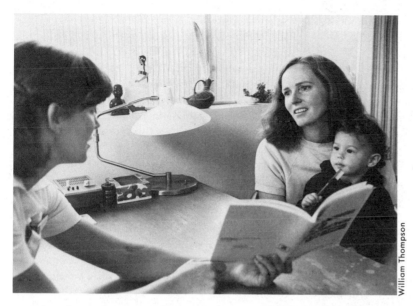

William Thompson

Anticipatory guidance, whether on nutrition, hygiene, development, or safety, is one of the health promotion activities of the community health nurse.

regarding the services received and the goals of care. In community health nursing practice, the term *client* is preferable to the term *patient,* which connotes an individual who is ill and more likely to be passive than active as a recipient of care.

Three general types of clients are recipients of community health nursing services: individuals, families, and groups. Groups may be communities, at-risk aggregates, or persons with similar problems or needs. The type of client largely mandates the types of nursing skills needed to serve the client and the type of role the nurse will implement.

The Individual Client   All community health nursing services provided to aggregates must eventually affect individuals in order to achieve their goals. Thus individual clients are frequent recipients of nursing services such as those provided by clinics and screening programs. Though the rationale for the clinic or screening service is derived from a community problem or need, frequent one-to-one encounters are required to achieve solutions to problems or to minimize risks.

The Family Client   With the recent development of alternate life-styles, the concept of family has become more broad (Gilliss, 1983). Chapter 2 presents various definitions of the family as well as conceptual frameworks for viewing the family. As a client in community health nursing the family can be viewed from many perspectives: as unit of service, as environment, as resource, or as a social group or system of at-risk individuals.

Often the community health nurse selects, or is referred to, a client who is at risk or who has a health problem directly related to that client's family environment. An example is the infant with symptoms of failure to thrive. The community health nurse's interventions would be directed to the total family unit so that an environment conducive to that infant's optimal growth and development can be achieved.

The family is often an important resource in situations where an individual's self-care abilities are insufficient for activities of daily living, but the family can be enlisted to provide home care. The nurse can teach a family to make the most effective and efficient use of its human and material resources to achieve its and the patient's optimal level of functioning.

Some families who are clients of community health nursing services contain members who share a common health problem or need. Examples are members of families who have experienced a sudden infant death, an episode of child abuse, a venereal disease, or who are at risk for malnutrition. In such situations the problem affects the family as a whole as well as each member individually and variably. Family interventions must reach and be acceptable to each family member as well as the family as a whole.

The Community Client   The concept of community as client originated in the early history of community health nursing. The health visitors in nineteenth-century Liverpool were assigned to districts, not only to promote efficiency of travel, but also to facilitate knowledge of community resources and problems and to maintain accountability for the analysis and solution of those problems. Most nurses working for governmentally sponsored health agencies are assigned to work within some specific geographic area. Analysis of the health resources, problems, and risks within that geographic area guide the choice of clients to be served and interventions to be applied within that community.

Although the concept of community is generally associated with a defined geographic area, community clients may be of other types. These include a subset of individuals sharing a common residence (e.g., the community of residents within a special housing unit), or persons who come together for specific collective activities (e.g., the children within a specific school). Often the community health nurse is simultaneously involved with various communities (Shamansky & Pesznecker, 1981). For example, the problem requiring intervention can be within one community, such as a factory with chemical hazards, while the solution to the problem requires intervention with a broader community, such as the state health department.

Whether community health nurses work primarily with individuals and families, or in a broader systems context, the understanding of the community client is fundamental to practice (Anderson, 1983). As the family is resource and environment to the individual, so is the community resource and environment to the family.

The At-Risk Aggregate Client   The concept of at-risk aggregate is becoming important in community health nursing practice. An aggregate is a subgroup within the community or population who are at greater risk of illness or poor recovery (Public Health, 1980). Using biostatistical data and epidemiology to determine factors associated with increased risk, the community health nurse can identify at-risk aggregates and develop service programs to eliminate or decrease risk in vulnerable individuals and families. Because risks and risk factors change over time and risks are minimized by intervention, the at-risk aggregate client groups of community health nursing services will change over time.

Putting Community Health Nursing into Practice

The previous portions of this chapter have included general discussions of the "whats" of community health nursing. This section contains an overview of the nursing process and its application to care for major client groups: individuals, families and communities. This overview is an introduction to more extensive discussions in subsequent chapters.

Box 1-1 Standards for Community Health Nursing

I. The collection of data about the health status of the consumer is systematic and continuous. The data are accessible, communicated, and recorded.

II. Nursing diagnoses are derived from health status data.

III. Plans for nursing service include goals derived from nursing diagnoses.

IV. Plans for nursing service include priorities and nursing approaches or measures to achieve the goals derived from nursing diagnoses.

V. Nursing actions provide for consumer participation in health promotion, maintenance, and restoration.

VI. Nursing actions assist consumers to maximize health potential.

VII. The consumer's progress toward goal achievement is determined by the consumer and the nurse.

VIII. Nursing actions involve ongoing reassessment, reordering of priorities, new goal setting and revision of the nursing plan.

SOURCE: Excerpted from ANA *Standards of Community Health Nursing Practice*. Published by the American Nurses' Association and reprinted with permission of ANA.

The Nursing Process

The nursing process is a useful framework for categorizing and analyzing the various components of nursing practice. Nurses apply their skills to clients through the nursing process, which is a problem identification and problem-solving process involving a series of steps. The steps of the nursing process vary among sources, but most models include the following:

1. Systematic client assessment
2. Identification of health problem(s) or health need(s) based on the assessment. This is equivalent to the Nursing Diagnosis step. See Chapter 10.
3. Development of a plan of action to solve the problem or meet the need
4. Implementation of the plan
5. Evaluation of the plan

These steps are discussed in detail in Part 2.

The nursing process is not the whole of nursing functioning, nor is the problem-solving method unique to nursing practice. The purpose of the nursing process is to provide a logical framework for client care (Henderson, 1982), as outlined in the American Nurses' Association's *Standards of Community Health Nursing* (1973) (see Box 1-1).

Care of the Individual Client Although the major theme of this book is family-centered approaches to community health nursing, the importance of understanding each individual family member contributes to understanding and working with the family as a unit. The nurse in community health practice must have skills in interventions on both the individual and family levels. Understanding the dynamic interactions between individuals and their families is fundamental to successful community health nursing practice.

Assessments of individuals can be very comprehensive or very focused depending upon the purpose of the initial nurse-client interaction and the comprehensiveness and duration of subsequent interaction. The amount of information that could be collected about an individual is potentially infinite. The nurse should collect sufficient information to provide safe, professional care based on scientific principles, but not information in excess of what is needed. Insufficient data could yield inaccurate conclusions; the collection of excess data is wasteful of nurse and client time. A good assessment includes specific information regarding the client's health history, family history, physical development, and psychosocial development. Malasanos et al (in press) provide a comprehensive list of specific items.

Nursing diagnosis in community health nursing is a developing area. One nursing classification system has been developed by the Omaha VNA and is being disseminated by them (Simmons, 1980). This system allows for the classification of individual, family, and environmental problems. Currently this system is undergoing intensive testing by the agency that developed it. This issue is discussed further in Chapter 10.

Planning for the health needs of the client should involve the client so that the most relevant and appropriate plan can be developed. Successful client involvement has several prerequisites: establishing an atmosphere conducive to client participation; teaching the client about the problem or need (i.e., providing the client with sufficient knowledge for informed participation); identifying alternative interventions; listening to the client to determine his or her perceptions of the various alternatives; and determining the most appropriate plan for the solution of the problem in collaboration with client. This client or consumer participation process is relevant for all types of clients.

Appropriate intervention techniques are based on the results of the assessment and diagnosis steps and are reflected in the planning process. The specific techniques selected vary according to the client's situation. These may include: teaching, counseling, coordinating care and resources, and acting as the client's advocate when the individual is unable to do so.

Evaluation of care, on the other hand, is often a neglected component of the nursing process. Research in the specialty is still sparse and has not provided the community health nurse with extensive data regarding relationships between nursing interventions and outcomes. The specification of projected outcomes on patients' charts and the comparison of projected with actual outcomes could be a useful method for evaluation of clinical care to individuals. Some general types of possible out-comes include: cure, comfort, prevention of a specific health problem, adequate knowledge for self-care, increase in well-being, optimal level of functioning, and decrease in health risks.

Care of Families A detailed discussion of the assessment of families is in Chapter 8. This section will provide an overview of the community health nurse's care of families.

As previously mentioned, the extent of influence between individuals and their families, families and their communities, and communities and individuals is extremely powerful. The family's influence on the health of its individual members is especially potent because the family generates, tolerates, or corrects health problems of its members. Also, the health problems of family members are interactive, and the family is a strong environmental influence. Because many health-related decisions are made within the family unit, nursing intervention must be of sufficient strength to counteract long-standing patterns. A strong nursing intervention must be based on a detailed assessment of the family, and the intervention must have some intensity and duration. Thus, care of the family as a unit is a complex, comprehensive, and costly endeavor.

It is impossible for the community health nurse to provide in-depth family care to many families or to all the families the nurse encounters. The nurse must, however, have skills in total family care and judgment in determining the families most likely to need and to respond to such care. An alternative to total family care is family-centered care in which the needs, strengths, and limitations of family units are considered in reference to an individual family member or a subset of the family.

The types of assessment data needed to support interventions with families will vary depending upon the health need or problem initiating the interaction of the nurse and the family. Family assessment, diagnosis, and evaluation are discussed in Part 2.

Care of Communities and Aggregates Community health nursing care to communities and aggregates will be discussed together because application of the nursing process to services for each unit is similar. There are several basic purposes for assessing a community: (1) identifying the health assets and liabilities of a community; (2) identifying high risk aggregates within a community; and (3) collecting data relevant to health planning for the community. Thus, assessments of communities must take into account those three purposes.

Community nursing is somewhat different from nursing diagnosis of individuals and families (Hamilton, 1983). In order to be useful, the community diagnosis should be a summary statement of the health status of the community in addition to an identification of the high-risk aggregates whose "problems" need to be addressed through intervention. A complete overall community nursing diagnosis includes: (1) a summary of the health status of the community; (2) a report of areas in which the health of the community is vulnerable; (3) a

specific listing of high risk aggregates of individuals or families; and (4) a summary statement of the community's competence, capability, or health resources (Goeppinger, Lassiter, & Wilcox, 1982).

The community health nursing diagnosis of any community is apt to identify both general health problems—such as lack of accessible primary care services for low income persons—and the problems of specific high-risk aggregates, such as adolescent mothers delivering low birthweight babies. The general health problem can be addressed directly. The high risk aggregate needs further assessment in terms of specific composition, location, and interaction with the community and its resources.

The interventions directed to community health problems are usually broadly directed toward the community system. Examples might include: program planning and implementation, consumer advocacy, policy formation, health education, and community development.

Community Health Nursing Roles

Community health nurses work in an assortment of positions, which vary according to whether the primary client focus is the individual, the family, or the community (Archer, 1976). For example, various types of nurse practitioners are primarily involved with individuals; community health nurse generalists in public health and home health agencies work primarily with families; and nurse planners and administrators work primarily with communities and at-risk aggregates. Several types of population-focused nurses, such as school health nurses, often work equally with individuals and aggregates.

Community Health (Public Health) Staff Nurses

The community health nurse generalist or staff nurse, who is prepared at the baccalaureate level, pro-

vides care to families and individuals within families in conjunction with a variety of community-based health services. Common roles for the community health nurse generalist include public health staff nurse and home health care nurse (also termed "visiting nurse").

The public health staff nurse commonly works for a political jurisdiction, such as a city, and provides nursing service in a variety of program areas and settings. The public health staff nurse's responsibilities may be extremely diverse (e.g., well child care, gerontological care, maternity care, school health, and home care) or may be limited to only several types of services. In any case, programs are designed to address health problems and/or meet health needs of the citizens within specified geographic communities. The public health nurse generalist has some skills in working with aggregates. However, usually the nurse is working to implement programs devised by others in response to aggregate need analysis and resultant program planning efforts. The settings for public health nurse interventions with families include clients' homes, clinics, schools, and community gathering places.

Home health care nurses or visiting nurses are employed in official and voluntary agencies. Often public health agencies, especially small ones, offer home health care services and utilize nurse generalists to provide home health services as their major role or a portion of their responsibilities. Most commonly, home health care services are provided by voluntary or proprietary agencies that are not components of governmental jurisdictions.

Historically, a distinction has been made among home health care agencies, commonly termed visiting nurse associations, not-for-profit, and for-profit or proprietary home health care agencies. However, these past distinctions are blurring because in most instances nurse roles in most types of agencies are similar. In home health care the primary site for nurse-client interaction is the home and the primary purpose is the nursing care of an individual. Because most individuals needing home health care reside within families and because the family is an important resource, the home health care nurse utilizes many family assessment and intervention skills.

The staff nurse in home health care does not generally work specifically with aggregates because clients are more often referred than selected for services. However, aggregate concepts should be utilized by those planning for home health services within a community.

Clinic Nurses

The clinic staff nurse role can be a community health nursing role, especially if the clinic is community-based, accountable to a defined community, oriented to health promotion, and involved with families. With the future development of community nursing centers, an increasing number of clients will receive community health nursing care in clinics.

Clinic nurses can provide a variety of preventive, screening, curative, and rehabilitative services to individual and family clients who come to a central site for services. In practice, many health departments run clinics and often public health staff nurses have clinic nursing responsibilities as well as field responsibilities.

Primary Care Nurse Practitioners

Many types of primary care nurse practitioners function in community health. They are usually differentiated according to their client group focus. A partial list of such practitioners includes pediatric nurse practitioner, adult nurse practitioner, obstetric-gynecologic nurse practitioner, nurse-midwife, school nurse practitioner, psychiatric-mental health nurse practitioner, and family nurse practitioner. These nurse practitioners provide primary care (including health maintenance and illness care) to individuals, usually in conjunction with physicians and other health care providers. This role is focused primarily on the individual because comprehensive care is being given to each individual client. Depending upon the type of practice and the clients' needs, nurse practitioners may also work with families as units of service. Minimally, nurse practitioners manage the health care of individuals within the context of their families, often involving the family as a resource in the treatment plan.

Nurse practitioners are also involved with aggregates in several ways. Their caseload is an aggregate and amenable to risk analysis as an aggregate. In addition, the nurse practitioner functions within a geographic community in order to provide appropriate preventive care and should be aware of the overall health and illness trends in the community to provide appropriate preventive care—to determine if the care being given within the health program is congruent with and appropriate to the health needs and problems in the total community.

Aggregate-Based Nursing Roles

Various community health nurses work with defined aggregates. The common examples are school health nurses and occupational health nurses. Each works with a preestablished client group composed of individuals sharing a common environment for a portion of their day. These two client groups may represent unique health problems and needs because of their developmental stage (school children) or their exposure to environmental stresses (employees). The group in which they are found may create an ideal situation for appropriate health intervention. (School nursing and occupational health nursing are discussed in Part 3.)

The school health nurse is most often prepared as a generalist, without practitioner skills. The primary role is monitoring the health of pupils within the school through a variety of screening methods, intervening directly with selected high-risk pupils and their families, and facilitating a school environment conducive to health and learning (Oda, 1982). Some school health nurses are prepared as teachers and can teach health in the classroom and conduct a health education program (Wylie, 1983). School health nurses are in an influential position for improving the total health and self-care of all children, especially those who may be living in unhealthy home environments (Stark & Siddons, 1983).

Nurses in occupational health may perform various roles. The nurse generalist is prepared to implement appropriate health screening and treatment procedures relevant to the industry and its employees. Several master's degree programs are preparing occupational nurse specialists who are able to plan, direct, implement, and evaluate comprehensive preventive, curative, and rehabilitative health programs in industry.

Community Health Nursing Specialists

Community health nurse specialists are prepared in graduate nursing programs for various leadership roles. Leadership roles range from provision of direct services at an advanced level to individual, family, and/or community clients to practices primarily concerned with systems and indirectly affecting client groups.

We just described the role of the primary care nurse practitioner in the care of individuals and families. The profession has conceived and implemented a parallel role for a community nurse practitioner. This community nurse practitioner has a community as the client and implements a broad range of activities to assist community members to improve the health status of the total community. The community nurse specialist role was designed not as an administrative role, but as a practitioner role. In reality, however, most nursing community care interventions are implemented by a nurse manager who plans and directs the nursing activities within a community-based health program.

The community health nursing clinical specialty is, therefore, largely an administrative specialty because the job's chief function is engineering and coordinating systems on behalf of the health of clients. Within this administrative specialty nurse leaders may be an advocate, collaborator, community organizer, consultant, coordinator, facilitator, educator, evaluator, manager, and director. The community health nurse specialist has the preparation and skills to provide leadership in most community-based health programs.

Thus community health nursing offers a gamut of roles and job opportunities for nurses interested in community-based practice that emphasizes prevention and health promotion.

Current Issues and Future Direction for Community Health Nursing Practice

Community health nurses face many issues concerning their current practice and future directions. These include the overall economics of community health nursing practice and the issue of third-party reimbursement, especially for preventive health care. Future challenges include the need for further research in the specialty.

The Economics of Practice

Reimbursement for community health nursing services is a major issue affecting the future of the specialty. Currently, reimbursement for home health care requiring skilled nursing is available through the Social Security, Medicare, and Medicaid programs, and health insurance plans. In general, reimbursement from third-party payers is not available for prevention and health promotion services. These services have commonly been provided by political jurisdictions and paid for through tax revenues. Thus in periods of economic difficulty, social and health programs supported by tax funding are seriously compromised, and the individuals most needing community health nursing services are often least able to pay for them. Indeed payment by the individual will always be a limited source of income for such services to high-risk persons.

Primary care nursing services are provided to individuals and families in different socioeconomic groups and are reimbursed through various mechanisms. In a health maintenance organization or a private practice, ambulatory setting clients often pay directly for services. Insurance companies and governmental agencies reimburse directly for nurse practitioner services in some programs or geographic jurisdictions. The services for other nurse practitioners are billed indirectly to third-party payers over the signature of a physician consultant.

Traditionally nurses have been salaried employees unaccustomed to understanding or dealing with health economics. As the practice of community-based nurses differentiates from that of other health care providers in the field, and as their practice autonomy increases, community health nurses will both want and need to develop economic autonomy including reimbursement mechanisms for services to clients across economic strata.

Cost-effective Approaches to Care

Although many primary care services must be given to individuals and families, a home visit is an especially expensive method for service delivery and may not be the most cost-effective method or site for interaction. Community health nurses may need to consider more extensive use of alternate methods of service delivery to groups of clients. Interaction with a group of clients not only increases the number of clients provided services per unit of time, but also may increase the effectiveness of such services. In peer groups having similar needs, clients often contribute much to each other. These contributions include information, understanding, and support. Often a client may perceive another client with a similar need or problem as more credible than the health care professional. Group interventions are obviously not appropriate for every type of client or client need, but this service technology has probably not been used to the extent that it could or should be used.

Media communications are major sources of health information for many individuals and families. Some nurses have been successful in publishing regular information columns in general circulation newspapers and magazines or in broadcasting health programs over radio or television. Unfortunately, however, such examples of nurse use of the media are not common. Much opportunity for media use exists, and community-based nurses would be a likely group to provide leadership in this area.

The Reality of Preventive Care

Public health largely developed in response to the need for control of communicable diseases through personal and environmental measures. With the development of effective pharmacologic intervention and the routine use of immunization, communicable disease prevention is no longer the primary focus of public health or community health nursing programs. Today the major threats to health originate from physical and psychological environmental hazards, such as chemical pollutants and stress, and from harmful life-style habits, such as smoking and overeating. Thus preventive measures that impact the total environment and change personal habits need to be developed. Biochemical, sociological, and psychological preventive interventions need to be added to existing biological interventions if prevention is to become a reality.

In a 1979 report published by the US Department of Health, Education, and Welfare, prevention was described as an idea whose time had come. Additionally the report stated:

Clearly, the American people are deeply interested in improving their health. The increased attention now being paid to exercise, nutrition, environmental health and occupational safety testify to their interest and concern with health promotion and disease prevention. . . . Prevention is an idea whose time has come. We have the scientific knowledge to begin to formulate recommendations for improved health. And, although the degenerative diseases differ from their infectious disease predecessors in having more—and more complex—causes, it is now clear that many are preventable (*Healthy People*, 1979, 6–7).

The development of preventive methodologies has been slow for various reasons. First, the cure of illness has been an unwritten, but explicit, priority service in most health programs, even those of health departments. Thus resources have been concentrated on developing technology and services to treat the sick. Furthermore, not all illnesses are amenable to primary prevention.

Second, the causes of some contemporary public health problems are not inherently evil or neg-

ative, and some are actually perceived as positive values. For example, smoking is a pleasure to many who smoke, and food is necessary to life. Chemical wastes are by-products of manufacturing processes that produce useful commodities. Most of today's public health problems result more from deliberate choices than from random, uncontrolled events and reflect value conflicts.

However, interest in prevention is increasing, and consumers are taking active, even leading, roles. For example, consumer groups have been successful in developing weight reduction, exercise, and substance abuse control programs. Because people are living longer, they recognize the importance of quality-of-life issues. Many have adopted general health promotion activities, such as adequate exercise, as general preventive action against a variety of chronic illnesses.

Community health nurses have long promoted health and wellness. They have the orientation and skills to provide leadership in this area. Although many community health nurses are making important contributions to prevention and health promotion, they are not perceived by either many consumers or health professionals as authorities in prevention or health promotion. A particular challenge to community health nurses is reestablishing their authority as leaders in this domain.

A contributing factor to nursing's current lack of leadership in prevention is the focus of nursing practice and education. Most of the population needs are in the primary and tertiary levels of health care, while most of nursing practice and education is focused on the secondary, acute care levels (see Figure 1-1). Perhaps a greater balance among these levels in the preparation for and the practice of nursing would effect the type of climate needed to make prevention a reality.

The Future of Community Health Nursing

Community health nursing has been a potent force in meeting the health needs of people. Innovations in community health nursing practice and educa-

Case Example 1-1: A Community Health Nurse's Day

Molly Jones is a community health nursing staff nurse in a public health department that has a home health care program as well as a school health program. The following activities are performed by Molly during one of her typical days.

Molly's first activity was a home visit to a newly discharged diabetic man who was learning to give himself insulin and to adjust his life-style to this chronic disease. The man's wife was present for the visit. Molly supervised the man's self-injection and talked with the couple about their eating habits, making suggestions regarding decreased calories and regularity of meals.

The individual as primary client

Care provided at tertiary level of prevention

Molly's next stop was a school in her community. The school is in a very low income neighborhood. The teachers had observed that some students had high rates of absence. Molly had recently read a research report stating that children with high absences are also at high risk for health problems.

Identifying individual, family, and at-risk aggregate clients

Molly then visited a senior citizen high rise apartment building to participate in an activity group session with ten residents and a physical therapist. While she was in the high rise, several residents asked her to teach them breast self-examination. One of the residents had recently been diagnosed as having breast cancer and the other women were concerned that they might have the problem also.

Screening through health teaching

---

tion hold much promise for important social benefit. Increasing numbers of community health nurses are being prepared as generalists, specialists, and leaders at the baccalaureate, master's degree, and doctoral levels. At no time have community health nurses been so well prepared to provide creative and relevant health services.

However, at no other time have there been so many constraints on practice. For example, studies have demonstrated that nurse practitioners can safely and effectively manage the majority of ambulatory health care needs, especially wellness needs (Chen et al 1982). Nevertheless, the major portion of this care is being provided by physicians at a higher cost. Governmental controls over the definition of skilled home nursing care for reimbursement restrict the full application of nursing skills in health promotion.

Nurses in all areas of community health nursing practice need to develop mechanisms of institutionalizing their roles, or in other words, making

their roles integral components of the systems in which they work. They also need to gain and to maintain more control in the management and delivery of their services in order to create an environment and a system that supports full demonstration and development of community health nursing skills (Dreher, 1982).

An important major trend in American health care is the increasing use of services in the community as an alternative to use of institutions, especially hospitals, for health care. When society fully perceives that community-based care is an alternative to institutionalization, an appropriate balance of health and illness care will be truly achieved. This movement is being accelerated by high costs of hospitalization and consumer interest in self-care.

Community health nurses can be in the forefront of a movement back to community-based care. The community health nurse knows the mechanism of mobilizing total systems on behalf of clients and can understand and work within each component of the overall health care system. For example, as patients with terminal illnesses move from hospital to hospice to home and back, a community health nurse can assist personnel in these systems and other practitioners to understand the patient's and the family's needs and adapt services to them.

An innovation in community-based nursing practice is the nursing center. A nursing center is a community-based program through which clients receive care managed by nurses (Lang, 1983; Reisch, 1980). The funding, sponsorship, and services provided by nursing centers are variable. However, the predominant themes are self-care and health promotion facilitated through nursing interventions. A strong and permanent funding base for nursing centers is a major issue; however, the nursing resources are currently present to provide such care and consumers are ready for it (Mezey, 1983). The second half of the 1980s will be an important developmental period for community health nursing.

Research in the Specialty

Although a number of studies demonstrate the effectiveness of community health nursing services, the quality and the quantity of the studies are insufficient to fully support current practice. Only recently have there been sufficient numbers of doctorally prepared nurses to begin development of a scientific basis for practice. Research is needed in all community health nursing practice areas. Priority areas for research are the documentation of practice, testing of the effectiveness of interventions, and measurement of the impact of services. These will be enumerated more specifically in various chapters of this text as "Topics for Nursing Research."

Summary

Community health nursing practice is a synthesis of nursing and public health knowledge and skill applied to a variety of client groups. These clients include communities, at-risk aggregates, families, and individuals. The basic unit of service within community-based health programs is, however, the family. The overall goals of community health nursing practice include disease prevention, general health promotion, and the promotion of an optimal level of functioning and self-care for clients. Community health nurses utilize an epidemiologic process to identify subgroups within a community who have particular health needs or health risks and provide services directly or indirectly to meet the needs or to reduce the health risks.

Community health nurses function in a variety of roles, from primary care provider to health services administrator, and implement numerous interventions in achieving their goals. The resolution of relevant economic issues will affect the future of community health nursing and its contribution to preventive care and the delivery of cost-effective health services.

Study Questions

1. Community health nursing practice differs from nursing practice in acute care settings in which of the following ways?
   (1) Community health nurses have discretion in selecting clients for services.
   (2) Community health nurses' involvement with clients extends over longer periods of time and exemplifies continuity of care.
   (3) The primary goal of community health nursing is health promotion and disease prevention.
   (4) Community health nursing practice involves interventions directed to client's environments.

a. 3 and 4 only
b. 2 only
c. All of the above
d. 1, 2, and 3 only

2. The notion of synthesis in community health nursing means that:
   a. Community health nursing is essentially the same as general nursing but practiced in community settings.
   b. Community health nursing is an integration of general nursing concepts and theories and public health sciences.
   c. Community health nursing is indistinguishable from public health practice.
   d. Community health nurses can plan and implement programs for various client groups.

3. Community health nursing originated in which of the following ways?
   a. As a result of war
   b. As a response to epidemics
   c. As a response to the need for family care in the home
   d. Because of the lack of institutions to care for the sick and the dying

4. Which of the following concepts do community health nurses most often use in applying their nursing practice to client groups?
   a. At-risk aggregates
   b. Nursing process
   c. Epidemiology
   d. All of the above

References

Aiken LH (editor): *Nursing in the 1980's: Crises, Opportunities, Challenges.* Philadelphia: Lippincott, 1982.

American Nurses' Association Division on Community Health Nursing: *A Conceptual Model of Community Health Nursing.* Kansas City, Mo.: Author, 1980.

American Nurses' Association: *Nursing: A Social Policy Statement.* Kansas City, Mo.: Author, 1980.

American Nurses' Association: *Standards of community health nursing practice.* Kansas City, Mo.: Author, 1973.

Anderson ET: Community focus in public health nursing: Whose responsibility? *Nurs Outlook* 1983; 31: 44–48.

Anderson ET et al: *The Development and Implementation of a Curriculum Model for Community Nurse Practitioners.* DHEW Publication No. ARA 77–24. Hyattsville, Md.: US Department of Health, Education, and Welfare, 1977.

Archer SE: Community nurse practitioners: Another assessment. *Nurs Outlook* 1976; 24: 499–503.

Archer SE: Synthesis of public health science and nursing science. *Nurs Outlook* 1982; 30: 442–446.

Archer SE, Fleshman RP: *Community Health Nursing: Patterns and Practice,* 2nd ed. North Scituate, Mass.: Duxbury Press, 1979.

Barkauskas VH: Public health nursing practice—An educator's view. *Nurs Outlook* 1982; 30: 384–389.

Benson ER, McDevitt JQ: *Community Health and Nursing Practice,* 2nd ed. Englewood Cliffs, N.J.: Prentice-Hall, 1980.

Brubaker BH: Health promotion: A linguistic analysis. *Adv Nurs Sci* 1983; 5(3): 1–14.

Chen SC et al: Health problems encountered by nurse practitioners and physicians. *Nurs Res* 1982; 31: 163–169.

Clemen SA, Eigsti DG, McGuire SL: *Comprehensive Family and Community Health Nursing.* New York: McGraw-Hill, 1981.

Commission on Professional and Hospital Activities: *International Classification of Diseases: Clinical Modification,* 9th rev. 3 vols. Ann Arbor, Mich.: Author, 1978.

Committee for the Study of Nursing Education: *Nursing and Nursing Education in the United States.* New York: Macmillan, 1983.

Delaney LL: Nursing assessment: Data collection of the family client. In Griffith JW, Christensen J (editors): *Nursing Process: Application of Theories, Frameworks, and Models.* St. Louis: Mosby.

Dickoff J, James P, Wiedenbach E: Theory in a practice of discipline. *Nurs Res* 1968; 17: 415–435.

Dreher MC: The conflict of conservatism in public health nursing education. *Nurs Outlook* 1982; 30: 504–509.

Duvall EM: *Marriage and Family Development,* 5th ed. Philadelphia: Lippincott, 1977.

Ervin N: Public health nursing practice—An administrator's view. *Nurs Outlook* 1982; 30: 390–394.

Extending the scope of nursing practice. *Am J Nurs* 1971; 71: 2346–2351.

Federal Register 1977; 42(229): 60886.

Fitzpatrick ML: *The National Organization for Public Health Nursing, 1912–1952: Development of a Practice Field.* New York: National League for Nursing, 1975.

Ford LC, Silver HK: The expanded role of the nurse in child care. *Nurs Outlook* 1967; 15(9): 43–45.

Freeman RB, Heinrich J: *Community Health Nursing Practice,* 2nd ed. Philadelphia: Saunders, 1981.

Fromer MJ: *Community Health Care and the Nursing Process.* St. Louis: Mosby, 1979.

Gilliss CL: The family as a unit of analysis: Strategies for the nurse researcher. *Adv Nurs Sci* 1983; 5(3): 50–59.

Goeppinger J, Lassiter PC, Wilcox B: Community health in community competence. *Nurs Outlook* 1982; 30: 464–467.

Griffith J, Christensen PJ: *Nursing Process: Application of Theories, Frameworks, and Models.* St. Louis: Mosby, 1982.

Hamilton P: Community nursing diagnosis. *Adv Nurs Sci* 1983; 5(3): 21–36.

Healthy People: The Surgeon General's Report on Health Promotion and Disease Prevention. Washington, D.C.: US Department of Health, Education, and Welfare, 1979.

Helvie CO: *Community Health Nursing: Theory and Process.* Philadelphia, Harper & Row, 1981.

Helvie CO: A proposed theory for nursing in community health; Part I: The individual, and Part II: The family. *Canadian Journal of Public Health* 1979; 70: 41–46, 266–270.

Helvie CO, Hill E, Bambino CR: The setting and nursing practice. Part I *Nurs Outlook* 1968; 8: 27–28. Part II *Nurs Outlook* 1968; 9: 35–38.

Henderson V: The nursing process—is the title right? *J Adv Nurs* 1982; 1: 103–109.

Henry OM: Perspectives of community health nursing practice. In: *Community Health Nursing: Education and Practice.* NLN Publication No. 52–1834. New York: National League for Nursing, 1980.

Hollen P: A holistic model of individual and family health based on a continuum of choice. *Adv Nurs Sci* 1981; 3(4): 27–42.

Jarvis LL: *Community Health Nursing: Keeping the Public Healthy.* Philadelphia: Davis, 1981.

Kalisch PA, Kalisch BJ: *The Advances of American Nursing.* Boston: Little, Brown, 1978.

King IM: *A Theory for Nursing: Systems Concepts, Process.* New York: Wiley, 1981.

Kurtzman C et al: Nursing process at the aggregate level. *Nurs Outlook* 1980; 28: 737–739.

Lang N: Nurse-managed clinics: Will they thrive? *Am J Nurs* 1983; 83: 1291–1293.

Leavell HR, Clark EG: *Preventive Medicine for the Doctor in His Community,* 3rd ed. New York: McGraw-Hill, 1965.

Levine ME: The four conservation principles of nursing. *Nurs Forum* 1967; 6(1): 46.

Malasanos L et al: *Health Assessment,* 3rd ed. St. Louis: Mosby, in press.

Martin K: A client classification system adaptable for computerization. *Nurs Outlook* 1982; 30: 515–517.

McLaughlin JS: Toward a theoretical model for community health programs. *Adv Nurs Sci* 1982; 5(1): 7–28.

Mezey MD: Securing a financial base. *Am J Nurs* 1983; 83: 1297–1298.

Miller JC: Theoretical basis for the practice of community mental health nursing. *Issues in Mental Health Nursing* 1981; 3: 319–339.

Nightingale F: *Notes on Nursing.* London: Harrison, 1859.

Norbeck JS: Social support: A model for clinical research and application. *Adv Nurs Sci* 1981; 3(4): 43–59.

Oda DS: School health services: Growth potential for nursing. In: Aiken LH (editor): *Nursing in the 1980's: Crises, Opportunities, Challenges.* Philadelphia: Lippincott, 1982.

Orem DE: *Concepts of Practice,* 2nd ed. New York: McGraw-Hill, 1980.

Pender NJ: *Health Promotion in Nursing Practice.* Norwalk, Conn.: Appleton-Century-Crofts, 1982.

Pesznecker B, Draye MA, McNeil J: Collaborative practice models in community health nursing. *Nurs Outlook* 1982; 30: 298–302.

Primary Health Care. Geneva: World Health Organization, 1978.

Public Health Nursing Section, American Public Health Association: *The Definition and Role of Public Health Nursing in the Delivery of Health Care.* Washington, DC: Author, 1980.

Reisch S, Felder E, Stauder C: Nursing centers can promote health for individuals, families, and communities. *Nursing Administration Quarterly* 1980; 4(2): 1–8.

Rogers ME: An Introduction to the Theoretical Basis of Nursing. Philadelphia: F. A. Davis, 1970.

Shamansky SL, Clausen CL: Levels of prevention: Examination of the concept. *Nurs Outlook* 1980; 28: 104–108.

Shamansky SL, Pesznecker B: A community is . . . *Nurs Outlook* 1981; 29: 182–185.

Simmons D: *A Classification Scheme for Client Problems in Community Health Nursing.* DHHS Publication No. HRA 80–16. Hyattsville, Md.: US Department of Health and Human Services, 1980.

Skrovan C, Anderson ET, Gottschalk J: Community nurse practitioners: An emerging role. *Am J Public Health* 1974; 64: 847–853.

Smith JA: The idea of health: A philosophical inquiry. *Adv Nurs Sci* 1981; 3(3): 43–49.

Spradley BW: *Community Health Nursing: Concepts and Practice.* Boston: Little, Brown, 1981.

Stark AJ, Siddons PJ: The public health nurses' caseload: Can we measure outcomes? One agency's experience. *Can J Public Health* 1983; 74: 208–214.

Stevens BJ: *Nursing Theory,* 2nd ed. Boston: Little, Brown, 1984.

Stewart MJ: Community health assessment: A systematic approach. *Nursing Papers* 1981; 14(1): 30–46.

Wagner DL: Nursing administrators' assessment of nursing education. *Nurs Outlook* 1980; 28: 557–561.

White C, Knollmueller R, Yaksich S: Preparation for community health nursing: Issues and problems. *Nurs Outlook* 1980; 28: 617–623.

White MS: Construct for public health nursing. *Nurs Outlook* 1982; 30: 527–530.

Williams CA: Community health nursing—what is it? *Nurs Outlook* 1977; 25: 250–254.

Winslow CEA: *Man and epidemics.* Princeton University Press, 1952.

Wylie WE: Cost-benefit analysis of a school health education program. *J Sch Health* 1983; 53: 371–373.

Chapter 2

The Concept of Family

Kathleen A. Knafl

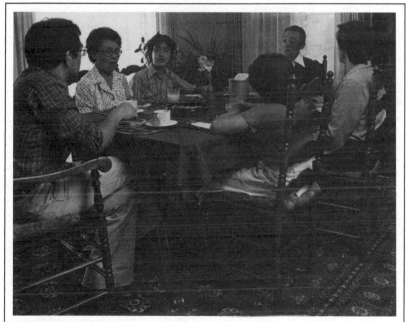

George Fry

The family is a network of emotional, economic, and biologic relationships. It is also the basic unit of care addressed by the community health nurse.

Chapter Outline

Chapter Objectives

After completing this chapter, the reader will be able to:

- Define what is meant by conceptual framework
- Explain how conceptual frameworks structure one's view of family
- Identify the major concepts associated with each of the frameworks
- Apply the major concepts to family situations
- Identify strengths and weaknesses of each of the frameworks

Nothing is or ever was more wonderful, more dreadful or more inescapable than families, nor are there many words more perplexing to define (Howard, 1978).

In community health agencies, acute or extended care facilities, and outpatient settings, nurses are likely to encounter a growing emphasis on family. They are admonished to be more family-centered or to "treat" the family, as opposed to the individual patient. They are encouraged to include family members in their teaching and planning activities. Too often, however, these global prescriptions to be family-centered lack realistic suggestions for translating this ideal into practice. While clinicians may agree that being family-centered is a worthy goal, they often are unsure about the practical implications of trying to achieve this goal in a particular setting. Does it mean a change in the usual routine, the nature of nurse-family interaction, or both? The term implies change, but the exact nature of the change may be difficult to define.

In a study of a newly instituted program of family-centered care, Rosenthal and her colleagues (1980) described changing patterns of family-nurse interaction as a result of the new program. Based on observations of family-nurse interaction in an acute care setting, these authors concluded:

The family and the nurse usually share the same overall goal of getting the patient well. However, the means required to attain this goal may be viewed differently by professional and client. Furthermore, the specific interests and goals of nurse and family are often very different.

. . . The family may want more information than it is getting, or may demand special privileges, different treatment, or more attention. . . . The nurse wants a smoothly functioning ward, without disruptive scenes, emotionally exhausting situations, unnecessary work, or loss of time. . . . To this end, the nurse seeks to control the work setting and the position of the family (p. 88).

Other authors have noted that working with family members can be fraught with difficult decisions and ambiguous situations for everyone involved. Knafl et al (in press) found that nurses and families often had differing notions about what constituted a family-centered approach: "Nurses evidenced a shared and rather narrow view of how parents *should* define and participate in their child's hospitalization. Parents' definitions, however, did not always coincide with those of nurses. They sometimes wanted more and sometimes less involvement than the nurses thought was appropriate."

Few authors have considered how intrafamily conflicts secondary to a health problem or family-nurse conflicts should be dealt with in the context of providing family-centered care. While few professionals would agree "family-centered" connotes that family members always should get their own way, the limits or boundaries of this philosophy of care seldom have been explored. In this chapter we present the concepts of the nature and functioning of the family as a foundation for family-centered community health nursing care.

The Nature and Use of Conceptual Frameworks

Conceptual Frameworks and Understanding Family Life

The task of presenting an overview of selected conceptual frameworks for understanding family life appears to be a simple matter. However, while several well-developed frameworks have been used extensively in nursing, actually applying conceptual frameworks to families turns out to be difficult for two reasons. First, most people grow up in families and, based on that lived experience, consider themselves "experts" in the field. We are family members of one sort or another for most of our lives and tend to be leery of a so-called expert who purports to expound on the nature and functioning of something that we are already acquainted with intimately. We all approach the subject of families with personal and emotional biases, but being intimately acquainted with one or even a few families does not make one an expert in the area. The amount of diversity across families is tremendous, and to understand that diversity it is sometimes useful to consider family life on a conceptual level as opposed to a subjective or feeling one. The specific frameworks presented in this chapter provide a range of perspectives for viewing and analyzing family life. Each presents a distinct view of the family and leads the clinician to focus on somewhat differing aspects of family life.

The second reason why presenting conceptual frameworks of family life is somewhat difficult has to do with "family" as an area of scholarly endeavor. As suggested by the quote introducing this chapter, families are perplexing and hard to define. There is little agreement among those who study families as to which of the available conceptual frameworks are the most helpful for understanding family life or the most appropriate for studying families. In fact, while most scholars subscribe to a favorite framework they acknowledge the need for a variety of frameworks with a variety of emphases. The need for multiple frameworks for understanding family life is not surprising in view of the myriad forms and functions of the contemporary family. Commenting on this diversity, Winch (1977) wrote:

"Family" is a word that may refer to a group of two people, husband and wife, or hundreds—as in the case of clans. Activities of the families may consist of little more than providing company and giving solace, as among the kibbutzim of Israel, or they may embrace virtually all of society's interaction, as among traditional Agrarian Chinese. A father may be unable to get his son to move a lawnmower, or he may determine the boy's occupation and life chances for all the latter's adult years (p. 1).

The numerous definitions of family, such as the following, are indicative of the diversity of thought in this area.

A *family* is a social group in which sexual access is permitted between adult members, reproduction legitimately occurs, the group is responsible to society for the care and upbringing of children, and the group is an economic unit at least in consumption (Zelditch, 1964, p. 680).

The *family* is a kin-based cooperative unit. The *consanguine* family is based on biological relatedness; it is the family of blood relatives and is the main basis of kinship. The *conjugal* family is the group formed by marriage (Broom & Selznick, 1973, pp. 315–316).

The Family Dynamics Measurement Group of the Midwest Nursing Research Society defines family in the following way in the family dynamics questionnaire they have developed:

A group of two or more people living together who have a commitment to each other. Often these people are related to one another by blood or marriage, but they may also be people who care about each other and who live together, such as friends.

As reflected in the preceding definitions, different authors use different criteria for defining family. While some, like Zelditch, emphasize the activities engaged in by family members, others, like Broom and Selznick, stress the composition of the family group and the relationship of the members to one another. The first is a "functional" definition of family; the second is a "structural" definition. Winch (1977) explains the difference between these two types of definitions as follows:

One option is that to qualify as a familial system, that set of individuals must present differentiated positions, the relation among which bear designations of kinship . . . of course, this is a *structural* definition (p. 2).

. . . One can impose the requirement that to qualify as a familial system, a social group must be engaged in one or more activities we recognize as familial, for example, sexual gratification, reproduction, child rearing. Of course, this is a *functional* definition (p. 2).

In contrast, the Family Interest Group of the Midwest Nursing Research Society has adopted a definition of family that includes the notion of commitment, a more subjective though not less important component of group membership. Like

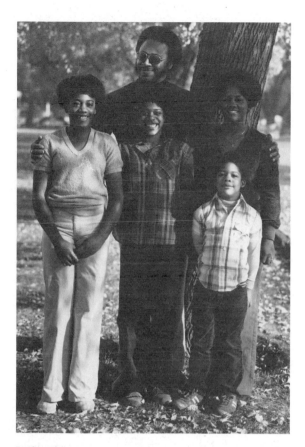

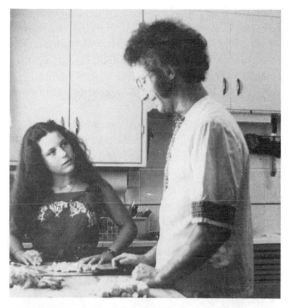

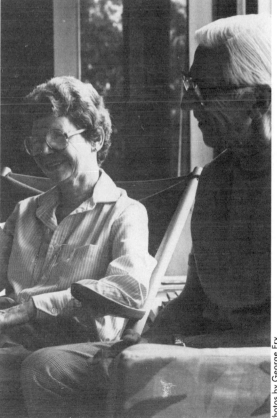

Defined by structure, these three families represent a nuclear family, a single-parent family, and a nuclear dyad. Discussed from a developmental perspective, these are a family with schoolchildren, a family with a teenager, and an aging family.

Winch's functional definition of family, the Family Interest Group's definition encompasses a wide range of alternative or nontraditional family systems. Definitions of family are consequential, since they direct our attention to very different aspects of family life (e.g., internal organization, activities, and mutual commitment).

Definitions are abstract conceptualizations of family. They are mental constructs devised to aid us in distinguishing the family from other social groups (e.g., a student body or a running club). Definitions such as those just cited are usually either part of a more encompassing conceptual framework or they are consistent with tenets of an existing framework. It is to these broader conceptualizations that we now direct our attention.

Conceptual Framework Defined

The term *conceptual framework* is used in this chapter to mean a series of related concepts used in analyzing or describing some aspect of reality. Some authors, such as Burr et al (1979), use the word *theory* rather than conceptual framework, but the concept is the same.

As suggested previously, such frameworks provide a filter or lens through which to view a given subject matter—in this case, the family. They direct our attention to certain phenomena while excluding others, and they provide an interpretive device for determining the meaning of a specific observation or piece of data.

For those who believe that the "facts speak for themselves," the last statement may seem confusing. However, consider the example of a community health nurse who is talking with a mother about her ten-year-old daughter's diabetes. The mother assures the nurse that over the twelve months since the initial diagnosis the family has learned how to handle the situation and that presently the child's illness is "no big deal." Depending on the nurse's frame of reference, the mother's comments may be interpreted as "denial" of the seriousness of her daughter's condition or evidence of successful

coping. In short, the same behavior (fact) can be interpreted in different, even conflicting ways, depending on the conceptual scheme the individual is applying in assessing the meaning of the event.

Often we make interpretations without explicitly linking them to a particular theory or conceptual framework. However, it is a generally held belief in nursing today that clinical nursing practice is enhanced to the extent that nurses can make explicit the rationales underlying specific interpretations, decisions, and interventions. Conceptual frameworks guide our observations and interpretations. As such, they can, in part, provide explicit rationales for action.

Overview of Selected Frameworks

Three social or social-psychological frameworks have been selected for presentation here: the symbolic interactionist framework, the family systems framework, and the developmental framework. While this selection is in no way exhaustive, it does provide a broad overview of the varying perspectives one can take on family life. Excellent references that describe and critically review a more inclusive range of theories are Burr et al (1979) and Nye and Berardo (1981).

In the *symbolic interactionist framework* the focus is on internal family dynamics and members' perceptions of these dynamics. In contrast, the *family systems framework* views the family as a subsystem of the larger society; it directs one's attention to the interchanges between the family and the larger social order of which it is a part. The *developmental framework,* which incorporates concepts from the other two, emphasizes changes in family structure, functioning, and internal dynamics across the family life cycle. The frameworks were developed to be broadly applicable to a wide range of family types and situations. As such, they stand in sharp contrast to those developed from a family therapy perspective, which focuses on therapeutic change. However, as Levant noted, "striking correspondences are observed between the major sociological models . . . and the major clinical models" (1980, p. 5). Thus, the frameworks presented also provide an excellent grounding for readers who also are interested in family therapy.

In order to facilitate comparison across frameworks, common topics will be covered for all. These include: (1) brief discussion of the framework's origin and its intellectual underpinnings, (2) presentation of the major concepts and view of family life presented in the framework, and (3) critique of the framework.

Symbolic Interactionism

Origin

Symbolic interactionism had its roots in the works of pragmatist philosophers who wrote in the late nineteenth and early twentieth century. Pragmatist scholars such as William James, Charles Cooley, John Dewey, and George Herbert Mead equated meaning with applicability, maintaining that things have meaning only if they have an application in the "real world." Building on the basic concepts of pragmatism, these philosophers developed a theory of social action or interaction that emphasized two concepts: self and definition of the situation. Consistent with this theory, individuals define themselves in relation to their situation. From its highly abstract beginnings, symbolic interactionism developed into a framework used to study and conceptualize basic social processes. Burgess (1926) was the first to apply the framework to the study of the family in an article entitled "The Family as a Unity of Interacting Personalities." Symbolic interactionism has subsequently been applied to family study by theorists and researchers in a variety of disciplines, including nursing.

Major Concepts

In general, the purpose of symbolic interactionism is to provide a framework for understanding human behavior on the interactional or microanalytical level by focusing on how individuals define their situation and the consequences of their definitions for action. The framework directs our attention to *internal* family dynamics, paying comparatively less attention to the relationship between the family and other social institutions. In addition, symbolic interactionism focuses on process—how definitions and interactions develop and change over time.

Stressing commonsense, conscious aspects of behavior, symbolic interactionists strive to describe and explain social interaction. Discussing the perspective and method of symbolic interactionism, Blumer (1969) stated that the approach is grounded in three fundamental premises:

1. Human beings act toward things on the basis of the meaning these things have for them.
2. The meaning of such things is derived from or arises out of the social interaction one has with others.
3. These meanings are handled in and modified through an interpretive process used by the people in dealing with the things they encounter (p. 2).

Thus, symbolic interactionism holds that human beings, through their capacity for self-interaction, selectively note and assess the world through a continuous process of interpretation that makes it possible for them to define their situation and construct their actions. For the symbolic interactionist, actions are more than unthinking reactions to stimuli. Rather, actions are *constructed* as the person defines and redefines the situation and makes and carries out decisions based on ongoing definitions. Social interaction is conceived of as a formative process in which individuals formulate and continuously revise their conduct through constant interpretation of each other's actions. To paraphrase Blumer (1969), action is built on the basis of what individuals note, how they assess and interpret what they note, and what kinds of projected lines of action they plan.

Burr and his associates (1979) differentiated between those variables or elements that symbolic interactionism emphasizes, and those it pays relatively less attention to. The framework leads investigators to consider how such things as feedback from others, broad social or demographic variables, and personal value systems contribute to the ongoing defining process all individuals engage in during the course of interaction. Symbolic interactionists pay less attention to intrapsychic phenomena, such as the id or the ego, and the concepts of reward and reinforcements as used by behaviorists. Moreover, they are more interested in understanding and explaining behavior on the interactional or interpersonal level than they are in developing laws applicable across all types of social systems or testing propositions derived from such laws.

The interactionist perspective on self, interaction, and role are especially salient to the purposes of community health nursing. The interactionist framework emphasizes the concept of self—the fact that human beings are organisms with selves. This means that the individual can be an *object* of his or her own actions and feelings. Just as we can be pleased or angry with one another, we can direct these feelings toward our "self."

The self is created by our relationships with others. It is not something established once and for all; it is a *process*, continually evolving out of interaction with others. The self image or sense of identity people have arises out of their ongoing perception of the definition others have of them. For the symbolic interactionist, self refers to an activity; organisms have a self to the degree that they view their own activities from the standpoint of others. The concept of the self is crucial to the

symbolic interactionist, since it is viewed as the mechanism by which individuals deal with their world.

Building on this conception of self, the framework defines human interaction as an emergent process wherein interactants interpret and reinterpret their situations, making and carrying out decisions on the basis of ongoing definitions of the situation and their notion of self. Wiseman (1975) has noted that from a symbolic interactionist perspective, any action entails the following elements: (1) perception of the situation; (2) definition of the situation; (3) consideration of alternative courses of action; (4) selection of a course of action; and (5) monitoring and adjusting a selected course of action.

Regarding roles, interactionists emphasize their emergent nature; they view roles as dynamic processes rather than established entities. Describing this viewpoint, Turner (1962) says:

Roles exist in varying degrees of concreteness and consistency, while the individual confidently frames his behaviors as if they had unequivocal existence and clarity. The result is that in attempting from time to time to make aspects of roles explicit, he is creating and modifying roles as well as merely bringing them to light; the process is not only role-taking, but *role-making* (pp. 22–23).

When undertaking the investigation of specific roles, interactionists do not at the outset attempt to define their parameters completely. Instead they focus on how role definitions emerge and evolve in the course of social interaction. Turner (1962) describes role-taking as "a tentative process in which roles are identified and given content on shifting axes as interaction proceeds. Both the identification of the roles and their content undergo cumulative revision" (p. 27).

The implications of this view of role can be highlighted with an example of how two community health nurses, each with differing notions of the concept of role, manage their initial interaction with a new, young mother. The first nurse, who is *not* a symbolic interactionist, has a well-defined view of what the role of "mother" entails.

His interaction with his client focuses on assessing the extent to which the woman is fulfilling this role. Following his assessment, he proceeds by planning interventions aimed at improving the client's enactment of the role.

In contrast, the nurse who subscribes to an interactionist view of role begins her encounter with a series of questions geared to finding out how this particular new mother defines her role and her more general situation. Further, she attempts to ascertain how these definitions are translated into action. Following this type of assessment, the nurse attempts to negotiate some mutually agreed-upon goals and ways to attain those goals with the mother. Her concern is not limited to her client's success or failure in her new role; rather, she wants to understand how the woman defines and subsequently enacts the role.

In sum, when adopting an interactionist perspective, the clinician or researcher is most likely to consider internal family processes from the comparative, subjective viewpoints of individual family members. This orientation does not imply that the nurse always accepts or takes these subjective views at face value. Nor does it mean that such views are necessarily accurate or in the individual's best interests. Symbolic interactionism does, however, imply that nurses will never be able to understand the family's situation unless they make a concerted, systematic effort to understand how the individuals define that situation.

Critique

Most critiques of symbolic interactionism address its adequacy as a scientific work. Evaluations have focused on such things as the clarity of the framework's major concepts and internal organization, and its usefulness as a conceptual framework in research. Meltzer, Petras, and Reynolds (1975) summarized the following major criticisms:

1. The major concepts are poorly defined and difficult to operationalize.

2. The framework pays inadequate attention to unconscious determinants of human behavior.

3. The framework pays inadequate attention to broader issues of social structure and organization.

On the other hand, various authors (Burr et al, 1979; Christensen, 1964; Hill & Hanson, 1960) have pointed out that symbolic interactionism has provided an organizing framework for a tremendous number of family studies covering such wide-ranging topics as mate selection, enactment of family roles, and family response to crisis situations.

Less attention has been paid to the potential of the framework for guiding clinical practice. Levant (1980) noted the influence of this framework on the work of family therapists such as Ackerman, Bowen, and Satir who subscribe to a process framework. He concluded:

Both models attempt to describe the *dynamic process* of family interaction. They both examine the family as a unity of interacting personalities. . . . In addition, both models tend to consider the family at two levels: The level of internal family processes, and the level of the relationship of the family and the individual family member. Finally, both models emphasize the homeodynamic features and change processes of the family (p. 18).

The applicability of the framework to community health nursing would seem to be to sensitize nurses or provide them an orientation, rather than to be a source of specific prescriptions for practice. In an article by Schroeder (1981) entitled "Symbolic Interactionism: A Conceptual Framework Useful for Nurses Working with Obese Persons," Schroeder provides a useful explanation of how nurses can use this framework. Schroeder writes:

Symbolic interactionism is a useful paradigm in exploring human behavior. It is theory that can be used by nurses in selective specialty areas. It looks at one aspect of human existence in an attempt to better understand dynamics of behavior. This framework adds to the repertory of creative nurses skillfully applying the nursing process. The more we know about each person, the more we know about everyone. The more we know and better understand other human beings, the greater the probability of understanding the world and ourselves. Symbolic interactionism can be one way to further that goal (p. 81).

Research emanating from symbolic interactionism may sensitize nurses to a perspective on their clients but will rarely suggest specific clinical interventions.

Stetler and Marram (1976) have differentiated between what they call "cognitive" and "direct"

application of research, saying that in the former the nurse uses "her knowledge of this study to enhance her understanding of various situations or to analyze the dynamics of practice" (p. 565). Direct application entails such things as using the findings as evidence for change, as impetus for further program evaluation, or as a model for action. Symbolic interactionism makes its greatest contribution in the realm of cognitive application.

The Systems Framework

Origin

In recent years there has been a growing interest in applying the principles of general systems theory to different types of groups and organizations. Associated with the work of Bertalanffy (1968), systems theory was intended to provide a language and framework that would be general enough to cut across scientific disciplines.

Buckley (1967) describes systems theory as a scientific world view with a "central focus on the principles of *organization per se*, regardless of what it is that is organized" (1967, p. 36). Systems theory provides us with a way of viewing people and their environments as an interrelated, interacting whole—a system of interrelated parts that interact within an identifiable boundary. Systems are defined in terms of their structure, the arrangement of the parts of the system, the system's function, the processes or activities in which the system engages, and the system's boundary or the demarcation between the system and its environment. Moreover, systems are characterized as interacting with their environment and being hierarchically arranged. They are hierarchical in that they can be arranged according to a point of reference and divided into both subsystems and suprasystems. For example, if the nuclear family is the point of ref-

erence, then the marital dyad can be viewed as a subsystem and the extended family can be viewed as a suprasystem.

As system theory developed, a point of controversy often raised regarding systems theory is whether or not the system itself is greater than or equal to the sum of its parts. In the area of family, this leads us to ask if we want to equate the family system with the individual members, or if we view the family system as having an identity that transcends that of its individual members. Clearly, community health nurses are concerned with individuals as members of families as well as with the dynamics and functions of the family system as a whole.

Another somewhat controversial point in the area of systems theory has to do with how systems change. While some theorists emphasize system stability and resistance to change, others have focused on its flexibility and adaptiveness. Buckley (1967), for example, distinguishes between homeostatic and complex adaptive systems. The homeostatic system, while it may be very complex, tends to resist change. When confronted with the need to change, such a system makes the least amount of change necessary to ensure its ongoing survival. On the other hand, complex adaptive systems are characterized as both initiating and thriving on change. The model of a complex, adaptive system is viewed by many as especially appropriate for characterizing family life (Aldous, 1978; Kantor and Lehr, 1975; Schwenk & Hughes, 1983; Taylor, 1979). The preceding comments, while introducing the reader to the systems theory perspective, also illustrate the highly general nature of systems concepts. The subsequent discussion of major concepts will focus on an examination of how systems concepts have been applied to the family.

Major Concepts

Aldous (1978, p. 26) cites the following as characteristics of a family social system:

1. The positions occupied by family members, the parts of the family system, are to varying degrees *interdependent.*
2. The family through *selective boundary maintenance* constitutes a unit.
3. The family is a *task performance* group, meeting the demands of other social agencies as well as those of its members.
4. The family is capable of change.

Discussing the applicability of systems theory to the discipline of family medicine, Taylor (1979, p. 101) presents a slightly different view of the family as a social system: "The family is comprised of a network of continually evolving interpersonal unions [structure]. It is linked by bonds of closeness, security, identity, support, and sharing [bonding], and is demarcated by genetic heritage, legal sanction, and interpersonal alliance [boundaries]. The family is perpetuated to fill individual biologic, economic, psychologic, and social needs [function]." Aldous's and Taylor's views have much in common. Both emphasize the concepts of structure, function, boundary maintenance, and change. Taylor's identification of bonding as a characteristic of the family system is somewhat analogous to Aldous's description of interdependency. Note that, ideally, the family as a social system simultaneously meets the needs of its individual members, the family system as an ongoing entity, and society in general.

Aldous's characteristics of the family as a social system will be discussed in greater detail in the section on the developmental framework, since the developmental framework encompasses systems theory concepts as well as sequential developmental changes over time. The characteristics will be introduced briefly here with the bulk of the discussion focusing on how, according to the systems perspective, families change or modify their structure.

Positions within the family and the patterned interactions that develop between and among the incumbents of the various positions constitute the structure of the family. While, in general, family positions are viewed as interdependent, Aldous (1978) describes how the degree and nature of these interdependencies vary over time. An obvious example of this is the dependency of children on their parents, which is often reversed during the parents' old age. In contrast, in a family with all members gainfully employed, members may be relatively independent of one another. The systems framework directs our attention to understanding the nature and intensity of family interdependencies at a given point in time.

Noting that families maintain control of their boundaries if they accomplish certain goals, Aldous (1978, pp. 41–42) lists the following as goals that the family is expected to achieve:

1. Physical maintenance of family members
2. Socialization of family members for roles in the family and other groups
3. Maintenance of family members' motivation to perform familial and other roles
4. Maintenance of social control within the family and between family members and outsiders
5. Addition of family members through adoption or reproduction, and their release when mature

Through the accomplishment of these goals families fulfill the needs of individual members, perpetuate the family as an ongoing entity, and meet society's need for an ongoing supply of appropriately socialized individuals. Similar to the structural interdependencies just discussed, family functions vary over time with certain goals being more or less important at different points in time. Thus, while socialization, the learning of appropriate social roles, is generally considered an especially important task in families with school-age children, social control, the ability to exercise self-discipline, may be the focal task in families with adolescents. On the other hand, physical maintenance is crucial regardless of the age configuration of family members.

Describing the family as a boundary maintaining unit, Aldous (1978) means that families constitute identifiable social entities. The family as a unit is recognizable through such tangible factors as shared residence and use of kinship terminology, as well as through less tangible factors like shared history and values. At the individual level we often associate family with a place (home), experiences held in common, and viewing the world in a particular way. Ideally, the family's structure contributes to its ability to fulfill essential goals and maintain its boundaries. Roles and tasks are fairly distributed, and the interactions among family members are sufficiently stable and cooperative to ensure that the five goals previously listed are, in fact, achieved. When this is the case, the family is capable of maintaining control of its own boundaries. When operating effectively, the family controls its own boundaries, granting access to outsiders such as police or social welfare agencies only when family members view such access desirable. Thus, an obvious indicator of family dysfunction or disintegration is the family's loss of control over its own boundaries.

Aldous also discusses how the systems framework can be used to describe how families adapt and change over time. Aldous (1978) describes this process in terms of information exchange and feedback processes. Families and their individual members constantly receive and transmit information. Such exchanges take place within the family and between the family and the community. Through such information exchange families evaluate their performance or progress toward achieving the pre-

viously listed goals. The perception by the family as a whole or by an individual family member that there is a poor fit between performance and goals can provide the impetus for change.

Family system theorists (Aldous, 1978; Broderick & Smith, 1979) have identified different ways families change. An important distinction is whether or not the family is viewed as a *reactive entity* that responds to internal or external pressure to change or if it is conceptualized as also capable of *initiating change.* Aldous (1978) terms the first change process *negative feedback,* saying: "Traditionally, in systems theory, these operations have been thought of in terms of negative feedback. Systems were conceptualized in organic terms as having only limited repertoires of responses to adapt to change. The emphasis was on homeostasis or relative stability. Such an approach sees families as changing over time through an accumulation of small changes" (pp. 37–38). The concept of negative feedback assumes that families attempt to avoid change and maintain existing structures. Change occurs only when these structures prove inadequate and the assumption is that the family will always attempt to minimize change.

In contrast, the concept of *positive feedback* emphasizes the family's ability to initiate change. Describing this process, Aldous (1978) says: "When the family initiates change, unlike situations in cases of negative feedback, there is no attempt to smother deviation. The family tries new behaviors and explores alternate goals so that there is a clear divergence from old ways and values" (p. 38).

An example of how two different families respond to the wife-mother's return to the work force should help distinguish between these two conceptualizations of change. Both are relatively stable families. Over the years, predictable patterns of interaction have developed among members. In particular, the husbands and wives have a well-defined and somewhat traditional division of labor. In the first family, the wife's return to the labor force is predicated on the assumption that it can be accomplished with minimal disruption to established routines. No attempt is made to alter long-standing patterns, and changes are made only after it becomes apparent that established patterns are no longer workable. For example, the usual dinner time may be moved up an hour when it becomes obvious that the wife-mother can no longer have dinner on the table at the usual time, or other family members may be called upon to assist the wife-mother with her usual responsibilities. In other words, family members attempt to *adapt* existing structures to the new situation. Only if these adaptations fail to work (e.g., the wife-mother finds the dual responsibilities of home and work unmanageable) will the family consider altering its existing structure.

Another family may deal with the wife-mother's return to the labor force in quite a different way. They, too, have a well-established and fairly stable division of labor. However, several months prior to the wife-mother's return to work, the parents call a family conference to discuss how members might change current ways of doing things in order to accommodate the impending change. Not only do family members negotiate a new division of labor, but they agree to "scale down" certain activities such as entertaining. This family is more concerned with *creating new structures* than it is with maintaining or adapting old ones. The first family illustrates negative feedback, the second is engaged in a positive feedback process. One can also conceive of situations where certain family members are struggling to maintain existing structures while others are striving to identify and initiate new, innovative structures.

A family's ability to initiate change is influenced by the number of options the family members identify as open to them, as well as by the amount of time the family has to plan and initiate an explicit change in family life. For example, it should be easier for families to initiate change when the situation in question is an impending birth, rather than a precipitous illness. Similarly, families who have contacts with others who have adapted to a given situation in a variety of ways are more able to initiate change than are families without such information.

Broderick and Smith (1979) identify another form of family change that they label reorientation or conversion. This type of change brings differences in the fundamental goals of the family system: "Little has been done to study dramatic reorientations such as occur when a black Baptist family becomes Muslim or a Protestant family converts to Judaism or members of a Catholic family become Jehovah's Witnesses. Analyses of these phenomena might shed light on the nature of family systems and the circumstances and preconditions that lead to this highest order of change" (p. 122).

The systems framework provides a useful scheme for determining the nature and magnitude of change in family life. Using this framework, the nurse can consider whether the family is primarily concerned with maintaining or altering existing structures or goals, or both, and can assess the appropriateness of the family's orientation in view of the situation at issue.

Critique

Broderick and Smith (1979, pp. 125–126) identify five general areas of family study that lend themselves to investigation using a systems perspective: patterns of interaction, communication and control, goal orientation, boundary maintenance, and complex relationships. They note that boundary maintenance typically has been a concern of family therapists; they include family response to crisis as part of patterns of interaction. All five areas are relevant to nursing practice.

In general, perhaps because of the relative newness of the systems approach in the area of family study, family scholars are more likely to emphasize its potential than to belabor its shortcomings. This stance is exemplified by Schwenk and Hughes (1983): "General Systems Theory helps to clarify an intimate, yet, confusing relationship between the family and its members . . . [it] provides an appropriate model by which the family can be analyzed in terms of its own structure, function, and the forces linking it to the individual, as well as other entities such as a family's community, culture, and society" (pp. 3 & 10).

Because it encourages considering both intra-family dynamics and family-community linkages, the framework, with its developing applications to the family, should prove especially useful to the community health nurse. Broderick and Smith (1979) conclude their chapter on the general systems approach to the family by saying, "what seems certain is that the contribution of systems theory to the study of the family is still in its infancy. The future holds promise of greater things" (p. 128).

Developmental Framework

Origin

The developmental framework was explicitly formulated to be of use to the professional who works with families. In her introduction Duvall (1977) emphasizes the applied orientation of the developmental approach: "The text in its previous editions has proven useful in such university departments as adult education, child development and family relations, home and family, home economics, human development, nursing, social work, sociology, and general education, as well as in pre-professional and paraprofessional courses" (p. xi).

The framework originated in the context of the First White House Conference on Family Life in 1948. Evelyn Duvall and Reuben Hill (cochairs of the conference) were charged with developing an organized framework for the conference that would contribute to the goal of summarizing research on the problems families face across time, and aid in describing and documenting the natural history of family life. Duvall (1977) described preparation for the conference in the following way:

As co-chairman of the Committee on the Dynamics of Family Interaction, Dr. Hill and I prepared a two-dimensional outline for plotting the developmental tasks of children and of parents for each stage of the family life cycle and anticipating the probable need for services arising out of the challenges, hazards, and problems involved in the achievement of each developmental task in our culture (p. 14).

Eight subcommittees of specialists at the various developmental levels were appointed by Duvall and Hill to prepare reports on the various life cycle stages. This led to the eventual production of several hundred pages of working papers that provided background material for the conference. The framework devised for this conference provided the basis for subsequent work on the developmental conceptual framework.

Describing the overall development of this framework, Burr (1973) pointed out that its origin and development were unique. For the first time a framework had been devised to look solely at family life with the intent of being both theoretically and clinically useful.

Duvall and Hill, who are usually acknowledged as the framework's originators, had their Ph.D.s in human development and sociology, respectively. Those attending the conference, as well as scholars who have been active in developing the framework since then, have continued to reflect an interdisciplinary interest in individual development and more general social processes. Thus, while most of the research based on the framework has been done by sociologists, the influence of developmental psychology on this perspective is evident. Moreover, the developmental framework incorporates and attempts to integrate several distinct, and in some cases competing, sociological orientations. Hill and Rodgers (1964) point out that it includes concepts from such diverse areas as rural sociology, symbolic interactionism, and sociology of professions.

The developers of the framework attempted to go beyond an exclusive focus on internal family dynamics, a goal that is apparent in Rodgers's (1964) definition of family. Rodgers expanded the definition of family beyond its focus on internal dynamics as he conceptualized the family as a semiclosed system of interacting personalities having the following characteristics (p. 264):

1. The family is not entirely independent of other social systems, neither is it wholly dependent. Thus, it is a semiclosed system.
2. The family as a small group system is interrelated in such a manner that change does not occur in one part without a series of resultant changes in other parts.
3. The family is composed of dynamic persons who are both group members and individuals, and, therefore, changes in both group relationships and individual personality factors must be taken into account.

Following the original White House Conference, which spurred the development of the framework, Duvall and Hill, along with their students, continued to refine and apply the framework. Their efforts continue today.

Major Concepts

Duvall (1977) described the basic premise on which the framework is based in the following way: "There is a predictability about family development that helps us know what to expect of a given family at any given stage. Much as each individual who grows, develops, matures, and ages undergoes the same successive changes and readjustments from conception to senescence as every other individual, the life cycle of individual families follow a very universal sequence of family development" (p. 141). In general, the framework's originators believed that our understanding of family life is increased by considering the family in the context of both individual human development and the larger social system.

Within the developmental framework the family is viewed as a social system and the framework itself contains elements of Aldous's four characteristics of the family as a social system discussed previously. For example, within this framework, the family is viewed as a social system characterized by the following: (1) interrelated, interdepend-

ent positions, (2) relatively closed boundaries, (3) ongoing adaptive processes, and (4) task performance. Thus, there is a great deal of conceptual overlap between the developmental and systems frameworks for viewing family life. In general, however, developmental family theorists have become increasingly explicit in relating systems concepts to the developmental approach. Hill (1974) has discussed the compatibility between the two frameworks. The developmental approach, however, emphasizes the nature of family development and change over time to a far greater extent than the other two frameworks discussed. Both the overlap with systems concepts and the unique life cycle focus are described in the following discussion.

To say that the family comprises interrelated positions means that it has an identifiable structure and that changes in one part of the system reverberate throughout the system as a whole. Describing family structure, Hill (1974) says: "The network of relationships that links family members together arises from shared normative expectations. These shared expectations unite family members and at the same time they also serve to differentiate the family unit from other associations" (p. 306). The family's structure is described as a series of paired positions (e.g., husband-wife; parent-child). At any given point in time, each position includes a number of roles that society generally expects of the individual in the position. For example, the roles of breadwinner, nurturer, and housekeeper typically are filled by persons in either or both of the parental positions. Patterned, relatively predictable interactions develop over time between incumbents of various positions. Such patterned interactions further define and determine the family's structure.

By characterizing the family as having *relatively* closed boundaries, Hill acknowledges the linkages between the family and other social institutions. He (1974) states, "The family is now viewed as neither wholly independent of other social systems, nor is it wholly dependent; thus, it is termed a "semi-closed system" opening up *selectively* to transact business with other associations" (p. 306). This view of family facilitates looking at the links and interchanges between the family and the community.

That it is characterized as an adaptive system means that, as a unit, the family is constantly confronting and dealing with change. Hill's colorful description of family life illustrates this point:

The family system is perhaps more subject to disturbance than other organizations because of its rapidly changing age composition and frequently changing plurality patterns. Its curious age and sex composition make it an inefficient work group, a poor planning committee, an unwieldy play group, and a group of uncertain congeniality. Its leadership is shared by two relatively inexperienced amateurs for most of their incumbency, new to the roles of spouse and parent. They must work with a succession of disciples having few skills and lacking in judgment under conditions which never seem to remain stable long enough to bring about a settled organization (p. 397).

In spite of the myriad sources of stress in family life, however, most families are capable of maintaining an identifiable structure over time. Although proponents of the framework recognize the possibility of family dissolution through divorce or death, the tendency has been to focus on stability in the face of changing circumstances.

Finally, the family is characterized as a task-performing unit that meets both the requirements of external agencies in the society and the internal needs and demands of its members (Hill, 1974). The family must accomplish certain tasks to continue as a viable unit. While different authors cite different family functions, the following are usually referred to as major ones: socialization, physical maintenance, and social control. Socialization entails communicating and teaching appropriate familial and societal roles to family members, especially during childhood and adolescence. It is a function shared with other social institutions such as the school system. Physical maintenance refers to achieving sufficient economic independence to maintain a household for one's family. In the United States it is generally assumed that individuals will establish households that are separate from their family of origin. The family social control function

refers to its ability to prevent members from disrupting family life, and from their causing disruptions in the community, as well.

In sum, the developmental approach views the family as a system of persons in well-defined positions who have well-defined role responsibilities. Families maintain an identifiable structure, which contributes to their ability to fulfill certain tasks or functions that, in turn, contribute to the survival of the family unit as a bounded, ongoing entity. Moreover, the family is viewed as adaptable and capable of accommodating change (both from within and without) while maintaining a relative stability.

As noted, this particular conceptualization of family contains elements of the systems perspective. However, the developmental approach is unique in its inclusion of concepts that are specific to family development and change over time. These concepts are "family life cycle" and "family developmental task," which Duvall (1977, pp. 137–186) defines as follows:

- *family life cycle:* Sequence of characteristic stages beginning with family formation and continuing through the life of the family to its dissolution
- *family developmental task:* Growth responsibilities that arise at certain stages in the life of a family, achievement of which leads to success with later tasks

While various authors have identified different numbers of stages in the family life cycle, ranging from as few as two (Duvall, 1977) to as many as twenty-four (Rodgers, 1962), Duvall's eight-stage breakdown, as noted by Burr (1973) is probably the most widely used. The eight stages and the period of time the "typical" family spends in each are as follows:

1. Married couples (without children): 2 years
2. Childbearing families (oldest child is aged birth to 30 months): 2.5 years
3. Families with preschool children (oldest child is aged 30 months to 6 years): 3.5 years
4. Families with schoolchildren (oldest child is aged 6 to 13 years): 7 years

Table 2-1   Major Developmental Task for Each Phase of the Family Life Cycle

Life Cycle Stage	Major Developmental Task
1. Married couple	Establishing a mutually satisfying marriage
2. Childbearing	Adapting to parenthood; establishing a satisfying home for parents and infant(s)
3. Preschool-age	Adapting to needs and interests of preschool child; coping with energy depletion and lack of privacy
4. School-age	Encouraging children's educational achievement; fitting into the community of school-age families
5. Teenage	Balancing teenage responsibility and freedom; establishing postparental interests
6. Launching	Releasing young adults while maintaining a supportive home base
7. Middle-age	Rebuilding marital relationship; maintaining ties with other generations
8. Aging	Adjusting to retirement, loneliness and bereavement

SOURCE:
Adapted from Duvall E: *Marriage and Family Development,* 5th ed. New York: Lippincott, 1976, p. 1979.

5. Families with teenagers (oldest child is aged 13 to 20 years): 7 years
6. Families launching young adult (first child gone to last child leaving home): 8 years
7. Middle-aged parents (empty nest to retirement): 15 years ±
8. Aging family members (retirement to death of both spouses): 10 to 15 years ±

This breakdown, grounded in the assumption that "families grow and develop as their children do" is based on a consideration of four factors: number of positions, age of oldest child, school placement of oldest child, nature of family before arrival and after departure of children (Duvall, 1977, pp. 1–5).

Duvall also identifies critical developmental tasks that must be accomplished if the family is to progress to the next stage successfully. Table 2-1 summarizes these tasks. Describing such tasks, Duvall says: "Stage critical family developmental tasks occur as the family enters each new stage of its development. Each new developmental crisis necessitates new adaptations and imposes new responsibilities at the same time that it opens up new opportunities and poses new challenges" (p. 178).

In general, the developmental approach provides us with a view of the family as a social system. It emphasizes the relationships of family structure to function and directs attention to families throughout the entire life span, which consists of a series of stages. According to this approach, during each stage of the family's life cycle there are specific tasks to accomplish.

Critique

Authors who have studied the family point out both strengths and weaknesses of this framework. Duvall maintains that the approach is relevant clinically for health professionals because "knowing where a family is in its life cycle makes it possible to anticipate a number of vital factors—its relative income level, its consumer practices, whether the wife works, the couple's probable marital satisfaction, areas of possible family conflict, and the nature of its parent-child relationships—for example" (Duvall, 1977, p. 157). Authors of nursing texts (Friedman, 1981; Janosik & Miller, 1980; Knafl & Grace, 1978) have included the framework as one having actual or potential applicability to nursing practice.

The framework is most applicable to traditional family forms. It is difficult, if not impossible, to apply to such nontraditional family forms as single-parent or blended family configurations. Moreover, it has been criticized for being overly child-centered and for having minimal applicability to those families whose progression through the family life cycle stages vary considerably from the norm.

Application of Frameworks

In the following discussion, Case Example 2-1 illustrates the point that one's conceptualization of the situation can have implications for clinical practice and that there are no absolutes when it comes to identifying the best framework to apply in a given situation. We compare how a community health nurse working from each of the frameworks would proceed. Table 2-2 presents a comparison of the three frameworks, which is also useful in understanding the case example.

The Symbolic Interactionist Nurse

Jean Bennett is a proponent of symbolic interactionism. After her initial interaction with Mrs. Allen, she is concerned that she has very little sense of how her client really defines her situation. She wants to know what meaning Mrs. Allen attaches to her son's birth, her thwarted plans to return to work, and her daughter's pregnancy. She "hypothesizes" that Mrs. Allen sees her family as significantly and irrevocably altered, but wants to know more about how family members define their situation before she considers possible interventions. Thus, her first concern is to spend more time talking with Mrs. Allen and to try to arrange to meet and talk with other family members. Jean doesn't think that her approach will necessarily make the appropriate intervention obvious, but she firmly maintains that unless she understands the viewpoints of the various family members, she will be severely limited in her attempts to help the family.

The Systems Nurse

Linda Ryan has always found it particularly helpful to view the family as a system. She has found the framework useful for understanding myriad family types and situations she encounters, and has no reason to think that the Allen family will be an exception. The focus of her discussion with Mrs. Allen is twofold. She first attempts to evaluate how the family has changed as a result of events taking place over the past year. This assessment includes evaluating the extent to which the family's usual functions have been altered and the family's overall orientation to change. She is especially interested in knowing if the family has a history of resisting change or if they are used to major changes and generally see them as an opportunity to grow. In addition, Jean wants to find out more about the family's ties to the community. She is interested in encouraging the family to reestablish ties that have lapsed since the birth of the impaired child and identifying community resources that may help the family to function more satisfactorily in spite of their difficult circumstances. Her aim is to identify resources that are appropriate to the family's needs and usual method of dealing with change.

Case Example 2-1: The Allen Family: A Clinical Application of Family Theory

Mr. and Mrs. Allen are a middle-aged couple (forty-five and forty-one years old, respectively) who have been married for twenty-two years. They have four children: a twenty-year-old daughter, Emily, who is a junior in college and lives at home; an eighteen-year-old daughter, Susan, who is a high school senior, pregnant, and trying to decide whether she wants to marry her boyfriend; a sixteen-year-old son, Jim, who is a junior in high school, an excellent student and athlete; and a one-year-old son, Jeff, who was "unplanned" and was born with multiple anomalies and is severely retarded.

Family in two life cycle stages

The community health nurse has been in contact with the family since soon after Jeff's birth. In her initial contacts with Mrs. Allen, she learned that Mrs. Allen had worked as a receptionist and bookkeeper in a dentist's office throughout her pregnancy and had looked forward to going back to work part-time after the baby's birth. However, given Jeff's numerous problems, this had not been possible. Soon after, Mr. Allen had taken a second job on a part-time basis. The three older children also worked part-time and contributed to household expenses, although they were generally unavailable to help care for Jeff, as was Mr. Allen. Mrs. Allen said she was worried about her daughter Susan, disappointed about the pregnancy, and hopeful that the community health nurse could convince her to get married. The two other children were described as "good kids," and Mrs. Allen said she didn't want them to be burdened by having to care for their impaired sibling at a time when they were anxious to have greater independence from the family.

Role responsibilities have changed

Mrs. Allen defines her own performance as inadequate

Mrs. Allen wants to minimize change

Mrs. Allen described herself and husband as regular church-goers who, until the birth of Jeff, had been active in several church groups. She also noted that both she and her husband had avoided usual contacts with friends and relatives since Jeff's birth and that the older children seldom brought friends home now.

Family's reliance on community support has changed

Mrs. Allen said she felt overwhelmed by her situation. She described caring for Jeff as a full-time job and felt that she had little time and energy left to do anything else. She felt she should be spending more time with other family members, especially her husband and pregnant daughter, but didn't believe this was possible. She said she was becoming more and more resigned to the fact that "the good times were over."

Mrs. Allen defines the family as negatively and permanently changed

The Developmental Nurse

Terry Simmons is fascinated by the Allen family. He has often found the developmental framework useful in his initial assessments of families and is challenged by the possibility of applying it to a family that seems to be in two family life cycle stages at once (childbearing and child launching). He uses the framework as a guide to asking questions that center on the tasks associated with both life cycle stages the family is in. He, too, is interested in how the family is functioning as a system, but he is sensitive to the fact that families function in different ways at different points in their life

Table 2-2 Comparison of Conceptual Frameworks

Framework	Origin	Major Concepts	Critique
Symbolic Interactionism	1. Pragmatist philosophy 2. Provide a framework for understanding social processes	1. Family as a unit of interacting personalities 2. Definition of the situation 3. Self 4. Interaction 5. Role	1. Major concepts vague and difficult to measure 2. Gives inadequate attention to psychic processes 3. Gives inadequate attention to social structure 4. Provides a guide for understanding, not a prescription for action 5. Sensitizes one to the family's viewpoint
Systems	1. Bertalanffy 2. Provide a common language and framework for science	1. Family as a social system 2. Structure 3. Boundary 4. Goal seeking 5. Negative feedback 6. Positive feedback	1. Major concepts understood and applicable across disciplines 2. Provides a framework for understanding change 3. Provides a framework for viewing family's relationship to the community 4. Relatively new approach with comparatively little research
Developmental	1. First White House Conference on Family Life 2. Provide a framework for understanding natural history of family life	1. Family as a semiclosed system of interacting personalities 2. Structure 3. Goal orientation 4. Orderly sequence (family life cycle) 5. Family developmental tasks	1. Developed to be clinically relevant and applicable 2. Difficult to apply to "nontraditional" families 3. Inadequate conceptualization of life cycle variables 4. Difficult to conduct longitudinal studies applying the framework 5. Provides a guide for assessing families at different stages of their life cycle

cycle, and concludes that many of the problems the Allens are experiencing are exacerbated by being in two life cycle stages at once. While he realizes that the Allens don't fit the traditional family situation for which the model was formulated, he sees the model, nonetheless, as a useful beginning point and guide for his assessment.

Summary

The frameworks discussed in this chapter should not be viewed as competing or mutually exclusive orientations. The reader is urged to view them instead as guides to conceptualizing, and therein, understanding. A given framework is neither good or bad, right or wrong, in any absolute sense. However, it may be more or less useful or appropriate, depending on the problem or situation to which it's applied.

The different frameworks emphasize, and thus direct attention to, different aspects of family life. Symbolic interactionism focuses on the emergence of subjective definitions of the situation during the course of interaction. The developmental framework focuses on sequential regularities, and the systems framework emphasizes interdependence, information processing, and change. All are likely to be useful in some situations and comparatively irrelevant in others. The practitioner is thus encouraged to pay close attention to the "fit" between a selected framework and the clinical or research problem at hand.

While there are important differences among the frameworks, it is also important to recognize that there is a good deal of conceptual overlap among them as well. Thus, while each has its own particular emphasis, it also shares common themes or emphases with the other frameworks. For example, an interest in interdependence and change characterizes each framework. It may well be that a given problem could satisfactorily be addressed by symbolic interactionism, the developmental framework, or systems theory, leaving the clinician or researcher free to fall back on his or her own personal favorite.

Finally, it is important to remind the reader that only an overview of each framework has been presented. The author's intent has been to provide the reader with a basic introduction to the frameworks. Numerous books and articles are available on each of them, and the reader who desires a more in-depth understanding is encouraged to seek out some of the reference material cited at the end of this chapter.

Study Questions

1. As a community health nurse you are especially interested in understanding the transition involved for parents as their adolescent children leave home. Which of the frameworks presented would be most suitable for understanding this situation?
   a. Developmental framework
   b. Symbolic interactionist
   c. Systems
2. As a home health nurse working with families who have a dependent elderly person living in the home, you are especially interested in ensuring that these families take advantage of available community support services. Which of the frameworks presented is especially suited for looking at the relationship of the family to other social institutions?
   a. Developmental framework
   b. Symbolic interactionist
   c. Systems
3. As a "budding" nurse theorist/researcher, you are concerned that current theories pay inadequate attention to the clients' viewpoint and want to conduct a study of families that

addresses this issue. On which of the frameworks presented would you ground your study?
   a. Developmental framework
   b. Symbolic interactionist
   c. Systems
4. You are a new graduate working for the Visiting Nurse Association and mention to a coworker that you are interested in family development and have been doing some reading of theories and research in the area. Your coworker suggests that you stop wasting your time, maintaining that theory and research are "ivory tower" endeavors that are never applicable to the real world. How would you respond to your coworker's accusations and justify your attempts to apply theory to practice?
   a. Tell your coworker that facts don't necessarily speak for themselves.
   b. Offer your coworker an example of how research findings contribute to theory development and understanding of behavior.
   c. Tell your coworker that you will wait until you have more experience to continue your interest in theory and research.
5. Which of the following statements is a useful way to view the conceptual frameworks presented?
   a. The frameworks emphasize and direct our attention to different aspects of family life.
   b. The frameworks are specific prescriptions for clinical practice involving families.
   c. The frameworks serve to interpret family behavior in the clinical setting.
   d. The frameworks have theoretical but not clinical relevance.

References

Aldous J: *Family Careers.* New York: Wiley, 1978.

Bertalanffy L von: *General Systems Theory.* New York: Braziller, 1968.

Blumer H: *Symbolic Interactionism.* Englewood Cliffs, N.J.: Prentice-Hall, 1969.

Broderick C, Smith J: The general systems approach to the family. In: Burr W et al (editors), *Contemporary Theories about the Family.* New York: The Free Press, 1979.

Broom L, Selznick P: *Sociology: A Text with Adapted Readings,* 5th ed. New York: Harper & Row, 1973.

Buckley W: *Sociology and Modern Systems Theory.* Englewood Cliffs, N.J.: Prentice-Hall, 1967.

Burgess EW: The family as a unity of interacting personalities. *The Family* 1926; 7: 3–9.

Burr W, Leigh GK, Day RD, Constantine J: Symbolic interaction and the family. In: Burr W et al (editors), *Contemporary Theories about the Family.* New York: The Free Press, 1979.

Burr WR: *Theory Construction and the Sociology of the Family.* New York: Wiley, 1973.

Christensen HT (editor): *Handbook of Marriage and the Family.* Chicago: Rand McNally, 1964.

Duvall EM: *Marriage and Family Development,* 5th ed. Philadelphia: Lippincott, 1977.

Friedman M: *Family Nursing: Theory and Assessment.* New York: Appleton-Century-Crofts, 1981.

Hill R, Rodgers RH: The developmental approach. In: Christensen HT (editor), *Handbook on Marriage and the Family.* Chicago: Rand McNally, 1964.

Hill RL: Modern systems theory and the family: A confrontation. In: Sussman MB (editor), *Sourcebook of Marriage and the Family,* 4th ed. Boston: Houghton Mifflin, 1974.

Hill RL, Hansen DA: The identification of conceptual frameworks utilized in family study. *Marriage and Family Living* 1960, 22: 299–311.

Howard J: *Families.* New York: Simon & Schuster, 1978.

Janosik E, Miller J: *Family Focused Care.* New York: McGraw-Hill, 1980.

Kantor D, Lehr W: *Inside the Family.* San Francisco: Jossey-Bass, 1975.

Knafl K, Grace H: *Families Across the Life Cycle.* Boston: Little, Brown, 1978.

Knafl KA, Cavallari K, Dixon D: *Perspectives in Pediatric Hospitalization.* Boston: Little, Brown, in press.

Levant R: Sociological and clinical models of family: An attempt to identify paradigms. *American Journal of Family Therapy* 1980; 8(4): 5–20.

Meltzer BN, Petras JW, Reynolds LT: *Symbolic Interactionism: Genesis, Varieties and Criticism.* Boston: Routledge and Kegan Paul, 1975.

Nye FI, Berardo FM (editors): *Emerging Conceptual Frameworks in Family Analysis.* New York: Praeger, 1981.

Rodgers RH: Toward a theory of family development. *Journal of Marriage and the Family* 1964; 26: 262–270.

Rogers R: *Improvements in the Construction and Analysis of Family Life Cycle Categories.* Kalamazoo, Mich.: Western Michigan University, 1962. Ph.D. dissertation from University of Minnesota.

Rosenthal CJ et al: *Nurses, Patients and Families.* New York: Springer, 1980.

Rowe GP: The developmental conceptual framework to the study of the family. In: Nye IF, Berardo FM (editors), *Emerging Conceptual Frameworks in Family Analysis.* New York: Macmillan, 1966.

Schroeder AMK: Symbolic interactionism: A conceptual framework useful for nurses working with obese persons. *Image* 1981; 13: 78–81.

Schwenk TL, Hughes CC: The family as a patient in family medicine—myth or reality? *Social Science and Medicine* 1983; 17: 1–16.

Stetler CB, Marram G: Evaluating research findings for applicability in practice. *Nurs Outlook* 1976; 24: 559–563.

Taylor RB: Family: A systems approach. *American Family Physician* 1979; 20(5): 101–104.

Turner R: Role taking: Process versus conformity. In: Rose A (editor), *Human Behavior and Social Processes.* Boston: Houghton Mifflin, 1962.

Winch RE: *Familial Organization: A Quest for Determinants.* New York: The Free Press, 1977.

Wiseman JP: The application of symbolic interaction theory and research findings to family behavior. Paper presented to the Theory Construction Workshop of the National Council on Family Relations, St. Louis, Mo., October 22–23, 1975.

Zelditch M Jr: Family, marriage, and kinship. In: Faris R (editor), *Handbook of Modern Sociology.* Chicago: Rand McNally, 1964.

Chapter 3

The Concept of Community

Cecilia E. Dawkins

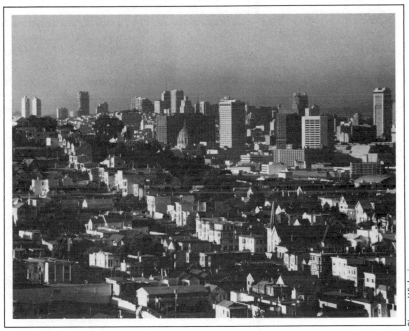

Communities are as varied in their structures and content as families are. Whether a residential neighborhood or bustling business district, communities encompass three dimensions: place, people, and social relationships.

Chapter Objectives

After completing this chapter, the reader will be able to:

- Explain ways that the community is defined
- Analyze the definitions for their relevance to community health nursing
- Describe the five functions of a community
- Describe three conceptual frameworks and explain how each can be a useful guide in a study of the community
- Apply the major concepts of the frameworks to a study of the community with relevance to community health nursing

Questions raised about the concept of family such as What is a family? and What are the functions of a family? are also appropriate to ask about the community. This is relevant because the family and community are interdependent entities.

Responses to the question What is a community? will probably include replies such as a small place where I grew up, a professional organization to which I belong, and a small group of people who live and work together. While the examples may be diverse, the common features of the concept seem to be at least intuitively obvious.

The community is also the arena in which community health nurses work to provide quality health care to individuals, families, and groups.

This chapter will discuss definitions of community, present an overview of the functions of a community, and describe three conceptual frameworks for the study of community. We will also explore the usefulness of these latter theoretical perspectives for the community health nursing practice. A case example concludes the chapter and demonstrates an application of the three conceptual frameworks.

A community can be examined and defined from two perspectives: descriptive characteristics and functional attributes. Descriptive characteristics encompass a three-dimensional view describing the community in terms of place, groups of people, and social systems. These characteristics are descriptions of what a community is. Functional attributes are descriptors of what is done in the community. The next section offers definitions of community based on descriptive characteristics. This is followed by an account of the functions performed in a community.

Definitions of Community

Defining the concept of community is a complex task because the perceptions of a community often vary with individual experience. Communities are simultaneously alike and different because of these experiences. Leading theories about community reflect a similar range of perspectives. Several key definitions of community, however, can assist the community health nurse in understanding community as it relates to community health nursing practice.

The many ways of thinking about the community are influenced by factors such as the (1) lack of formally structured organizations corresponding to the unit labeled as community; (2) the lack of clear geographic boundaries to delineate a community; and (3) the spilling over of social relationships beyond political or municipal boundaries (Warren, 1976).

A three-dimensional conceptualization of the community, which encompasses what most definitions include, defines the community as a place, a collection of people, and a social system (Sand-ers, 1972). This three-dimensional concept of a community provides a useful approach to understand community in general and as it relates to public health.

Place, the first dimension, refers to the physical and social environment and is important to health for three reasons. First, in epidemiological study, there is some reliance upon the physical mapping or pinpointing of areas to locate and explain types of illness. (See Chapter 6 for a fuller discussion of epidemiology.) Second, place affects the availability of health services and how they are used. Third, the place dimension is important to public health because it is the physical environment where people spend their lives (Sanders, 1972).

The second dimension entails a view of the community as a collection of people. This dimension allows observation of such characteristics as population size, ethnic or cultural compositions, and predominating family structure. These characteristics can be further specified by such data as proportion of white-collar to blue-collar workers, the population's general level of education, the relative proportion of poor and affluent residents, and the influence that the practice of cultural traditions and values has on the population's health status and use of health resources.

One of the responsbilities of community health nurses is the identification of population groups at risk to health problems in the community. This is one of the purposes for the assessment of a community. (See Chapter 9.) Activities that facilitate the identification of population groups at risk can be categorized under this second dimension.

Social system is the third dimension in this concept of community. The community is viewed as a system with interaction among individuals and groups of individuals and families within the community. These interactions can be grouped around broad concerns, which include systems in the community such as health, the economy, politics, religion, and education. Community health nurses are especially concerned with the health system in the community. Because health does not exist in a vacuum or in isolation of other systems, the linkages with other systems in the community must be understood for community health nursing to be effective.

Shamansky and Pesznecker (1981) posit an operational definition of community, offering the community health nurse a pragmatic approach to define a community and begin assessment activities. Since they believe a definition of community minimally should consider (1) the individual; (2) the system of people and social organizations; and (3) time and space aspects, they cite Moe's (1977) definition of community as "people and the relationships that emerge among them as they develop and use in common some agencies and institutions and a physical environment" (p. 129). After considering community as the "what," Figure 3-1 delineates the three fundamental areas of their operational definition of community: people factors (the "who"); space and time factors (the "where" and "when"); and purpose (the "why" and how").

The people factor component permits the community health nurse to answer the salient question of who are the people—their sociodemographic characteristics, their perceptions, and attitudes about health in particular and their community in general. The space and time factors refer to the reality that people factors coexist in a time-space framework (Shamansky & Pesznecker, 1981). Accordingly, the space or geographical area and the passage of time affect the people factors. The third area of the definition of community in Figure 3-1 is the "why and how" component and refers to the purposes of the particular community.

If, for example, a team of community health nurses in a neighborhood health center propose to conduct health education programs to community residents, the operational definition depicted in Figure 3-1 could serve as a framework in formulating questions to identify the kinds of data needed to begin both defining and assessing the community in terms of the feasibility of conducting health education programs for the community. The "who" component may lead them to ask the following types of questions to uncover "people factors":

- What is the demographic profile of the people in the community?
- Which group(s) perceive themselves as a "community"?
- Does the municipal, geographical area designated by governmental and health authorities coincide with residents' perceptions of the community?
- Who will be the target group for the health programs?
- Will the target group be a young or elderly group of people?

Drawing from the "where and when" component, the community health nurses would see the need to determine:

- What is the location of the people to be served by the various health education programs (e.g., in schools, in neighborhood block clubs, their current clients)?
- When is the best time to conduct the health education programs?

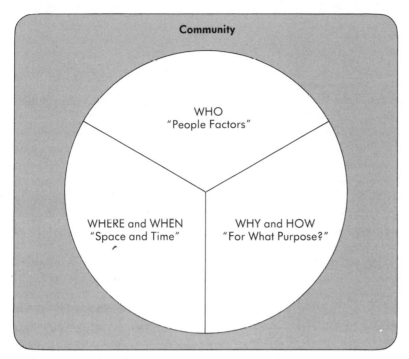

Figure 3-1 Operational Definition of Community. (By Shamansky and Pesznecker. Reproduced with permission from *Nursing Outlook,* March, 1981. Copyright © 1981, American Journal of Nursing Company.)

The "why and how" component could lead the community health nurse to formulate the following general questions:

- What are the purposes and goals of this community?
- What are the resources already available to the community?
- What kinds of health education programs are needed by this particular community?
- What do the residents perceive as the kinds of health education programs that are needed?

While this is not an exhaustive list, it illustrates that the "who, why, how, where, and when" dimensions of this operational definition of community can serve as a framework for the community health nurse to begin the process of defining and assessing a community. Understanding the functional attributes of the community also helps in the process of community assessment.

Functional Attributes

People historically have found that living in groups enabled them to survive and started them toward the development of high civilizations. The major functions of a community are also plausible explanation of why people have formed communities. The five functions are (1) production-distribution-consumption; (2) socialization; (3) social control; (4) social participation; and (5) mutual support (Warren, 1978).

Production-distribution-consumption refers to the ability of the community to provide for the economic welfare of its members. The community participates with the other communities and society in general in the production, distribution, and consumption of goods and services needed in daily activities. Hence, there is an interdependency with businesses, industries, and organizations outside the community. The impact of these activities is felt by the residents at the local level.

Socialization is the process of providing for the transmitting of social values, culture, knowledge, and skills to the members of a community. This is usually accomplished through traditional institutions such as the family, school, and the church, as well as social organizations and voluntary associations.

Social control refers to the manner in which order is maintained in the community. This is generally achieved through the establishment and enforcement of laws that provide for the safety of residents—for example, from crime. Social control may also be achieved through the norms of the groups in the community. In addition to the governmental entities, social control is accomplished through other institutions such as the family, school, and the church.

Social participation is the way the community provides the informal and formal channels to satisfy the need of its residents for companionship. Traditionally, the church has provided the opportunity for people to interact with each other to affect social issues as well as to express a mutual religious affinity. The family also serves to help satisfy its members' need for companionship. Public and private social organizations also perform this function.

Mutual support is the ability of the community to provide for the specialization and the organization of essential tasks needing more than one individual, especially in time of illness or economic distress. The family can help to provide for this function. It may also be necessary to seek the assistance of public or private agencies in the community or external to the community. Consider, for example, an elderly widow living alone who suffers a serious illness that prevents her from performing usual activities of daily living such as personal hygiene, meal preparation, and housekeeping. Relatives and close friends were able to assist her for a short time during the initial phase of her illness. However, it was also necessary to turn to health and social services to augment the social support network of family and friends during her recovery.

An awareness of the functions community serves for its residents provides a foundation to examine various approaches to study community.

Conceptual Frameworks for the Study of Community

Three theoretical perspectives can be helpful to community health nurses in examining and assessing communities. The first perspective uses concepts in an evolving framework called the competent community. The second and third perspectives make use of concepts from symbolic interaction and systems theory, respectively. While there are other conceptionalizations and approaches,

Table 3-1   Essential Conditions of the Competent Community

Essential Condition	Explanation
1. Commitment	There is an attachment and loyalty to the community among the residents.
2. Self-other awareness and clarity of situational definitions	Different community groups are aware of their own identity and positions on issues and also the identity and position on issues of other groups in their midst.
3. Articulateness	Community groups have the ability to formulate and state their interests and concerns to each other.
4. Communication	Community groups have the ability to talk to each other with mutual understanding. In other words, there is two-way effective communication.
5. Conflict containment and accommodation	Community has the ability to develop formal and informal procedures to keep conflict from getting out of control.
6. Participation	Residents are involved in community activities.
7. Management of relations with the larger society	Community has knowledge and capability of how to use and manage external resources and social supports to ensure a viable community.
8. Machinery for facilitating participant interaction and decision making	Community has rules and regulations that will result in the consensus needed for decision making.

SOURCE:
Adapted from Cottrell L: The competent community. In: Warren RL (editor), *New Perspectives on the American Community*. Chicago: Rand McNally, 1977.

the perspectives of the competent community, the interactional concept, and systems theory are especially applicable to aggregates, groups, and individuals.

The Competent Community

Definition A competent community has members with the ability to identify the problems and concerns in their community. They are able to prioritize problems so that strategies for solving them are possible. Finally, the members of a community can collaborate effectively in the implementation of these strategies (Cottrell, 1977).

Accordingly, Cottrell posited eight conditions that are necessary for community competency: (1) commitment, (2) self-other awareness and clarity of situational definitions, (3) articulateness, (4) communication, (5) conflict containment and accommodation, (6) participation, (7) management of relations with the larger society, and (8) machinery for facilitating participant interaction and decision making. (See Table 3-1.)

Explanations of the eight conditions are as follows:

1. Commitment to the community is shared by the residents. The residents' sense of loyalty to

their community translates into an interest and concern about community issues and activities.

2. Clarity of identity and interests refers to the self-knowledge that the different interest groups within the community have about their own needs and behavior and how clearly they can relate new situations to those needs. Interest groups also are aware of the identity and interests of other groups located in their midst. They must understand how each group's agenda affects them.

3. Articulating their interests and concerns is a necessary ability for each group in the competent community. This attribute ensures that each group can formulate and state their issues.

4. Communication skills must be strong so that discussion and problem solving are possible among groups in the community. The groups must be able to talk and listen to each other with mutual understanding. Hence, strong communication skills are needed to guarantee effective dialogue.

5. Conflict containment and accommodation refers to the ability of the community to develop formal and informal procedures that serve to keep conflicts from getting out of control. Examples include basic procedures to prevent everyone from talking at the same time at community meetings or using abusive language as well as the arrangements to notify residents of public hearings so that they can offer their input on issues.

6. Participation by residents in the attainment of community goals is an extension of the commitment attribute.

7. Managing relations with the larger society is the ability to deal with the numerous activities taking place at the local, state, and national or federal levels that affect a community in such areas as health, education, economics, etc. The competent community is able to relate to these various systems effectively.

8. Machinery for facilitating participant interaction and decision making refers to the ability to maintain rules and regulations that will result in the consensus needed for decision making.

This is not an exhaustive list of conditions denoting a competent community. These are characteristics and conditions that Cottrell (1977) observed in communities that successfully implemented community-based programs. These characteristics were also absent among the communities that were unsuccessful in the implementation of their programs.

Implications for Community Health Nursing
Because community health nurses work with individuals, families, groups, and diverse organizations and agencies in communities, they should be knowledgeable about the decision-making processes and capabilities of the communities in solving problems. The conceptualizations in the competent community framework offer guidance for the nurse to learn about such processes that have applicability to poor and affluent communities.

There has been limited research in community health nursing using the competent community framework. Goeppinger and her associates (1982) at the University of Virginia are involved in research to develop a practitioner's guide to assess community competence. This will be beneficial to community health nurses and others who provide community services.

Although the competent community framework is an evolving conceptionalization, we can make use of its perspectives to provide guidance in defining and assessing a community. For example, one community health nursing agency desired to train laywomen residents to be able to educate other women in their community in self-care preventive behavior, such as breast examinations. The women lived with their families in a low income housing development with a resident as a president of each building. This individual acted as a gatekeeper for his or her building in terms of what kinds of groups and communications were available to the residents in the buildings. Hence, the community health nurses from the agency desired to use the focus of the competent community framework as a way to determine the decision-making processes in the various buildings in this housing development to gain and maintain access to the women. They had targeted a group for assessment and would explore framework concepts such as commitment, participation, communication, etc., to determine the group's strengths and weaknesses, and their needs and desires—and, ultimately, the feasibility of conducting the self-care project.

Interactional Conception of Community

Definition An interactional conception of community is concerned with what happens in a community rather than what a community is. The community is viewed as an arena or interactional field with the focus on community action or interaction. The theoretical grounding for Kaufman's (1977) interactional conception of community is symbolic interactionism, which is discussed in Chapter 2. The focus in Chapter 2 deals with major concepts of symbolic interactionism as applied to the family. Kaufman's efforts are directed at reconceptualizing aspects of symbolic interactionism to permit its applicability in explaining interactions in the community.

The unit of study at the interactional level is action (Kaufman, 1977). The three elements of the action are (1) the persons involved in it, (2) the groups or organizations through which the action occurs, and (3) the sequences of time of the action (e.g., occasional, periodic, or continuous). Actions may be called projects, activities, or events. Examples of community actions include such activities as building a community hospital, operating a local park district, or planning a community's annual charity dance.

A major concern in this interactional model is to distinguish community from noncommunity activities and, hence, determine the criteria for what constitutes community action in the community field. Criteria that distinguish community activities from noncommunity activities include: "(1) the degree of comprehensiveness of interests pursued and needs met, (2) the degree to which the action is identified with the locality, (3) relative number, status, and degrees of involvement of

local residents, (4) relative number and significance of local associations involved, (5) degree to which the action maintains or changes the local society, and (6) extent of organization of the action" (Kaufman, 1977, p. 84).

The explanations of the six dimensions provide the rationale for their inclusion in the criteria. The first dimension concerns the range of interests in a community. If the activity is to be considered as one of community, it must be identified with the locality and encompass a number of interests of the residents of that locality. For example, the project of building a community hospital in a low income, black community has been initiated as a result of an informal and formal assessment involving continuous dialogue between residents of the locality and health providers. The check of the status of workers reveals a high unemployment rate as compared with other communities. In conjunction with local groups and associations, the community hospital plans programs to train and hire some local residents for openings in the new hospital facility. Community outreach programs are planned to integrate the interests and needs of the residents with the goals of the community hospital. The results include health education programs and innovative health care delivery systems sensitive to the needs of the residents in the locality. The hospital project now addresses not only the needs related to building an acute care facility, but also those related to community employment and health promotion. A broader spectrum of community interests are incorporated into the project, which encourages residents to identify the project as their project, and the hospital as their hospital.

The second dimension refers to the degree to which the activities have identification with the locality. In the example, the community hospital project was oriented toward the local community, rather than toward the society at large.

The third and fourth dimensions concern the degree of involvement of local residents and local associations in activities. A high level of participation by residents and associations does not automatically mean that the action is highly community in character. The nature of the participation has to be perceived by the residents as significant to the project. In our example of the project of building the community hospital, we can surmise that local residents would have a low affinity toward the project if their participation has been minimal to nil. This could result in an underutilization of the community hospital's services, which would affect its viability.

The fifth dimension addresses whether or not the action will change the locality or maintain the status quo; the sixth dimension is concerned with the extent of the organization of the action. While changes within the locality would take place in the instance of the community hospital project, it would be desirable to be responsive to the values and cultural themes that the residents desire to have in their locality. This is of paramount importance in an interactional conception of community. Also, if the extent of the organization of the community hospital project becomes too institutionalized and bureaucratic, and participation of residents and local associations decline, the project could become unstable and less viable. It would also cease to be a community activity.

Implications for Community Health Nursing Kaufman's (1977) framework of an interactional conception of community is more an enumeration of the elements or components of the interactional perspective rather than a precise, definitive explanation or theory. However, it offers a perspective that is beneficial to community development. In this respect, Kaufman's framework is similar to that of Cottrell's competent community in its need for development of indices for its various dimensions. Among the implications for community health nurses of the interactional conception of community are the following:

- The interactional perspective's focus on "what happens" in a community is the continuous concern of community health nurses because of the nature of their practice with individuals, families, and groups.
- The interactionist seeks to delineate the elements of action, which includes the identifica-

tion of community participants and associations and their roles in activities in the community. Community health nurses work collaboratively with other agencies and organizations to deliver quality health services to residents. A "people"-oriented framework is desirable because it facilitates the development of assessment tools for the study of the community, especially regarding community organizations.

- Community health nurses work in and develop programs, events, and projects, which they would want to be considered as community activities and reflective of the value complexes and cultural themes of community residents. The interactional perspective provides a framework to facilitate this goal.

Systems Theory

Definition Systems theory and its application to the family have been discussed in Chapter 2. However, since this complex, powerful perspective can also guide the study and understanding of community, we'll discuss the theory itself again here and highlight its usefulness to community health nursing.

An assumption of general systems theory is that similar principles occur across living and nonliving systems (Broskowski, 1983). Hence, one sees explanations of this theory that have applicability in both the physical and social sciences. Our concern is with living systems—i.e., individuals, families, groups, and communities—versus nonliving systems, which are generally concerned with inanimate objects such as stones or machines.

A system can be defined as "a whole which functions as a whole by virtue of the interdependence of its parts" (Braden & Herban, 1976, p. 5). Accordingly, "systems theory studies the patterns of interactions among the system's parts, derives from these interaction patterns laws of their functioning, and organizes classes of systems from wholes whose patterns of interactions are governed by the same laws" (Braden & Herban, 1976, p. 5).

One of the first questions that one would ask to illustrate the relevance of the key concepts of systems theory to entities such as the community is, How do you go about determining a social system? At least six criteria are essential for determining a social system: a boundary, a focal unit, proximity of members, similarity of members, resistance of members to intrusion, and internal communications.

The boundary of the system is the initial component that must be determined in defining a system. The boundary stands between the system and its environment (Helvie, 1981). Examples of questions that assist in defining a community's boundary are: Is it one neighborhood? Is it a specific census tract? Is it a place of work? Is it the membership in a particular profession? These and similar questions assist in establishing the scope.

A second criterion that must be defined is the focal unit. When defining this component, one would seek to answer questions such as: Is the focal unit of study at the micro-, mezzo-, or macrolevel? Because a system involves many variables, it is difficult to know when one system ends and another begins. Braden and Herban (1976) posit the notion of three focal units of study: micro-, mezzo-, and macrolevels. If the focal unit of study is small, such as between two persons in a family, or a small group, it is called a microsystem. When several microsystems are the focal unit of study and the focal unit is more complex, this is a mezzolevel. Examples at the mezzolevel include a community or a large complex organization such as the department of health in a large urban city. The macrolevel has as its focal unit of study more complex systems and may entail systems at the local, state, and national levels. The United States as a society is an example of a macrolevel study unit. If one studied the health system or any of the social systems in society (such as economics, religion, education, politics, etc.) in a broad scope, this would be at the macrolevel. In the final analysis the complexity of the particular system determines whether the focal unit of study is at the micro-, mezzo-, or macrolevel. However, the focal unit of study has to be delineated before an assessment of the particular social system can be made.

Once the boundary and the focal unit within that boundary have been established, a determination has to be made about the proximity of members and the extent of similarity among the system members. Questions that assist in determining the proximity include: Are they at home? Are they in the neighborhood? Are they members employed at the same community health nursing agency? The knowledge of the proximity of the members permits us to assess in what arena or situation their interaction takes place. Questions concerning the similarity of the system's members include: Are they all family members? Are they members of the same profession or organization? Are they individuals engaged in community health nursing? Information on the similarity of the members tells us about characteristics of the system members.

Finally, it is important to assess resistance to intrusion from the outside and the nature and effectiveness of internal communications. The degree of resistance to intrusion would be determined from answers to questions such as: How are you as a nursing student in a community health nursing practicum accepted into a particular organization? How readily is a new family accepted into a neighborhood? An estimate of the strength of the relationships among members of an organization can be made from observations of the type and amount of resistance that outsiders experience upon entrance to the organization.

The nature and effectiveness of the internal communication channels is assessed in evaluating questions such as: Is there an internal communication transfer so that members of the system have access to similar information? For example, is the individual the first or the last person to know of program plans or changes in the organization? A person's role in a system may be indicated by the types and amount of information he or she receives as well as when the information is received.

These criteria do not constitute an exhaustive list of questions to help delineate a social system, but these are minimum factors to consider. Once you have delineated the social system, there are additional selected concepts within the purview of

Case Example 3-1: Proposal for a Neighborhood Health Center

A multihospital corporation proposes to build a neighborhood health center in a community composed of predominantly low income, black residents. The corporation operates ten community hospitals, five neighborhood health centers, and a health maintenance organization. The decision to construct and operate an ambulatory care facility reflects the philosophy of this corporation to provide community-based health programs that are also focused on health promotion and health maintenance for high-risk groups. Community health nurses are employed in the various centers. They hold leadership positions in the administration of health care delivery systems.

Although there has been dialogue between several residents who were perceived as community leaders and key health providers of the corporation, a formal community assessment has not been done to determine the feasibility of having the neighborhood health center in the community. During these conversations between the residents and health providers, the residents have asked for the employment of local residents in the construction of the facility as well as in the completed center to help ease the high unemployment rate in their community.

The community health nurses have been requested to work closely with the team of health care providers and administrators and community leaders to begin the plans for the neighborhood health center project.

Everyone is in agreement that the first thing to do is to select a framework so that this can guide them for an assessment of the community for subsequent plans.

The corporation's delineation of community may or may not be the same as the residents' perception of community.

The corporation is a subsystem of the health care delivery system.

There is evidence of community involvement in the project.

This is an example of the potential interrelationship of the health system with the economic sector.
Community health nurses work with diverse groups.

---

systems theory that are important to the study of community.

For our purposes in analyzing the community, systems also can be characterized as having two dimensions: openness and equilibrium. The system can be open or closed depending on how it processes input of information from the environment outside of its system. An open system is able to exchange positive and negative feedback via feedback loops. Feedback loops are channels that allow the exchange of data to enter and leave the system. Negative feedback is information that maintains stability or the status quo, while the positive feedback is information that will result in a change within the system. Both types of data are important to the system's ability to function. Closed systems do not have an exchange of data with the environment.

Closed systems are typically found in the physical science field as classic chemical or physical models. Thus when social scientists refer to closed systems, they are referring to open systems that accept feedback slowly. These systems tend to be inflexible and rigidly organized (Braden & Herban, 1976). A community must be able to exchange information with other organizations and institutions outside of its parameters and effectively process the information in order to be an open system.

The second dimension on which systems can be analyzed is the extent to which the system's components are in equilibrium. A system tends to strive for equilibrium to reduce tension as much as possible. Here equilibrium is defined as a selective balance between input, transformation, and feedback. Accordingly, a key question in examining the community from the perspective of this dimension is, What is the relationship between disorganization and equilibrium within the system? Because systems have different capabilities for assimilating and transforming information and feedback, the system is in a continuous state of disorganization or disequilibrium. Additionally, there are probably always varying degrees of tension in a system. Nonetheless, the state of equilibrium in the system can be determined by (1) cataloging the sources of input or communication channels; (2) determining what is being communicated from the external environment to the system and within it; (3) assessing how information is transformed and processed within the various components; and (4) determining what is being offered back as feedback. For the systems to survive, according to Auger (1976), there must be a degree of harmony between input, transformation, and feedback. This process is highly dynamic.

Implications for Community Health Nursing
Systems theory can provide a meaningful, pragmatic theoretical perspective to assist the community health nurse in the delivery of health services to clients. It provides a framework for viewing not only individuals, families, and communities but also interrelationships among these systems as they influence health (Helvie, 1981). An additional benefit of the systems approach is that it enables the community health nurse to more clearly conceptualize how other subsystems within the health care system interact to influence the nature of community health nursing practice. Since other health and social services providers also deliver community services to clients in a community, a systems approach facilitates the community health nurse's ability to practice in communities. An ultimate goal and an important attribute distinguishing community health nursing from other nursing specialties is its nursing of communities (Hamilton, 1983). That is, the community becomes the client. Systems theory provides a perspective for study at the individual, group, and aggregate levels.

Application of the Frameworks

Case Example 3-1 ends with the decision to select a framework to guide them in their community study. This section discusses the application of the frameworks based on the Case Example 3-1.

The Competent Community Nurse

Mr. P. is the community health nurse who thinks the framework of the competent community would provide an effective approach to study this low income black community. He would be especially interested in determining the residents' commitment to their community and previous health-related projects. This information would have implications for the potential success or failure of their enterprise. This competent community framework would guide them in analysis of the strengths and weaknesses of the community's ability to implement community programs in general. An equally important focus of the study would be on this community's decision-making processes. These goals would be accomplished by exploring the concepts from the competent community framework and constructing the inquiries to be specific to this community.

The Interactional Conception Nurse

Ms. H. thinks the approach for the study should be based on a knowledgeable understanding of what happens in this community. This means knowing what organizations and groups are involved in activities and events in that community, knowing the persons who are usually involved, and knowing how often the activities and events occur. More importantly, if the multihospital corporation's goal to make the proposed neighborhood health center a community affair is to be achieved, the corporation would need to determine the residents' perceptions of what happens in their community. This is Ms. H.'s rationale for recommending the interactional conception of community as their framework for the study.

The Systems Nurse

Mrs. B. strongly recommends a systems approach to study this community. This would enable an analysis of the community as a social system with an emphasis on examining subsystems in the community such as health, economics, religion, politics, and education. There is the opportunity to analyze the interrelationships of these subsystems in the community. Mrs. B. shares that the systems approach will even provide guidance for studying patterns within the health subsystem of the community.

The reader can note that each framework has a different theoretical thrust. The corporation will have to decide which of these will best satisfy its needs for guidance in the study of this community. It is also possible to use a combination of approaches.

Summary

The community is a complex entity. It is possible to use the conceptualizations of social scientists, in addition to our own personal experiences as members of communities, in order to understand the concept of a community. Community health nurses can contribute to the definitions and study of the community by the development of approaches that are most applicable to community health nursing practice. We saw examples of this in Shamansky and Pesznecker's (1981) operational definition of community and in Goeppinger and her colleagues' (1982) work with the concept of a competent community.

Community health nurses may be guided by at least three common frameworks in their study of a community: the competent community with its emphasis on determining the decision-making ability of a community; an interactional conception of community with its emphasis on what happens in a community and its distinction between community versus noncommunity action; and systems theory with its focus on the analysis of the community as a social system with subsystems. Community health nurses function in different communities with diverse populations. Hence, knowledge of the concept of community in general can enable them to be sensitive to and aware of the differences and similarities of individuals, families, and groups in different communities. These attributes of knowledge, sensitivity, and awareness can translate into action through community health nurses' commitment and involvement to improve and change unhealthy situations in communities. One way to achieve this is by working with community groups as well as within professional health organizations to support legislation, ordinances, and practices that maintain and promote healthy environments and life-styles for community residents.

Study Questions

1. A three-dimensional view to understand the community defines a community as:
   a. A place, people, and a social system
   b. People, health organizations, and health professionals
   c. A place, people, and community health agencies
   d. None of these
2. In a competent community
   a. Groups with opposing ideas do not talk with each other
   b. Residents are informed of the time and location of community meetings
   c. Residents participate in community activities
   d. b and c
3. An understanding of the decision-making ability of a community can be best obtained by use of
   a. An interactional conception framework
   b. Systems theory
   c. The competent community framework
   d. None of these
4. A community functions to
   a. Provide for the transmitting of culture and knowledge to the members
   b. Provide a means for members to meet their financial needs
   c. Provide for the safety of its members
   d. All of these

References

Auger JR: *Behavioral Systems and Nursing.* Englewood Cliffs, N.J.: Prentice-Hall, 1976.

Braden CJ, Herban NL: *Community Health: A Systems Approach.* New York: Appleton-Century-Crofts, 1976.

Broskowski A: The application of general systems theory in the assessment of community needs. In Bell R et al (editors), *Assessing Health and Human Service Needs.* New York: Human Sciences Press, 1983.

Cottrell L: The competent community. In: Warren RL (editor), *New Perspectives on the American Community.* Chicago: Rand McNally, 1977.

Goeppinger J et al: Toward the assessment of community competence: The development of a practitioner's guide. Paper presented at the annual convention, American Public Health Association, Montreal, Canada, November 15, 1982.

Hamilton P: Community nursing diagnosis. *Adv Nurs Sci* 1983; 5 (3): 21–36.

Helvie, CO: *Community Health Nursing: Theory and Process.* Philadelphia: Harper & Row, 1981.

Kaufman H: Toward an interactional conception of community. In: Warren R (editor), *New Perspectives on the American Community.* Chicago: Rand McNally, 1977.

Moe EO: Nature of today's community. In Reinhardt AM, Quinn MD (editors), *Current Practice in Family-Centered Community Nursing.* Vol. 1. St. Louis: Mosby, 1977.

Sanders IT: Public health in the community. In: Freeman H, Levine S, Reeder L (editors), *Handbook of Medical Sociology.* Englewood Cliffs, N.J.: Prentice-Hall, 1972.

Shamansky SL, Pesznecker B: "A community is . . ." *Nurs Outlook* 1981; 29 (3): 182–185.

Warren RL: The good community: What would it be? In Warren RL (editor), *New Perspectives on the American Community,* 3rd ed. Chicago: Rand McNally, 1977.

Warren RL: *The Community in America,* 3rd ed. Chicago: Rand McNally, 1978.

Chapter 4

Family and Community Health

June Crayton

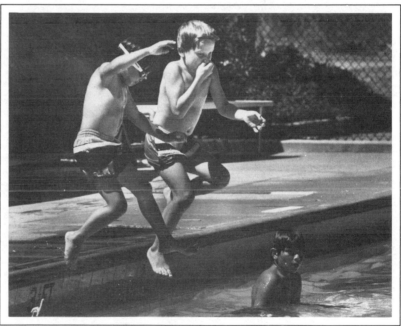

A public swimming pool provides a place for exercise, social interaction, and play for these children and their families; it can also be a health hazard. Both health promotion and disease prevention are goals for family and community health nursing.

Chapter Outline

Chapter Objectives

After completing this chapter, the reader will be able to:

- Define the concept of health as a continuous level of adaptation related to the underlying assumptions about the nature of the human being
- Describe the factors influencing health and their interrelatedness
- Discuss the implications that major health influences have for primary preventive and health promotional services
- Discuss the adequacy of the health care system based on the levels of preventive services and the quality, access, appropriateness, and costs of services provided
- Discuss the validity of various approaches to health care—i.e., medical, nonmedical and self-help activities
- Relate the implications of the major multifactorial health influences for community nursing practice

Consistent with other aspects of civilization, developments in community health evolved slowly throughout the ages. However, theoretical and practical trends related to community health advanced by leaps and bounds during the twentieth century. Rapidly growing scientific knowledge and technology, changing social values, unfolding world events, and shifting resources contributed to ever-broadening concepts of health. Within the last fifty years, state of the art health care shifted from an emphasis on disease control to prevention and health promotion, from concerns with equity of access to health services to cost containment and individual responsibility for health. These are only a few of the issues that must bear upon any discussion of the subject.

This chapter brings together a number of ways of looking at family and community health and also surveys the historical developments that shaped and defined family and community health in the United States.

Theoretical Perspectives of Family and Community Health

Historical Overview of Community Health

Although traditional health practices focused on the individual as the unit of concern, community health practices were evident in the earliest civilizations. In their struggle for survival, people have always been concerned with birth, death, illness, and health. The prestigious status enjoyed by priests, medicine men, or physicians of various societies reflects the high priority assigned to health throughout the ages. Therefore, the history of community health begins with the history of ancient civilizations.

Archeological excavations have revealed that the ancient Egyptians had community systems for collecting rainwater and disposing of sewage. These and other community health practices of the Egyptians were the basis of the Mosaic Codes, which provided for personal and community responsibility for health, communicable disease control—seg regation of lepers, decontamination of buildings, supplies of fresh water, and so on—and maternal health practices (Anderson, Morton, and Green, 1978).

The rediscovery of the Egyptian papyri, some of the oldest historical records, confirmed the Egyptians' detailed medical and surgical treatment protocols for hundreds of diseases and injuries (Cot-trell, 1964; ben-Jochannan, 1972). The treatment of specific diseases among individuals obviously influences community health. Some speculate that Imhotep, living approximately 2000 years before Hippocrates was born, and known to the ancient Egyptians as the father of medicine, formulated a single master text from which the Egyptian papyri were derived.

Very little attention was given to environmental or community health during the classic period of Greece. Emphasis during this period was placed on individual physical aesthetics. However, the Greeks were innovators in gymnastics, athletics, and the concept of the well-developed physique (Anderson, Morton, and Green, 1978).

The state, rather than the individual, held significance for the Romans. In their efforts to secure the well-being of the state and military during the rising empire (100 B.C.–A.D. 745), the Romans registered citizens and slaves, took periodic censuses, regulated the construction of paved streets with gutters, and controlled the removal of garbage and sewage (Anderson, Morton, and Green, 1978).

The period from the fall of the Western Empire (A.D. 476) to the Italian Renaissance (A.D. 1000), known as the Dark Ages, were characterized by extreme backwardness in health care. Religious dogma superceded general aesthetic practices. Filth and neglect of personal hygiene were associated with epidemics of plague and communicable diseases.

Severe pandemics occurred during the later medieval period (A.D. 1000–1453). In 1348 the world was devastated by the bubonic plague. Approximately 25 million people in Europe died from the plague. Three guardians of public health were appointed in Venice in 1374, and entry to the city was denied to anyone suspected of carrying the disease. Returning crusaders were isolated in 1377 to rule out the possibility of them carrying the plague. However, in the absence of scientific knowledge, these measures had very little effect (Anderson, Morton, and Green, 1978).

The Renaissance period of Western and Northern Europe (A.D. 1453–1600) emphasized the return to individual, scientific inquiry and facilitated the understanding and knowledge of infectious diseases. Scholars began to differentiate communicable diseases such as influenza, smallpox, bubonic plague, and tuberculosis. Unfortunately, growth of cities, expanding trade, improved transportation, and concentration of people in urban areas accelerated the spread of communicable diseases beyond the potential for control during this period.

The period 1600 to 1800 was a time of tremendous illumination concerning infectious diseases and community health in Europe. Increased knowledge of the circulatory system, innovations in the use of the microscope, the collection of vital statistics, and the discovery of smallpox vaccine led to considerable advancements in community health. However, community health received very little attention in America during this period. Although epidemics of smallpox, yellow fever, and other diseases crippled many rapidly industrializing American cities, ignorance and superstition regarding the origin and spread of disease pervaded and impeded communicable disease control efforts.

Public health was officially recognized in England in 1837 when legislation related to community sanitation was enacted. Two innovators in the modern public health movement were English-born Edwin Chadwick and an American named Lemuel Shattuck. Chadwick's *Reports on Inquiry into the Sanitary Conditions of the Laboring Population of Great Britain*, published in 1842, aroused concerns regarding child labor conditions and stimulated the formation of a general board of health. In 1850 Lemuel Shattuck submitted his *Report of the Sanitary Commission of the Commonwealth of Massachusetts*. This report, which served as a guide in the field of health for the next century, made specific recommendations regarding the establishment of state and local health boards, sanitation codes, sanitary inspections, collection of vital statistics, and programs for school health, tuberculosis, alcohol, mental illness and environmental nuisance.

Shattuck's 1850 report coincided with the beginning of the modern era of health, as defined by Anderson, Morton, and Green (1978). Anderson outlined four phases of the modern era of health (1850 to the present). The *first phase,* the miasma phase (1850–1880), was characterized by beliefs that disease is caused by dirt, noxious odors, and lack of cleanliness. For example, diphtheria and malaria were thought to be associated with bad air. Therefore, disease control was directed toward garbage collection and street cleaning. The first modern state board of health, established in Massachusetts in 1869, and the American Public Health Association (APHA), founded in 1872, were milestones of this period.

The *second phase,* disease control (1880–1920), witnessed the demonstration that disease is caused by specific organisms. Pasteur disproved the theory of spontaneous generation and developed a method of vaccinating against rabies. Koch discovered the tubercle bacillus, *Streptococcus,* and cholera vibrio. Theobold Smith of the U.S. Department of Agriculture demonstrated that Texas fever is transmitted by ticks—consequently, introducing the concept of the intermediate host. By 1900 insect vectors for malaria, yellow fever, and other diseases were identified. Community-wide application of this and other scientific knowledge made control of fatal diseases, such as smallpox, diphtheria, and tuberculosis, an obtainable goal.

The *third phase* was health promotion (1920–1960). The discovery that 34 percent of American youth were unfit for military service during World War I stimulated concerns about the neglect of other preventable health hazards. Chronic degenerative diseases such as hypertension, heart disease, stroke, cancer, diabetes, and mental illness received increased attention. State, county, and city health departments expanded and broadened their efforts to include health promotion among their services and functions.

In 1956 the National Health Survey Act and the Health Amendments Act were enacted, providing for on-going comprehensive, national health surveys and financial support for the education of public health personnel. Additionally, considerable legislation was enacted during this period providing government enforcement, entitlement to government financed and/or provided health services for the elderly and poor, food and substance control, research, and education.

The *fourth phase,* social engineering (1960–present), generated awareness of the inequitable distribution of health benefits among the social strata of the world. Large segments of the population were and are denied access to the technological health care advances due to poverty, geographic location, or inadequate education. Economic and psychosocial aspects of health gained maximum priority. In 1964 Congress passed national legislation—Title VI of the Civil Rights Act—assuring all American citizens health care, regardless of race, color, or national origin. In 1965 Social Security Amendments established health insurance for the aged and grants to states for medical assistance programs for the poor—Medicare and Medicaid. This and other legislation related to the study and prevention of heart disease, cancer, and stroke provided impetus for the development of community health services and primary prevention. Although the modern community health programs addressed issues related to citizens of all economic strata, they continued to target the underprivileged population for higher penetration.

During the 1970s, states shifted their emphasis from the provision of health services in public institutions to private services with government reimbursement. Arguments supporting the funding of private institutions and programs were centered around assumptions that public institutions could not provide services as competently and efficiently as the private sector, and that the promotion of private programs would eliminate the two-class system of health care by ensuring private services to all patients (Mollica, 1983).

Certain policy contradictions were inherent in the proliferate funding of private institutions. Community health centers found themselves in competition with private hospitals and outpatient programs. Additionally, the government retained responsibility for monitoring quality, effectiveness, and efficiency of services supported by tax dollars. However, numerous contracts to private health care providers resulted in more contracts than the government could effectively evaluate. Consequently, adequate effective health care continued to elude lower income patients as government spending for health care increased by leaps and bounds (Mollica, 1983).

Increased federal spending for health care services provoked or was accompanied by a backlash of sentiments for health care cost containment and emphasis on individual responsibility for wellness and health. While the 1960s to mid-1970s was a period of economic expansion and growth for the health care industry, the late-1970s and 1980s were described as a period of maturation within the industry (Goldsmith, 1981). During the 1960s to mid-1970s values concerning the right to health, and the availability and equity of access to quality health care services for the poor and elderly gained emphasis in the United States (Aday & Andersen, 1981; Aday & Andersen, 1983; Robert Wood Johnson Foundation, 1983). However, those values are undergoing reconsideration in the early-1980s as emphasis shifts to policies related to cost containment. These rapidly changing developments present complex challenges for the definition and scope of community health.

Concepts of Health

Concepts of health evolved in response to the changing values and resources, and the scientific and social state of the art in public health. Over the last fifty years, concepts of health as the absence of disease have been replaced by positive concepts related to wellness, vitality, and self-actualization.

In Chapter 1 the concept of health was introduced in terms of four models of health: (1) eudaimonistic; (2) adaptive; (3) role performance; and (4) clinical. On the other hand, Dever (1980) analyzed health concepts, values, and assumptions as an emerging historical process. A natural consequence of the "germ theory" was the ecological concept of health as a balance between people, organisms, and the environment (Dever, 1980). Health was sought through the treatment and prevention of infectious diseases. Within this framework, health was measured in terms of mortality or morbidity from infectious diseases. The weakness of this concept was its sole focus on the environment's impact on health.

With the eradication of communicable diseases and the increase of chronic diseases, the ecological model was broadened to include sociological concepts that recognized personal behavioral influences on health (Dever, 1980). Again, health was measured in terms of morbidity, mortality and disability rates. Efforts to achieve health included not only treatment of illness, but also nutrition and life-style changes.

The World Health Organization's definition of health as "a state of complete physical, mental and social well-being, and not merely the absence of disease or infirmity" (WHO, 1964) added the dimension of mental well-being and broadened our framework in preparation for holistic and wellness concepts.

The holistic definition of health emphasized unity of mind, body, and spirit. The health field in the holistic framework includes an environment, life-style, human biology, and health systems that are conducive to healing. Proper balance in these four areas creates psychosocial and somatic health or well-being. Efforts to achieve holistic health include use of the best traditional and nontraditional approaches to care.

However, still oriented toward treatment, holism has been challenged by high-level wellness concepts (Dever, 1980). Wellness stresses physical exercise, stress management, nutrition, and self-responsibility. Wellness involves a self-designed life-style that allows the individual to be one in mind, body, and spirit in order to practice nutritional awareness, physical activity, stress management, and self-responsibility, and to have potential for healthful life-style and well-being (Dever, 1980).

In addition to temporal variations, concurrent variations in the definition of health existed. Some concepts focused on the relative functional capacity of the individual given preexisting illness and the disability of biological makeup (Patrick et al, 1973). Other models defined health as a continuum with wellness on one end and illness on the other (Benson & McDevitt, 1976), or as a state of integrated biopsychosocial functioning oriented toward maximizing the individual's potential within his or her environment (Byrne, 1972).

As these concepts of health became more complex, they also became less measurable in terms of achievable goals. However, increasingly, health has been conceived as an illness-wellness continuum with health—a state of integrated biopsychosocial functioning that enables people to achieve their maximum potential within their environment and have reasonable freedom from undue pain or disability—on one end and illness or disease on the other (Benson & McDevitt, 1976; Kinlein, 1978).

Underlying this definition is the assumption that a person is an integrated biopsychosocial system striving for equilibrium through mutual adaptation with the environment. This definition will contribute to a conceptual framework for our discussion of community health.

Within this framework the factors influencing health are generally agreed to include environment, human biology, personal and behavioral characteristics, and adequate health care services. Environmental factors may be thought of as natural, people-caused, biological, or psychosocial, and may be supportive or harmful. Personal and behavioral characteristics include life-style, nutrition, age, sex, and genetic factors. As a contributor to health, health care services may be viewed in terms of type, quality, availability, accessibility, adequacy, efficiency, and effectiveness—which, in turn, are dependent on the overall health care delivery system.

As noted earlier, values regarding life and health also determine health status and the extent to which it is achievable for all. The recent focus in the 1980s on human rights around the world had a positive impact on public, professional, and individual aspirations for health. However, the value placed on health changes periodically in response to increased knowledge, changing costs, resources, and priorities.

Family Health

A meaningful definition of family health must be prefaced by a conceptual definition of family. The reader is referred to Chapter 2 of this text for definitions and conceptualizations of the family. For the purposes of this chapter it is sufficient to note that families fulfill for their members such basic functions as boundary maintenance or regulation, resource attainment, communication, energy release, and self-care. Fulfillment of these functions increases the general well-being and health of the family. Other family functions directly determine health and are related to nutritional behavior, exercise, and other life-style patterns; use of health services, and self-care and preventive activities; and environmental practices (Friedman, 1981).

The healthy family regulates its boundaries and uses energy, communication, and power, the resources of health services and self-care to achieve the biopsychosocial functioning that enables the family and its members to have reasonable well-being. Based on this logic, it follows that environment, genetic factors, familial and behavioral characteristics, the health care system, and self-care practices also influence family health.

Ideally, members of the healthy family are well-nourished, have achieved mental or spiritual well-being, are free from diseases, or are adapted to handicaps in such a way as to achieve optimal daily functioning in such areas as work, recreation, education, self-care, and expression of affection for each other. Homes of the healthy family are safe,

secure and comfortable. Positive health behavior, intelligent self-care or health services, e.g., periodic health assessments, are utilized. Members are trustful, creative, productive and content. As a whole, the healthy family is cohesive and cooperatively works to maximize its goals. The healthy family would be located on the wellness end of the illness-wellness continuum. Actual families move along the continuum in response to periodic changes in their own health determinants.

Friedman (1981) proposed a two-level focus on the whole family and its individual members as the basic unit of community nursing services. Health and illness behavior are learned, and the family is the primary teacher. An individual's family is in many ways affected at every point along the illness-wellness continuum. Strong interdependent relationships among family members are such that the health of its members affect other members and the family as a whole. Illness disrupts basic family functions resulting in impeded role fulfillments.

Community Health

In 1966 the National Commission on Community Health Services stated: "Health services, operated to meet the health needs of every individual, should be located within the environment of the individual's home community." However, what is meant by "community health" is also obscured by varying definitions of community. Chapter 3 of this text presented various frameworks of community. Classic definitions of community included such concepts as unit or solidarity based on consensus, interdependence, informal relationships, and common interests (Hawley, 1950). Consistent with the assumptions that a human being is an integrated, open social system, many theoretical frameworks viewed the community as a relatively autonomous and enduring social system, field, or network comprised of interacting individuals, groups, or organizations (Arensberg, 1959; Clark, 1968; Effrat, 1974; Parsons, 1959). The community was usually conceived to have boundaries related to territory, shared interests, goals, customs, or values. The interests, goals, or values of the community were usually thought to be expressed through collective policies and actions (Kaufman, 1959). Therefore, *community* can be defined as an enduring, interacting social system of individuals, families, groups, and organizations sharing common interests, goals, and values, which are expressed through collective policies, actions, and institutions. The health status of aggregates making up the community also forms an illness-wellness continuum, affected by natural, people-caused, and psychosocial environmental risks or supports; by biological, demographic, and life-style characteristics of the individuals, families, or groups comprising the community; and by the performance and adequacy of health care services available to the community.

The healthy community has safe and adequate housing, relatively clean air and water, safe streets, transportation, and sanitation. Its members are trusting, cooperative and productive, and they are relatively free from premature mortality and morbidity. Educational, recreational, occupational, health promotional, and health care services are sufficient to meet the needs of the population. Again this is more of an ideal standard against which to assess community health. Actual communities may be located at any point along the illness-wellness continuum.

Factors Influencing Family and Community Health

The determinants of health status do not share equal importance in terms of their impact on the individual, family, or community's location on the illness-wellness continuum. It is important to note that the environment, personal health characteristics, health care system, and human biology, respectively, have decreasing impact as determinants of health. Figure 4-1 illustrates this point. The size of the health influence arrows indicate commonly held assumptions about their relative degrees of impact on health status (Dever, 1980; Longest, 1979). Supporting or positive environments, healthy personal and behavioral characteristics, supportive health care systems, and human biological characteristics move the individual, family, or community toward the wellness end of the continuum. If the factors influencing health status are negative, the person, family, or community moves toward the illness end of the continuum.

Environmental Factors

The environment is a source of resources (i.e., foods, water, air, and raw materials), the extraction of which enables people to live and create. To the extent that environmental resources are available and accessible to the community in adequate quality and quantity, life and health are enhanced. However, the environment is also a source of risks and constraints. People constantly engage in mutual adaptation with the environment to maintain equilibrium and health. Environmental factors influencing community health may be categorized as natural, people-caused, or psychosocial. As Figure 4-2 illustrates, positive or supportive interactions with the environment move individuals, families, and communities toward the wellness end of the continuum. Negative interactions with environment move them toward the illness end of the continuum.

Natural Environmental Factors The natural environment usually supports life and enhances health. The air, water, food, and scenery we enjoy are part of our natural environment. However, natural phenomena sometimes threaten life or health when, for instance, the weather becomes inclement and the sunshine or rainfall are inadequate to support life. Other natural phenomena such as droughts, severe storms, or weather conducive to

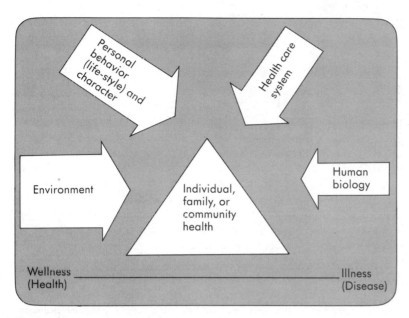

Figure 4-1 Factors influencing health status. (Adapted from Dever, 1980.)

the growth of pollens or the overgrowth of insects, microorganisms, or vegetation may seriously threaten people's health and survival.

People-caused Environmental Threats Our technological development has been our greatest advancement in the last 200 or 300 years. Technology has made it possible for people to live in greater comfort and leisure, and has brought to ordinary people material and intellectual advantages that kings could not enjoy a few hundred years ago. Unfortunately, the danger of thermonuclear war, depletion of natural resources, exponential population growth, inadequate urban design and organization, poverty, and pollution are major costs of advanced technology (Eisenbud, 1981). Changes, which are occurring more rapidly than people's capacity for hereditary, intellectual, or social adaptation, present ecological threats to humankind and the environment. This has led to raging debates between environmentalists and industrialists over the need for ecological wisdom. One side argues for increased emphasis on environmen-

tal protection, resource conservation, public health and welfare to ensure present and future ecological balance, while the other promotes industrial growth, and continued scientific and intellectual advancement (Dubos, 1972; Eisenbud, 1981; Terry, 1972).

Probably the most important environmental resource to people and their community is the air they breathe. Air pollutants such as liquid and solid particulates, sulfur and nitrogen oxides, carbon monoxide, hydrocarbons, ozone, acid rain, and photochemical substances are hazardous to plant life, buildings, fabrics, and other materials (Purdom, 1980). Unfortunately, the deleterious effects of air pollutants on health are difficult to assess because such effects occur over long periods of time. However, worsening symptoms of bronchitis, respiratory irritation, and increased rates of lung cancer and broncheo-constriction in test animals were associated with increased levels of sulfur oxides. Carbon monoxide levels higher than safety standards are known to interrupt oxygen transport in human beings and to cause cardiovascular changes and decreased visual acuity. Effects of long-term

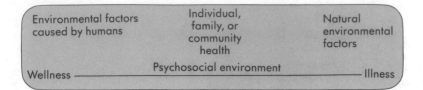

Figure 4-2 Impact of Environment on Health Status. A supportive, positive environment moves the individual, family, or community toward the wellness end of the continuum. A negative environment moves them towards the illness end.

exposure to unsafe nitrogen oxide levels have been associated with increased frequency of bronchitis in school children. Nitrogen oxides and hydrocarbons also deteriorate fabrics and plants (Purdom, 1980).

The adequacy of drinking water may also be questionable, since water quality in the majority of the nation's streams, lakes, reservoirs, and estuaries has not improved much since 1972 (Miller, 1984), although the cost of water pollution control was estimated at $250 billion for the period 1975–1984 (Eisenbud, 1981).

Other people-caused environmental factors that impact on health are hazardous wastes, natural resources depletion, housing deterioration, population growth, and noise pollution. Hazardous wastes include chemicals from industrial processing, nuclear waste, and other sources. These waste products may be buried in the soil, dumped in surface waters, or dumped in the air as particulates. An estimated 2500 lb of hazardous wastes per person is generated each year. A major vehicle for hazardous wastes is groundwater contamination by leaking underground storage tanks. Another source of hazardous waste is radiation from nuclear reactors. However, consistent with other environmental disputes, supporters and detractors of atomic reactors disagree on every important point. Proponents claim a need for its development to ensure military security. Opponents insist that it be stopped in the interest of safety (Thompson, 1984).

Population overgrowth and diminishing raw materials are other problems related to our tech-

nological and industrial growth. Eisenbud (1981) proposed that environmentalists should also address these issues.

Housing is a private and public health responsibility. It is known to be an important factor in people's health. However, the impact of housing on health is difficult to isolate from the interrelated influences of income, education, and access to social support services. Nevertheless, it is generally known among public health experts that crowded or substandard living conditions increase the chances of accidents and communicable disease transmission. Inadequate toilet facilities, lack of sunshine, and inadequate ventilation and heating can have adverse effects on physical and mental well-being. Crowded living conditions have also been associated by some investigators with increased stress, hypertension, and cardiovascular heart disease (D'Atri & Ostfeld, 1975). Regulation of housing construction and maintenance is a local government function. However, the federal government has taken a role in implementation of legislation and resources to improve housing.

The Psychosocial Environment The psychosocial environment is integrally related to community, family, and personal health. Ciocco (1940) found that married males and females live longer than single males and females. Marriage is a powerful social institution that provides established routines related to nutrition, sleep, and other health patterns (Mechanic, 1982). Emile Durkheim (1967) pioneered investigations showing that family ties and social integration provide psychological support that seems to enhance and reinforce the individual's ability to handle demanding and uncertain social and industrial experiences. Based on the findings of Durkheim and others, divorced, single, or widowed individuals are, therefore, at greater risks of suicide and other adverse health conditions. Marital status, fragmented associations, poverty, and crowded living conditions were also found to be associated with higher incidents of cancer among males of Massachusetts (Jenkins, 1983). We may deduce from these findings that industrialized, urban communities may experience higher rates of certain health problems related to isolation, population concentration, and social disintegration than rural communities.

Race, ethnicity, and social class are related to health status. However, it is quite difficult to explain common behavior in one racial or ethnic group on the basis of racial or ethnic factors alone because, in various ways, ethnicity, class, and race are inseparable in the American social system (Harwood, 1981). However, in spite of the difficulties of isolating ethnicity from the effects of socioeconomic status and acculturation, ethnicity has been shown to be particularly relevant to health beliefs and behavior. (See Chapter 5.) Whether due to biases in the collection of vital statistics, unequal access to treatment, genetic predisposition, or shared risks, ethnic groups have been found to vary in morbidity and mortality rates, concepts of health, health maintenance and illness behavior, or utilization patterns (Harwood, 1981). However, the relationships between minority membership, income levels, access to health care, and health status have been frequently documented (Gary, 1982). Diseases such as hypertension, stroke, diabetes, cancer, and mental illness are considerably more prevalent among lower income minorities than dominant counterparts (Jackson, 1981; Schreibner & Homiak, 1981).

Income, occupations, and general socioeconomic status were empirically demonstrated to have positive relationships to general health status (Pratt, 1973) and longevity (Anderson, Morton, and Green, 1978), and an inverse relationship to stress (Dohrenwend, 1969). Again, it is difficult to sort out the impacts of class and occupation from the impacts of personal health maintenance practices or hazards associated with the workplace. To illustrate, nearly half of the one million workers surveyed in Chicago in 1970 by the U.S. Department of Health and Human Services' Bureau of Occupational Safety and Health reported urgent and serious health hazards on their jobs. At least four million workers contract occupational diseases every year (Navarro, 1976).

Inequitable distributions of resources in most societies create conditions leading to poor nutritional status, and impaired physical and mental health. Specifically, in the United States, discrimination in housing, educational and job opportunities impede societal role fulfillment and the pursuance of life and happiness among blacks, some Spanish-speaking Americans, and other minorities (McFarland, 1982).

Personal and Behavioral Characteristics

Personal characteristics such as age, sex, life-style, and values affect health to various degrees. Virtually all standards for health shift with age according to many experts. Blood pressure readings of 140/90 are not only normal, but good, for some fifty-year-old persons. On the other hand, this reading would be indicative of problems in nine- to ten-year-olds. Therefore, age is a factor that should not be overlooked in the consideration of health. It logically follows that the age distribution of a community reveals information regarding the nature of its health problems.

Weight, nutritional habits, and life-style also have considerable influence on health. Nutrition is a specific factor in the prevention and control of many chronic diseases. Weight control, for example, is the primary preventive factor in such diseases as diabetes, hypertension, and heart disease. The majority of state and local health agencies employ a nutritionist in their chronic disease programs. Nurses teach nutrition in the clinic and home. The emphasis placed on individual responsibility for healthy behavior by wellness-oriented and cost-conscious experts signals an unlimited horizon for nutrition education.

Life-styles involving stress reduction or management, physical exercise, and social and emotional stimulation are other factors related to health and wellness. Public education regarding the importance of healthy life-style behavior is a major responsibility of the community health nurse. Family and cultural beliefs and norms are important predictors of health-seeking behavior and, therefore, must be considered by health care providers in the planning and delivery of care (Friedman, 1981).

Values influence health at the personal, family, cultural, and community level. Personal or individual values determine the relative value placed on health at various stages of life and in various situations. For example, the value placed on health may be different during illness than during health, or for youth than for the elderly. Nutrition, lifestyle, utilization of health care services, and the perceived costs of such utilization are also determined by personal values. Likewise, family and cultural values also determine the acceptability of specific health practices for specific groups in the community.

Community or public values influence health policies, resource allocation, general life-style behavior, and the extent of community support or involvement in health programs. The current health care cost containment movement illustrates the value placed on health relative to other publicly financed goods or services.

The Health Care System

The health care system is another factor influencing health status. It is usually the source of intervention when illness occurs related to environmental, biological, or behavioral determinants. The health care system is a vital link in the maintenance and improvement of health. The scope of the health care system is quite broad, however, and

will be treated more extensively in the next section of this chapter.

At this point it is important to note that the factors influencing health and illness are integrated and multifactorial. Usually, a combination of the factors act in concert to affect a healthy or detectably pathological state. Therefore, a man with a family history of heart disease (genetic tendency) who consumes an excess of saturated fats and cholesterol in his diet, lives a sedentary life-style (behavioral and life-style factors), works in a stress-provoking managerial position (psychosocial environment), and lives in a community that places little emphasis on primary preventive and health promotional services (appropriate health care services) is at greater risk of acquiring heart disease than a man with any one of these risks.

Human Biology

Human biology is the science and study of the origin, reproduction, structure, functioning, and distribution of human life. It is comprised of many subdivisions (e.g., cytology, embryology, biochemistry, biophysics and genetics). Genetics is one of the newest and most vigorous branches of biology. It has grown to be one of the most fruitful branches of the biological sciences concerned with the differences among individuals.

The characteristics of organisms are determined by their genetic constitution and forces of the environment. At any time only a small percentage of the genes are active. The environment sets certain physical processes into motion that determine which aspects of the genetic code are activated. Therefore, the genetic endowment of the individual determines the potential expression of that individual. However, the environment regulates the extent to which the potentials are expressed. For example, selective environmental influences molded innate differences in body shapes, skin pigmentation, and hair texture, and consequently, the evolution of separate biological or racial groups. Genetic codes determine the predisposition for diseases such as sickle-cell anemia and Tay-Sachs. Other diseases such as breast cancer, hypertension and diabetes are associated with occurrences in immediate family members and, therefore, might be biologically linked.

The genetic evolution of the human species has been supplemented by other biological, social, and technological controls that make it possible for people to live and adapt to their environment. Examples include tanning of the skin, which increases its resistance to solar radiation; immunity acquired through early exposure to disease; the use of fire, tools, clothing and shelter as protective and food-getting measures; and control of ventilation and temperature. Through the complex feedback that governs our lives, our biological endowment influences culture and in turn, is also modified by our cultural environment (Dubos, 1965).

Dubos (1965) contends that humankind's propensity for physiological adaptation, and social and environmental control has resulted in minimal genetic development throughout the millennia. However, over the last 100 years, manipulation of man's biological nature has become an increasing reality. Today people have the capacity for genetic selection in the reproduction of their offspring. Genetic diseases and the gender of unborn children can be determined early enough to terminate pregnancy if undesirable problems are foreseen. Consequently, we have the capacity to eliminate carriers of undesirable genetic diseases from society.

Family and Community Health Care Delivery Systems

The health care delivery system has been defined as the resources (money, people, facilities, and technology) and organizations necessary to transform these resources into health services (Longest, 1979). Over the last forty years the health care system has experienced tremendous growth and change in response to changing priorities, new technology, new delivery methods, changing illness, and social trends. With the growth and concentration of populations in urban areas, health needs and demands have increased and become more complex. Society has come to accept responsibility for the delivery of increasingly more comprehensive services for the community. The effectiveness of the health care system can be analyzed in terms of the objectives and outcomes of services.

The quality of health services became a major public issue in the 1960s and 1970s as third-party payers emerged as regular purchasers of services. Funding of health care services were usually contingent upon documentation that services met certain quality standards. Standards regarding outcomes of services, process of delivery, credentials of professionals, and structure of equipment and facilities are typical variables for measuring the quality of health services.

Access and costs of services became health care issues of the 1970s and 1980s as the nation first focused on equity of access to services and later on cost of services. Community health systems are networks of resources and organizations interacting to plan, support, and provide effective and efficient family and community health services. The complex nature of today's organizations and social institutions requires collaboration among medical and medically oriented groups, as well as nonmedical and self-help organizations. The access and cost of services depend upon cooperation and sometimes competition among these entities.

Levels of Prevention

Given the relative impact of the factors influencing health, another way of measuring the effectiveness of the health care system is to evaluate the types of preventive services. Health services are sometimes classified according to their primary, secondary, and tertiary preventive impacts. (See Chapter 1.) The reader should recall that primary prevention promotes optimum health and provides protection against specific diseases. Physical fitness activities, premarital counseling, or stress management are examples of health promotional activities. Cholesterol reduction, avoidance of smoking, or weight control are specific protection against cardiovascular heart disease.

Secondary prevention involves early diagnosis and treatment after diseases do occur. Regular checkups, weight loss, and adherence to treatment regimens facilitate early diagnosis and treatment.

Tertiary prevention includes restoration and rehabilitation after late manifestations or complications develop. Examples of tertiary prevention are coronary bypass, cardiac rehabilitation, and gradual return to regular activities.

Ideally, effective health systems should promote health and wellness. That means that services provided through the health care system should prioritize efforts to improve environmental and behavioral health. Family living workshops, parenting classes, and nutritional awareness and recreational programs are examples of promotional activities geared toward family environmental and behavioral improvements. Setting standards for safe air, water, and housing or promoting economic growth (i.e., jobs, education, and general welfare) are examples of health promotional programs geared to enhance the environment at the community level. Such services move the community toward the wellness end of the spectrum.

It is possible for benefits of health promotion and disease preventive programs to include improved health, reduced medical costs, reduced loss of time from work, improved quality of life and creativity. Unfortunately, in spite of the growing emphasis on preventive health care and health promotion, obstacles to health promotion and disease prevention exist and include limited allocations for prevention (only $.02 of each health care dollar), ambiguous health policies that reward higher cost treatment of illness, personal freedom regarding unhealthy life-styles (such as cigarette smoking),

and conflicting interests related to public welfare and industrial production (Knobel, 1983).

The purpose of the health care system is to provide services intended to improve, maintain, or promote health. Ironically, expenditures on health services are not consistent with the general assumptions about the relative impact of the factors influencing health. While environmental and life-style factors are thought to have greater impact on the individual, family, or community's health status, 91 percent of all federal health care expenditures are consumed by the health care system (Longest, 1979).

Medical and Medically Oriented Systems

The health care system in the United States is predominantly a medical system. The resources, health care delivery, and the planning and regulating organizations that comprise the health care system support the scientific-based medical model of care. The medical model is a scientific-based model that focuses on disease as an abnormal biological process involving alterations in human structure or functioning (Orem, 1971). The predominant influence of the medical model on the health care system has been criticized for fostering illness and sick role behavior (Bloom & Wilson, 1979) rather than promoting wellness and patient responsibility for health. However, the system has evolved to encompass values and activities related to prevention of disease and promotion of health, particularly with regards to communicable and chronic disease prevention.

The medical model assumes that disease is a multicausal process engendered by living and nonliving agents, personal characteristics, and responses to stimuli in the environment (Orem, 1971). The medical model is distinguished from unconventional models on the basis of societal assumptions that the medical model uses proven techniques in the provision of care (Gillespie, 1979), and on assumptions that nonmedical and traditional systems involve quackery. The physician is the recognized, primary practitioner of scientific medicine. "Medical care" generally refers to care given by physicians. However, sometimes the term is used in reference to services provided by agencies and members of various other health professions, such as nurses. The physician's functions include the diagnosis and treatment of disease and its effects. This distinguishes the physician's practice from those of other members of the medical team (Orem, 1971).

Nurses traditionally practiced under the aegis of the medical model. However, health promotion and primary and secondary prevention have long been the basis of nursing practice. The nurse assesses and diagnoses individual, family, and community health status, utilizing a psychosocial and biological framework. Nurses also plan and deliver educational counseling and referral and hands-on, therapeutic services and coordinate medical services and services of other disciplines. One can classify medical and medically oriented systems according to governmental resources and organizations, private systems, and independent practices.

Federal, State, and Local Government Resources and Organizations The basic resources enabling the health care system to fulfill its mission are money, manpower, technology, and facilities. In 1982 expenditures for health care in the United States totalled $322.4 billion, an average of $1,365 per person, and constituted 11.5 percent of the Gross National Product. Eighty-nine percent of the $322.4 billion expenditures was for personal health services such as hospital care, physicians' services, dentists' services, and other health professional services. The remaining 11 percent was for insurance costs, research, construction, and governmental public health activities (U.S. Bureau of the Census, 1983). Overall, this profile of health care expenditures illustrates the magnitude of the health care industry in the United States.

Traditionally, health care was delivered to individuals and families by private physicians or institutions. However, the realization that some services are met more effectively and efficiently through collective action led official organizations to supplement services provided through private sources with community services to promote and protect the community's health. These community programs receive input from federal, state, and local health care resources and organizations.

Official health agencies such as the U.S. Department of Health and Human Services, and state and local health departments are tax supported and accountable to the citizenry through official boards and legally mandated responsibilities. These agencies interact to provide services, set standards, regulate other community organizations, and collect and disseminate statistical and educational information.

Prior to 1960 the federal government's involvement in health care delivery was usually limited to supporting and regulating health services of state and local agencies and providing services that were beyond the scope of the states. Health activities of the federal government usually included maintaining health statistics and other data related to communicable disease control; supporting or conducting research and providing technical consultation to the legislature or to state or local areas; setting national health policy through legislation and supporting states or local agencies through grants, contracts, and other funding sources; and providing direct services to special groups such as American Indians, members of the military, and veterans of the military (Freeman, 1970).

In the mid-1960s Congress passed legislation that expanded the federal government's role in the field of health care. Title VI of the 1964 Civil Rights Act assured all United States citizens the right to health care, regardless of race, color, or national origin.

In 1965 the Social Security Act was amended to provide third-party payments by the federal government for health care to the poor and elderly—Medicare and Medicaid. Maternity and Infant Care projects, Children and Youth Programs, Comprehensive Health Planning and Regional Medical Programs were other efforts to strengthen the nation's health services. Regional health plans cut across state and local geographic boundaries to attack problems such as air and water pollution, food and drug regulation, and health resources utilization.

During the late-1960s and early-1970s the U.S. government, through the Maternal and Infant Care Programs and Office of Economic Opportunity, bypassed state channels and directly funded local community projects—such as comprehensive community health centers and community mental health centers—in an effort to respond more effectively to the needs of people at the grass roots level (Benson & McDevitt, 1976).

As government spending approached approximately $100 billion, the 1970s and early-1980s witnessed a reversal of some of the preceding trends, and a shift toward greater accountability and efficiency, cost containment in health care, revenue sharing, and increased emphasis on state responsibility for health care.

The state retains ultimate responsibility and authority for the public's health. The state's authority originates from the sovereign powers granted it by the U.S. Constitution.

Each state establishes its own public health services, primarily, under the state health department. The major functions of the state health department include analyzing public health needs and planning programs to meet those needs; providing financial assistance to local areas and health services to areas not otherwise served, such as in emergency situations; setting standards through public health laws, codes, or licensure; collecting vital statistics and maintaining a liaison with the federal health agencies (Benson & McDevitt, 1976; Freeman, 1970).

The local health department coordinates and mobilizes resources and activities to meet the needs of the community. Typically, the role and function of the local health department depend on the mandate from the state and local government and the resources available in the community. Usually the functions include communicable disease investigation, provision of services through clinics, supervision of milk and water supplies, supervision of the quality and safety of meat and other foods, investigation and supervision of the sanitary conditions in public restaurants, provision of health education, provision of services related to maternal and child health, communicable disease prevention, chronic disease control, and provision of laboratory services for physicians.

Private Health Care Systems and Independent Practices Physicians, nurses, dentists, pharmacists, optometrists, podiatrists, and other health professionals who work in private hospitals, ambulatory clinics, physicians' offices, health maintenance organizations, nursing homes, and similar settings constitute the various configurations that make up the private sector of the health care industry. Many of these professionals, such as physicians and dentists, are private profit-making entrepreneurs, providing services on a fee-for-services basis.

Generally, over 715 million persons were employed in the health services industry in 1981. The U.S. Department of Health and Human Services (1982) reported over 440,000 active physicians, 1,165,000 registered nurses, 121,000 dentists, 22,300 optometrists, 142,700 pharmacists, and 8,880 podiatrists in the United States in 1980. It was estimated that the number of physicians would increase by almost 50 percent by the year 2000. However, due to the uneven distribution of health professionals throughout the country, primary health services are still not available to many citizens. National legislation, such as the Health Professions Educational Assistance Act of 1976, was enacted to produce more primary care professionals and improve health care services in underserved areas. However, projections of oversupplies of health care professionals, particularly, physicians and nurses, led to cuts of federally supported health education programs during the last few years.

Services provided by private hospitals and professionals are largely funded through third parties, which developed in response to the rising costs of health care and the rising financial risks to individuals. Over half of all third-party payments now come from either Medicare and Medicaid payments or Blue Cross and Blue Shield plans. Another component of third-party payers are the several hundred private insurance companies in the United

States (i.e., Prudential, Aetna, Equitable, Metropolitan, and Connecticut General). Philanthropic sources of health care financing virtually disappeared by 1976 (Longest, 1979). However, Lightle and Plomann (1981) predicted that the current cost containment movement will force hospitals to solicit philanthropic funding more aggressively in the next few years as an alternative source of debt financing.

Social values regarding the relative price the public is willing to pay for health care have changed. Prior to the mid-1970s, the health industry enjoyed the benefits of generous federal support through the Hill Burton Act, Medicare, and Medicaid. While the government previously funded extensive construction of hospital facilities and beds, regulatory policies have recently been enacted to limit construction as well as the expanding utilization of medical technology.

Until recently the health care industry was essentially comprised of not-for-profit structures. Private physicians, a small number of private hospitals, and the health professionals employed within hospitals and other health organizations were the few exceptions. However, increased competition among hospitals for clients, especially those with private insurance, and decreased financial support from governmental sources triggered strategies aimed at survival on the part of many community hospitals. One of the most significant changes was the development of multiinstitutional, investor-owned arrangements among private hospitals. Through sharing of manpower expertise, technical resources, and other costs, and the provision of more profitable services to the more lucrative, private paying customer, these investor-owned corporations earn dividends for their stockholders.

Over 18 percent of all American hospitals are investor owned. These organizations led the industry in efforts to expand and diversify their services. Some not-for-profit hospitals have set up for-profit divisions to subsidize their costs. Consequently, the health care industry has experienced an increase in profit-making hospitals, ambulatory care services, and after-care facilities (Kuntz, 1982; LeRoux, 1982). In order to survive in a period of con-strained resources many of the profit-making and not-for-profit hospitals are adopting strategies to serve fewer Medicaid and Medicare patients in favor of private paying patients. There is concern among some people that these strategies will restrict access to health care services for persons in lower socioeconomic status groups.

Health Maintenance Organizations   Another approach to the delivery of care in the health care system is through Health Maintenance Organizations (HMOs). They are present in the public and private sectors, but are most often found in the private sector. HMOs are based on the idea of delivery of health services on a prepaid, rather than fee-for-service, basis. They have been in existence for over half a century but may become more important in the future as they are restructured to contain medical costs, while at the same time maintain quality of medical care (Luft, 1982).

HMOs are defined as organizations that assume "contractual responsibility to provide or ensure the delivery of a stated range of health services including physician or hospital services, to a voluntarily enrolled population in return for a fixed periodic payment with minimal co-payments (or additional charges) related to utilization" (Luft, 1982, pp. 317–318). Luft concludes that this definition is broad enough to include several types of HMOs.

While each HMO has its own characteristics, Deeds (1985, p. 2) identifies four distinct types:

1. Staff. Services are delivered through a group practice established to provide health services to members. Physicians are salaried.
2. Group. An HMO contracts with a group practice to provide health services, and the group is compensated on a capitation basis.
3. Network. An HMO contracts with two or more group practices to provide health services.
4. Individual Practice Association (IPA). An HMO contracts with physicians from various settings, both solo practitioners and groups, to provide services.

Furthermore, Deeds (1985) maintains that HMOs are well suited to provide health promotion and patient education services. Potentially these health systems have a key role in performing health monitoring functions for healthy adults and children.

The desire and necessity to curtail health care costs in the future is likely to have a favorable effect on the growth of HMOs. As these health systems grow and subsequent competition develops among them, they are likely to increase advertisement of their services so that more people will know about them. Therefore, they have the potential to provide innovative services to families and community residents. Examples of such services in the health promotion and health maintenance arena include: weight control, stress reduction and management, exercise and fitness, and smoking cessation (Deeds, 1985). Factors such as available sources of funding, federal and state regulations, and the need for cost containment of health services will influence the future viability of HMOs.

HMOs are generally thought to promote health and primary prevention to a greater extent than the earlier mentioned, private medical systems. Nurses have played expanded roles in the delivery of health service through HMOs. Through the use of nurse practitioners as patient-care managers, HMOs provide high quality at lower costs than private hospitals. Case Example 4-1 illustrates the nurse practitioner's role in the HMO.

Nonmedical and Self-Help Approaches

Nonmedical Approaches Nonmedical approaches to health are usually referred to as traditional or natural health practices. Many traditional health practices had their roots in religious philosophy. In some cultures religion reinforced resignation to misfortune and offered opportunities for dignified suffering—for example, in Christianity an opportunity for closer association with the Savior on the Cross. However, historically, all cultures also endorsed some organized school of beliefs and practices related to prevention or cure of illness. Although the use of pharmaceuticals and surgery was evident as early as the ancient Egyptian period,

many of these approaches involved nonmedical theories and practices.

Uncertainty about the motives, efficiency, and effectiveness of medical treatment and practitioners; movements towards self-responsibility for health and self-sufficiency; and the emphasis on freedom of choice have generated an upsurge of interest in unconventional or traditional health care (Gillespie, 1979). However, some consumers and professionals harbor reservations and myths about unconventional or traditional health care practices. These reservations remain in spite of evidence that traditional practitioners are not usually quacks and that their patients are satisfied with their services. Gillespie noted that lack of objective knowledge exists concerning traditional health care and its widespread use. She and other investigators have stressed the positive benefits to be gained through collaboration among conventional and unconventional providers. Benefits associated with traditional health practices result from the nature of the care—its focus on the whole person—and gaps within the conventional health care system.

Many unconventional, traditional, and natural approaches are extensively practiced in Western culture today and include such specialties as chiropractic, naturopathy, homeopathy, acupressure, and various cultural folk practices.

Chiropractic is based on beliefs regarding the relationship of bones and nerves. Displacement of any part of the skeletal frame may press against the nerves and cause disturbances or disease. In order to alleviate pressure on the nerves, the chiropractor manipulates by hand all of the 200 bones, especially those of the vertebral column. The chiropractor also advocates sound hygienic habits and good nutrition as part of the treatment regimen. Conditions said to respond to spinal adjustments are sacroiliac strain, neuralgia, neuritis, migraine headaches, lumbago and other back pains, asthma, and numerous other conditions (Clark, 1978).

Naturopaths diagnose and treat patients through natural practices to restore body processes. They utilize diet, exercise, manipulation, chemical substances naturally found in or produced by living

Case Example 4-1: Family Nurse Practitioner Functions in Health Care System: Health Maintenance Organization (HMO)

Ms. Bond is a family nurse practitioner employed in a large HMO. She has a regular caseload of families (parents and their children) whom she sees for routine checkups and for treatment of episodic minor health problems, the common cold being a typical example.

Nurse practitioner monitors and manages health of families (adults and children).

Mid-mornings twice per week Ms. Bond conducts a class on self-care for the older (mostly retired) adults enrolled in the HMO. She teaches the group members about managing chronic conditions and maintaining healthy life-styles—managing activities of daily living such as sleep, rest, and exercise.

Nurse practitioner addresses self-care needs of older adults.

Ms. Bond discovered that a significant number of the women in the HMO were overweight and many worked in the nearby medical center. She began a noon weight-reduction seminar focusing not only on weight reduction and diet management but also on stress reduction and management. In addition Ms. Bond discusses with the women the importance of regular exercise and physical fitness to physical and emotional well-being and encouraged them to enroll in an exercise program taught in the evenings in the HMO facilities.

Nurse practitioner plans and implements health education and health promotion program.

Two afternoons per week, Ms. Bond conducts seminars for adolescent males and females whose parents are enrolled in the HMO. She facilitates discussion on sex education, alcohol and drug abuse, school adjustment, and family communications.

Nurse practitioner addresses health needs of a particular group (adolescents).

Once per week in the evening, Ms. Bond chairs a community relations committee, where HMO representatives and community leaders and consumers exchange ideas about the community and the HMO. Community residents and leaders discuss community activities, needs, and concerns; and HMO staff describes HMO programs, particularly those free to the community. They also distribute information about membership in the HMO.

Nurse practitioner assumes leadership and collaborates with community representatives to address community health needs.

---

bodies, and healing properties of the air, light, water, heat, and electricity. Naturopathy excludes use of major surgery, X-ray, radium and nonassimilable drugs for therapeutic purposes (Clark, 1978).

Homeopathy was discovered by Samuel Hahnemann, a physician trained in the 1770s who proved the beneficial use of minimum dosages of drugs in treatment of disease. There are three fundamental laws in homeopathy: the law of similars, law of proving, and law of potency. The law of similars states that the same substance that causes

problems or diseases will cure them if given in small dosages. The law of proving involves systematic verification of the first law by giving people small dosages of certain herbs daily and recording the observed symptoms as proof that this herb caused these symptoms or effects. The law of potency posits that the power of remedy lies, not in large quantities of the herb, but in its qualities or subtle aspects (Anderson, Bulgel and Chervin, 1978). Homeopaths use natural sources and seek to stimulate the body's vital forces to effect natural healing. They

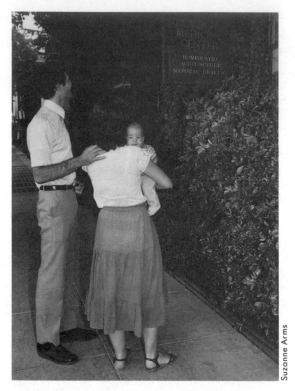

Suzanne Arms

Concerned over the efficiency and motives of medical practices, some families are seeking out alternative forms of health care. Homeopathists, for instance, emphasize minimal dosages of drugs in disease treatment.

treat the patient as a whole and use microscopic doses of drugs.

Although some practitioners learn homeopathy through self-study or preceptorships with established practitioners, homeopathy is also available to physicians as an elective postgraduate course following a medical doctor degree. There is only one homeopathy school in the United States today, the National Center for Homeopathy in Falls Church, Virginia (Clark, 1978).

Cultural practitioners, or medicine men, apply physical or spiritual (or psychological) treatment that assures the sufferer that all will be well. Medicines are made from substances such as herbs, powders, seeds, juices, and minerals. In many cul-

tural settings illness and misfortune are religious experiences and require religious approaches to treatment. Therefore, medicine men may apply needles, massages, incantations, rituals, and physical medicine. They may make sacrifices or ask the patient to sacrifice chickens, goats, or other animals. While many of these activities may not have any overt value, they have enormous psychological value in treating the illness, including the patient's perception of illness (Mbiti, 1970).

Medicine men are also responsible for providing preventive measures. By providing people with charms or conducting rituals in the home or field, the medicine men provide counterprotection against potential misfortune. They also give advice on how to increase productivity or improve marital relationships. They detect sorcery, remove curses, and control the spirits. They symbolize the hopes of society. They are the friends, pastors, psychiatrists, and doctors of traditional communities. Like conventional physicians, they have access to knowledge that is unknown or little known by the public. Therefore, they are entrusted with the duty of protecting the community from harm (Mbiti, 1970).

Cultural practitioners or medicine men undergo formal or informal training under the scrutiny of established medicine men. Training is long and expensive, often starting as young as five years of age. Payment for the training varies and often is made periodically as candidates acquire their knowledge. This may consist of learning one medicine a month (Mbiti, 1970).

Other traditional approaches such as acupressure are based on either proven physiological effectiveness and/or spiritual beliefs. The broadened definition of health with its emphasis on life-style, diet, and physical, spiritual, and mental balance has also broadened the horizon for nonmedical approaches to health care. No longer can medical and medically oriented health professionals, including nurses, afford to overlook the effectiveness of vegetarian diets, acupuncture, herbs, and psychological approaches to health.

Self-Help Approaches Self-help approaches include a broad range of activities including voluntary organizations, consumer action groups, mutual aid or support groups, ethnic self-help activities, or individual life-style behavior. Although some of these activities do not fall within the conventional definition of self-help activities, each, in effect, reflects the consumer's active attempt to have an impact on factors that influence his or her own health.

Self-help groups provide a variety of educational and mutual support services for their members and/or members' families. Alcoholics Anonymous is an outstanding example of a self-help group that was founded on the grounds of mutual support. Other examples are groups organized to support families experiencing sudden infant death syndrome or victims of cancer or mastectomies.

Self-help groups traditionally originated outside the medical system. However, with the emergence of primary prevention and prepaid health programs, the concept of self-help or self-care has increasingly become integrated within established health programs. The organization of self-help groups to stop smoking is an example.

Individuals practice self-help through a variety of ways that are reinforced by current health promotional and wellness-seeking trends. Numerous primary preventive measures such as breast self-examination, weight control, or stress management are individual approaches to health maintenance. In some cultural groups, particularly ethnic immigrant groups, there is heavy reliance on informal support systems such as the extended family for assistance with health maintenance (see Chapter 5). People also rely upon other groups such as voluntary organizations to assist them maintain and promote their health.

Voluntary organizations originate as an expression of public concern with problems or needs not satisfied through personal or government effort. Their mission and function are determined by their boards of directors. However, they are regulated by laws governing incorporation, fund-raising activities, taxation, and general public welfare. Also, they must work within the framework of the total community effort and avoid duplication of services (Benson & McDevitt, 1976).

Voluntary organizations may act to influence environmental conditions, specific health problems, or standards and practices related to health care delivery. Examples of voluntary health organizations are professional organizations such as the National League for Nursing and the American Public Health Association, which collaborate to accredit home health agencies; health foundations such as the Rockefeller Foundation or the Milbank Memorial Fund, which seek to improve the condition of mankind through a variety of philanthropic activities; and problem-related organizations such as the American Red Cross, American Heart Association, or the American Cancer Society.

Consumer action groups also seek to impact on environmental, behavioral, or health care delivery factors. Through concerted effort, consumers try to influence the type, quality, availability, accessibility, effectiveness, and cost of services they receive. Consumer activity in the health care community has essentially been of two types: participation in planning and service organization, and activity related to health behavior, such as smoking cessation, medical checkups and self-help (Reeder, 1978).

According to Reeder (1978):

The mere use of the term 'consumers' to replace 'clients' initiates a different perspective. . . . As a client, on the one hand, the individual delivers himself into the hands of the professional who presumably is the sole decision-maker regarding the nature of the services to be delivered. On the other hand, when the individual is viewed as a consumer, he is a purchaser of services and tends to be guided by caveat emptor. . . . Thus in consumer-provider relationships caveat emptor implies that the consumer has considerably more bargaining power than formerly (pp. 113, 114).

Reeder (1978) argues that the relationship between professional and client has and will continue to change as a result of structural changes in society related to health care. For example, as consumers increase their awareness and participation in health care organizations, health care systems will become more responsive to consumer concerns. Questions have been raised, however, regarding the validity of the positive impact of citizen participation on the health care delivery system. In spite of the strong demand for citizen participation in the 1960s and 1970s, the concept is not a new one. Citizen advisory groups have been used by government and private organizations for quite some time. How-ever, some of these groups have had merely sym-bolic or legitimizing functions for maintaining the status quo. Some citizen's groups have had sub-stantive functions. However, often the goals of such groups have tended to be quite vague (Davis, 1978).

Summary

Advancements in community health evolved parallel to the general history of civilization. Throughout history people have always been con-cerned with health and have assigned high esteem to groups or individuals who guarded and protected the community's health. As scientific knowledge increased, emphasis shifted from control of disease to promotion of wellness and health; from equita-ble access to care to individual responsibility for health. Along with these changes the definition of health broadened to encompass an illness-wellness continuum. Underlying this definition was the assumption that the individual is an open, inte-grated biopsychosocial being engaged in mutual adaptation with the environment in an effort to achieve equilibrium.

Family and community health can be concep-tualized along the illness-wellness continuum. Ill-ness and wellness behavior are learned in families. The health status of individual family members affects the health of other members and the family as a whole. The health status of the community is affected—in order of importance—by environ-mental factors, personal behavior and character-istics, the health care system within the commu-nity, and human biology. Therefore, preventive and promotional services are crucial to health main-tenance, and nurses are in excellent positions to work with families and communities toward achieving their health goals. Nurses may deter-mine the health status of families and communities by analyzing the multifactorial influences on health—the conditions within the environment, life-styles, and health care systems. Problems iden-tified in these areas will help the community nurse delineate health problems that may be targeted for solutions at the family, individual, or community level.

Study Questions

1. The major factors influencing health status of the family and community in their relative order of impact are:
    a. National historical trends, values of the community, human biology, and envi-ronment.
    b. Environment, values of the community, human biology, and adequacy of the health care system.
    c. Environment, life-styles (and personal demographic characteristics of families and groups constituting the community), the health care system, and human biology.
    d. Environment, human biology, the health care system, and the life-styles and personal demographic characteristics of the fami-lies or groups that make up the community.
2. Increasingly health has come to be viewed, not as a dichotomous variable, but as:
    a. An illness-wellness continuum with opti-mum functioning on one end and disability on the other.
    b. A state of equilibrium that enables individ-uals to function to their fullest potential and have reasonable freedom from undue pain or disability.

c. An illness-wellness continuum with health—a state of integrated biopsychosocial functioning that enables people to achieve their maximum potential within the environment and have reasonable freedom from undue pain or disability—on one end, and illness or disease on the other.

d. A state of complete physical, mental, and social well-being, not merely the absence of disease or infirmity.

3. One way of measuring the performance and adequacy of the health care delivery system is to evaluate the quality, appropriateness, accessibility, and efficiency of the services provided. Given the relative impact of the determinants of health, another way of measuring the adequacy of the system is to assess the various levels of:

a. Preventive services provided
b. Community support
c. a and b
d. Neither a nor b

4. Which of the following are environmental threats to health?

a. Severely hot and dry weather, air pollution, noise pollution, substandard housing conditions and disintegrated living conditions.

b. Inclement weather, high socioeconomic status, ethnic majority membership, and substandard housing.

c. Living surroundings characterized by detached social relationships only.

d. Genetic makeup of the individual.

References

Aday LA, Andersen RM: Equity of access to medical care: A conceptual and empirical overview. *Med Care* 1981; 19: Suppl to No. 12: 4–27.

Aday LA, Andersen RM: National trends in access to medical care: Where do we stand? Center for Health Administration Studies Graduate School of Business, University of Chicago, November 16, 1983.

Anderson D, Bulgel D, Chervin D: *Homeopathic Remedies*. Honesdale, Pa.: Himalayan International Institute, 1978.

Anderson C, Morton R, Green LW: *Community Health*. St. Louis: Mosby, 1978.

Anderson CL, Green LW: *Community Health*. St. Louis: Mosby, 1982.

Arensberg CM: Community as object and as sample. In: Friedrick CJ (editor), *Community*. New York: Liberal Arts Press, 1959.

Ben-Jochannan Y: *Black Man of the Nile and his Family*. New York: Alkebu-Ian Book Associates, 1978.

Benson E, McDevitt J: *Community Health Nursing Practice*. Englewood Cliffs, N.J.: Prentice-Hall, 1976.

Bloom SW, Wilson RN: Patient-practitioner relationships. In: Freeman HE, Levine S, Reeder LG (editors), *Handbook of Medical Sociology*, 3rd ed. Englewood Cliffs, N.J.: Prentice-Hall, 1979.

Byrne ML, Thompson LF: *Key Concepts for the Study and Practice of Nursing*. St. Louis: Mosby, 1972.

Ciocco A: On the mortality in husbands and wives. *Proceedings of the National Academy of Sciences* 1940: 26: 610–615.

Clark L: *Get Well Naturally*. New York: Arco, 1978.

Clark TN: *Community Structure and Decision-making: Comparative Analyses*. San Francisco: Chandler, 1968.

Coe R, Brehm H: *Preventive Health Care for Adults: A Study of Medical Practice*. New Haven, Conn.: College & University Press, 1972.

Cottrell L: *Life Under the Pharoahs*. New York: Grossett & Dunlap, 1960.

Crawford CO: *Health and the Family: A Medical Sociological Analysis*. New York: Macmillan, 1971.

Davis JW: Decentralization, citizen participation, and ghetto health care. In: Schwartz HD, Kart CS (editors), *Issues in Medical Sociology*. Reading, Mass.: Addison-Wesley Publishing Company, 1978.

D'Atri, DM, Ostfeld, AM: Crowding: Its effects on the elevation of blood pressure in a prison setting. *Preventive Medicine*, 1975: 4: 550–566.

Deeds S: Health-promotion activities in selected HMO settings. *Family and Community Health* 1985; 8(1): 1–17.

Dever GEA: Community health analysis. *Family and Community Health*. Germantown, MD.: Aspen Publications, 1980.

Dohrenwend BP, Dohrenwend BS: *Social Status and Psychological Disorder: A Casual Inquiry*. New York: Wiley, 1979.

Dubos R: Human Ecology. In: Hafen BQ (editor), *Man, Health and Environment*. Minneapolis: Burgess, 1972.

Dubos R: *Man, Medicine, and Environment*. London: Pall Mall Press, 1965.

Durkheim E: *Suicide: A Study in Sociology*. New York: The Free Press, 1967.

Effrat MP: *The Community: Approaches and Applications*. New York: The Free Press, 1974.

Eisenbud M: *Environment, Technology and Health: Human Ecology in Historical Perspective*. New York: New York University Press, 1978.

Freeman RB: *Community Health Nursing Practice.* Philadelphia: Saunders, 1970.

Friedman MM: *Family Nursing: Theory and Assessment.* New York: Appleton-Century-Crofts, 1981.

Gary LA: A social profile. *Black Men.* Beverly Hills: Sage, 1982.

Gillespie K: Unconventional health care: A positive alternative? *Family and Community Health* 1979; 2(3), 41–46.

Ginsberg E: The competitive solution: Two views. *N Engl J Med* 1980; 303 (1): 1112–1115.

Goldsmith JC: *Can Hospitals Survive? The New Competitive Market.* Homewood, Ill.: Dow Jones-Irwin, 1981.

Gori GB, Richter BJ: Macroeconomics of disease prevention in the United States. *Science* 1978; 200: 1124–1130.

Harwood A: *Ethnicity and Medical Care.* Cambridge, Mass.: Harvard University Press, 1981.

Hawley AH: *Human Ecology.* New York: Ronald Press, 1950.

National Commission on Community Health Services: *Health Is a Community Affair. Report of the National Commission on Community Health Services.* Cambridge, Mass.: Harvard University Press, 1966.

Jackson JJ: Urban black Americans. In: Harwood A (editor), *Ethnicity and Medical Care.* Cambridge, Mass.: Harvard University Press, 1981.

Jenkins CD: Social environment and cancer mortality in men. *N Engl J Med* 1983; 308 (7): 395–398.

Kane RL: *Challenges of the Community.* New York: Springer, 1974.

Katz AH, Felton JS: *Health and the Community.* New York: The Free Press, 1965.

Kaufman HF: Toward an interactional conception of community. In: Friedrick CJ (editor), *Community.* New York: Liberal Arts Press, 1959.

Kinlein LM: Point of view on the front: Nursing and family and community health. *Family and Community Health* 1978; 1 (1): 57–68.

Knobel RJ: Health promotion and disease prevention: Improving health while conserving resources. *Family and Community Health* 1983; 5 (4): 16–27.

Knutson AN: *The Individual, Society and Health Behavior.* New York: Russell Sage Foundation, 1965.

Kuntz EF: General Medical to take on American Supply Corporation. *Modern Health Care* 1982; 12 (5): 138–142.

Lee JS, Rom WN, Craft FB: Preventing disease and injury in the work place. *Family and Community Health* 1983; 12 (2): 10–18.

Lehman EW: Social class and coronary heart disease: A sociological assessment of the medical literature. *J Chronic Dis* 1967; 20: 381–391.

LeRoux M: Health hospital insurers grapple with commercial firms. *Modern Health Care* 1982; 12 (9): 83–84.

Lightle MA, Plomann MP: Hospital capital financing entering phase four. *Hospitals* 1981; 55 (15): 61–63.

Longest BB: The U.S. health care system. In: Albrecht GL, Higgins PC (editors), *Health, Illness and Medicine.* Chicago: Rand McNally, 1979.

Luft H: Health maintenance organization: Implications for nursing. In: Aiken L, Gortner S (editors), *Nursing in the 1980s.* Philadelphia: Lippincott, 1980.

Mbiti JS: *African Religions and Philosophy.* Garden City, N.Y.: Doubleday, 1970.

McFarland CE: The impact of crisis, race and class: A dual perspective on the American family. M.S.W. thesis, State University of New York, Stonybrook, 1982.

Mechanic D: Disease, mortality, and the promotion of health. *Health Affairs* 1982; 1 (3): 28–38.

Miller S: State of the environment. *Environmental Science Technology* 1984; (18) 8: 250A–251A.

Mollica RF: From asylum to community. *Public Policy and Psychiatry* 1983; 308 (7): 367–373.

Navarro V: The underdevelopment of health of working America: Causes, consequences and possible solutions. *Medicine under Capitalism.* New York: Prodist, 1976.

Nelson EC, Simmons JJ: Health promotion—the second public health revolution: Promise or threat? *Family and Community Health* 1983; 12 (2): 1–12.

Olphuls W: *Ecology and the Politics of Scarcity.* San Francisco: W. H. Freeman, 1977.

Orem DE: *Nursing: Concepts of Practice.* New York: McGraw-Hill, 1971.

Parsons T: The principal structure of community. In: Friedrick CJ (editor), *Community.* New York: Liberal Arts Press, 1959.

Patrick DL, Bush JW, Chen MM: Toward an operational definition of health. *J Health Soc Behav* 1973; 14 (1): 6–22.

Pratt L: *The relationship of socioeconomic status to health.* In: Reinhart AM, Quinn MD (editors), *Family-Centered Community Nursing.* St. Louis: Mosby, 1973.

Purdom PW: *Environmental Health,* 2nd ed. New York: Academic Press, 1980.

Reeder LG: Patient client as consumer: Some observations on the changing professional-client relationship. In: Schwartz HD, Kart CS (editors), *Dominant Issues in Medical Sociology.* Reading, Mass.: Addison-Wesley Publishing Company, 1978.

Robert Wood Johnson Foundation: Updated report on access to health care for the American people. *Special Report* 1983; (1).

Schreiber JM, Horniak JP: Mexican Americans. In: Harwood A (editor). *Ethnicity and Medical Care.* Cambridge, Mass.: Harvard University Press, 1981.

Selby P: *Health in 1980–1990: A Predictive Study Based on an International Inquiry.* New York: S. Karger, 1974.

Shekelle RB et al: Social status and incidence of coronary heart disease. *J Chronic Dis* 1969; 22: 381–394.

Terry LL: Pollution. In: Hafen BQ (editor), *Health and Environment.* Minneapolis: Burgess, 1972.

Thompson PB: Need and safety: The nuclear power debate. *Environmental Ethics* Spring 1984; (6): 57–67.

US Bureau of the Census: *Statistical Abstract of the United States: 1984,* 104th ed. Washington, D.C.: US Government Printing Office, 1983.

US Department of Health and Human Services: *Health United States 1982.* DHHS Publication No. (PHS) 83–1232. Hyattsville, Md.: US Department of Health and Human Services, December 1982.

US Department of Health, Education, and Welfare—US Public Health Service, Health Resources Administration: 1976. *Health in America, 1776–1976.* DHEW Publication No. (HRA) 76–616.

WHO: Constitution of the World Health Organization, 1948. In *Basic Documents* 15th ed. Geneva: WHO, 1964.

Chapter 5

Culture and Ethnicity

Barbara Bryan Logan and Clovis E. Semmes

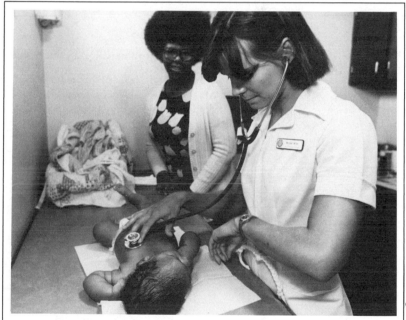

With the diversity of ethnic groups in American society, community health nurses must be sensitive to the cultural values of their clients and aware of their own biases and beliefs.

Chapter Outline

Overview of Concepts
 Culture
 Ethnicity
 Culture, Ethnicity, and Health
Ethnic Families
 Irish American Families
 Mexican American Families
 Black American Families
 Native American Families
 South Vietnamese Families

Implication and Strategies for Community Health Nurses
 Self-awareness
 Acceptance
 Professional Traditions and Values
 The Client's World View
 Functioning in Ethnic Communities
 Functioning as Client Advocates
Summary
Study Questions
References

Chapter Objectives

After completing this chapter, the reader will be able to:

- Describe the concepts of culture and ethnicity and their relationship to health
- Identify cultural dimensions that are essential to nursing assessment
- Discuss the nursing profession as a unique culture
- Describe the ethnographic interview
- Discuss family values, health beliefs, and practices of selected ethnic families
- Analyze how their own ethnic and cultural background affects interactions with clients
- Identify strategies community health nurses can use to increase their effectiveness with clients

We are all members of a culture. How we interpret the reality around us, what we consider to be reasonable statements and behavior, and what we believe to be health and illness all stem from the culture we share with some people and not with others. Those whose cultural experiences differ from our own will also differ in their beliefs and interpretations of reality.

We are all rooted in an ethnic group as well, even if this group is simply the so-called "majority" of white, middle-class, protestant heritage. The degree to which we identify with an ethnic past will vary according to the strength with which family tradition has maintained that identity, and to the degree that the family chooses to assimilate into the larger society. The extent of an individual's or a family's identification with an ethnic heritage is as important as the specific features of that heritage.

American society is ethnically and culturally diverse, and community health nurses will find themselves practicing in communities that reflect this diversity. A particular family or a whole community may belong to an ethnic or cultural group very different from the nurse's own. Those community health nurses who are most sensitive to variations in clients' beliefs and behaviors will be most effective in promoting their wellness.

Community health nurses can achieve this sensitivity by examining their own culture in order to understand how it colors their world view and their interactions with individuals, families, and communities. Recognizing that clients are individuals as well as members of a larger culture, nurses will reject stereotypical views of clients' ethnic groups that can impede communication and diminish their effectiveness. Indeed, culture mediates all social encounters, including those between nurse and client, and its study can enhance the effectiveness of health care services.

This chapter will present an overview of the concepts of culture and ethnicity, and explain how these concepts relate to variations in health beliefs and practices. A brief discussion of selected ethnic families in the United States will illustrate these variations in specific instances with the understanding that significant differences exist *within* cultures. The concluding discussion of implications for the community health nurse should serve to sensitize the student to the importance of culture and ethnicity in all nurse-client encounters.

Overview of Concepts

Culture

Culture is the distinctive way of life characterizing a given community. It includes the community residents' beliefs, values, customs, and institutions. Culture develops as people adapt to their environment and thus consists of a community's solutions to the problems of life. For example, in different cultures people have found various solutions to such problems and questions as: How do you construct effective shelter against the elements? What is the purpose of life? What is beauty? How do you live together without warfare? How do you communicate? and What causes diseases?

The products of culture—language, architecture, religion, philosophy, and so on—form a structure that is both enduring and dynamic. Culture is learned and is preserved by society's institutions, but it also evolves and changes as it is passed on to subsequent generations. Thus culture provides order but at the same time permits human creativity.

Culture can be divided into two broad categories: material culture and nonmaterial culture.

Material culture consists of objects and techniques created and used by a given group. Television sets, automobiles, clothing, and eating implements are examples of material culture. Nonmaterial culture consists of how people perceive, understand, and order their world. It is what people consider to be knowledge, which they then use to construct a social reality. Nonmaterial or cognitive culture includes beliefs (what people think is true), values (what people think is important), and norms (what people expect regarding social behavior). It also involves how people perceive cause and effect, and how they order time and space. For example, in some Asian cultures illness is viewed as an imbalance of the body's vital energy, and in traditional African cultures time is reckoned based on events rather than increments as in Western cultures. Also, different ethnic groups have different concepts of space with respect to social distance and the way they conceive of space as public and private. The elements of cognitive culture collectively form what may be called a *world view*. This world view represents the broad frame of reference through which people perceive and understand events.

An understanding of cognitive culture and its impact on behavior is crucial to the delivery of health services to individuals, families, and community groups and underlies successful planning and implementation of these services.

Cultural Assessment Comprehensive and accurate health assessments are necessary antecedents to the planning and implementation of health services. An important dimension of the health assessment is the cultural assessment, which includes a systematic examination of the cultural beliefs, values, norms, and practices of individuals, groups, and communities within their social context (Leininger, 1977). In some instances, the nursing literature presents the cultural assessment as an activity that nurses do especially when they encounter clients from cultures different from their own. However, since *all* clients belong to a culture, nurses should routinely assess the cultural dimensions as they influence the health status, beliefs,

and behaviors of clients. In other words, a nursing assessment is incomplete unless it includes the cultural dimensions.

The cultural component of the health assessment involves examining the material and nonmaterial aspects of the client's culture. One way for community health nurses to discover the cognitive culture of the people they serve is to explore in-depth how their clients perceive their experiences with given health problems. This means that the nurse's own values must be put aside temporarily in order to elicit the perspective of the client. Nurses must also ask questions that reveal clients' social and physical environment as well as their various health beliefs and practices. Box 5-1 lists examples of cultural dimensions that are essential to a good health assessment.

In the assessment process, probing or encouraging clients to elaborate their point of view is very important. For example, if clients do not view a particular activity as destructive to health, they will take no action to correct it. Similarly, clients' beliefs about the cause of disease will determine whether they feel a particular treatment or health practitioner is appropriate.

At times, the community health nurse may find it necessary to construct unique treatment strategies that accomplish the goal of promoting health without violating the beliefs and values of the client. This approach may be needed, for example, in cases where people consider certain foods to be taboo. The community health nurse may be able to help clients identify alternative foods or nutritional sources. Thus assessment of clients' cultural backgrounds as they relate to health and life-style contribute to effective planning and implementation of nursing care.

The nature of the assessment and the cultural dimensions included may differ depending upon whether the client is an individual, family, or community. The ethnographic interview, however, is one tool that can be used in conducting a cultural assessment on an individual or group level. This is because the interview can be used to obtain the perspective of a specific individual or to obtain facts about the group to which the individual belongs.

Box 5-1 Cultural Dimensions: Essential Content in Nursing Assessment

Material Culture
- Food and diet
- Dress
- Residence or neighborhood
- Physical characteristics—hair, skin color, body features, etc.
- Language—dialect, accents
- Ethnic group affiliation—level of participation in ethnic community
- Family activities—folkways
- Community "ethnic" organizations

Nonmaterial Culture
- Values
    Family
    Health
    Human nature
    Social interaction
- Beliefs
    Wellness or health promotion
    Causes and treatment of sickness

Time and space; privacy
    Family relationships
    Child-rearing
- Norms or Customs
    Family traditions
    Rituals including personal habits (e.g., hygiene, sleep patterns, modesty, responses to life events such as births or deaths)
    Communication patterns—verbal or non-verbal
    Religion or religious beliefs

Client-Nurse Cultural Interface
- Client's culture
- Nurse's culture
- Client's health care system
- Nursing professional health care system
- Communication process
- Level of differences
- Potential conflict areas

The Ethnographic Interview The ethnographic interview is an in-depth, open-ended interview designed to obtain information from the interviewee's perspective. This means that questioning does not force the client to select from predetermined answers, but allows for detailed answers. When using this technique, the community health nurse encourages clients to speak openly and freely about their health problems, status, history, beliefs, and practices. Thus, the nurse attempts to obtain a picture of the client's concept of health, illness, and treatment. It is important that clients be allowed to frame their responses in their own words and describe situations based upon how they perceive them. Thus, the nurse elicits the definitions and meanings the client attaches to phenomena or events.

The ethnographic interview is conducted from a natural history approach and is tailored to fit the specific client-nurse encounter or health problem. Using a natural history approach means that the community health nurse brings the client back in

time to some point prior to the onset of a given health problem and moves forward in time to the present. Thus, the community health nurse allows the client to relate what has happened, who has been involved, what was done, and what the client seeks to have done surrounding the health problem. Furthermore, the nurse elicits from the client the meanings attached to the experience thus far. In this process the nurse discovers the client's self-care and self-treatment activities, the extent to which these have been combined with professional intervention, and whether or not the client's experiences with other health care professionals have been successful or unsuccessful, positive or negative. It is important that this information be obtained because (1) what people have done or continue to do concerning their health will influence any subsequent nursing intervention, (2) self-treatment almost always occurs despite professional intervention, (3) formal or professional treatment may have been modified by the client in some way and for various reasons, and (4) clients who have had a history of negative or unsuccessful relationships with formal treatment or health care professionals may be inclined to reject further professional intervention. Thus, in the course of the ethnographic interview the nurse can discover the client's perspective and better understand the social environment, life stresses, and support networks that affect the client's life-style and response to health and illness. Case Example 5-1 (p. 104) is an excerpt taken from an ethnographic interview.

The direction of the ethnographic interview is determined by the purpose of the nurse-client encounter and to a certain degree by the actual experiences of the client. The goal is always to understand fully the cultural milieu of the client in order to deliver health care services effectively. In Case Example 5-1 the parents felt that the health professionals had misunderstood them in their initial encounters. They wanted to be in control of their life-style and health practices but felt health care professionals undermined their authority by exerting their own personal and professional biases.

Nursing as a Culture   All people are organized in ways that affect their cognitive orientation and their behavior and thus can be said to function within the framework of a culture. Nursing and other professions represent distinctive forms of social organization. Social organizations, or structures in which people interact on a regular basis, give rise to specific beliefs, values, and conventions that are shared to varying degrees by its members. Thus, one can say that nurses function within the framework of a professional culture. They become socialized into the professional culture in much the same way that individuals become socialized into their family structures.

In the professional socialization process, nurses learn to adopt the values and traditions of the nursing profession. Since nursing emerged as a profession rooted in the European traditions, these value orientations are likely to reflect mainstream Anglo-American values. Unconscious adoption of such values can bias the nurse's perception of how people ought to behave and how the therapeutic process ought to proceed. For example, as professionals,

nurses generally expect clients to show interest in their own health, to trust and value the opinion and expertise of the professional, and to comply with prescribed treatment regimens. However, some clients may rely more on self-treatment in the context of their families, friends, or religious institutions, and they may question or even distrust the expertise of the health professional. This does not mean that clients are not interested in their health, as exemplified in Case Example 5-1. Community health nurses need to be sensitive to these factors and alert to how family and other community-institutional bonds shape the nurse-client encounter. Misfitting expectations in the professional-client encounter may contribute to noncompliant behavior by the client and even rejection of the client as hopeless by the professional. It is important that community health nurses minimize this potential conflict in their practice.

Ethnicity

Although many definitions of *ethnicity* exist, the term is generally used to define groups within a larger society on the basis of (1) social ties such as common ancestry, shared geographical locale, and historical past; (2) shared and learned standards of behavior such as language, communication patterns, food patterns, celebration of holidays, and sex-role patterns; and (3) shared focus on one or more symbolic elements such as language or dialect, tribe affiliation, nationality, and phenotypical features (Schermerhorn, 1970).

The concept of ethnicity is very relevant in the United States because it has a heterogeneous population. To varying degrees ethnic groups view themselves as culturally distinct in significant ways. Instead of blending totally into the dominant American culture, they hold on to their cultural heritage. This heritage, in turn, influences their attitudes, values, and personal behaviors. Certain categories have been developed to describe the extent to which ethnic groups have been acculturated into the larger society. Whereas some groups are almost totally assimilated into the dominant culture, other groups maintain their own cultural and ethnic traditions within the larger society (Harwood, 1981).

The category *behavioral ethnicity* applies to people who are well socialized into the distinctive values, norms, and customs of their ethnic groups. These values, norms, and customs serve as a basis for interaction within the larger society. Maintenance of, and participation in, ethnic customs and behaviors is conscious, obligatory, and systematic. On the other hand, *ideological ethnicity* refers to the situation in which ethnic groups' customs are practiced voluntarily rather than automatically. These customs are not central to the person's daily life and are not necessarily learned from early socialization.

These two concepts are helpful for community health nurses since the clients they encounter will run the gamut from behavioral to ideological ethnicity in terms of how they manifest their ethnic identity. For example, some clients may rely on ethnic values and customs to guide most aspects of their lives (behavioral ethnicity), while others may only celebrate their ethnic holidays (ideological ethnicity). Whether or not individuals and families lean more toward behavioral or ideological ethnicity depends on their degree of socialization in the larger culture and the extent to which they remain insulated within a subculture.

The designation *categorical ethnicity* explains cultural differences in terms of the degree to which different ethnic groups manifest distinctive cultural traits such as skin color, food preferences, language, and religion. This aspect of ethnicity, which concerns objective characteristics such as how people look and behave, is usually the focus of attention in the United States when people informally discuss ethnic groups. On the other hand, *transactional ethnicity* focuses on interaction between individuals from different ethnic groups, and regards ethnicity as a "situational phenomenon" (Barth, 1969; Green, 1982). In these cross-ethnic encounters people's sense of cultural distinctiveness becomes important; they signal their intracultural identity through the way they behave and interact in ethnic transactions. In such situations cultural traits can be used as criteria for inclusion or exclusion as cultural groups attempt to define boundaries around themselves. For example, health professionals may view clients who speak nonstandard English as unintelligent and may use this as a reason not to communicate with them, thus indirectly excluding them from participation in health care systems. The more rigid the boundaries established, the more stereotyped intergroup encounters will be.

Green (1982) postulates that one can be more or less acculturated as the situation demands, and, consequently, the degree to which a person is acculturated is situational rather than absolute. Therefore, it is important for community health nurses to realize that the importance of ethnic identity is partly a function of the nature of the encounter or interaction in which people of the same or different ethnic groups are engaged.

Culture, Ethnicity, and Health

Culture and ethnicity are relevant to health and the health care process because ethnic groups vary both within groups and across groups with respect to their life-styles, health beliefs and practices, and use of health services. Ethnic groups have also varied in terms of morbidity and mortality for different diseases (Harwood, 1981).

One social scientist who is also a physician (Kleinman, 1980) has identified three culturally determined arenas that intersect to influence people's health practices: the popular arena, the folk arena, and the professional arena. The popular arena involves health beliefs and self-help practices determined within the context of family, social networks, and community activities. The folk arena consists of nonprofessional healing specialists (sacred or secular) such as faith healers, lay midwives, and herbalists. The professional arena involves practitioners of Western scientific medicine or professionalized indigenous healers if outside of the Western context.

Community health nurses, like other professionals, are trained to act within a professional arena, which holds the values of Western scientific med-

(text continued on p. 106)

Case Example 5-1: An Ethnographic Interview

The Abdul family—Mr. and Mrs. Abdul; Cara, age 6; James, age 5; and Tanya, age 3—is black and middle class. They are vegetarians, eat natural foods as much as possible, and are very health conscious. Their experiences with mainstream health systems began when Cara required a medical examination in order to enter school.

Brief description of family background and life-style.

Mr. and Mrs. Abdul took Cara to the outpatient department of a large medical center for the physical examination because a friend of Mrs. Abdul's mother works in the center. In the process of the examination, the physician discovered that Cara had a hairline fracture of the leg, which had apparently healed.

The physician determined that Cara's fracture was due to a vitamin deficiency. He and other hospital personnel alleged that the Abdul children were being neglected. After several weeks of conflicts and misconceptions between the Abduls and health practitioners at the medical center, and a regimen of vitamin replacements for both Cara and her siblings, the family was referred to their neighborhood health center for follow-up. A concerned and distrustful father, Mr. Abdul is the spokesperson in the following segment of the ethnographic interview conducted by Ms. Banks, a registered nurse prepared at the B.S.N. level.

Ms. Banks: Tell me what brings you here today?

Nurse begins with an openended, nonproblem-focused question that encourages further discussion.

Mr. Abdul: Cara is supposed to have a checkup. They said she had a vitamin deficiency.

Ms. Banks: When did this happen?

Nurse explores for natural history of events.
Nurse obtains client's account of previous experience with health care setting and health care providers.

Mr. Abdul: It all started when we were going to put Cara in school. They said she had to have a medical exam. We want to get the physical. We waited at the hospital all day. So they did x-rays on Cara. They wanted to check her leg out. Then they wanted us to take Cara to the hospital, so we did. It turned out that Cara's leg wasn't broken, but she had a hairline fracture, which probably happened a long time ago when we went on a trip. He [doctor] wanted to put a cast on it to make sure she wouldn't reinjure it. We told the doctor we didn't want to hospitalize Cara, but we would deal with the hospital out-patient services.

Ms. Banks: What happened next?

Nurse continues to explore natural history of events from family's perspective.

Mr. Abdul: Well, the doctor agreed but then they thought . . . our diet must have had something to do with why Cara got injured so easily, and with my mother-in-law's interference—God knows what she told them—they wanted us to write down our diet, what we ate everyday. Eventually they diagnosed her [Cara] as having a vitamin deficiency—rickets. But they had this attitude that it was due to our neglect of the children. They wanted them all tested.

Ms. Banks: What's your understanding of why all of this happened?

Mr. Abdul: Well, we are vegetarians. We are into natural health. The medical people and others like my mother-in-law don't really understand what natural health is all about. They are all skeptical, so they put us through all these changes. Just like they prescribed vitamin D pills for the children. It didn't work too good. The kids couldn't hold it on their stomachs . . . so we had to find natural sources of vitamin D—like raw coconut. We put raw coconut in their cereal.

Ms. Banks: How can we help you now?

Mr. Abdul: Well, you know, we think we are doing the right thing. We want people to understand us. Sometimes when you are black, people don't take you seriously. They think you are ignorant and don't know what you are doing. We want to be healthy. We just want to do it our way.

Ms. Banks: Tell me about your way, what works for your family?

Mr. Abdul: Our way? The natural way; we try to get our nutrients from natural foods.

Ms. Banks: We are very much concerned about your family's health as you are, so I would like to bring in our dietitian consultant to talk this out—with you, Mrs. Abdul, the children, and myself.

Mrs. Abdul's mother was also brought into subsequent meetings because of her love for, and involvement with, the family, as well as her misunderstanding of their dietary patterns and life-style.

Conclusion:

With some assistance from the dietitian and their own natural health consultant, Mr. and Mrs. Abdul devised a diet plan consisting of natural foods the children liked but that were also rich in natural sources of vitamin D and other essential vitamins and food values. They were happy with the plan because it was not contradictory to their beliefs and life-style and enthusiastically agreed to periodic follow-up at the health center.

Nurse seeks client's perspective.

Nurse elicits family's input in order to devise a solution to their problem.

Opportunity given to family to present their perspective and provide input in the health care process resulted in positive outcome.

icine. However, people in general are more likely to adopt only varying aspects of the approach or values of scientific medicine. Internalization of Western scientific medicine, or the mainstream biomedical model of health care, is itself a cultural phenomenon and may reflect levels of acculturation to mainstream America. Likewise, rejection of biomedical approaches can symbolize efforts to maintain and preserve ethnicity (Harwood, 1981).

Individuals, groups, and families may use one arena predominantly or may interchange or use different approaches simultaneously. A comparative study of different ethnic groups illustrates this point. Scott (1975) studied nonwhite ethnic groups: Bahamians, Haitians, Puerto Ricans, and American-born blacks. She found that all the ethnic groups in the study exhibited patterns of using their own folk systems as well as orthodox scientific medicine. Variable use of orthodox and folk systems were affected by language and transportation difficulties, social distance factors, and a lack of cultural "fit" with the health beliefs and practices of the health practitioner. Furthermore, Scott's (1975) study illustrated cultural divergence from mainstream American culture and cultural similarities across nonwhite ethnic groups. All the ethnic groups in her study attributed certain symptoms and conditions to social and interpersonal conflict and supernatural activity. In many instances, because of their beliefs about the causes of disease, orthodox medical practitioners were viewed as inappropriate.

Based on her data, Scott (1975) developed several hypotheses that are relevant to this discussion: (1) where medical treatment is quickly effective, dramatic, and evident, it will prevail over others; (2) modes of curing are arranged in hierarchies of resort and depend on the progress of the illness and the acculturation process; (3) choice of health care alternatives depends upon the perceived appropriateness of the institution; (4) people are bicultural in their choices; (5) orthodox medicine supplements, rather than replaces, folk counterparts, and variation depends upon belief concerning the etiology of disease; (6) the type of disease is crucial

in influencing choice; and (7) the reliance on one therapy, therapist, or system of health care may be viewed by patients as too precarious. These findings dramatize the need for community health nurses to have a complete understanding of their clients' health beliefs and practices.

Of course, there is also substantial variation within ethnic and racial groups regarding etiological interpretations of health and disease. For example, among Afro-Americans there is a persistent spiritual (or metaphysical) orientation in interpreting the causes of illness (Semmes, 1983). Nevertheless, various segments of this community express these beliefs differently depending on the context. Involvement with specific religious groups and adherence to specific spiritual philosophies are often important factors affecting variation. Thus, it is necessary for the community health nurse to discover the specific beliefs of clients and the social context in which they are maintained.

The beliefs of the client and the context in which they are maintained are made evident by the way that clients go about interpreting symptoms and seeking care. This process has been described by social scientists as the client's "help-seeking career" (McKinlay, 1981).

This help-seeking career has recognizable and predictable stages: a beginning, a middle, and an end. These stages are generally sequential as follows: (1) onset of the problem; (2) response to symptoms; (3) lay consultations, lay referrals, and self-medication; (4) client expectations and the encounter with a medical practitioner; (5) aftermath of the patient-practitioner encounter; (6) rehabilitation or death and bereavement.

While this formulation of a help-seeking career is generally applicable, there are variations in individual cases. For example, the outcomes (rehabilitation or death and bereavement) may be replaced by effective management of a chronic condition. Further variations might involve how some people select among professional nonmedical (e.g., chiropractic) systems of health care (Semmes, 1983) in addition to the mainstream system. Others may select among folk practitioners (e.g., spiritual advisors, lay midwives, or herbalists) to address their health problems and seek mainstream professional health services only when they deem it appropriate to do so.

Different cultural groups may vary in the intensity to which they use informal support networks at various points in their help-seeking career. For example, one study of help-seeking (Lin et al, 1982) found that black and Asian-American clients used more informal networks in their pathways to help-seeking than did Caucasian clients. An earlier study of ethnic variations (Zola, 1966) documented the role of ethnicity in the response to symptoms and in reporting of illness. In his comparative study of Italians and Irish presenting complaints, Zola found that the Irish, more than Italians, tended to locate their primary problems in the eye, ear, nose, or throat, and more often denied pain as a feature of their illness. Italians complained of more symptoms, more bodily areas affected, and more kinds of dysfunctions than did the Irish. Whereas Zola's and subsequent studies provide general impressions of the differences in response to pain and other symptoms among ethnic groups, one should not expect that all members of the ethnic groups will display the behaviors mentioned.

In a study of physically ill patients of Jewish, Italian, Irish, and white Anglo-Saxon protestant (WASP) background, Zborowski (1966) found significant differences in each group's reaction to pain. Whereas Jewish and Italian clients complained greatly about their pain, Irish and WASP patients did not. WASP and Jewish patients were specific in describing their pain, while Irish and Italian patients were nonspecific. Italians worried about their pain to the extent that it affected life situations such as work, family, and finances, and easily forgot their symptoms when they were no longer suffering. On the other hand, Jewish patients were not so concerned about the symptoms as they were about the "real" source of the pain. Consequently, they wanted complete explanations of the meaning of the pain, and they did not want to take pills to relieve symptoms. Irish patients tended to be fatalistic. They complained little, failed to mention pain, and did not expect relief. The Irish saw pain as a result of their own sinfulness and held themselves responsible for it (Zborowski, 1952, 1966). From these examples we can see that the description of a help-seeking career is useful for identifying critical points where cultural variation comes into play. Such variation contributes to the understanding of how symptoms may be interpreted by different populations.

Help-seeking is closely related to one's concept of health and sickness. That is, in order for people to declare themselves sick and begin to seek help, there must be some preexisting notion about what it means to be healthy, so that deviation from that normal state can be assessed (Zola, 1966). These deviations, changes, or symptoms then must be determined to be significant. For example, the "sick" person determines whether the symptoms are transient or indicate a more serious disorder. Cultural variation is thus an obvious component of what has been called the "sickness career" because it necessarily involves interpretive processes within the context of preexisting beliefs, values, and norms and includes interaction with significant others. Twaddle (1981, p. 116) put it succinctly, "a sickness career takes place for any individual in specific *settings* in interaction with *other people*, who in accordance with their assessment of the problem and taking into account their own needs and the *opportunities* for alternative courses of action which are available, apply the *social norms* of their particular groups and set expectations for behavior."

Help-seeking and management of symptoms are also influenced by the dynamics of communication within subcultures. Networks of significant others become important factors. People generally tend to contain deviations from normal states within everyday social situations involving networks of family and friends and only seek care when such deviations can no longer be ignored. Moreover, people have symptoms of various types for which they do seek professional help. Some of this variation can be accounted for by the input of family and/or friends. Individuals frequently consult others, primarily those who constitute their social networks, in managing illness and seeking legitimation for their claims to illness (Alonzo, 1979; Telles & Harris, 1981; Zola, 1973).

Social networks generally function as ways through which people maintain social identities, gain social support, material aid, services, and information; and acquire new social contacts. Social networks influence how people formulate responses to illness, choose self-medication, select specific health practitioners, and develop expectations regarding encounters with formal health providers. They also affect expectations about these encounters—whether people experience feelings of satisfaction, for example, and whether or not they comply with treatment regimens.

Ethnic Families

The family is the primary organization in society that preserves and transmits culture. Family values account for much of the variation in the life-styles, health beliefs, and practices of different ethnic groups. The family is also a critical support system because whenever there is ill health, it maintains an important role in determining the type of treatment sought. Thus, the ethnic values of a family and its ability to function effectively are of great significance for determining the health status of individuals, the family itself, and whole communities. The following descriptions of several ethnic families illustrate the importance of their differences in structure and value orientation for community health nursing.

The various ethnic families in America have been affected by differing historical and social circumstances. For example, from the country's earliest days religion has been a strong distinguishing feature. Anglo-Saxon protestants represent the first and most culturally dominant European group. Catholics and Jews were later European immigrants and so had to adjust to Anglo-Saxon protestant cultural, political, and social dominance. They were at one time objects of discrimination by the former group. Later Asian immigrants such as the Chinese, also suffered discrimination from various European groups, in part because of racial and cultural differences. Among American ethnic family groups are nonwhite, non-European, and oppressed minorities such as Afro-Americans, Native Amer-

icans, and Hispanics. The ancestors of most Afro-Americans were brought to America as slaves, and subsequent generations of Afro-Americans continue to suffer social injustices including racism that has become institutionalized in American society. A disproportionate number of Afro-Americans suffer from poverty and related social problems. Native Americans also have a history of oppression even though they were indigenous to America. Their land was taken away, and they were relegated to an inferior political, economic, and cultural position in American society. Hispanics vary in their experiences, but most have emerged from a legacy of European oppression. The common experience of these groups is that they have continued to be victims of systematic discrimination in American society. Despite individual gains and achievements of some members of the groups, on the whole, members of these ethnic groups are not truly assimilated to the point where they interact with members of the dominant white culture on the primary group level (Greeley, 1974). Significantly, African Americans, Hispanics, and Native Americans continue to be at greatest risk with respect to health problems.

Recent immigrants including Asians, especially Southeast Asians, Hispanics such as Mexicans and Salvadorans, and some Middle Eastern groups, primarily those of non-Christian religions such as Islam, are rapidly increasing their population in certain areas of the United States. For example, a recent article (Maurine, 1983) reported a growing influx of such groups in Southern California, particularly the Los Angeles area.

Unlike earlier European immigrants who attempted to assimilate quickly into the larger American culture, these new immigrants tend more to preserve their customs, language, and sense of ethnic identity, and it is reasonable to assume that they will pose unique challenges to community health nurses as their numbers increase.

Ethnic families in American society are, therefore, products of a host of historic, social, economic, and political factors. Religion, minority status, immigrant status (recent or early), and race are some of the important factors affecting family values and family functioning.

In the descriptive overviews of ethnic families that follow in the next section, the role of these factors is explained. For example, Irish American families are presented here as an example of an early immigrant white ethnic group, strongly influenced by a dominant religion, Catholicism. Mexican Americans or Chicanos and Black American families are presented as examples of differing immigrant groups whose primary position in American society is their relative poverty and the level of racial discrimination, oppression, and inequality they suffer compared to other ethnic groups. Native American families are presented as an example of a nonimmigrant group existing in America before other ethnic groups, but who are in similar positions as Blacks and Hispanics. South Vietnamese families are presented as an example of a recent Southeast Asian immigrant group.

The discussion will provide a general overview of traditional family values and health beliefs and practices that may be reflected in the life-styles of different ethnic families. (The information should serve only as a guide or hypothesis to be tested on a case-by-case basis because clients are unique and vary considerably in terms of their behaviors both within and across ethnic groups.) An individual client's ethnic identity may tell nothing about the client's personal experience of family values and health practices. The overview can, nevertheless,

serve as a beginning point to help community health nurses understand what impact adherence or non-adherence to such values and beliefs have on families.

For example, strong kinship bonds, considered to be a traditional strength of black families, carry additional responsibilities to provide for members of the extended family when resources are low. These obligations may be a source of added stress on a family system already strained by economic hardships. Similarly, a newly immigrant South Vietnamese family may experience stress as a result of intergenerational conflict between younger and older generations. Younger family members are likely to adjust more rapidly to American ways, acculturate faster, and therefore, clash in values as they begin to interpret family role obligations differently from their older relatives. Such conflicts have the potential to erode the family system.

Irish American Families

Irish immigrants came to the United States during the mid-nineteenth century. About four million Irish immigrants came between 1820 and 1900 (Biddle, 1981). The history of the Irish people is complicated in part because of colonization by the British, long-standing British rule, religious dividedness, and a political situation characterized by "a turbulent history of battle, rebellion, intrigue, settlement, suffering, terrorism and pauperism" (Biddle, 1981, p. 92).

Their immigration to the United States was propelled by these factors as well as by the Great Potato Famine of Ireland, which occurred between 1845 and 1848. Irish immigrants came primarily to American cities: Boston, New York, New Jersey, Philadelphia, Chicago, St. Louis, and San Francisco. They established the Catholic church as the center of family and community life.

Traditional rural families of Ireland were organized in a "stem" family, which is the practice by parents of passing on their farms intact to a favorite son (or sometimes a daughter). This favorite son

Box 5-2   Traditional Family Values and Health Beliefs and Practices of Irish American Families*

Traditional Family Values

General
- Concern for economic welfare of total family
- Stem family characteristics (favorite son, or if there are no sons, daughter, inherits family land, which causes potential sibling rivalry and family conflicts)

Kinship Patterns
- Kin recognized as people associated by blood or marriage; sibling loyalty emphasized
- Male as well as female roots recognized
- Family obligated to care for one another and maintain strong emotional ties; family loyalty emphasized over individual concerns

Child-rearing
- Children are:
  Accepted as inevitable outcome of marriage
  Expected to be respectful and obedient
  Handled with firmness
  Expected to be subordinate, obedient, and respectful
  Tendency to prefer boys over girls

Traditional Health Beliefs and Practices

- Health beliefs closely related to life experiences
- Belief in sin and guilt, long suffering

- Possible use of denial as a defense mechanism to deny illness
- Denial of illness may result in:
  Reluctance to admit symptoms
  Limiting symptoms to specific locations: usually eyes, ears, and throat

Religious
- Catholic church as dominant force
- Church reinforces traditions and is important force in maintaining community stability through structures as the Parish and the Catholic schools, etc.

Sex-Role Behavior
- Husband or father considered head of household, required to be good provider, may be emotionally detached but still dominant decision-maker
- Mother in charge of the household; expected to stay home and raise children
- Unmarried daughter may leave the home to work

SOURCE:
Biddle E: The American Catholic Irish family. In: Mandel C, Haberstein R (editors), *Ethnic Families in America: Patterns and Variations.* New York: Elsevier, 1981.

*A general overview may not be applicable to all group members encountered.

was usually, but not always, the oldest. Parents remained on the farm as dependents of the chosen son or daughter, and though other sons or daughters also remained on the family farm, they were not considered full-fledged adults. This practice often caused bitter disputes among family members (Biddle, 1981; Greely, 1974), and many "unchosen" sons migrated to the United States to escape this situation. The tradition of identifying a child as "favorite" may still influence family relationships. Today, compared to other ethnic groups who are considered minorities, Irish American families are well integrated into mainstream American life. However, the Irish are fiercely proud of their

heritage and maintain a strong sense of ethnic identity. The Catholic church is a central force in preserving their ethnic traditions, values, and family structure (Biddle, 1981). Box 5-2 provides a summary of selected traditional family values, and health beliefs and practices of Irish Americans.

Mexican American Families

Mexican American families in the United States represent a blending of various cultures, primarily Spanish and Indian. Indian ancestors include the Aztecs and Mayans who built great civilizations in

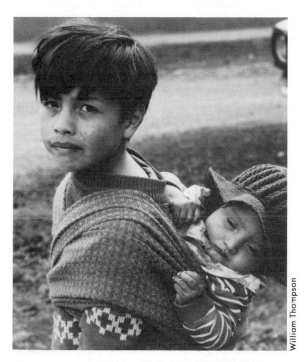

At an early age, Mexican American children often take on responsibility for younger siblings. This practice stems from the high value placed on strong family cohesion in Mexican American culture.

Mexico prior to the arrival of the Spanish Conquistadors in the 1500s. Mexico originally included territory now part of the southwestern United States. However, with the discovery of gold in California in 1848 Easterners of white Anglo background poured into the Southwest, and conflicts erupted between the two groups as a result of economic competition and racial and cultural differences. Gradually, the Mexicans lost their land and most of their rights to the English-speaking Anglo-Americans from the East. Many remained in the Southwest under the political and economic dominance of the Anglo-Americans (de Valdez & Gallegos, 1982).

Substantial Mexican migration to the United States began in the early 1900s and has occurred in several waves since then. High unemployment in Mexico coupled with high birth rates leads many Mexicans to migrate to the United States in search of greater economic opportunities. They have constituted a significant proportion of the manual labor force in farm work, on railroads, and in similar industries (de Valdez & Gallegos, 1982). Each wave of Mexican immigrants has become acculturated to the dominant white American culture in varying degrees, but many have maintained their traditional beliefs and customs.

Today Mexican Americans, or Chicanos, are considered the fastest growing ethnic minority group in the United States. Regional, socioeconomic, generational, educational, and other situational factors account for variations within the group. However, like Puerto Ricans, the next largest Spanish-speaking ethnic group in the United States, many Mexican American families reside in high density, poverty areas; they experience communication problems because of language difficulties and suffer from racial injustices. Unlike Puerto Ricans who are born United States citizens, most Mexican Americans have alien status until they achieve United States citizenship. Some are undocumented (illegal aliens) and as such lack health insurance to pay for health services and are unable to receive public services because of inability to establish residence and citizenship. Yet, like other ethnic minority groups, Mexican Americans on the whole are at disproportionately higher risk to health problems compared to whites. They devise various strategies for meeting their health care needs, which include their traditional folk methods of caring. As in the case of Irish Americans, Mexican American culture and traditions are strongly intertwined with the Catholic church. Box 5-3 presents a summary of selected traditional family values and health beliefs and practices of Mexican Americans.

Black American Families

Black Americans are of African ancestry and derive various aspects of their culture from the African context.

They were brought to the United States and other regions of the Western hemisphere primarily

Box 5-3   Traditional Family Values and Health Beliefs and Practices of Mexican American Families*

Traditional Family Values

General

- Family serves as natural supportive network—buffers its members from outside stresses
- Personal courtesy and respect for one another emphasized
- More oriented to cooperation than competition
- Family cohesion extends beyond nuclear and extended family to communal awareness
- *Machismo*—patriarchal family system associated with honor, dignity, and respect

Kinship Patterns

- Familism; tendency to extend kinship ties beyond nuclear family
- Generational interdependence and loyalty to the family of origin
- Strong emotional ties and kinship bonds in families

Child-rearing

- Divided among parents—father disciplines and controls; mother provides nurturance and support
- Godparents and extended family members such as grandparents, uncles, and aunts perform many parental functions of nurturance, guidance, and support for children; parent-child relationship warm and nurturing, but children are expected to respect both parents and manifest good behavior

Sex-Role Allocation and Division of Labor

- Family structure hierarchical: with ascribed status and roles arranged around age and sex—male dominance—eldest male is central authority figure; older dominates younger in both sexes, although more equalitarian sex-role patterns are emerging
- Children expected to participate in age-appropriate family duties

Religious Influences

- Catholic religion dominant: its doctrines and the church play an important role in daily life; not as unifying a force and support structure as in the case of the Irish, except in areas where Chicanos are the majority and the parish priest is also Chicano
- Religious rituals may be practiced when there is illness in the family; rituals include:
  Promise making
  Visiting shrines
  Offering candles
  Offering prayers

---

as slaves by Europeans who used them as cheap sources of labor. Some blacks existed outside of slavery as "freed" descendants of indentured servants, and/or as mulatto offspring of white slaveowners, and some escaped or bought their way out of slavery. Forced migration from Africa created involuntary separation from families; such separations continued during slavery and served to seriously disrupt black American family patterns.

After Emancipation, blacks were systematically discriminated against and racially excluded from almost every aspect of life in the dominant society including work, housing, education, and main-

stream health service. Many such injustices and inequalities persist and influence the health status of black Americans (Leigh & Green, 1982; Lewis, 1975; Staples, 1981). Box 5-4 presents selected traditional family values and health beliefs and practices of black American families.

Native American Families

Native Americans are a diverse group consisting of approximately 280 different tribes, speaking

Traditional Health Beliefs and Practices

- Disease and illness viewed as having spiritual and social as well as biological ramifications
- Suffering (i.e., disease) often regarded as punishment *(castigo)* for having sinned
- Folk medicine includes various herbs and plants used as cathartics, diuretics, and for other medicinal purposes
- Several folk ideas and practices singled out as important:

  Mal ojo, "bad eye"—believed to result from influences outside the family such as excessive admiration and desire on the part of another because of envy of the victims who are usually babies and young children. Symptoms include tiredness and headaches

  Caida de la Mollena—occurs in infancy and is associated with neglect of the child; caused by the child having a fall; or being purposely "dropped" by someone; usually has emotional or psychological implication because it implies parental neglect; also regarded as originating from dislocated organs

  Mal de Susto, "fright"—associated with a traumatic situation at some point in early childhood or adulthood; could be precipitated by loss of a favored one through death;

symptoms include indigestion, anorexia, anxiety, insomnia, and palpitations

  Mal Puesto—disease brought about by the requests or "bad deed" of another person (i.e., *brujos,* or "sorcerers" and *brujas* or "witches") who have the power to cause illness to befall another person; such evil forces can also come from the devil

  Empacho—believed to be caused by the wall of the stomach curling in the form of a ball; symptoms include stomach cramps

- Treatment of disease and illness may take following forms:

  Extra human prayer to God and the Saints, pilgrimages to holy places, and use of holy water

  Use of lay practitioners (e.g., family, friends and specialists such as *medicos* and *curanderos*)

  Use of scientific medicine often in combination with traditional practices

SOURCES:

Kay M: Health and illness in a Mexican American barrio. In: Spicer E (editor), *Ethnic Medicine in the Southwest.* Tucson: University of Arizona Press, 1979.

Martinez R: *Hispanic Culture and Health Care: Fact, Fiction and Folklore.* St. Louis: Mosby, 1978.

*General overview may not be applicable to all group members encountered.

approximately 252 different languages. Many live in cities and have integrated values and traditions of the dominant American culture, while others live in rural areas or on reservations, know little English, and maintain their traditional cultural values and behaviors (Miller, 1982).

Unlike other ethnic groups who migrated to the United States, Native Americans were indigenous to North America, and so were here when the Europeans arrived. Today identity as a Native American is determined by self-declaration, based on these criteria: enrollment as a member of a recognized tribe, residence on an Indian reservation, or ability to declare at least a quarter Indian blood. Most Native Americans live in Oklahoma, Arizona, and Alaska on reservations or in rural areas, although some live in cities as well. High unemployment rates, persistent negative stereotypes, and lack of adequate numbers of Native American health professionals (including nurses) are stubborn problems within this ethnic group, which continues to be one of the population groups at high risk to health problems. For example, otitis media among children under two years old with resulting hearing impairment is one of the group's most serious health problems, along with alcoholism and high suicide

Box 5-4   Traditional Family Values and Health Beliefs and Practices of Black American Families*

Traditional Family Values

General

- African world view at base of black culture (i.e., all things are interrelated, interconnected, and reinforced by a deep sense of family)
- Strong work and achievement orientation in terms of occupation and education

Kinship Patterns

- Extended family central (whether as an African tradition or as a response to oppressive conditions in the United States)
- Strong kinship bonds and kinship obligations often extend to several individual households with lines of authority and support transcending any one household unit

Child-rearing

- Family is child-oriented, individual uniqueness, independence, and assertiveness are stressed
- Boys and girls generally treated equally; preference for children usually not displayed based on gender
- Multiple parenting may exist; grown children expected to contribute to parents in times of need

Sex-role Allocation and Division of Labor

- Shared decision-making and household tasks
- Flexible and interchangeable family role definitions and performance
- Degree of authority linked to economic provider not necessarily to gender

Religious Orientation

- Church has strong influence; strong commitment to religious values and church participation

Traditional Health Beliefs and Practices

- Health viewed holistically (e.g., feeling good; having good luck, wealth, and success)
- Interwoven remnants of African folk medicine and selected beliefs from modern scientific health system
- Illness viewed as a result of *natural* forces (e.g., impurities from air, food, and water enter the body and cause illness) and *unnatural* forces (e.g., witchcraft, voodoo, a "fix," rootwork, etc.)
- Symptoms often associated with eating, loss of appetite, and stomach pain
- Self-treatment often instituted (i.e., roots, herbs, potions, oils, powders, tokens, rituals, and ceremonies)

SOURCES:

Snow L: Folk medical beliefs and their implications for the care of patients. A Review based on studies among black Americans. In: Henderson G, Primeaux M (editors), *Transcultural Health Care.* Menlo Park, Calif.: Addison-Wesley, 1981.

Staples R: The black American family. In: Mendel CH, Haberstein R (editors), *Ethnic Families in America: Patterns and Variations.* New York: Elsevier, 1981.

*General overview may not be applicable to all group members encountered.

rates. The high rate of alcoholism among American Indians has been used to negatively characterize and stereotype the group. This attitude has somewhat undermined the seriousness with which alcoholism is viewed as a health problem for young as well as older adults.

Native Americans generally place a high value on maintaining their ethnic and cultural identity.

This emphasis and their social isolation on Indian reservations have curtailed their level of acculturation and assimilation in the dominant white culture. However, factors such as intertribal relations, adoption of Christianity, formal education, and experiences with the dominant culture outside of Indian reservations are bringing about some cultural changes within the group. Such changes are

Box 5-5   Traditional Family Values and Health Beliefs and Practices of Native American Families*

Traditional Family Values

General
- Harmony with nature
- Present or short-term orientation
- Consciousness of time not based on clocks but on completion of tasks
- Cooperation and group responsibility stressed as opposed to individualism and competition
- Shyness and sensitivity with strangers

Kinship Patterns
- Strong family orientation; respect for aged members
- Extended family focus; three generations with relatives on both sides may live in one household
- Distant blood relatives such as cousins and nonblood relatives such as tribal members may be incorporated into the family structure at any given time
- Family obligations and interests are primary

Child-rearing
- High fertility rate
- Respect for child's individuality, as well as duty and responsibility for sharing are emphasized
- Discipline (especially force) not used to enforce control because of belief in noninterference and taboos against controlling other people's behavior
- Grandparents, aunts, and uncles assume parental functions

Sex-Role Allocation
- Strong role for women
- Female households may share family functions

Religion
- Religious beliefs totally interwoven with life-style and health practices; may vary across tribal groups

Traditional Health Beliefs and Practices

- Health and illness viewed in a holistic way, as functions of the entire person
- Medicine men and herbalists of different types are used
- Preventional measures include warding off the effects of witchcraft; health maintenance and curing through various healing ceremonies; performing acts such as witchcraft and poisoning and use of spells against another person have the potential to cause harm
- Treatment a combination of rational and religious practices
- Going to a hospital or clinic may be associated with illness and disease; therefore, family members may not seek health care for what they consider normal processes (e.g., pregnancy)
- Food restrictions and preferences influence health practices
- Foul-tasting medicines, emetics, and purges may be used because of the belief that they can rid the body's system of demons present in the body and causing disease

SOURCES:
Primeaux M, Henderson G: American Indian patient care. In: Henderson G, Primeaux M (editors), *Transcultural Health Care.* Menlo Park, Calif.: Addison-Wesley, 1981.

Vogel V: American Indian medicine. In: Henderson G, Primeaux M (editors), *Transcultural Health Care.* Menlo Park, Calif.: Addison-Wesley, 1981.

*General overview may not be applicable to all group members.

likely to be reflected in the level at which families maintain cultural traditions (Wilson, 1983). Box 5-5 provides a summary of selected traditional family values and health beliefs and practices of Native Americans.

South Vietnamese Families

Compared to other Asian American ethnic groups such as the Chinese and Japanese, South Vietnamese families are new immigrants to the United States. Their immigration was impelled by political and economic forces in their own country. Many came following the fall of the Saigon government to the North Vietnamese. Early immigrants were mostly young, well-educated Catholics who initially came as refugees to various camps or temporary shelters. They came in almost equal numbers of males and females, many as parts of extended families.

A second group of South Vietnamese families came to the United States after 1975. Compared to earlier Southeast Asian immigrants, they were less well educated, less urban, and less well acquainted with Western ways. As some were illiterate, they were generally poorly equipped to live in a technologically advanced society. They came with few belongings, and most had no compatriots to greet them—unlike some earlier immigrant groups, particularly Europeans.

As new immigrants from a very different culture, South Vietnamese families have experienced acculturation and adjustment problems. Many have language and communication difficulties, and some required sponsors to supply them with food, clothing, and shelter until they became self-supporting. As a result of exposure to many years of war, some may distrust strangers including health professionals. Some may experience cultural shock as they learn to live in the United States and adjust to American customs and values (Orque, 1983). Box 5-6 describes South Vietnamese traditional family values and health beliefs.

Implications and Strategies for Community Health Nurses

Familiarization with the cultural traditions and health beliefs of different ethnic families can help community health nurses work more effectively with them. Effectiveness with families is enhanced by (1) avoidance of *ethnocentrism*, the belief that one's own culture is right and better than other cultures, and (2) avoidance of *stereotyping*, which is inaccurate assessment of others based on preconceived notions rather than on nonprejudicial facts. Applying the preceding descriptions to all members of an ethnic group would be an example of stereotyping that individual. Each individual or family should be viewed as unique with special sets of values and traditions based on their personal experiences in their cultures of origin as well as in the American culture. Whereas these descriptions can serve as a guide, their applicability to specific families or individuals should be evaluated on a case-by-case basis.

The information presented on selected ethnic groups should serve as a starting point for further study, and is intended to increase the awareness of community health nurses to culture, ethnicity, and ethnic families. The culturally aware nurse will be able to make more effective use of the nursing process with ethnic and culturally diverse clients. The nurse's ultimate goal is to assist clients to reach and/or maintain optimal states of health. Achievement of this state requires focus on the client as a whole person. Attention to the ethnic and cultural aspects of the client's life is, therefore, crucial. This does not mean that community health nurses devise specific techniques, skills, or formulas for dealing with specific ethnic groups (given the uniqueness

Box 5-6 Traditional Family Values and Health Beliefs and Practices of South Vietnamese Families*

Traditional Family Values

General
- World views originate from indigenous religion and from Taoism, Confucianism and Buddhism, which have also influenced Chinese philosophical and religious beliefs
- Duty to others rather than individual rights are important
- Belief in ever-present deities and spirits that control the entire universe
- Belief that spirits of dead relatives continue to dwell in the home to protect living relatives

Kinship Patterns
- Kinship system patrilineal; males are dominant; mother has some voice and usually manages family funds
- Generational continuity emphasized
- Extended family central
- Family name usually given before middle and first names

Child-rearing
- Children socialized to value family; family interests and harmony prevail over individual needs
- Children taught to maintain family name and participate in ancestor worship; expected to be industrious and obedient toward parents, ancestors, and authorities

Sex-Role Allocation and Division and Labor
- Father major decision-maker, although both parents considered leaders of the family

- Traditional roles changing due to migration and acculturation

Religious Orientation
- Religion has strong influence on family life (e.g., Buddhist and Confucian principles encourage passivity, stoicism and personal reserve)

Traditional Health Beliefs and Practices

- Disease thought to be caused by natural physical forces, or by disruptions of harmony
- Cosmic forces believed to influence individual behavior; consequently, physiognomy, astrology, fortune-telling, and divine instruction used to determine cosmic forces
- Health viewed as being in harmony with existing universal order; harmony obtained by pleasing good spirits and by avoiding evil ones
- Principles of yin and yang, "hot and cold," part of the concept of harmony; health results from balance between yin and yang, and the interaction between the elements composing the body: wood, water, fire, and earth
- Treatment of symptoms includes home remedies, cultural herbs, and special diets

SOURCES:
Muecke M: Caring for Southeast Asian refugee patients in the U.S.A. *Am J Public Health* (April) 1983; 73 (4): 431–438.

Orque M: Nursing care of South Vietnamese patients. In: Orque M, Black B, Monroy L (editors), *Ethnic Nursing Care: A Multicultural Approach.* St. Louis: Mosby, 1983.

*General overview may not be applicable to all group members.

---

of each individual and the variations that exist within ethnic groups). Instead, community health nurses should adopt an orientation to health care that includes sensitivity to the cultural needs of all clients.

Community health nurses can utilize knowledge of ethnic and cultural variations to develop and implement strategies that reflect such knowledge.

The following are examples of strategies useful to community health nurses.

Self-awareness

Nurses are trained to be objective, and some nurses may interpret objectivity to mean keeping one's

Case Example 5-2: Cultural Bias

Mrs. Baker, a nurse of upper middle-class Anglo-Saxon protestant heritage, recently gained employment with the Visiting Nurses' Association (VNA) in a multiethnic neighborhood. On her caseload was Mrs. Ragusco, a 65-year-old widow who has been having chronic back pain, which has interfered with her ability to do household chores. Mrs. Baker's assignment was to evaluate Mrs. Ragusco's back pain and to see if she was continuing to take the medications and do the exercises prescribed for her by her doctor. After a few visits to Mrs. Ragusco, Mrs. Baker discovered that the woman was living with her son and daughter-in-law, taking care of their two children, and doing most of the household chores while the parents worked. Mrs. Baker concluded that Mrs. Ragusco's problem was that she was overburdened with child care and household activities that she could no longer manage and that the best solution for her was to move out of her son and daughter-in-law's household into a small senior citizen's apartment, where she would have freedom, independence, and more leisure. She could visit her children and grandchildren, but would be free from heavy domestic responsibilities.

Nurse works in multiethnic community; encounters client of different ethnic background.

Client is part of an extended family system.

Nurse makes an assessment without considering family's cultural dimensions.

Nurse's decisions are influenced by own cultural values.

Mrs. Baker discussed these plans with Mrs. Ragusco who seemed to agree, but once the plans were set in motion, Mrs. Ragusco became very distraught. Mrs. Baker was unable to get a good understanding of why Mrs. Ragusco was so upset, so she brought the case up for discussion at one of her team conferences involving her supervisor and the psychiatric nurse consultant.

Recommendations from the team conference were for Mrs. Baker to explore Mrs. Ragusco's family situation further, including learning about

Nurse uses team conference to evaluate her decision and explore feelings.

true feelings from showing, particularly to the client, and preventing personal matters from influencing patient care. Carrying this notion to the extreme, some nurses ignore or pay little attention to the influences of their own ethnic background and/or cultural values. By trying to be objective they sometimes show little awareness of the extent to which these factors affect their lives and color their perceptions of the world. This can be a grave error since ethnic orientations and cultural values can influence attitudes, behaviors, and motives. Case Example 5-2 illustrates these points.

By systematically examining their motives for working with clients of different cultural backgrounds and by examining possible linkages between their values and these motives, community health nurses can further increase their self-awareness. Leininger (1972) has provided descriptions of various types of health practitioners who work with culturally different groups. Based on a study of attitudes or orientations such practitioners have toward the groups with whom they work, she described practitioner types as follows: (1) those who are *genuinely interested* in the cultural group, (2) those who cultural values and traditions, and to explore her own feelings about wanting Mrs. Ragusco to move out in order to gain more freedom and independence. Mrs. Baker discovered that Mrs. Ragusco was from a very close-knit Italian family. She and her late husband were born in Italy. She was very close to her son and daughter-in-law. They all had a very strong sense of family solidarity and believed in the Italian family tradition of the women being the center of home and providing nurturance for the children. However, there had been some underlying conflicts in the home between Mrs. Ragusco and her daughter-in-law. Although her daughter-in-law loved, respected, and valued Mrs. Ragusco, she felt threatened by the central position Mrs. Ragusco had in the family. At the same time, she also felt guilty that she was not living up to her traditions—that is, providing the nurturance and home-making functions as a "good" Italian wife-mother should. Examining her own motives for wanting Mrs. Ragusco to move out, Mrs. Baker discovered that her hasty decision was based on biases she had internalized from her own background and family values. Within her tradition, high value is placed on the nuclear family as an autonomous unit having responsibility for itself, and on personal freedom and individuality. Once Mrs. Baker had a better understanding of the family's cultural background, and her own values and motives, she worked more effectively with Mrs. Ragusco and her family. She talked with mother and daughter-in-law together and helped them to clarify their roles and to divide household responsibilities so that they each felt fulfilled and at the same time not overburdened. Mrs. Ragusco's daughter-in-law was able to help her with her back exercises, which gradually subsided as the stress from the underlying conflict decreased.

Nurse explores family's cultural traditions.

Nurse gains insight into how her own cultural background biased her perception of the family and her behavior.

Nurse action results in positive outcome.

are isolated and *non-involved* with the cultural group, (3) those who are *curious* about the cultural group, (4) those who view the cultural group as *hopeless*, (5) those who are *exploitive* of the cultural group, (6) those who find *refuge* in the cultural group, and, (7) those who are *overprotective* of the cultural group. Although this typology cannot describe or predict all possible types of practitioner attitudes or orientations toward culturally different clients, the typology is useful as a guide to exploring one's inner feelings and promoting greater awareness and sensitivity toward clients. Each type, their char-

acteristics, and possible outcomes as a result of the practitioner-client encounter are described in Table 5-1.

Acceptance

Facing cultural differences can sometimes be threatening. Whereas people are similar in some ways, they are also different, with unique health beliefs and cultural practices and different ways of dealing with life experiences. The tendency in
(text continued on p. 122)

Table 5-1 Typology of Nurse Practitioners

Practitioner Types	Characteristics	Possible Outcomes
Type I (Ideal Type) Genuinely Interested (in client group)	*Attitude* Manifests positive, healthy attitude toward culturally different groups and is genuinely interested in their health beliefs and practices and what they think will help them most	Professional growth; expression of insights, confidence, and skills; development of trust and comfortableness between client and health practitioners
	Helping Pattern Takes learner-facilitator role; open to learn about different cultures' beliefs, values, and ways of living; constructively responds to help people and devise healthy programs within the context of their own resources and social structure and in light of their own values, beliefs, and health practices, while comfortably using own strengths and skills	Positive acceptance of practitioner by culturally different group
	Personal Attributes Able to become involved with and adjust to life-styles of culturally different people; flexible, intellectually astute, patient, tolerant, and willing to learn from others	
Type II Isolated and Non-Involved (with client group)	*Attitude* Feels superior to clients; feels that they should be glad to receive anything from a professional person and be appreciative that something is being done for them, whatever it is, and however it is given, because anything is better than what they have—nothing!	Practitioner isolated and insulated from cultural group; mutual withdrawal
	Helping Pattern Task-oriented; sails through expected physical work "tasks" in routine "professional" manner without bothering with client psychosocial and cultural concerns; follows own cultural norms, values, and practices and seldom evaluates how his or her services are meeting people's needs and how people are accepting him or her	
	Personal Attributes Withdrawn and nonresponsive; does not permit self to become involved in lives, values, and beliefs of the culturally different; remains emotionally detached and socially isolated from people	

Table 5-1 *(continued)*

Practitioner Types	Characteristics	Possible Outcomes
Type III Curious (about cultural group)	*Attitude* Highly curious about seeing and working with people who are markedly different from own culture; curiosity dissipates when strangeness disappears and practitioner sees humaneness and similarities between self and seemingly strange, exotic, and different cultural group *Helping Pattern* Appeals to the perceived exotic and primitive nature of cultural group *Personal Attributes* Desires distinctly different behavior and cannot tolerate the possibility of being more alike than different from a group he or she perceived to be exotically different from own group; fears similarities between self and others	Practitioner seldom stays long with cultural group
Type IV Hopeless (views cultural group as hopeless)	*Attitude* Consciously or unconsciously views culturally different group as hopeless and as inferior to own group, and believes it is impossible to change their health practices *Helping Pattern* Apathetic to clients because of feelings that it is impossible to change their health practice; uncomfortable working with people who are culturally different but feels he or she must perform expected duty or assignment; conveys hopeless image of them in nonverbal communication *Personal Attributes* Feels superior to people who are culturally different; uncomfortable around them	Work is unpraiseworthy; practitioner fails to help people with their health problems or concerns Clients' feelings of not wanting outsiders to come to them are reinforced; mutual relief when practitioner leaves
Type V Exploitative (of cultural group)	*Attitude* Concerned with own self-interests and needs *Helping Pattern* Motivated to help culturally different groups because of self-needs and for self-gains—to achieve purposes such as special experiences, financial gains, research opportunities, or other similar reasons	Culturally different groups (i.e., minorities usually feel and basically *are* exploited) Cultural group become uneasy; suspicious and usually ask practitioner to leave. Practitioner may become threatened by group and leave on own accord

(continued)

Table 5-1 *(continued)*

Practitioner Types	Characteristics	Possible Outcomes
	Personal Attributes Selfish and exploitive	
Type VI Escapist (finds refuge in cultural group)	*Attitude* Views cultural group as a way to escape from personal failures in own cultural group or environment	Practitioner experiences cultural shock
	Helping Pattern Personal problems and concerns limit his or her ability to consider needs and problems of the new setting in which he or she finds self	His or her survival is questionable and doubtful
	Personal Attributes Has personal problems that he or she attempts to work out through escape in new setting; therefore, motives are questionable and not always overt until work is begun in the new setting	
Type VII Overprotective (of client group)	*Attitude* Extremely empathetic to the cultural group; wants to be a strong protector of their rights, ideas, and norms from outside changes and external influences	Cultural group may be denied opportunities to try new modes of living or cultural values
	Helping Pattern Overprotective; as a result, may block cultural group from new opportunities they desire	
	Personal Attributes Extremely empathetic and overly protective	

SOURCE:
Adapted from Leininger M: Becoming aware of types of health practitioners and cultural imposition. In: *Becoming Aware of Cultural Differences in Nursing.* Speeches presented during the 48th Convention, ANA, 1972.

American society to view everyone as the same and to think that underneath the skin we are all alike can obscure important differences that set people apart from one another. Whereas the notion that we are more alike than different is often appealing, the tendency to emphasize sameness causes us to minimize, or even ignore, differences. This is partly due to belief in the melting pot theory that American society is a homogeneous group of people from various cultures who have blended together to form one new fairly homogeneous culture. Consistent with this view, early immigrants of varying ethnic groups were expected to become Americanized— that is, to learn American values and habits and to adopt and practice them. Some nurses may still hold such views, and thus instead of adjusting professional expectations to meet clients' needs, they expect clients to adapt to institutional rules and to the beliefs and values of the profession.

Nurses who have the ability to deal with differences show respect for clients' uniqueness, avoid labelling clients who are different as deviant or

Case Example 5-3: Overcoming Stereotypes

A group of nursing students in a BSN nursing program were assigned to a Hispanic community for their clinical rotation in community health nursing. When discussing their clients at a post-conference session, one of the students reported very casually that her client, the Rosario family of Mexican descent, had recently lost a child, who died shortly after birth. It was the sixth child for Mrs. Rosario, who was thirty-four years old. The instructor asked the student to tell the group how the family was dealing with the loss and the student said, "I really didn't go into it. I didn't think it was a big thing with them . . . I read somewhere that Hispanics had many children . . . that it was a burden to take care of so many children. I thought that losing one was like a relief. . . . Like they wouldn't miss it so much since they have so many."

Student nurses are assigned to Hispanic community for clinical rotation in community health nursing.

Student nurse's judgment is influenced by stereotype of family.

The instructor was appalled at the student's comments but realized that, as a whole, the group of students were all white, from middle-class backgrounds, and had little or no contact with Hispanics and other culturally different ethnic groups. Therefore, in a supportive way, the instructor encouraged the student to discuss the sources and accuracy of her feelings.

Instructor assists nursing student to examine stereotype of Hispanic client.

The student came to realize that her feelings about the Rosario family were based on stereotypical images she had of Hispanic people, that they were unchecked assumptions, and that she really knew and understood very little about members of that ethnic group. The instructor recommended that the student return to Mrs. Rosario with this new insight and allow the woman to express her feelings concerning the death of her child.

Upon recommendation from instructor, student takes different action.

The student was overwhelmed by the deep sense of loss and outpouring of grief from Mrs. Rosario. She realized that the entire family was in mourning for the loss of the baby. She was unaware of this fact at her initial visit because she had been blinded by cultural stereotypes. She had been dealing with the family at the level of categorical ethnicity—that is, dealing with stereotypes rather than entering into meaningful interactions with the family. With the support and encouragement of the instructor, the student nurse was able to help the family work through the grieving process. She gained a deeper appreciation of them as real people and was able to penetrate ethnic group boundaries. The entire student group profited from this experience.

Transactional ethnicity: student confronts stereotypes and interacts meaningfully and effectively with client of different ethnic background.

---

negative (i.e., lazy, uncooperative, uncommunicative, and troublesome), accept differentness without viewing it as negative, avoid imposing their own value systems on everyone, and maintain open, effective communication. By overcoming barriers to effective communication, community health nurses can maintain a high level of therapeutic competence with clients of varying cultural backgrounds. They can avoid interactions shaped by

cultural stereotypes and can transcend cultural barriers. Case Example 5-3 illustrates these points.

The more culturally different nurses are from clients, the more nurse-client transactions are likely to be shaped by stereotypes, mistrust, and discomfort. On the other hand, it is also a mistake to assume that interpersonal transactions between nurses and clients from similar cultural backgrounds are always easy. For example, a nurse of

African American descent with strong Anglo-American values and a high level of acculturation in the dominant society may have difficulty communicating with African American clients who more fully embrace and participate in the Afro-American culture. Communication in this situation is likely to be even more difficult if the nurse and client are from different socioeconomic backgrounds.

Utilizing good interpersonal techniques, which include listening, showing empathy, manifesting a nonjudgmental attitude, and exercising creativity and flexibility, will greatly enhance the nurse's ability to deal with cultural differences. For example, a culturally sensitive nurse who is aware that persistent eye contact may be interpreted as aggressive behavior by some Native American clients (Wilson, 1983) understands and accepts clients of that background who avoid eye contact. The nurse will continue to maintain a friendly, nonjudgmental attitude toward them and not assume that the clients aren't interested if they look down or away during an interaction.

Professional Traditions and Values

Sociologists have pointed out that increased social distance between clients and professionals may serve as a barrier to client utilization of health services. Professionals consistently show preference for clients who are more like them and who reflect the ideals of their profession. Clients from minority ethnic groups, the masses of whom are from the lowest socioeconomic levels compared to other ethnic groups, are likely to be of greatest social distance from the health professional, and least likely to match the ideal of what a client should be. Yet they are also most likely to be in need of health services. The very process of becoming acculturated into their profession may blind nurses to the specific problems and needs that different clients may have. It is, therefore, important for community health nurses to be sensitive to this inherent conflict in the health care system.

The Client's World View

Community health nurses need to know about their clients' world views. Consistent with their ethnic and cultural background, clients hold certain beliefs and values, such as what they believe to be true, what they think is important, and what they expect from self and others. Community health nurses are particularly concerned about how these beliefs and expectations influence health behaviors and health status. Because of this it is important for nurses to assess the cultural dimensions (see Box 5-1) that affect or have the potential to affect their clients' care.

Clients' world views will determine their health maintenance strategies; whether they utilize regular checkups from mainstream health systems, traditional healers, folk medicine, or a combination; their pathways to health care—who they consult when they experience symptoms, and the purpose, timing, and sequence of their consultation and their expectations in treatment encounters. Successful encounters with health professionals such as community health nurses will increase the frequency of such experiences. Community health nurses can acquire a knowledge of culture to increase the probability of successful client-nurse encounters. This is especially important in initial encounters, since clients are more likely to return for services if their initial contact with health care professionals is positive.

Functioning in Ethnic Communities

American communities, particularly those for which community health nurses are likely to be responsible, are increasingly composed of one predominant ethnic group or another. Blacks and Hispanics usually populate inner-city urban areas while Appalachian whites and Native Americans are more likely to be concentrated in rural than in urban communities. These ethnic groups usually suffer disproportionally higher incidences of ill health and greater inequities in the health care delivery system. Often they have no voice in the type or quality of care they receive or in the quality of the practitioners who provide such care. Despite the great need for health services in such communities, practitioners, including community health nurses, tend to avoid working in these areas because of fear for their safety. These communities are usually viewed as having high crime rates and other social pathologies that make them dangerous and unattractive work environments, particularly to outsiders who are likely to be from different ethnic and cultural backgrounds. Professionals may harbor a "blame the victim" attitude, whereby, as members of the dominant society, they blame the inequities on the people themselves.

However, the tremendous need for services to ethnic minority and oppressed communities still exists, and community health nurses can play a significant role in fulfilling this need. To be effective in such communities, it is crucial that community health nurses confront their fears and devise realistic ways for ensuring their safety in communities where they feel unsafe. Barnes (1979) has suggested taking sensible safety measures such as these: become familiar with community residents and their life-styles; note stores, housing, gathering places, and social agencies, etc.; show interest in the neighborhood by being friendly but alert; dress properly; travel in pairs when necessary; travel familiar routes; park as close as possible to the point of destination and avoid placing self in compromising situations.

Community health nurses can also work with community leaders to learn about the community—its neighborhoods, houses, schools, and people. Utilizing the input and cooperation of community groups, community health nurses can more effectively assess community health needs and develop health programs specific to these needs. Also, nurses can encourage community residents to provide input concerning their health needs and encourage them to participate in meeting these needs when appropriate. Case Example 5-4 is an illustration.

Functioning as Client Advocates

Community health nurses work with clients who are primarily well and uninstitutionalized but who live in their own territories—homes and communities. Community health nurses are often guests in these territories, and their main function is to facilitate their clients' efforts to maintain maximum health rather than to care for them directly. They can improve their functioning by adopting a customer approach (Burgess & Lazare, 1976) to clients and by functioning as client advocates. In this approach the initial nurse-client practitioner encounter (interview) is a negotiated process whereby the clinician elicits client's requests, collects relevant clinical data, and enters into a negotiation process that facilitates a mutually beneficial relationship. Once this mutually beneficial relationship is established, the nurse can then help to assist clients to meet their needs by acting on their behalf or as their advocates.

This advocacy role is most important when clients who have disproportionately greater health needs compared to other groups are also disproportionately underrepresented as professionals in the health care system. Acting as advocates on behalf of such clients means that community health nurses are ready to support clients' rights to improved standards of health services, and includes assisting them in learning how to use health services and how to increase their level of participation in decision-making concerning their own health. Nurse advocates serve as liaison and referral agents between the individual, the family, and the community; collaborate with other professionals and community representatives to obtain better health care for individuals and families in communities; and document and report inadequacies in health care services.

The six strategies that we've just discussed will greatly increase community health nurses' effectiveness in working with culturally diverse clients. Effective cross-cultural communication is essential in the negotiation process when clients and clini-

Case Example 5-4: Community Participation

Mrs. Clark, a community health nurse, works in a neighborhood health center of a low income, black inner-city community. She participated in organizing a network of local service providers consisting of teachers, business representatives, ministers, health care social service providers, police officers, and other concerned residents. The group met regularly and discussed a variety of community issues including health concerns. Mrs. Clark learned that community residents were concerned about the incidence of hypertension among many families. She participated with the network group and utilized health resources in the community to initiate a blood pressure screening program, which was conducted in the community's schools. Based on the incidence of hypertension found and the level of interest among community residents, Mrs. Clark developed education classes for families with a member who has hypertension. The classes were taught in the evening in one of the local schools. Mrs. Clark provided factual information concerning the causes and treatment of hypertension, including dietary and stress factors. She also used her group skills to facilitate discussion of feelings concerning their fears, misconceptions about the condition itself, and about the frustrations related to instituting life-style changes that are necessary to control hypertension.

Community health nurse works with community group to identify health needs of a particular ethnic group.

Nurse institutes program in response to community health needs.

The program was highly successful and significantly increased the community health nurses' credibility, acceptance, and rapport with residents of the community. Above all, the program was a direct response to a community health need.

Nurse establishes rapport and works well with community.

cians are of different cultural and ethnic backgrounds. Aspects of categorical ethnicity, such as skin color and language differences, and of transactional ethnicity, such as the nature of interpersonal interactions between the two parties, will affect the client's and clinician's degree of comfort and openness with one another. When there are rigid boundaries between racial and ethnic groups,

both sides are likely to relate to one another according to stereotypes and protective maneuvering (Green, 1982). It is essential that community health nurses be aware of the possible difficulties that might occur in cross-ethnic and cross-cultural encounters and work through them in order to reach a negotiated consensus about clients' health needs.

Summary

Community health nurses encounter individuals and families from various ethnic and cultural backgrounds, and they are often responsible for the health care of diverse ethnic communities. To enhance

the community health nurse's ability to deal more effectively with diverse client populations, this chapter provided an overview of the concepts of culture and ethnicity. It is important that nursing assessment include the role of culture and ethnicity in the health beliefs, practices, and status of clients. Self-awareness is important too: nurses and the nursing profession have their own unique cultures, which may become sources of conflict in nurse-client encounters. Culture and ethnicity are closely related to the help-seeking process in part because of cultural variations in the definition of health and illness.

Whereas there are great variations within ethnic groups, there are also striking similarities based on shared values, health beliefs, and practices. Descriptive overviews of selected ethnic families were presented to sensitize nurses to group variations and to provide guides to be tested on a case-by-case basis. Generalizations cannot be made since there is variations within ethnic groups.

The overall purpose of this chapter is to raise the awareness of community health nurses and increase their sensitivity to cultural and ethnic differences, as well as to illustrate how such differences can affect the delivery of health care services. It is important for community health nurses to learn about, be sensitive to, and respect the cultural heritages, traditions, and customs of the people they serve.

Study Questions

1. Which of the following statements best describes the distinction between culture and ethnicity?
   a. Culture refers to all people while ethnicity refers to minority groups.
   b. Culture refers to distinctive ways of life of a group of people while ethnicity refers to participation in a group on the basis of symbolic elements.
   c. Culture refers to the esthetic elements in a given society while ethnicity refers to racial characteristics of individual groups of people.
   d. There is virtually no distinction between culture and ethnicity.
2. A characteristic of the ethnographic interview is that it: (1) encourages clients (interviewees)

to speak openly and freely, (2) allows clients (interviewees) to describe their own perspective, (3) forces clients to select responses from predetermined answers, (4) focuses only on ethnic content.
   a. 1, 2, and 3
   b. 3 only
   c. 1 and 2
   d. 2 and 4
   e. 1 only
3. The W family lives in a Jewish community characterized by a Jewish synagogue and several Jewish stores and businesses. Like other Jewish families in the community, the Ws are identifiable in the community by their different style of dress and regular attendance at the neighborhood Jewish synagogue. They shop in local Jewish stores and eat only Jewish foods. They also visibly socialize their young children in the roles and customs of the group. This description is an example of:
   a. Ideological ethnicity
   b. Behavioral ethnicity
   c. Categorical ethnicity
   d. Transactional ethnicity
4. Ms. A, an R.N., has been assigned to a community clinic with a multiethnic patient population. Which of the following behaviors is likely to be most helpful to Ms. A in establishing good relationships with her clients?
   a. A good sense of her own ethnic-cultural background and value orientation
   b. An exceptional ability to communicate clearly
   c. A thorough knowledge of the history and health beliefs of the community clients
   d. None of the above
5. Which of the following statements best explains the concept of transactional ethnicity?
   a. Emphasis on interpersonal relationships when members of ethnic groups interact
   b. Emphasis on the noncognitive aspects of culture
   c. Tendency to view one's ethnic group as unique and better than others
   d. Tendency to behave and think in terms of ethnic group values on a regular basis
6. Ethnic families maintain varying degrees of their cultural traditions and values. Which of the following factors is likely to account for

the extent to which ethnic families maintain traditional health beliefs and practices?
(1) Socioeconomic status
(2) Length of time since family migrated from country of origin
(3) Exposure to mainstream medical system
a. All of the above
b. None of the above
c. 1 only
d. 3 only

References

Alonzo A: Everyday illness behavior: A situational approach to health status deviation. *Social Science and Medicine* 1979; 13A:397–404.

Barnes S: Your safety first. *Nursing '79* 1979; 9 (4):86–90.

Barth F: *Ethnic Groups and Boundaries.* Boston: Little, Brown, 1969.

Biddle E: The American Irish-Catholic family. In: Mendel CH, Haberstein RW (editors), *Ethnic Families in America.* New York: Elsevier, 1981.

Burgess A, Lazare C: *Community Mental Health: Target Populations.* Englewood Cliffs, N.J.: Prentice-Hall, 1976.

deValdez T, Gallegos J: The Chicano familia in social work. In: Green J (editor), *Cultural Awareness in the Human Services.* Englewood Cliffs, N.J.: Prentice-Hall, 1982.

Dowd, M: The new Ellis Island. *Time* (June 13) 1983: 18–27.

Greeley A: *Ethnicity in the United States.* New York: Wiley, 1974.

Green J: *Cultural Awareness in the Human Services.* Englewood Cliffs, N.J.: Prentice-Hall, 1982.

Harwood A: *Ethnicity and Medical Care.* Washington, D.C.: Howard University Press, 1981.

Kay M: Health and illness in a Mexican American barrio. In: Spicer E (editor), *Ethnic Medicine in the Southwest.* Tucson, University of Arizona Press, 1979.

Kleinman A: *Patients and Healers in the Context of Culture.* Berkeley, Calif.: UC Press, 1980.

Leigh J, Green J: The structure of the black community: The knowledge base for social services. In: Green J (editor), *Cultural Awareness in the Human Services.* Englewood Cliff, N.J.: Prentice-Hall, 1982.

Leininger M: Becoming aware of types of health practitioners and cultural impositions. In: *Becoming Aware of Cultural Differences in Nursing.* Kansas City, Mo.: American Nurses' Association, 1972.

———: Culturological assessment domains for nursing practices. In: Leininger M (editor), *Transcultural Nursing: Concepts, Theories and Practices.* New York: Wiley, 1977.

Lewis D: The black family: Socialization and sex roles. *Phylon* 1975; 36 (3): 221–239.

Lin K et al: Sociocultural determinants of help-seeking behavior of patients with mental illness. *J Nerv Ment Dis* 1982; 170 (2): 78–85.

Martinez R: *Hispanic Culture and Health Care: Fact, Fiction and Folklore.* St. Louis: Mosby, 1978.

McKinlay J: Social network influences on morbid episodes and the career of help-seeking. In: Eisenberg L, Kleinman A (editors), *The Relevance of Social Science for Medicine.* Dordrecht, Holland: D. Reidel, 1981.

Miller N: Social work services to urban Indians. In: Green J (editor), *Cultural Awareness in the Human Services.* Englewood Cliffs, N.J.: Prentice-Hall, 1982.

Muecke M: Caring for Southeast Asian refugee patients in the U.S.A. *Am J Public Health* (April) 1983; 73 (4): 431–438.

Orque M: Nursing care of South Vietnamese patients. In: Orque M, Black B, Monroy L (editors), *Ethnic Nursing Care: A Multicultural Approach,* St. Louis: Mosby, 1983.

Schermerhorn R: *Comparative Ethnic Relations: A Framework for Theory and Research.* Chicago: University of Chicago Press, 1970.

Scott C: Competing health care systems in an inner-city area. *Human Organization,* 1975, *34,* 108–110.

Semmes C: Toward a theory of popular health practices in the black community. *West J Black Studies* 1983; 7: 206–213.

Snow L: Folk medical beliefs and their implications for the care of patients. A Review based on studies among black Americans. In: Henderson G, Primeaux M (editors), *Transcultural Health Care.* Menlo Park, Calif.: Addison-Wesley, 1981.

Staples R: The black American family. In: Mendel CH, Haberstein RW (editors), *Patterns and Variations.* New York: Elsevier, 1981.

Telles J, Harris M: Feeling sick: The experience and legitimation of illness. *Social Science and Medicine* 1981; 25A: 243–251.

Twaddle A: Sickness and the sickness career: Some applications. In: Eisenberg L, Kleinmen A (editors), *The Relevance of Social Science for Medicine.* Dordrecht, Holland: D. Reidel, 1981.

Vogel V: American Indian medicine. In: Henderson G, Primeaux M (editors), *Transcultural Health Care.* Menlo Park, Calif.: Addison-Wesley, 1981.

Wilson V: Nursing care of American Indian patients. In: Orque M, Black B, Monroy L (editors), *Ethnic Nurs-*

ing Care: A Multicultural Approach. St. Louis: Mosby, 1983.

Zborowski M: Cultural components in response to pain. Journal of Social Issues 1952; 8: 16–30.

———— : People in Pain. San Francisco: Jossey-Bass, 1966.

Zola I: Culture and symptoms: An analysis of patients presenting complaints. American Sociological Review 1966; 31. 615–630.

———— : Pathways to the doctor—from person to patient, Soc Sci Med 1973; 7: 677–689.

Chapter 6

Epidemiology

Dixie W. Ray

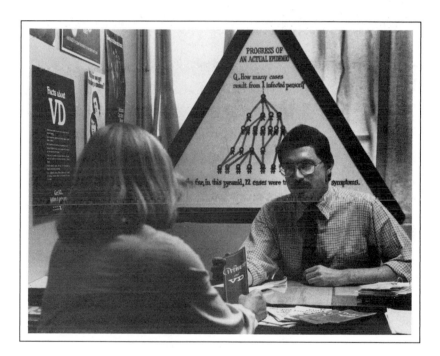

The concepts of epidemiology play an important role in all aspects of community health nursing, including targeting and implementing health teaching programs.

Chapter Objectives

After completing this chapter, the reader will be able to:

- Discuss the major epidemiologic concepts
- Describe the sources and nature of data appropriate for use in epidemiologic studies
- Define the various rates and explain their use
- Differentiate between the types of epidemiologic studies and their use
- Relate the use of epidemiology to community health nursing practice

Epidemiology provides one of the scientific bases for the practice of community health nursing. There are many definitions of *epidemiology,* but all agree that it is concerned with the distribution of health, disease, and health behaviors in human populations (Slome et al, 1982). Epidemiology, which addresses health at an aggregate or population level, is concerned with the extent and types of illnesses in groups of people and the factors affecting their distribution. This description acknowledges that health is not randomly distributed throughout the population, and that groups vary in the frequency of different diseases (Mausner & Bahn, 1974). Using the epidemiologic process, the community health nurse can identify these variations and related factors and apply this information to developing appropriate interventions that reduce risk in the population and improve its health status.

The emphasis on *health* is an important feature of the definition of epidemiology. The World Health Organization (1964) defined health as "a state of complete physical, mental, and social well-being and not merely the absence of disease and infirmity." The definition stresses the idea that the health status of an individual, family, or community includes at some time all the elements of well-being (mental, physical, and social). Although attempts have been made to develop measures of health, it is still measured mainly through its converse—death and disease.

History of Epidemiology

Statistics about the population and its health are an essential element of epidemiology. Collection of population statistics began in the early seventeenth century in England. Using these data, John Graunt constructed the first life tables from which he derived inferences about mortality and fertility in the human population (Graunt, 1662). He also observed a seasonal variation in mortality. At the same time mathematical principles were being developed and refined. These quantitative methods were necessary to the analysis and understanding of epidemiologic data.

As these developments were occurring, there was growing concern about public health and identification of factors affecting it. In the 1850s John Snow conducted his classic epidemiologic study of the occurrence of cholera in London. Snow noted that cholera rates were particularly high in an area of London supplied with water by three companies that drew their water from the Thames River at a heavily polluted point (Snow, 1855). When one company moved to a less polluted point in the river, the incidence of cholera declined in the area of the city it served. Snow identified the houses receiving water from each of the three companies calculated the cholera death rates among each company's customers and compared them to death rates in the rest of London. His findings clearly identified the companies with the highest rates. Snow integrated these findings with his findings from other investigations and inferred that there was a "cholera poison" transmitted by polluted waters.

Both Graunt and Snow recommended action to improve the health of the population based on their data on mortality rates and the distribution in the population. That tradition continues today. Epidemiologic data are collected and studies conducted as a part of efforts to improve health, not just as research exercises.

The relationship between nursing and epidemiology also has a long history. Florence Nightingale worked closely with William Farr, a founder of epidemiology, in the analysis of data from a survey she conducted by mail in London (Woodham-Smith, 1950). Today school nurses and community health nurses take an active role in the reporting and follow-up of communicable disease and participate in research studies.

Epidemiologic Concepts

The epidemiologic triangle has served as a framework for studies for many years. Three factors—agent, host, and environment—interact and determine susceptibility and exposure to disease (see Figure 6-1). Development of this triangular model reflected an understanding of the interrelationships among infectious etiological agents and hosts and environments (see Table 6-1). Although it is sometimes difficult to separate the host (intrinsic) variables from the environmental (extrinsic) variables, the distinction continues to be made in delineating the factors related to a health problem. For example, when studying malnutrition, one cannot easily separate the host's diet, an intrinsic factor, from biologic and socioeconomic extrinsic factors, which affect production of food. Although these factors can be examined separately, the interaction among them must also be considered.

Cause and Relationship

Epidemiologic studies frequently identify factors that occur together with certain health problems. For example, epidemiologic studies helped to show that smoking is associated with lung cancer and to identify public health implications. However, this was not sufficient evidence to prove cause in the strict scientific sense. Controlled laboratory experiments were conducted to verify the inferred relationships from the epidemiologic studies.

In epidemiology a causal relationship may be defined as "an association between categories of events or characteristics in which an alteration in the frequency or quality of one category is followed by a change in the other" (MacMahon & Pugh, 1970, pp. 17–18). Attributing a health condition to a cause requires a meticulous and thorough study of facts. To confirm that a given factor is a cause, the health condition must exist in the population where the presumed causal factor exists. Alternative explanations of the association must also be evaluated and discarded as not useful. A conservative approach should be used in attributing cause when there are no experimental data available. The following are considerations to be used in evaluating the causal nature of associations:

- *Time sequence.* The event that is considered causal must precede the effect.
- *Strength of association.* The more often the events occur together, the more likely the association is causal. Decisions should not be made on findings unique to one study.
- *Consistent with current knowledge.* The causal association should be supported by knowledge in the relevant sciences.

Multiple Causation

In recent years epidemiology has increasingly been used with problems other than infectious disease, such as coronary heart disease or teenage pregnancy. In many cases it is not possible to identify a single agent leading to the problem. Instead there are a multiplicity of events, some independent, others responses, to earlier events. Interacting with the host factors, these events result in the health problem. No single agent can be said to cause problems such as coronary heart disease or teenage pregnancy. They are instead the result of multiple interactions between the host and the environment. Several models have been developed to address the problems of multiple causation, including the "web of causation" (MacMahon & Pugh, 1970) and the "wheel" (Mausner & Bahn, 1974). These models stress the need to identify multiple etiologic factors of a health problem rather than emphasizing a single disease agent.

In the "web of causation" model, effects never depend on a single cause (MacMahon & Pugh, 1970). The model considers all the predisposing factors and their complex relations with each other and with the disease. When their relationships are graphically presented, they resemble a "web."

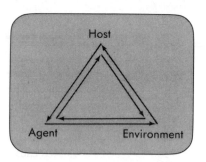

Figure 6-1 Epidemiologic triangle.

Knowledge of the relationships allows one to select alternative interventions.

The "wheel" model focuses on the interactions of the host (a person) and the environment. The host is conceived as the hub of the wheel, while the environment is a ring around the hub. The ring is divided into three segments, each containing a type of environment representing the biologic, social, and physical environments. The relative size of the components of the wheel depends on the particular health problem under study.

Classification of Disease

To study a state of disease or health over time and among large numbers of people, epidemiologists use two kinds of criteria to assign people to disease categories: causal criteria and manifestational criteria. *Causal criteria* are used to group persons according to experiences believed to be the cause of their illness. For example, pica is associated with lead poisoning in children, and therefore, children with pica would be a key group to study when working to prevent lead poisoning. With *manifestational criteria*, on the other hand, persons are grouped according to their symptoms or changes in physiologic function. An example of such a grouping would be all people with diabetes mellitus.

Congruence between causal criteria and manifestational criteria is often lacking. Within a population, people grouped by causal criteria may not be exactly the same group of people resulting from selection based on manifestational criteria, even though the disease being studied is the same. An example of this is lung cancer. Although cigarette smoking and lung cancer have a demonstrated relationship, not all carcinomas of the lung are associated with cigarette smoking, nor do all cigarette smokers develop lung cancer.

There are other problems with disease classifications. Classification based on similarities may mask individual differences among patients. Classifications also have a way of influencing and narrowing thinking. In some situations the disease, rather than the individuals who have the disease, may become the point of interest. A final complication is that disease names are transitory and may change as knowledge of the condition increases.

Because knowledge of causal factors is often lacking, manifestational criteria provide the primary basis for disease classification. The epidemiologist frequently has no alternative but to develop studies based on manifestational criteria and hope that certain associated factors can be identified as causes.

An internationally accepted classification of disease entities is the International Classification of Diseases (ICD). The origins of this classification system go back more than 100 years. Currently published by the World Health Organization and revised every ten years, the ICD is in its ninth revision (1978). The ICD allows the exchange of comparable data from region to region and country to country. Thus, comparisons of one population to another and the study of disease over long periods of time are possible.

In an adapted version, the ICD-A, the United States has extended the classification to use with morbidity data. It is used extensively in indexing hospital records and by local health departments, visiting nurse associations, and home health agencies.

Table 6-1 Agent, Host, and Environmental Factors Affecting the Health of Human Populations

Agents of Disease (Etiologic Factors)

Infectious agents	Viruses, bacteria
Physical agents	Radiation
Chemical agents	Poisons, allergens

Host Factors (Intrinsic Factors)

Genetic characteristics	Sickle cell trait
Physiological states	Fatigue, pregnancy, obesity, stress
Specific immunities	Prior infection, immunization
Human behavior	Personal hygiene, diet, exercise, substance abuse, food handling, use of health resources

Environmental Factors (Extrinsic Factors)

Physical properties	Geology, climate, water, air, and chemical agents
Biologic entities	Viral particles Groups of human beings Animals, plants, food, drugs, vectors (flies and mosquitos)
Socioeconomic factors	Socioeconomic and political organization Institutions Social customs Culture Integration into society Occupation Mobility Wars

Rates and Other Measures

The simplest quantitative measurement in epidemiology is the *count* of the number of persons who have a particular condition or characteristic. Much information is reported in this way by practicing community health nurses. For example, community health nurses report the number of clients seen in a clinic. This information is useful for administrative purposes in assigning staff and planning facilities. However, to determine the relative importance of the number of cases of a disease, the proportion of cases to the total number in the group must be considered.

In epidemiology the proportions frequently used are *rates.* In addition to descriptive uses, rates allow comparisons of groups across time in a meaningful and useful way. A rate has three components: a measure of some event, a referent population, and some specification of time. In most situations the referent population is also the population at risk—that is, individuals capable of developing a specific health state. They become the denominator for calculating the rate of the health state. The two most common rates are *incidence rates* and *prevalence rates*. Incidence rates provide a measure of *new* cases of disease over a period in time. For example, how many new cases of measles (numerator) are there in a school population (denominator) during the year (period of time)?

$$\text{incidence rate} = \frac{\text{number of persons developing a disease}}{\text{total number at risk}} \text{ over a period of time}$$

In contrast, the prevalence rate describes the *total* number of cases at a point in time and includes new cases and previously existing cases. For example, on the fifth day of school (point in time) how many children are absent with measles (numerator) out of a school population (denominator)?

$$\text{prevalence rate} = \frac{\text{number of persons with a disease}}{\text{total number in group}} \text{ at a point in time}$$

Rates are used by health agencies at all levels to describe the health of populations of various geographic areas. This information is helpful to the community health nurse in identifying the community's strengths and its problem areas. The most frequently used rates are shown in Table 6-2. Since definitions of the components occasionally vary, it is important to check the definitions when using rates calculated by other persons. Note that the multiplier (e.g., 1,000, 10,000) varies across the different rates, its size depending on the relative magnitude of the numerator and denominator. The value selected should be large enough that the rates produced are equal to or greater than one. The fewer the number of cases relative to the population, the larger the multiplier must be. Rare events, such as maternal mortality, will require a large multiplier.

The rates just described are characterized as *crude rates*. They encompass people with various characteristics and make no attempt to distinguish

between them. Crude rates are useful because they are summary rates and can be constructed from a minimum of information. An example may help to clarify calculation of rates. In Indiana in 1980, there were 47,300 deaths in a population estimated at 5,497,600. Using the formula for Crude Death Rate from Table 6-2:

$$\frac{47,300}{5,497,600} \times 1,000 = 8.6$$

Cause-specific rates are probably the most important epidemiologic index. They estimate the risk of death from a specific condition and can help identify major health problems in a population. One limitation of cause-specific death rates is the low reliability of reporting of multiple causes of deaths.

Rates can be expressed in terms of subgroups as well as for the total population. Rates specific for age, socioeconomic status, and other demographic characteristics add to our understanding of the health of a community. For example, it is useful to know if coronary heart disease is occurring among women aged 35–44 at the same rate as men of this age. To do this, one must calculate a rate that is age-, sex-, and cause-specific. The basic formula for specific rates is given in the following example of a sex-specific rate.

$$\text{sex-specific death rate} = \frac{\text{number of deaths among men}}{\text{estimated number of men}} \times 10,000$$

For this calculation the multiplier is increased. Use of both cause and sex to limit the population reduces the number of events. If 1,000 had been used, the resulting rate would have been less than one. Caution should be exercised in using rates when the population is small. For example, much community health data are collected for census tracts, a geographic area defined by the U.S. Census Bureau and usually containing 2,000 to 5,000 persons. At this level it may be more appropriate to use actual numbers. Rare events may produce a rate that is extremely high because of a small denominator and will be misleading if viewed by

Table 6-2 Frequently Used Rates

Natality

Crude Birth Rate	$\dfrac{\text{Total Number of Live Births}}{\text{Total Population}}$	× 1,000
Fertility Rate	$\dfrac{\text{Total Number of Live Births}}{\text{Number of Women 15–44 Years of Age}}$	× 1,000

Morbidity

Incidence Rate	$\dfrac{\text{Number of New Cases of a Specified Disease Reported During a Given Time Interval}}{\text{Estimated Mid-Interval Population at Risk}}$	× 1,000[a]
Attack Rate	$\dfrac{\text{Number of New Cases of a Specified Disease Reported During a Limited Time Interval}}{\text{Population at Risk During Same Time Interval}}$	× 100
Prevalence Rate	$\dfrac{\text{Number of Cases (New and Old) of Specified Disease Existing at a Given Point in Time}}{\text{Estimated Population at the Same Point in Time}}$	× 1,000

Mortality

Crude Death Rate	$\dfrac{\text{Total Number of Deaths}}{\text{Estimated Mid-Interval Population}}$	× 1,000

itself. By examining vital statistics data from one area over a period of time, one can usually identify this problem by the highly unstable rates that fluctuate widely over time.

Once the rates for a condition are known, they can be compared to rates for other areas to determine the relative magnitude of the problem. For example, a community health nurse from Elkhart, Indiana, can compare infant mortality rate for the area, 18.4, to the national rate, 13.8 (U.S. Bureau of the Census, 1982). The difference between the two rates suggests infant mortality is a problem in Elkhart. Comparisons can also be made among the rates for various conditions—for example, between different age- and cause-specific rates to determine health problems among different age groups. These comparisons can be used in determining priorities and designing programs of a preventive nature.

Table 6-2 *(continued)*

Crude Cause-Specific Death Rate	$\dfrac{\text{Total Number of Deaths From a Specific Cause}}{\text{Estimated Mid-Interval Population}}$	× 1,000
Case Fatality Rate	$\dfrac{\text{Number of Deaths from Specified Disease}}{\text{Number of Cases of the Disease}}$	× 100
Fetal Death Rate	$\dfrac{\text{Number of Fetal Deaths of 28 Weeks or More Gestation}}{\text{Number of Live Births}}$	× 1,000
Neonatal Mortality Rate	$\dfrac{\text{Number of Deaths Under 28 Days of Age}}{\text{Number of Live Births}}$	× 1,000
Post-neonatal Mortality Rate	$\dfrac{\text{Number of Deaths from 28 Days to 1 Year}}{\text{Number of Live Births}}$	× 1,000
Infant Mortality Rate	$\dfrac{\text{Number of Deaths Under 1 Year}}{\text{Number of Live Births}}$	× 1,000
Material Mortality Rate	$\dfrac{\text{Number of Deaths Assigned to Causes Related to Pregnancy}}{\text{Number of Live Births}}$	× 10,000[b]

[a]May be expressed per 10,000 or 100,000 when the number of cases is small.
[b]May be expressed per 100,000 when the number of cases is small.

Sources of Data

Community health nurses rely on epidemiological data for their practice with aggregate populations. Epidemiology often relies heavily on data that have been collected by agencies for purposes other than the study of health and disease. For instance, when Graunt published his *Bills of Mortality* in 1662 he used data collected by parish clerks. In the United States, government agencies at the national, state, and local levels are excellent sources of data.

Information about the population's health is available from many sources. National health data are collected by the National Center for Health Statistics (NCHS). They conduct an ongoing sur-vey of a sample of households in the country using a core of health-related questions. Other NCHS research involves physical examinations and hospital records as well as surveys. The NCHS also conducts research on nutrition, fertility, and health services. Preliminary reports of NCHS projects are published in *Advance Data* on a monthly basis. Full reports appear later in the *Vital and Health Statistics Series* of the NCHS.

Another major source of information related to the health of the population is vital statistics, including records of births and adoptions, deaths, marriages, and divorces. Use of standard birth and death certificates across the United States has improved reporting of these data, which are recorded at local health departments and then sent on to the state health department. From the state the information is sent to the NCHS. Reports are generally available at all three levels of government. Although most local health departments publish annual reports for their areas, small local health departments may not retain any data for local statistical reports. However, state health departments also publish annual health and vital statistics, which summarize data for the state as well as for cities, towns, counties, and other geopolitical jurisdictions in the state. The NCHS publishes national and state data and describes trends in birth and death rates in the *Monthly Vital Statistics Reports* and *Annual Summaries.*

Communicable disease reports are disseminated in a similar manner. The selection of diseases to be reported is primarily a state matter. However, International Sanitary Regulation requires reporting on six diseases: cholera, plague, louse-borne relapsing fever, smallpox, louse-borne typhus fever, and yellow fever. Most states require the reporting of about forty infectious diseases. There is serious underreporting of most communicable disease, and this should be taken into consideration when using these data. Reports are made to local health officials, and the reports are transmitted to state health departments and, subsequently, to the U.S. Public Health Service, Centers for Disease Control (CDC). The CDC publishes weekly summaries of these reports in the *Morbidity and Mortality Weekly Report (MMWR).* Annual summaries are also published.

Population description is also essential to epidemiology. At the national level, the Bureau of the Census conducts a census of the population every ten years. Information about demographic characteristics of the population and their housing are included. Partial results of these surveys are published and are available at public libraries and university libraries. Since these data are collected only once every ten years, they may not always provide current information about a highly mobile population. Cities that believe there have been major population changes between censuses may request a special census to document the change.

Since the problems confronting community health nurses frequently go beyond the traditional bounds of health services, they may need data relating to other sectors of the community. Local data can be obtained from official records from several sources. For example, community health nurses working with school populations can use information from school records in problem identification and program planning. Data relating to crime and safety can be obtained from local police and fire departments. Local housing authorities frequently have information about the clients they serve and the condition of housing in a community. City planning departments are a good source for information about the characteristics of the city, as well as the population.

Data from the sources just described can assist the community health nurse to identify populations at risk. For example: Is there a high proportion of elderly? Is there a high rate of deaths from coronary heart disease? Is there a high rate of adolescent pregnancy? Once a population at risk has been identified, it may be necessary to conduct a special survey of the population to obtain other information used in developing services for the population at risk.

Methods of Study

The concepts and principles of epidemiology can be applied in several different types of study. Because it is a science that addresses the health of humans, epidemiology typically uses an observational rather than an experimental approach (Slome et al, 1982). Researchers observe events occurring in the population rather than manipulating a factor or causing an event to occur. Use of the nonexperimental mode means there is less control of the factors of interest and detracting factors may be included. However, epidemiologic studies can identify the nonrandom variations of health and disease in the population and point to areas where experimental studies are needed and are possible.

There is a logical progression in the types of epidemiologic studies. The progression starts with simple description (*descriptive studies*) and then searches for relationships among health conditions and other factors (*cross-sectional studies*). Based on ideas about these relationships, tentative hypothesis are developed and tested (*case control studies*). Next, the hypotheses are refined and tested to confirm the causal association (*cohort studies*). For many topics of epidemiologic study this is the final test. However, some relationships are appropriate for additional study to confirm cause and effect by more rigid testing (*experimental studies*). Each of these studies will be discussed in this section.

Descriptive Studies

The descriptive study is considered by many epidemiologists to be the starting point for all epidemiologic research because it identifies the areas appropriate for further study. This method of study relies primarily on existing data. From examining pertinent data, the community health nurse can identify the types of persons most likely to be affected by a condition, the geographic area in which it will occur, and when it will occur. Since these dimensions are utilized in all the other types of studies, considerable attention will be given to them in this discussion. We'll look at the following dimensions of health and disease:

- *Person*—who is affected?
- *Place*—where does it occur?
- *Time*—when does it occur?
- *Population*—what is its overall effect?

Sheer description of this information may seem trivial when compared to more sophisticated studies of the etiology of disease. However, descriptive studies can provide insights into the interactions among the host, agent, and environment that would otherwise be undiscovered.

Person   The most important personal determinant of health is age. Since cause-specific mortality and morbidity vary by age, different programs are needed to handle the problems of different age groups. Although accidents in the home are a problem for preschool children and persons over 65 years, different community health nursing interventions are required for the two populations at risk (NCHS, 1980).

Analysis of disease and death rates also show differences by sex. Although there are higher mortality rates for males, females have higher morbidity rates. Women report more illnesses, yet men die at a greater rate. This differential between males and females has been observed for more than 300 years. Graunt (1662) noted that although more women were observed at physicians' offices, there were higher death rates among men. In our society this continues to be true. Recent studies suggest there may be differences in the way in which men and women recognize and label symptoms, which then results in higher utilization by women (Cleary, Mechanic, & Greenley, 1982). As a result of the higher mortality rates among men, women may be faced with many years without a partner. The difference in mortality rates persists at all ages and is likely related to a combination of sex-linked inheritance, environment, and life-style. In recent years women's death rates for some diseases have increased to near the level of men's rates. This may be due to change in women's life-styles as they increasingly participate in the work force and are confronted with the additional stresses (Haw, 1982). More research is needed to understand the complex relationships between work force participation, role responsibilities outside of work, and stress-related disease.

Women have also continued to increase cigarette consumption, which has resulted in a dramatic increase in deaths from lung cancer among women. The death rate has climbed from 4.6 per 100,000 in 1950 to 20.9 in 1982 (Stolley, 1983). This almost equals the rate for men.

Marital status is another factor of interest as married persons live longer than singles. Several explanations have been offered for these differences (MacMahon & Pugh, 1970). First, self-selection into marriage may occur among healthy persons, while those who are in poor health remain single. Second, persons who choose "dangerous" life-styles and are exposed to disease-producing agents and situations tend not to marry. Last, differences in life-style of single and married persons are related to development of certain diseases. The sex differences for mortality continue across marital status. However, impact of the social support associated with the marital state is more pronounced for men than for women (Cohen & Brody, 1981).

The use of race or ethnicity for classification of health data is controversial but continues to be used in reporting of health data (Terris, 1973). Because many diseases occur at different rates among ethnic groups, collection of health data by ethnic group helps to identify these problems. For example, examination of data related to hypertension and race clearly shows a higher rate of hypertension among black persons (29.1 per 100) than among white (10.2 per 100) (U.S. Bureau of the Census, 1981). Some conditions that occur at different rates among ethnic groups may do so as a result of socioeconomic factors.

The family into which a person is born or spends the formative years also affects health. Family factors are highly interrelated, and it is difficult to establish significance for them individually. Despite this difficulty, their effects should be considered. Although the number of children per family has decreased, large families occur more frequently among the poor (Moore, 1978). Already scarce resources, such as money, space, and food, must then be spread across more family members. Birth order certainly affects a person's life experiences. However, its relationship to health has not been clearly established. Maternal age, on the other hand, is known to be of distinct importance in relation to a baby's health. Births occurring among women at either extreme of maternal age carry higher risks for the mother and baby (Fingerhut, Wilson, & Feldman, 1980). Knowledge of the relation of maternal age and birth outcomes is a factor community health nurses should consider in identifying the high-risk population among referrals.

Since an increasing number of children in the United States are in single-parent homes, we must look at the effects of this circumstance on their health. Reports of the effects of parental deprivation through death, divorce, or separation on a child's health are conflicting; however, this factor still deserves consideration (Hetherington, 1979). In addition, single-parent homes are frequently economically deprived and do not function as well as other homes—both of which can have harmful effects on the child's health (Blotcky & Tittler, 1982).

Other personal factors that have been shown to be related to health include education, occupation, income, religion, and life-style. These data are not always collected or reported with the usual vital statistics. When available, they can enhance the community health nurse's ability to identify more closely the populations at greatest risk.

Health effects are experienced several ways in the workplace including accident, exposure to contaminants, stress, and so forth. Some occupations, such as logging, farming, and welding, are more hazardous than others and expose workers to more life-threatening situations. Workers are affected by the materials they handle—for example, asbestos, benzopyrene, or radiation. In addition, they may carry home residues on their clothes that affect the health of the entire family.

Religions have varying views toward health, illness, and health-related factors, and these affect the health of the group. A group frequently discussed in this context is the Seventh-Day Adventists. Their unique life-style, especially dietary practices and views regarding substance use, has a positive affect on their health. In particular, they have been found to have lower rates of cardiovascular disease (Berkel & deWaard, 1983).

Place   Knowledge of the distribution of geographic events that affect health is important for administrative purposes as well as for understanding the etiology of diseases. When this information is known, additional health resources can be directed to the area. The unit of place varies depending on the condition being studied and the intended use of the data. Nations, states, counties, cities, neighborhoods, schools, and buildings are all appropriate places of concern.

Comparison of rates from different places offers a perspective on the relative significance of any particular rate. Frequently used comparisons are between: countries, states, counties within a state, neighborhoods in a city, and a unit and a larger unit of which it is a part (for example, comparing a county rate to a state rate).

Within the United States there is geographic variation in infant mortality among the states. For example, the infant mortality rate in New Hampshire in 1980 was 9.2 as compared to 10.4 in Utah (Hartford, 1984). Comparing these rates to the national infant mortality rate of 12.5, these states appear to have low infant mortality rates. However, when these rates are compared to infant mortality rates in other industrialized countries, another view emerges. The lowest rate in 1980 was 6.9 in Sweden and the United States ranks sixteenth in comparison to other similar countries.

Some caution should be exercised in international comparisons because there is not standardization of statistics worldwide, even in industrialized countries. In general, international comparisons should be reserved for the more general crude rates. Although the ICD is used by most countries, there may be differences in diagnostic and reporting practices that influence the number of cases used in calculating rates.

Urban and rural differences in the distribution of health and disease have been identified. Garcia-Palmieri and associates (1978) reported statistically significant higher rates of coronary heart disease (CHD) among urban men compared to men in rural areas. Among men in urban areas there is a trend of increasing incidence of CHD with degree of urbanization.

Within cities there is variation in the occurrence of disease. Many older cities in the northeastern and north central part of the United States developed in a zonal system—an industrial zone with slum housing next to a central business core (Park & Burgess, 1925). Remnants of these patterns still exist; low income housing is placed adjacent to industrial areas, while higher income homes are further away in a more healthful environment. Newer cities, developed after the introduction of automobiles, have developed in a more sprawling manner, although the relationship between housing type and industrialization persists. Sprawling cities with "bedroom" communities have introduced additional factors related to health. The necessity of automobile travel for all family activities has led to increased mortality and morbidity from automobile accidents. In addition, persons (especially children) who live near heavily traveled streets can be adversely affected by the high levels of lead and carbon monoxide (Caprio, Margulis, & Joselow, 1974).

Health differences in the various areas can be expressed as a function of socioeconomic status; however, this may mask environmental factors that affect health within the areas. Health problems may affect the socioeconomic status of individuals and their selection of a place to live. Although statistical correlations may exist between type of area of the city and incidence of a health problem, one must be careful about assuming a causal relationship. Families with low incomes may not be able to pay the price of housing in a healthy physical environment and may be forced to live in close proximity to heavy industries or other areas with less desirable characteristics. It is difficult to separate the effects of residence from socioeconomic status.

To study the distribution of disease within an area, it is useful to plot the cases on a map. Cases can be represented on the map by pins or dots. Then one may determine their proximity to each other and to environmental factors. For example, mapping the cases of histoplasmosis occurring in Indianapolis, Indiana, in 1979 led to the identification of an abandoned amusement park as a potential source of the disease. Control measures were then introduced to eliminate the problem.

When an association is found between a geographic location and occurrence of a disease, five criteria are used to determine if the characteristics of the place are probably responsible for the problem (MacMahon & Pugh, 1970, p. 153):

1. High frequency rates exist among all inhabitants of the area.
2. High frequency rates do not occur among similar inhabitants of other areas.
3. Healthy immigrants into the area become ill at a rate similar to indigenous inhabitants.
4. Migrants from the area do not show high rates.
5. Species in the same area other than man show similar manifestations.

Only *one* of these criteria must be met to suggest a relationship between characteristics of place and the condition.

Time   Time is an essential element in epidemiologic analysis and is included in every epidemiologic measure. There are three major kinds of change that can occur: short-term fluctuations, secular trends, and cyclic change.

Short-term fluctuations occur when a number of cases cluster at a point in time. Clustering in time indicates that a certain preceding event and the onset of disease are associated in time. However, it does not establish the causal nature of the association. An *epidemic* occurs when the number of cases exceeds the number of cases usually found in that population. The term *endemic* is used to describe the normal number of cases.

Secular trends refer to changes that occur over long periods of time—years or decades. An example of a secular trend can be seen in the crude death rates for the last twenty years (see Table 6-3). The crude death rate has been decreasing for many years now. Although in some years there is an increase in the rate, the overall trend is to lower rates. For the past few years, the rates have not changed. Economic conditions have been described as the primary cause of this phenomenon. However, this has not been substantiated by empirical studies and the trend appears to be resuming its downward slope.

Table 6-3   Death Rates in the United States, 1940 to 1981

Year	Rate[a]
1940	10.8
1945	10.6
1950	9.6
1955	9.3
1960	9.5
1965	9.4
1966	9.5
1967	9.4
1968	9.7
1969	9.5
1970	9.5
1971	9.3
1972	9.4
1973	9.4
1974	9.2
1975	8.9
1976	8.9
1977	8.8
1978	8.8
1979	8.7
1980	8.7
1981	8.7

[a]Per 1,000 population
SOURCE:
US Bureau of the Census: *Statistical Abstract of the United States.* Washington, D.C.: US Government Printing Office, 1983.

Some secular trends may be the result of social, biologic, physical, and chemical changes that occur with the passage of time. Other such changes may be related to adequacy of diagnoses and reporting.

Cyclic changes are alterations in disease frequency that recur on a regular basis. A common cycle is the seasonal variation that occurs among mortality rates for diseases such as pneumonia and influenza. The number of cases through the year is rather consistent with peaks at epidemic levels in January, February, and March. Other cyclic trends are the increased number of drownings during summer months and higher death rates from automobile accidents on weekends (Friedman, 1980).

Population   In combination the preceding factors have an impact on the characteristics of the population of an area. The population can be described in terms of the increase and the dependency ratio. These terms, which we'll define in a moment, are generally used in describing large areas such as countries or states. With this information one can address questions about the ability of an area to be self-sufficient. For example, is there a sufficient number of persons of working age to provide food for those who are dependent? Or, is the population growing so rapidly that necessary resources, such as schools and health care, will be inadequate?

Increase in population can be described in two ways. The *natural increase* is the difference between the number of births and the number of deaths. The *total increase* adds the effect of migration into and out of the area. Since data are regularly collected on births, deaths, and migration, no new data collection is needed.

The effect of births is evaluated through the fertility rate. This rate uses the number of women in the childbearing ages rather than the total population as the denominator (see Table 6-2) and adjusts for the proportion of women in the relevant age group. Fertility rates vary around the world. For example, the fertility rate ranged from 8.0 in Kenya to 1.4 in Denmark and West Germany, with a rate of 1.8 in the United States (Population Reference Bureau, 1984).

The effect of deaths is evaluated through the crude death rate for the area. Death rates follow a pattern similar to births with lower rates in industrialized countries and higher rates in less developed countries. The rates vary from 28 per 1000 in Gambia to 3 per 1000 in Kuwait. The United States rate is 9 per 1000 (Population Reference Bureau, 1984). In addition to the usual factors affecting births and deaths, the number of births or deaths in an area can be influenced by natural and human-made events. Natural disasters such as drought, earthquakes, and famines can drastically increase the number of deaths in an area. Wars also introduce changes in fertility and death rate patterns. Death rates increase among young men and, depending on the nature of the war, may increase across the entire population. On the other hand, fertility rates tend to increase when order is restored.

Migration is a change of residence in which a boundary of some type is crossed. Examples of this are movement from one country to another or from one region to another (e.g., from north to south). Migration can be described as *immigration*, moving into an area, or *emigration*, moving out of an area. When large migrations occur, there can be serious consequences for both the area left behind and the new home. If many young people emigrate, it may deplete the human resources needed for production. On the other side, immigration of large numbers of persons into one area may create crowded substandard living conditions and low wages, which could lead to health and social problems.

Some general statements can be made about the relationship between births and deaths. Countries at different stages of development have populations that represent different rates of fertility and death. In countries at an early stage of development, there is a high fertility rate and a high death rate. In countries where industrialization is beginning to occur and there are improved health services, death rates tend to decrease while birth rates stay high. Kenya is a country where the death rate has decreased (13 per 1000) while the fertility rate continues to be high (8.0) (Population Reference Bureau, 1984). Historically, as countries have continued to develop, the fertility rate has decreased.

Another way of characterizing the population of an area is the *dependency ratio*. This is the relationship between the number of potentially self-supporting persons (usually ages fifteen to sixty-four) and those older and younger. Dependency ratios tend to be higher in developing countries than in industrialized countries. This means that a smaller proportion of people is providing for the needs of persons in developing countries than in industrialized countries. In developed countries, increases in longevity have been offset by decreases in fertility, thereby maintaining a favorable dependency ratio.

Cross-Sectional Studies

Cross-sectional studies are also characterized as observational studies. They describe the distribution of health characteristics in populations and the associations of the health characteristics with other variables (Slome et al, 1982). These studies can also be called *prevalence* studies, because all cases of the disease (both old and new) are noted.

The cross-sectional method usually addresses a sample rather than the total population. Data are collected and the presence or absence of disease is determined. Information is collected on other variables believed to be related to the condition of interest. For analysis, the population is usually divided according to suspected predisposing factors, and comparisons are made among subgroups. These types of studies develop associations, thereby generating hypotheses. However, they do not tell us *why* health differentials exist.

An example of a cross-sectional method is a study conducted in California to explore the relationships between lung function and pollution levels (Detels et al, 1979). Data from residents were collected through physical examinations and a survey of health behaviors. Residents were categorized as living in low or high pollution areas. Initial results suggested there was a relationship between pollution level and lung function, especially among residents with long-term exposure. However, when smoking and other factors were introduced, the effects of pollution were decreased.

Case Control Studies

The case control method also examines the relationship of existing conditions to other factors. Individuals are selected who have the condition. Other persons who do not have the condition but are similar to the cases on factors believed to be relevant to the disease are selected as "controls." The two groups are *not* matched on the particular factor that is hypothesized to be related to the condition. Case control studies are *retrospective* studies, since the existence of the disease has been documented before the study begins.

The case control studies are easy and relatively inexpensive to conduct. They are useful when the disease is rare or when resources for other types of studies are not available. The choice of an appropriate control group is crucial to this type of study but is frequently problematic. Case control studies are usually the first approach to testing hypotheses before more expensive incidence studies are conducted.

Case control studies have been used with conditions of interest to community health nurses. In a case control study of accidental childhood poisoning, cases admitted to a hospital were compared with community controls and hospital controls matched for sex and age (Basavarj & Forster, 1982). Being in a family with four or more children was significantly associated with the cases. Behavioral factors significant for the cases and not the controls were roughness, aggressiveness, noisiness, and pica.

Cohort Studies

The cohort method looks more directly at factors related to the development of a health condition. It establishes time relationships between presumed antecedents and effects. These are *prospective* studies, which start with a population that does not have the condition and follows them across time. As time passes, the cohort is divided into subgroups according to the presence or absence of the condition. Cohorts may be obtained in several ways. A birth cohort includes all persons born at a certain time, usually within certain years. Sometimes special exposure cohorts are studied—for example, all Vietnam veterans exposed to "Agent Orange."

The cohort method is the most potent method available for use in analytic epidemiology. It not only provides cause and effect information but reduces biases that confound results of other study methods. Information on the health state comes from objective classification rather than selective recall. However, the length of time required for cohort studies creates some disadvantages. The long time period required for these studies means results are achieved slowly and the studies are very expensive. Despite follow-up, there will be some loss of participants. This type of study is not appropriate for rare events because few persons will ever manifest the condition. Despite these problems, cohort studies remain the most powerful strategy to be used in epidemiology.

Factors related to the health of newborns are especially amenable to study by the cohort method. A birth cohort study of neonatal mortality was conducted in Utah (Woolley, Schuman, & Lyon, 1982). The cohort consisted of all births for a six-month period. Membership in the Mormon church served as a proxy for parental health practices. A high level of activity in the Mormon church was shown to be significantly related to lower neonatal mortality rates. This suggests the parental health practices of Mormons active in the church lead to healthier babies.

Experimental Studies

In an experimental study the researcher studies the impact of some factor that has been manipulated.

The outcome is compared to outcomes for a control group where the factor has not been altered. Experimental studies are useful in establishing causal relationships. For example, fluorides can be added to drinking water and the rate of dental caries in the population after an appropriate time period compared to the rate in a population with unfluoridated water. If the rate decreases among the population with fluoridated water, a causal relationship can be said to exist. Although experimental studies in epidemiology are primarily concerned with measures to *prevent* health problems, ethical issues may arise. If a researcher sincerely believes treatment would reduce the incidence of disease, it is difficult to justify withholding treatments to maintain the scientific rigor of a study. In some situations data are collected from experimental studies, analyzed sequentially, and the experiment terminated as soon as statistically significant results are achieved. If the treatment is shown to be beneficial, it can then also be given to the control group.

In some circumstances, conditions may create opportunities for natural experiments. In the case of fluoridation it was possible to compare the rates of dental caries in areas that were similar but had naturally different concentrations of fluorides in the water.

Epidemiology and Community Health Nursing

The community health nurse has many opportunities to use the epidemiologic process. In fact, epidemiology plays a central role in every phase of the community health nursing process—assessment, nursing diagnosis, planning, implementation, and evaluation. Delivering care to families, aggregates, and communities can also assist the nurse in contributing to the epidemiologic research of others. This contribution "may range from iden-

tifying situations requiring further investigation or research . . . to full involvement as a specially employed team member at all stages of a study" (Barnard, 1982, p. 175).

The nurse uses epidemiology in assessment by identifying population characteristics such as age, sex, race, income, education, and life-style, and relating them to the distribution of health status. Birth rates, death rates, morbidity, and other measures derived from vital statistics are also important tools of community assessment (see Chapter 9). From a thorough assessment, the community health nurse can begin to identify specific problems (nursing diagnoses) in need of nursing intervention, and can help identify the target populations that merit further investigation.

In nursing diagnosis and planning the community health nurse uses epidemiologic concepts to (1) analyze the data on the distribution patterns of health and illness in the community or client population; (2) identify areas and factors of risk as well as behaviors that promote health; (3) identify populations at risk that will be the source of cases for nursing intervention; and (4) identify appropriate nursing measures that will achieve specified goals for the client population.

Using epidemiology to study the characteristics of the population can help the nurse to choose implementation strategies that will be most readily accepted by the client families and aggregates. The nurse supplements epidemiologic data with personal observations of the nature, style, and behavior patterns of community members.

Epidemiologic analysis is an important means of evaluating the effectiveness of health promotion programs and other community health nursing measures. By keeping meticulous records on all health problems and preparing reports, the community health nurse contributes to a broader perspective on the status of health and disease in the community and on the effectiveness of existing community health programs.

Examples of the contributions of epidemiology to the analysis of community health abound in both the professional literature and the public press. In the field of communicable diseases, for example, where the epidemiologic model of host-agent-environment seems to fit most neatly, the monitoring of sexually transmitted diseases such as gonorrhea and herpes is common practice in public health agencies. A recently discovered health problem that is often sexually transmitted is the acquired immune deficiency syndrome (AIDS). AIDS has become a major focus of attention for both health professionals and the lay public. The problem of AIDS is a highly charged issue in part because of the controversy surrounding the major population at risk (homosexual men), because of the particularly devastating nature of the diseases known as AIDS-related conditions (ARC); and because of the medically baffling nature of the syndrome itself. Although a specific agent (human T-cell lymphotropic virus, Type III, or HTLV-III) seems to have been identified, medical research is still some distance away from either curative treatment or preventive vaccination.

The epidemiologic process has been instrumental in identifying population characteristics associated with the incidence of AIDS such as life-style, gender, and specific medical conditions. In the absence of definitive medical interventions, AIDS can be seen as primarily a nursing problem, one in which community health nurses have played and will continue to play a central role. Community outreach, preventive education, and identification and coordination of services and resources are all activities for which community health nurses are uniquely qualified. The information provided by the epidemiologic process is crucial to the nurse's ability to provide these services.

Community health nurses can also use epidemiologic concepts with school populations. Student health records contain information that assists the nurse in identifying potential problems. For example, determining the immunization levels among the different age groups facilitates identification of classrooms most susceptible to outbreaks of communicable disease. Action can then be taken to increase immunization levels in the classroom. Nurses have also helped to study the incidence of injuries in schools and school districts, with the aim of identifying school characteristics that are potentially important to the injury rate of individual schools (Boyce, 1984).

Epidemiology, and specifically behavioral epidemiology, can be used to study not only disease in populations but also health-promoting life-styles. *Behavioral epidemiology* is "the identification of behaviors that are causally linked to disease" (Mason & Powell, 1985). The Centers for Disease Control conducted a Workshop on Epidemiologic and Pub-

Case Example 6-1: Epidemiologic Process

Alice Miller, a community health nurse in northern Indiana is concerned about what appears to be a large number of deaths from coronary heart disease (CHD) among middle-aged men in the county. To learn more about the potential problem, she reviews the vital statistics to determine the sex- and age-specific death rate for CHD in the county. She compares the rate to the state rate, which is considerably smaller.

Rates are compared to determine magnitude of the problem.

Ms. Miller uses other existing data to learn more about the nature of the problem. In the search for the reasons for the higher death rates, she compares these data to similar data from adjacent counties and the state. She uses census data to obtain demographic information on the men in the county population. She collects data on race, ethnic background, occupation, marital status, educational level, and other factors of interest. The men are predominantly of Eastern European backgrounds and work in management. As much as possible, she notes characteristics of the county, such as degree of urbanization, type of employers, unemployment rate, crime rates, and health care resources. The data reveal a very high unemployment rate in this county.

The population at risk (person) is described.

The location (place) of the problem is described.

Comparison of local area population characteristics to the larger area population characteristics identifies difference between the two groups. Factors where there are differences suggest relationships and possible intervention points. Research has shown linkages between unemployment and morbidity and mortality. In addition, literature and research on life-style of Eastern Europeans should be reviewed.

Further research is needed to establish cause.

Ms. Miller decides to develop stress reduction programs aimed at men who might be concerned about unemployment. In addition, she initiates a more general program for the whole family directed at life-style practices that are related to CHD.

Intervention based on the data.

lic Health Aspects of Physical Activity and Exercise in September 1984 to explore the connections between physical activity and public health. This line of research is a most appropriate one for community health nurses, since it supports nursing's philosophical focus on wellness and health promotion.

Summary

If the focus of community health nurses is to be on public health, it is essential that they concern themselves with the aggregate problems of the community (Williams, 1977). Epidemiologic concepts and measures provide the analytical tools that community health nurses need to study the community as a whole, evaluate its health status, identify health problems and populations at risk, and implement strategies that address those health problems.

Study Questions

1. Rates are a basic element of epidemiology. When should crude rates, rather than specific rates, be used?
    a. International comparisons and in small population areas
    b. Comparisons across time
    c. Comparisons across communities
    d. None of the above
2. What kind of epidemiologic study would be appropriate to test hypotheses regarding factors related to AIDS?
    a. Descriptive
    b. Case control
    c. Cohort
    d. Experimental
3. In an upper-class suburban community (population 10,000) adjacent to a large metropolitan area, seven children ages 5 and 6 who live in the same neighborhood have developed leukemia in the past year. Using the epidemiologic approach, what is the first step the community health nurse should take?
    a. Institute a search for toxic waste disposal sites
    b. Develop a program for the families
    c. Compare the cause-specific rates to rates in other areas
    d. Design a cohort study to determine the cause
4. Health and vital statistics vary greatly in their reliability, completeness of reporting, and standardization. Which of the following would provide the most accurate information?
    a. Communicable disease reports
    b. Death and birth reports
    c. Morbidity reports
    d. All of the above
5. There appears to be a decrease in the mortality rates from coronary heart disease over the past thirty years. Although this may be a true decrease, what other factors could affect the number of cases reported?
    a. Changes in medical technology
    b. Changes in diagnostic classifications
    c. Use of single cause on death certificates
    d. All of the above

References

Barnard JM: The occupational health nurse's contribution to epidemiology. *Scan J Work Environ Health* 1982; 8 (Suppl 1): 172–175.

Basavarj DS, Forster DP: Accidental poisoning in young children. *J Epidemiol Community Health* 36: 31–34.

Basco D et al: Epidemiologic analysis in school populations as a basis for change in school nurse practice—Report of the second phase of a longitudinal study. *Am J Public Health* 1972; 62(4): 491–497.

Berkel J, deWaard F: Mortality pattern and life expectancy of Seventh-Day Adventists in the Netherlands. *Int J Epidemiol* 1983; 12(4): 455–459.

Blotcky AD, Tittler BI: Psychosocial predictors of physical illness: Toward a holistic model of health. *Prev Med* 1982; 11: 602–611.

Boyce WT et al: Epidemiology of injuries in a large urban school district. *Pediatrics* 1984; 74: 342–349.

Caprio RJ, Margulis HL, Joselow MM: Lead absorption in children and its relationship to urban traffic densities. *Arch Environ Health* 1974; 28: 195–197.

Cleary PD, Mechanic D, Greenley JR: Sex differences in medical care utilization: An empirical investigation. *J Health Soc Behav* 1982; 23: 106–119.

Cohen JB, Brody JA: The epidemiologic importance of psychosocial factors in longevity. *Am J Epidemiol* 1981; 114(4): 451–461.

Detels R et al: The UCLA population studies of chronic obstructive respiratory disease. I. Methodology and comparison of lung functions in areas of high and low pollution. *Am J Epidemiol* 1979; 109(1): 33–58.

Dowdle WR: The epidemiology of AIDS. *Public Health Reports* (July–August) 1983; 98(4): 308–312.

Fingerhut LA, Wilson RW, Feldman JJ: Health and disease in the United States. *Annu Rev Public Health* 1980; 1: 1–36.

Friedman GD: *Primer of Epidemiology*, 2nd ed. New York: McGraw-Hill, 1980.

Garcia-Palmeri MR et al: Urban-rural differences in coronary heart disease in a low incidence area. *Am J Epidemiol* 1978; 107(3): 206–215.

Graunt J: *Natural and Political Observations Made upon the Bills of Mortality.* London, 1662. In: MacMahon B, Pugh TF (editors), *Epidemiology: Principles and Methods.* Boston: Little, Brown, 1970.

Hartford RB: The case of the elusive infant mortality rate. *Population Today* 1984; 12(5): 6–7.

Haw MA: Women work and stress: A review and agenda for the future. *J Health Soc Behav* 1982; 23: 132–144.

Hetherington EM: Divorce, a child's perspective. *Am Psychol* 1979; 34: 851–888.

MacMahon B, Pugh TF: *Epidemiology: Principles and Methods*. Boston: Little, Brown, 1970.

Mason JO, Powell KE: Physical activity, behavioral epidemiology, and public health (editorial). *Public Health Reports* (March–April) 1985; 100(2): 113–115.

Mason SF: *A History of the Sciences*. New York: Collier Books, 1962.

Mausner JS, Bahn AK: *Epidemiology: An Introductory Text*. Philadelphia: Saunders, 1974.

Moore MJ: *Perspectives on American Fertility*. Current population reports, Special reports, Series P-23, No. 70. US Government Printing Office, 1978.

NCHS: *Vital Statistics of the United States, Vol. II—Mortality, Part A, 1977*. DHSS Publication No. (PHS) 81-1101. Hyattsville, Md.: Author, 1980.

Park RE, Burgess EW: *The city*. Chicago: University of Chicago Press, 1925.

Population Reference Bureau: *1984 World Population Data Sheet*. Washington, D.C.: Author, 1984.

Slome C et al: *Basic Epidemiological Methods and Biostatistics: A Workbook*. Monterey, Calif.: Brooks/Cole, 1982.

Snow J: *On the Mode of Communication of Cholera*, 2nd ed. London: Churchill, 1855. In: MacMahon B, Pugh T (editors), *Epidemiology: Principles and Methods*. Boston: Little, Brown, 1970.

Stolley PD: Lung cancer in women—five years later, situation worse. *N Engl J Med* 1983; 309(7): 128–129.

Terris M: Desegregating health statistics. *Am J Public Health* 1973; 63(6): 477–480.

U.S. Bureau of the Census: *State and Metropolitan Area Data Book, 1982*. Washington, D.C.: US Government Printing Office, 1982.

U.S. Bureau of the Census: *Statistical Abstract of the United States, 1981*, 102nd ed. Washington, D.C.: US Government Printing Office, 1981.

Williams CA: Community health nursing—What is it? *Nurs Outlook* 1977; 25: 250–254.

Woodham-Smith C: *Florence Nightingale 1820–1900*. London: Constable, 1950.

Woolley FR, Schuman KL, Lyon JL: Neonatal mortality in Utah. *Am J Epidemiol* 1982; 116(8): 541–546.

World Health Organization: Constitution of the World Health Organization, 1948. In: *Basic Documents*, 15th ed. Geneva: WHO, 1964.

World Health Organization: *International Classification of Disease*, 9th rev. Geneva: Author, 1978.

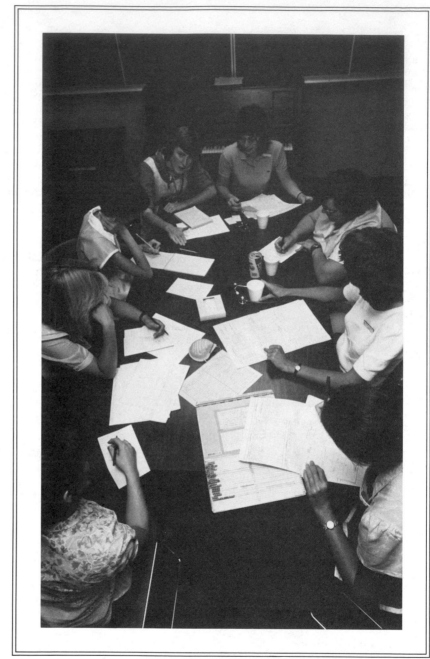

William Thompson

"Consumers generally perceive nurses as friends and allies who are supportive and caring in their struggle to maintain some control over their own health status. Because of this, nursing—in addition to providing services—can often serve as a bridge between consumers and other providers." (Edwards LH: Health planning: Opportunities for nurses. Nursing Outlook *(Nov/Dec) 1983; 31(6): 323.)*

2 The Community Health Nursing Process

Chapter 7

The Nursing Process
in Community Health

Wealtha M. Alex and Carol G. Klint

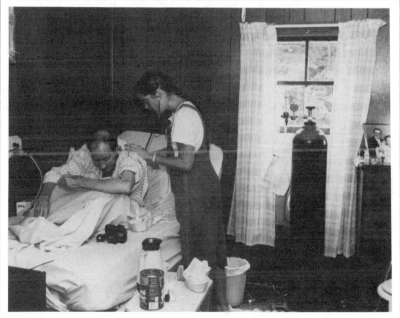

Gabrielle Beasley

*Clients in the community retain more autonomy than those entering
the hospital. Preventive services as well as continuing care are
matters of choice and availability.*

**Chapter
Outline**

**Chapter
Objectives**

After completing this chapter, the reader will be able to:

- Identify similarities and differences between use of the nursing process in hospital and community settings
- Explain why the nursing process is a valuable method of practicing community health nursing
- Describe how each component of the nursing process is applied in community health nursing practice
- State how the nursing process was used in a community nursing case study

This chapter will provide an overview of the nursing process as used in community health nursing. The nursing process provides a systematic foundation for practice that links community nursing to other nursing specialties and settings.

Using the nursing process in community nursing is essential because: (1) The nursing process is endorsed by professional nursing for use in all nursing specialties; as indicated by Barkauskas in Chapter 1, the *Standards: Community Health Nursing Practice* (American Nurses' Association, 1973) are built on the components of the nursing process. (2) The nursing process is a common framework for care delivery on the three client levels: individuals, families, and communities. (3) The nursing process provides an anchor for practice amid the flux and controversy of contemporary community health nursing practice. (4) The nursing process bridges theory and practice. Although the nursing process provides a general framework for practice, judgment about what to do with specific clients comes with experience based on the application of the theory. As a systematic intellectual endeavor, the nursing process replaces the idea that nursing is done by tradition, habit, intuition, or common sense.

Since nurses have been exposed to the process as applied in a hospital setting, this chapter begins with a comparison that differentiates its application in community settings. Then the components of the process: assessment, diagnosis, planning, implementation, and evaluation are discussed in terms of their application to community health nursing.

Comparing the Nursing Process in the Hospital and the Community

Table 7-1 compares variables affecting nursing practice in hospital and community settings. Suggestions are given for applying the nursing process in the community. Though comparisons in the table are simplistic, the generalizations are intended to help readers adapt the nursing process from the hospital to the community.

The following common variables influence the application of the nursing process in both settings: the client, client health state, client autonomy, goal of health care, nature of nursing care, client outcome, physician influence on nursing care delivery, and payment for nursing care. They appear in the left column of Table 7-1, and each is discussed briefly here.

The Client

One of the first decisions to make when using the nursing process in the community is to identify the client. Community health nursing emphasizes care of the family and community groups, because many of the problems nurses encounter are best solved by family and/or community action. Facilitating family and community action is done most effectively when the family or community is viewed as larger systems that can affect individuals' health behaviors.

Client Health State

Since client health state in the community ranges from terminal illness to optimal health, community nursing requires a broad knowledge of health and disease, including health promotion, disease prevention, and rehabilitation. Clients' perception of health and illness, self-care practices, and use of traditional (folk) as well as biomedical systems of health will help to determine their health status.

(text continued on p. 160)

Table 7-1   The Influence of Setting on Use of the Nursing Process in Community Nursing

Variable	Hospital Setting	Community Setting	Nursing Process in the Community
Client	Individual	Individual, family, community	Identify the client before proceeding through process. Apply theory to the process based on client selection. Look for relationships between individual, family, and community clients.
Client health state	Acutely ill	Ranges from optimal wellness to severe illness. Diverse chronic health conditions among clients.	Draw upon broad knowledge of health and disease.
Client autonomy	Limited due to institutionalization. Consent to hospitalization implies consent to nursing services.	Retains autonomy. Client may not have asked for or consented to nursing service.	Obtain client consent to interact before beginning the process.
Goal of health care	Institutional goal is treatment and recovery of acute illness. Nursing care goals collaborate or compete with medical care goal of institution. Less client input into goal setting.	Goal of community health is prevention. Prevention ranges from health promotion to rehabilitation. Nursing care competes with non-health-related goals of clients and institutions. Client goal-setting imperative.	Recognize that the process competes with other client-related interests. Tailor the content of the process to compete favorably with other interests by providing care the client wants. Use the process to personalize the reasons for and benefits of prevention, since the value of prevention is not always self-evident. The concept of prevention is addressed during each component of the process.

Table 7-1 *(continued)*

Variable	Hospital Setting	Community Setting	Nursing Process in the Community
Nature of nursing care	Predictable client population segregated by disease entity and/or age. Responsibility for planning nursing care is rotated with nursing staff assignment. Care provided directly by nurse or delegated to auxiliary nursing personnel (i.e., social worker, chaplain, etc.) and is facilitated by institutionalization.	Diverse client population. One nurse usually responsible for care planning because nursing staff assignments are not rotated. Care provided indirectly through others. Coordination of care via multiple institutions and resources. Work with health- and nonhealth-related personnel.	Review references frequently and consult with resource people in order to apply theory to the process. Generalist practice requires a broad theory base. Work with and through others. Identify client strengths.
Client outcomes	Nursing care results are more readily observable to client, nurse, and others.	Nursing care results are less apparent to client, family, and coworkers.	Involve the client in documenting goal achievement. Break long-term goals into small steps. Reinforce client progress by recognizing small steps toward goal.
Physician influence on nursing care delivery	Influence is direct (i.e., medical diagnosis and treatment orders provide the framework for many nursing activities). Hospital admissions (by physicians) dictate caseload. Physicians more readily available. Each patient has a physician.	Influence is less direct but remains substantial since clients may refuse nursing care because their physician did not recommend it. Nurse has more control over caseload. Physician is less available. Some clients do not have a physician.	Recognize that many clients view the physician as the decision-maker for any health-related problem or concern for which they seek professional care. Use the state's nurse practice act as a guide for deciding which services require physician collaboration. Decide who does and does not need nursing (admit to caseload) as a part of nursing diagnosis. Screening for disease and physician referral is a necessary part of the community nurse role.

(continued)

Table 7-1 *(continued)*

Variable	Hospital Setting	Community Setting	Nursing Process in the Community
Payment for nursing care	Nursing care is frequently an unidentified part of the hospital bill. Insurance covers hospital nursing care. Clients have little control of expenditures for nursing.	Service costs and funding are unknown to most clients. Insurance payment for community nursing services other than home health care is rare. Clients have more control of expenditures for nursing care, especially services not paid by insurance or public funds. Out-of-pocket payment is difficult to obtain because the public has little experience shopping for nursing care. The cost-benefit ratio of nursing service is largely unknown. Payment sources greatly influence care delivery.	Use the nursing process to market nursing so as to explain nursing as a way to mutually resolve client health problems and concerns. Name nursing services and point out the benefits of nursing care to clients. Consider the cost-benefit ratio of nursing services for all clients. Recognize that efficient client progress is extremely important since funding sources help decide whether the service is worth the cost. The nursing process facilitates efficient, effective, nursing practice. Be alert to recognize how payment sources influence care delivery.

SOURCE:
Selected ideas comparing settings from Helvie CO, Hill AE, Bambino CF: The setting and nursing practice. *Nurs Outlook* 1968; 16: 27–29.

Client Autonomy

Clients in the community retain more of their autonomy or self-determination whereas people entering the hospital tend to assume that nurses will care for them and that insurance will help pay for nursing service costs. Persons in the community also may not have asked for or consented to nursing service, as in the case of a person named as contact for a sexually transmitted disease.

Factors such as travel time, cost, client availability, agency, or program mandates all influence client autonomy. For example, regarding cost, an elderly community resident with congestive heart failure and diabetes might need health promotion nursing services but may decide not to seek such services if she must pay for such services out-of-pocket because they are not paid for by Medicare. (Medicare generally does not reimburse health promotion types of health care costs.) Thus the client exercises her autonomy in choosing not to pay for services she needs.

Goal of Health Care

The health care goals of the hospital and community differ in their primary focus. Hospitals exist to treat acute illness; the goal of community health is prevention. The need for nursing care is usually self-evident to the hospitalized client, but clients in the community may be unsure whether they need or want nursing service, especially preventive care. The nursing process may be used, therefore, as a strategy to market nursing. Nurses can explain to clients how they will work with them to help them solve or prevent health problems. They can personalize the reasons for and benefits of prevention.

Nature of Nursing Care

Nursing in hospital and community settings differs according to the way nursing care is planned, coordinated, and delivered. In hospital settings, responsibility for care planning may be rotated among staff (except in institutions with primary nursing). Community nurses usually do not share care planning with other nurses. Coordination of care in hospitals involves relating directly to other hospital personnel, whereas coordination of care in the community is frequently done by phoning or sending letters to persons outside the agency. Geographic distance, agency turf, and confidentiality requirements complicate this collaboration. Nursing care in hospitals is done by nurses themselves or auxiliary nursing personnel. In the community, nursing is frequently provided indirectly through others. For instance, a community health nurse may teach one family member to provide self-care or various family members to provide health care to other family members, such as when a mother is taught how to institute positive life-style changes for the whole family through institution of good dietary practices, and when a daughter is taught to give insulin injections to her sick mother.

Community nurses are more dependent on client participation during the nursing process than are hospital nurses. For example, clients must be willing to keep an accurate twenty-four-hour diet record if the nurse is to be able to analyze the diet, whereas hospital nurses can check meal tray contents. Since much of community nursing involves fostering client self-care, community nurses must

identify client strengths. Client strengths provide the energy and resources to tackle health problems.

Client Outcomes

Community client outcomes attributable to nursing care may be less apparent than are hospital client outcomes, because disease entities are usually in less acute stages and client improvement may occur more slowly in the community. Sometimes the nursing care goal is simply to maintain health or slow its deterioration. Thus it is important to involve the clients in documenting goal achievement. This means showing the client what to monitor and how to interpret results. For example, to improve diabetes control, the nurse teaches the diabetic client how to do home monitoring of blood glucose and helps the client relate blood sugar results to a factor such as diet. Since client change is gradual, it is important to break long-term goals into small steps. Feedback on the progress helps motivate self-care.

Physician Influence on Nursing Care Delivery

Physicians exert influence on nursing care delivery in both hospital and community settings. This influence is less direct in community settings. The nurse has more control over the management of client caseloads, whereas the physician's influence is more direct in the hospital setting. Physicians also influence the formulation of health policies and laws that affect the delivery of health care in hospitals and community agencies. Collaboration among health professionals is a legal and practical necessity for dealing effectively with client situations.

Payment for Nursing Care

Whether in hospital or community settings, nursing services are rarely itemized and are usually reimbursed indirectly by a third party, such as through insurance or public funds. Insurance payment for nursing is usually limited to disease-related care; public funds for health promotion and disease prevention nursing services are largely controlled by health departments. There are few community health nurse entrepreneurs, in part because their clients must pay for most care out-of-pocket. Obtaining direct payment is difficult because clients are unfamiliar with the cost-benefit ratio of specific nursing services such as, for example, the worth of having a nurse teach family planning.

By describing the nursing process to clients, nurses can market nursing care as a way to mutually identify and resolve client health problems and concerns. Sharing assessment information, validating nursing diagnosis, involving clients in goal setting, implementing care, and evaluating its success are all ways of fostering client self-responsibility and teaching people what nursing is and does. Having an understanding of nursing is crucial if people are to consider buying community nursing services as an alternative to other health care services.

Components of the Nursing Process

Assessment

The goal of assessment in community health nursing is to collect information to identify accurately the existing or potential health problems of individuals, families, or communities.

Community health nurses tap data sources used by other nursing specialties, but they are also more likely than nurses in other clinical areas to obtain information from referrals and community residents. Examples of data sources for individual assessment are self-reports, family perceptions of the individual's health behavior, and nursing observation of self-care. Data sources for family assessment include nurse observation of the home and family interaction. Information about the community is gleaned from interviewing key community residents, attending health-related community events, and using statistical data from the local health planning agency.

Methods for data collection are:

- *Interaction*—interviewing
- *Observation*—use of the senses of sight, touch, hearing, smell, and taste
- *Measurement*—quantifying general observations or using tools to make precise observations (Griffith & Christensen, 1982).

Use of multiple data collection methods during assessment increases the likelihood of an accurate assessment.

Assessment guides are used to collect data needed to practice nursing. Nursing lacks a universal or standardized data collection format such as those used for the medical history and physical examination. A universal assessment guide would be valuable because it would organize data needed to apply any nursing theory and it could be used with any client. Community health nurses would find a universal assessment guide particularly useful because of the variety of client situations and the need to practice at multiple client levels.

Table 7-2 is the product of integrating several community health nursing assessment guides. Gordon's (1982) functional health patterns are named and defined on the left. Examples of data to collect for individual, family, and community assessment are in their respective columns. Table 7-2 shows the similarity of data collection across client levels and presents an overview of data collection for all nursing practice.

When looking at the integrated assessment guide, consider the following:

- Compare Gordon's functional patterns with previously used data collection guides. Look for

(text continued on p. 166)

Table 7-2   An Integrated Individual, Family, Community Assessment Guide

Functional Health Patterns and Definitions[a]	Examples of Data to Collect for Three Client Levels		
	Individual	Family[b]	Community[c]
1. Health Perception-Health Management: Describes client's perceived pattern of health and well-being and how health is managed	Individual's definition of health and illness and his or her level of knowledge Individual's drug habits Individual's self-care practices Use of personal and other resources for health	Family's definition of health and illness and their level of knowledge Family's drug habits Family's self-care practices Medically based preventive measures Dental health practices Use of health resources in the community	Community's definition of and meaning of health; health behaviors for prevention—exercise, nutrition, use of health resources, immunization levels, and hygiene practices; rates for drug abuse, crime, and juvenile delinquency; economic and educational resources; and quality of work opportunities. Management of illness: private and public medical resources; acute and chronic institutions; community support systems—ambulatory services and home care services; consumers' and providers' patterns of responsibility and accountability
2. Nutritional-Metabolic: Describes pattern of food and fluid consumption relative to metabolic need and pattern indicators	Individual dietary practices such as typical diet and meal schedule; medically based measures including condition of teeth and mucous membranes; height and weight	Family dietary practices such as adequacy of family diet; attitudes toward food and mealtimes; shopping and food preparation	Cultural beliefs related to foods; knowledge of nutrition; availability of quality foods and water; cost of nutritional goods relative to other communities
3. Elimination: Describes patterns of excretory function	Care of bowel, bladder, and skin, including presence of prosthesis	Environmental sanitation, including pets and pest control; laundry facilities and hygiene practices	Environmental sanitation such as management of debris, waste disposal, and water drainage

(continued)

Table 7-2 *(continued)*

Functional Health Patterns and Definitions[a]	Examples of Data to Collect for Three Client Levels		
	Individual	Family[b]	Community[c]
4. Activity-Exercise: Describes pattern of exercise, activity, leisure, and recreation	Activities of daily living; mobility status; participation in sports	Family's recreational and leisure-time activities Mobility status	Transportation and recreational resources; mobility status; accommodations for elderly and handicapped
5. Cognitive-Perceptual: Describes sensory and cognitive pattern	Status of special senses (e.g., vision, hearing) Cognitive functional abilities, including decision making, language, and education	Health-related decision making	Educational levels— elementary, secondary, college; pupil-teacher ratio; reading levels; responsiveness of schools to community needs; and opportunities for adult education Health-related decision making
6. Sleep-Rest: Describes patterns of sleep, rest, and relaxation	Usual sleep-wake schedule Perception of ability to sleep and rest	Sleeping and resting practices (e.g., usual sleeping habits); adequacy of beds; appropriateness of sleeping locations of family members	Usual sleep-wake schedule of community Environmental noise
7. Self-Perception/Self-Concept: Describes self-concept and perceptions of self	Attitude toward self, perception of abilities, body image, identity, general sense of worth and emotional pattern	Affective function: Family's need-response patterns, mutual nurturance, closeness, and identification; separateness and connectedness	Community image, status, and sense of "pride" Positive-negative views of community and specific groups; stigmas
8. Role Relationships: Describe pattern of role-engagements and relationships	Current perception of major roles and responsibilities (e.g., satisfaction or dissatisfaction with family, work, or social relationships)	Formal and informal role structure; communication patterns, including characteristics of family communication network and areas of closed communication; socialization patterns (e.g., family child-rearing prac-	Communication patterns: Verbal and nonverbal to outsiders; network within community (e.g., newspapers, government officials, and politicians). Relationships: Social patterns, openness and attitudes toward

Table 7-2 *(continued)*

Functional Health Patterns and Definitions[a]	Examples of Data to Collect for Three Client Levels		
	Individual	*Family[b]*	*Community[c]*
		tices); family's associations and transactions with the community	strangers, evidence of level of trust, family and community attachment or separation, and inclusion of elderly in community affairs
9. Sexuality-Reproductive: Describes client's patterns of satisfaction with sexuality pattern; describes reproductive patterns	Pattern of sexual activity; fertility	Sex education of children; contraception practices	Prevailing views of male-female roles; relatedness between sexes; acceptance of sexuality in young and old; birth rate; contraceptive practices
10. Coping-Stress: Describes general coping pattern and effectiveness of the pattern in terms of stress tolerance	Recognition of personal stressors; stress management abilities and resources	Family social support network; family coping abilities; functional and dysfunctional coping strategies (present and past)	Support systems—family, churches, health agencies, senior citizen centers, peers, volunteers, government; information centers (e.g., political, economic, health, recreational, and religious); community stressors (e.g., crime, inadequate housing, absent landlords, and poor self-image; ways of dealing with stressors (e.g., community organizations, newsletters, denial, and hopelessness); resources such as mental health centers, churches, and support groups

(continued)

Table 7-2 *(continued)*

Functional Health Patterns and Definitions[a]	*Examples of Data to Collect for Three Client Levels*		
	Individual	*Family[b]*	*Community[c]*
11. Value-Belief: Describes patterns of values, beliefs (including spiritual), or goals that guide choices or decisions	Personal values, goals, and beliefs that influence outlook on life and decision making	Cultural (ethnic) and religious orientation, (e.g., stated ethnicity and religious preference); dietary habits; dress, home decor. Family values regarding health, education, religion, and cleanliness	Community value system (e.g., political affiliations, religious influence, and community support of the "less fortunate")

SOURCE:
The table is an integration of several nursing assessment guides.
[a] From Gordon M: *Nursing Diagnosis Process and Application*, New York: McGraw-Hill, 1982, p. 81. Copyright 1982 by McGraw-Hill Book Company. Used with permission.
[b] Adapted from Friedman MM: *Family Nursing: Theory and Assessment*, New York: Appleton-Century-Crofts, 1981, pp. 312–313. Copyright 1982 by Appleton-Century-Crofts. Used with permission.
[c] Adapted from Lunney M: A framework to analyze a taxonomy of nursing diagnoses. In Kim MJ, McFarland GK, McLane AM (editors), *Classification of Nursing Diagnosis: Proceedings of the Fifth National Conference*, St. Louis: Mosby, 1984, p. 407. Copyright 1984 by C. V. Mosby Co. Used with permission.

relationships between past knowledge and new content.

- Compare family and community data collection information presented in Chapters 8 and 9 of this text to that in Table 7-2. These chapters provide more detailed content on these topics.
- Compare data categories for three client levels within each pattern. An appreciation of similarities across client levels will allow you to recognize important interrelationships between individual, family, and community clients. This recognition of relationships is needed to practice across client levels.
- Include additional and more detailed assessment tools in specific categories as needed. Gordon's patterns and definitions are fairly broad. More specific information may be needed. For example, if a sexual history is required because of client difficulties in this area, a detailed sexual history assessment guide can be incorporated into the ninth section, entitled "Sexuality-Reproductive." Knowing where to fit more detailed tools in the assessment guide enables the nurse to obtain comprehensive data as well as to organize data collection for all client levels and nursing specialties.

- Although community health nurses work across client levels, they usually select either a family or community client focus at any given time. Thus, Table 7-2 would not be used to assess all client levels simultaneously. Also, since the integrated guide is quite comprehensive, a screening approach would be more useful in practice to identify problematic functional patterns. More detailed investigation of these pattern areas may require additional data collection beyond the examples in the Integrated Assessment Guide.

Diagnosis

The purpose of nursing diagnosis in community health nursing is to reach accurate conclusions about the health status of individuals, families, and communities. These conclusions are based on the data collected during the assessment phase of the nursing process.

The importance of nursing diagnosis in nursing practice is confirmed by its inclusion in professional and societal practice mandates. Nursing is defined in the American Nurses' Association's *Social Policy Statement* (1980, p. 9) as "the diagnosis and treatment of human responses to actual or potential health problems." Note the centrality of diagnosis to the definition of nursing. Nursing diagnosis is included in the practice standards for nursing specialties, including *Standards: Community Health Nursing Practice* (American Nurses' Association, 1973) and in many state nursing practice acts. Nursing diagnosis is a crucial point in the nursing process, because it summarizes and interprets assessment data and forms the basis for nursing intervention. If the nursing profession is to realize its definition of nursing, individual nurses must assume the role of diagnostician as well as the roles of advocate, teacher, caregiver, assessor, planner, manager, coordinator, protector, comforter, healer, counselor, communicator, and rehabilitator (Mallick, 1983).

The role of diagnostician should be a primary rather than a secondary nursing role for two reasons. First, the profession has accepted the nursing process (which includes nursing diagnosis) as the foundation of nursing practice. Second, for nurses to be able to perform independent nursing activities, they must be able to make nursing diagnoses that are relevant to nursing care and distinct from those made by other health professionals (Mallick, 1983). Community health nursing practice necessitates identification of the nursing role in varied client situations and the ability to perform competently and comfortably in independent nursing activities.

Diagnosis has always been a part of nursing practice, but professional activity related to nursing diagnosis increased dramatically during the last decade. Its application to community health nursing is introduced in this section and developed more fully in Chapter 10.

There are multiple definitions of nursing diagnosis. Some definitions describe the act of diagnosing and other definitions refer to the conclusion reached. One author's description of the act of diagnosing is "to store in memory a 'template' for each diagnosis, to search the patient for as much information as possible, and to match the signs and symptoms with the template in the memory. The diagnosis is that . . . which best matches the data" (Mallick, 1983, p. 457). One definition of nursing diagnosis as a conclusion is "a clear, concise, and definitive statement of the client's health status and concerns that can be affected by nursing intervention" (Griffith & Christensen, 1982, p. 111). This definition does not limit nursing diagnosis to problematic or potentially problematic conditions but can include health promotion and disease prevention concerns that are important in community health nursing.

Although "client" refers to individuals, families, and communities, it is particularly useful to clarify what is meant by family and community nursing diagnoses. A family nursing diagnosis refers to problems or concerns experienced by the family as a whole or by at least two of its members. Common family health problems are parenting, role conflicts or role change problems, affectional problems, lack of preventive health care, and inadequate nutritional, sleeping, or cleanliness patterns (Friedman, 1981).

Hamilton (1983) states that the distinguishing feature of a community nursing diagnosis is the implied idea of the community as the direct client or recipient of care. Diagnoses derived from thinking of the community as the direct client reflect (1) assessment of the community as a physical, sociocultural, and experiential entity and (2) intervention directed toward instituting change at a community level. Examples of community nursing diagnoses could include increased infant mortality rate related to teenage pregnancies, lack of neighborhood participation in community events related to apathy, and increased number of respiratory diseases related to air pollution (Griffith & Christensen, 1982). When the community is the client, services may ultimately be delivered by working with individuals and families who are viewed, in this instance, as indirect clients. However, the target for the delivery of community health nursing is the community client.

The match between data collected and the signs and symptoms of a likely nursing diagnosis will usually be imperfect; however, it must be close enough to warrant use of the diagnostic label. Nurses seek to make a "best bet" diagnosis. "A best bet diagnosis is that which will be correct in the long run—the diagnosis that will be correct in a large number of cases" (Mallick, 1983, p. 457).

Published nursing diagnosis labels along with their definitions, signs, and symptoms, and possible etiologies are the "templates" nurses can use to make nursing diagnoses. Several lists of nursing diagnoses applicable to community health nursing are included in Chapter 10. Although published nursing diagnoses are imperfect and incomplete, they offer the novice diagnostician in community health nursing a legitimate place to start. Current nursing diagnoses will change, but skill in using existing nursing diagnoses will enhance the reader's ability to use future nursing diagnoses.

There are few published family or community nursing diagnoses. Health promotion and disease prevention nursing diagnoses are almost nonexistent in current classification systems. Consequently, community health nurses frequently need to develop their own diagnosis. Nursing diagnosis for the family and community will be discussed more fully in Chapter 10.

Planning

Planning "is a future-oriented process in that it lays out an orderly design for reaching a prospective destination" (Broden & Herban, 1976, p. 97), as when a plan of care is designed to resolve client health problems. Planning attempts to anticipate and avoid future problems as well as to solve existing problems. The underlying rationale for planning is to order change. If orderly change occurred naturally, planning would be unnecessary. Ordering change requires a systematic approach and the participation of persons responsible for making the change.

The purpose of planning within the nursing process is to design a system of nursing intervention that will incorporate client input and provide a framework for nursing care evaluation. The planning process consists of

1. Arranging problems by priority
2. Setting goals
3. Writing client-centered objectives
4. Selecting nurse and client intervention strategies
5. Developing plans for evaluation and follow-up

(See Chapter 11 for a detailed presentation of the planning process.)

Client-centered planning in community health nursing is necessary to provide a way for clients to participate in their care, to resolve client health problems effectively and, to teach clients how to problem solve. Including the client in care planning not only helps the client deal with the immediate situation but also enhances future client problem-solving abilities. Werner (1976) asserts that unless families learn independent problem solving, the effect of the nurse is short-lived. Client-nurse planning, therefore, supports effective intervention.

One method to accomplish nurse-client planning is contracting. In community nursing a contract may be defined as any working agreement, continuously renegotiable, between nurse and client. The agreement may be formal or informal, written or verbal, simple or detailed, and it may be signed or unsigned by client or nurse (Sloan & Schommer, 1975).

Sometimes it is helpful to develop a formal written contract. The major advantage of formalizing the contract is to increase the likelihood that both parties understand and agree with the plan. There

Statement of Health Goal: <u>Decreased feelings of stress and tension</u>

I <u>Jim Johnson</u> promise to <u>use progressive relaxation techniques</u>
     (client)

<u>(four-muscle-groups) upon arriving home from work each day</u>
         (client responsibility)

for a period of <u>one week</u>, whereupon, <u>Nancy Turner</u>
                  (nurse)

will provide <u>a copy of Herbert Benson's book, Relaxation Response</u>
         nurse responsibility

on <u>Saturday, March 7th</u> to me.
     (date)

If I do not fulfill the terms of this contract in total, I understand that the designated reward will be withheld.

Signed: *Jim Johnson*
                (client)

           February 2, 1986
                (date)

           Nancy Turner
                (nurse)

           February 2 1986
                (date)

Figure 7-1 Example of a contingency contract (Adapted from Pender NJ: *Health Promotion in Nursing Practice.* Norwalk, Conn.: Appleton-Century-Crofts, 1982, p. 188. Copyright 1982 by Appleton-Century-Crofts. Used with permission.)

are two types of written contracts used in community health nursing: contingency contracts and noncontingency contracts. The major differences between these two is that contingency contracts state a reward to be granted to a client for performance of a specific behavior (Steckel & Swain, 1977) and noncontingency contracts do not mention a reward. Noncontingency contracts reward behavioral change through such means as the positive consequences of the behavioral change itself, such as decreased blood glucose following improved adherence to the diabetic diet. In contingency contracting clients select their own reward, which

may or may not be related to the consequences of behavioral change. For example, an obese client on a weight loss program purchased a special dress after reaching her goal weight in her contingency contract. See Figures 7-1 and 7-2 for examples of a contingency contract and a noncontingency contract.

Contingency and noncontingency contracts require "skill training"—that is, applying general information to the client's own particular environment and social circumstances (Swain & Sterkel, 1981). The nurse and client must discuss long-term and short-term client behavioral goal(s), and set

Contract for Service

1. Goals: M. M. will develop adequate parenting skills

2. Length of contract: Spring semester 1986

3. Client responsibilities: M. M. will read and discuss the pamphlet "You and Your New Baby."

   M. M. will incorporate suggested parenting skills into her daily activities.

4. Nursing responsibilities: Complete B. Caldwell's Assessment Tool, Home Observation for Measurement of the Environment.

   Provide a parenting pamphlet suitable for M. M.

5. Fee determination: Services reimbursed through Title XX grant.

Date: January 14, 1986

Signatures: Mary Mother _____ Client

Nora Nurse _____ Community Nurse

Figure 7-2 An example of a noncontingency contract (Adapted from Sloan MR, Schommer BT: The process of contracting in community nursing. In: Spradley B (editor), *Contemporary Community Nursing*. Boston: Little, Brown, 1975, p. 222. Copyright 1975 by Little, Brown. Used by permission.)

time limits for goal achievement. The contracts must be signed and dated, and the client should be given a copy of the contract.

Differences between contingency and noncontingency contracts are:

- Contingency contracts are developed as a series during successive visits. Noncontingency contracts may outline nurse-client behavior for the expected duration of their relationship.
- Long- and short-term goals may both appear on noncontingency contracts, but a contingency contract contains only one short-term goal. The long-term goal will have been agreed upon by nurse and client, but it is not written in the contract.
- Contingency contracts do not outline nurse

responsibilities unless the client chooses a reward that involves the nurse. Noncontingency contracts usually list nurse and client responsibilities.

- In the literature, contingency contracts were presented as individual contracts, but noncontingency contracts are either individual or family contracts. Specifying which family member(s) are responsible for a behavior and which member(s) are entitled to a reward is imperative for family contracts.

The nurse must exercise judgment in use of contracting as a planning approach. Johnson and Hardin's (1962, p. 101) research cautioned against "uniform rules prescribing how nurses are to behave in households across the board." They state that community health nurses need to be flexible in their contacts with diverse families and households if they are to be effective.

Two problems that impede nurse-client planning or contracting are client apathy and indecision (Dyer, 1973). Client apathy or lack of interest may be due to a client's feelings of hopelessness about the situation, futility due to lack of available resources, or rejection of the idea that change is needed. Such rejection usually results from differences between nurse and client value systems. Further nurse action depends on the probable reason for client apathy and the projected consequences of no nursing intervention.

Another impediment to successful nurse-client planning is indecision. Client indecision is the inability of clients to make decisions about their health situation. "Indecision often results from the inability of the person or persons making the decision to see any real advantage to the consequences of one decision over another" (Dyer, 1973, p. 151). It may also result from unexpressed fears and concerns. One suggested nursing approach to working with the indecisive client is to discuss the indecision and review the pros and cons of the situation in a nonthreatening atmosphere.

The plan is written to communicate the results of nurse-client planning and decision making. Plan formats vary according to the setting, client level, planning method (i.e., whether or not a nurse-client contract is used), and the purpose of the plan. Plans usually include the nursing diagnosis, client-centered goals and objectives, and the criteria for evaluation. Nursing student care plans may require scientific rationale. When contracting is done, the contract is a plan. Written plans should be part of the client's or agency's permanent record, since both the plan and actual records of care delivery are needed to describe and evaluate the care process.

Implementation

Implementation is the execution of the plan of care. Client and nurse are active participants in the implementation phase since both carry out the responsibilities delegated to them during the plan-ning process. Thus, the care plan is implemented within the nurse-client relationship.

This discussion of the implementation phase of the nursing process will briefly describe several intervention strategies used in community health nursing. The intervention strategies to be described are:

- Group process
- Health promotion
- Partnerships.

(See Chapters 12, 13, and 14 for detailed discussion of these strategies.)

Group Process *Group process, group interaction,* and *group dynamics* are all terms that describe what goes on within a group—the group's life. Group interaction may be related to task accomplishment (i.e., getting the work done) or to group maintenance (i.e., fostering good working relationships). Although groups vary in membership, purpose, and size, their common life together can be analyzed using concepts of group dynamics. Community health nurses assist diverse groups, such as families, committees, teams, and organizations to work together to complete their tasks.

Group interaction and nurse-individual client interaction have similarities and differences. For example, both kinds of interaction are concerned with roles, communication, perceptions, and functions. Working with groups can be more complex than working with individuals. Nurses' ability to capitalize on knowledge and skill in group dynamics enables them to participate effectively in group situations.

Health Promotion This area is significant because of its role in preventing chronic disease. Many chronic diseases are either caused by or aggravated by unhealthy life-styles, which have high morbidity and mortality rates. Since chronic diseases are incurable, they must be prevented or controlled. Moreover, health care of chronic disease consumes personal and societal resources. Some potential benefits of health promotion and prevention are an improved quality of life, decreased health care costs, and increased national productivity through reduced illness and absenteeism (Pender, 1982).

Community health nurses have historically worked to prevent disease and promote health, but the demands of illness care continue to vie for their time and energy. The task is twofold: to assist clients to achieve competence in self-care and to promote the establishment of a national health policy supportive of healthful life-styles (Pender, 1982).

Teaching is one way of providing clients with the knowledge and skills they need to improve their health. Since health promotion requires engaging in lifelong positive health behaviors, helping clients learn desirable self-care practices is the only way health promotion can be accomplished.

Partnerships The concept of partnership in community health nursing involves activities of goal-directed interaction, exchanging perceptions, mutual planning, joint decision making, and shared responsibility. Partnerships are formed at all client levels, with other nurses, and other health- and nonhealth-related community organizations.

Establishing partnerships is difficult but rewarding. Some of the impediments to establishing partnerships include professional turf issues and cultural, educational, and socioeconomic differences among participants. One major reward of partnerships is effective nursing practice. Partnerships are frequently the best way to achieve nursing care goals. For example, when clients participate in service design, they are more likely to use the services.

Nurses need to believe in the value of partnerships and consciously acquire the knowledge and skills necessary to use partnerships in practice. A clear understanding of the nature, scope, and mission of community health nursing is essential for establishing effective partnerships.

Evaluation

This discussion describes evaluation as a component of the nursing process and the nursing process as a method of care delivery. As a component of the nursing process, evaluation involves making judgments about the process and outcome of nursing care. What transpires during care is called "process," and client behavior upon termination of care is referred to as "outcome." The term "process-outcome" describes evaluation of the link between nurse action and client response.

Evaluation is done by comparing at least two entities. Selecting which comparison to make depends upon the reason for the evaluation and available resources. If one wanted to know how well the nursing process was implemented with a client, one could compare the method of care delivery with the *Standards: Community Health Nursing Practice* (American Nurses' Association, 1973). The effect of care on client health status can be determined by comparing client behavior at termination with the client-centered goals and objectives generated during planning. Asking the client why he or she made a health-related change is a way of linking client change with the stimulus for change. Acquiring and reviewing information relevant to the desired comparison leads to an evaluative judgment about the nature and results of care delivery.

Evaluative judgments provide input for making decisions about current client care and guide future action. Evaluation enables the nurse to decide whether to continue care delivery as planned, change the plan, or terminate care. Awareness of a predictable link between a specific nurse action and a client response within a given set of circumstances will enhance the efficiency and effectiveness of future nursing practice.

Little research has been done to confirm or disprove the value of using the nursing process in care delivery despite widespread opinion that it is an important development for improving client care worldwide (International Council of Nurses, 1981). Perhaps one explanation for the lack of research on the nursing process is due to the apparent validity of its close relationship to the scientific method and the problem-solving method. Research on evaluation of the nursing process is summarized here for each component of the nursing process.

Using a systematic method of data collection helps ensure that data are relevant to identifying client health problems. Cianfrani (1984) studied the influence of the amounts and relevance of data collected on health problem identification. He found that accuracy in the identification of health problems declined with increased amounts of data and with irrelevant data. Community health nurses are exposed to a wide variety of client situations with innumerable opportunities for data collection. Research is needed to assist community health nurses in refining data collection methods.

Use of nursing diagnosis was encouraged. Gordon (1980) studied the use of nursing diagnoses on hospital discharge referrals to community health nursing agencies. When they had discharge referrals containing the nursing diagnosis, etiology, signs and symptoms, and suggested plans, community nurses reported such referrals saved assessment time and made continuity of care possible. Saving time and improving the continuity of care are important concerns in community health nursing.

Client-centered care planning has been endorsed as the way to plan care. Blair (1971) described the changes that occurred in a community health nursing staff after they began "contracting." Contracting was defined as a mutual understanding of the reason for the service and the problems or areas that would be discussed during visits. She reported that an "overwhelmed, physically exhausted and thoroughly frustrated nursing staff were able to serve more families, felt more productive in terms of patient progress and achieved high levels of job satisfaction after contracting was instituted" (p. 588). The effect of contracting on community health nurse productivity and client response is a prime area for continuing health nursing research.

Perry (1974) studied the process, purposes, and outcomes of contracting with ten patients and their families receiving home health care. She found that when contracts were used, client problems were identified sooner, more options for solutions became available, clients felt confident in their own problem-solving ability, clients were at home for their appointments, and nurse and family felt confident of client self-care ability upon nursing service termination.

Effective nursing practice requires using the most productive intervention strategy in any given client situation. Swain and Steckel (1981) studied clients with hypertension being treated as outpatients. They compared the effects of using contingency contracting and patient education on client knowledge of hypertension, discontinuation of medical treatment, and blood pressure control. Their research indicated that contingency contracting was a more effective intervention strategy than patient education for improving client knowledge, preventing treatment dropout, and improving blood pressure control. There were no contract failures.

Evaluation involves comparing client response to the goals and objectives of the plan of care. One way to improve the evaluative ability of community health nurses is to specify what client changes, or expected outcomes, should occur and how these changes will be manifested in terms of outcome criterion.

The Visiting Nurses Association of Omaha is developing expected outcome and outcome criterion schemes to accompany their classification system of problems in community health nursing. The schemes are designed to reflect reasonable, measurable client behaviors that can be observed and monitored by the community health nurse (Martin, 1982). (See Chapter 15 for further information on evaluation as a component of the nursing process.)

Case Example 7-1: Illustration of the Nursing Process in Community Health Nursing

Weca County is a rural community located near a large midwestern city. The authors (university nursing faculty members) became associated with the Weca County Board of Health through their work in a university nursing center. When we arrived in Weca County, there were no public health nurses, but the need for public health nursing was evident to us. However, the county board of health administrators wanted evidence of the kinds and extent of unmet health needs that existed in Weca County before they would agree to having new services provided. Establishing a contractual relationship between the university (our employer) and the county health department enabled us to provide nursing services in the community.

Nursing faculty establish a base for community health nursing practice in a rural community.

We ultimately developed a program for pregnant teens after first conducting an assessment of the health needs of Weca County residents. Assessment and subsequent components of the nursing process are illustrated in this case example.

University faculty collaborate with county board of health officials: Mutual goals and benefits are identified; contract is established; groundwork for partnership is laid: These activities facilitate assessment.

Assessment

Our first activity in the county was to interview key persons from fourteen community agencies. These persons identified common needs: (1) family planning, (2) Women, Infants, and Children (WIC) food supplement program, and (3) pre- and postnatal education and support for pregnant adolescents. The accuracy of this data was verified through our more detailed needs assessment.

Interviews provide data, facilitate interaction with community representatives, give community health nurses visibility, and help them establish rapport.

Community health nurses are politically astute: Their political awareness allows them to make decisions that lead to acceptance of their program.

To conduct this needs assessment we decided to use an assessment outline from the *Illinois Department of Public Health: Standards for Local Health Departments in Illinois*. This decision was made because using the state's outline made it easier for us to gain state certification as a local health department. The assessment outline requested sociodemographic data and information about the health characteristics and resources relating to maternal health and family planning. In areas where the outline was sketchy, we substituted information from other assessment guides about which we were knowledgeable.

Different sources of information are combined for better needs assessment.

Major sociodemographic information sources were 1980 census data obtained via local Health Systems Agency, vital statistics (e.g., birth certificates obtained through the county courthouse), and income information acquired from the County Public Aid Office. It was found that 11 percent of county births in 1981 were to single women. There were 99 births to county teenagers in 1980, and 32 percent, or 960 teens, in the county were at risk of unintended pregnancy (Illinois Caucus on Teenage

Pregnancy, 1980). We also learned that 31 percent of county families had incomes of less than $8000 per year.

Sources of information on the health characteristics of pregnant adolescents included results of observations of pregnant adolescents in the WIC Clinic, a graduate student assessment survey, and our Nursing Center work with pregnant and postpartal teens. (Our work was through the WIC program already established in Weca County.)

Data sources and methods

About 30 percent of county pregnant adolescents participated in the WIC program. During WIC Clinics, we particularly noted (1) their health behaviors such as smoking, (2) the interaction between the adolescent and persons accompanying them to the clinic, usually their mothers, and (3) behaviors relevant to their self-concept like eye contact and personal hygiene. Frequently, the interactions between adolescents and their mothers were strained. The mothers talked for the adolescents and made decisions for them. Many adolescents smoked, had poor personal hygiene, and looked apprehensive.

A part of the assessment data is direct observation of adolescents' health behaviors during their participation in a WIC program.

The data collection method here is observation of health habits guided by knowledge of pregnant adolescents.

A graduate community health nursing student with faculty assistance developed a questionnaire based on risk factors for adolescent pregnancy identified in the literature. Risk factors concerning the adolescent relate to child spacing, unplanned pregnancy, socioeconomic status, educational achievement, maternal age, medical risk, and child abuse. Pregnant teens at WIC were asked if they were willing to have the graduate student interview them. Twenty-seven pregnant or postpartal adolescents were interviewed. The risk factors and questionnaire results are presented in Table 7-3.

Data collection by a questionnaire is especially useful because quantifiable data for program planning are needed.

Sources of data about resources for the needs of pregnant adolescents were: our knowledge of community resources in counties bordering Weca County, the local Health Systems Agency, a directory of Weca County community resources, interviews with agency personnel serving the county, the nurse-to-nurse network, and clients. We found community resources for the pregnant adolescent to be as follows: private physicians, obstetrical clinics at two hospitals, family planning services at a public agency in an adjoining county, two adoption agencies, an abortion clinic, and limited educational and support services from the county schools. Services were somewhat fragmented and needed coordination.

Examples of data sources

Community health nurses identify and assess community health resources for pregnant adolescents.

Diagnosis

Collected data were processed to identify the health needs of and resources for pregnant adolescents in Weca County.

Data collected from the community needs assessment was interpreted by comparing the findings to norms, standards, and theories. For example, data in Table 7-3 about unplanned and repeat pregnancies were interpreted in terms of child and pregnant adolescent welfare and socioeconomic impact. These data revealed that children of teenage parents are at greater risk of child abuse and neglect; repeat pregnancies among teen mothers are high; repeat pregnancies too soon after delivery increase the risk of premature or low birthweight babies; the financial assistance single mothers receive from Public Aid is inadequate. Even with the Med-

Unplanned and repeat pregnancies place adolescents at high risk for physical, economic, and psychosocial difficulties. Knowledge of these factors helps nurses to intervene effectively.

(continued)

Case Example 7-1   *(continued)*

Table 7-3   Pregnant Adolescents Attending a WIC Clinic: Assessment Survey Results

Risk Factors of Adolescent Pregnancy	Results	Functional Health Pattern[a]
Child spacing	48% of the teens were having their second or third child.	Sexuality-Reproductive
Unplanned pregnancy	About one-third of the pregnancies were unplanned. One-half of the adolescents with unplanned pregnancies had not received any birth control information and some had unanswered questions. 21% of the adolescents who wanted birth control had no affordable source available to them.	
Marital status	60% of the pregnancies were to unmarried women.	Self-Perception/Self-Concept
Low socioeconomic status	85% were unemployed. 15% were employed. (About 8% of all mothers receiving welfare in the county are under age 20.)	Coping-Stress
Low educational achievement	38% completed high school. 70% did not attend prenatal classes. Only 48% had received some information about parenting and child care.	Cognitive-Perceptual
Young maternal age	Only one birth reported in the past two years to female under age 15.	Sexuality-Reproductive
Medical risk	96% were receiving prenatal care. 70% sought prenatal care during their first trimester.	Health-Perception/Health-Management
Child abuse	52% lacked parenting and/or child care education. 43% did not leave home without the child at least once a week.	Role Relationships

[a] Names of Functional Health Patterns from Gordon M: *Nursing Diagnosis Process and Application.* New York: McGraw-Hill, 1982.

icaid card and food stamps, their standard of living is substantially below poverty level.

After the data were collected and interpreted, we looked for a published diagnosis matching our data. Gordon's nursing diagnosis "Knowledge Deficit (specify)," defined as the "inability to state or explain information or demonstrate a required skill related to disease management procedures, practices, and/or self-care-health-care management" (1982, p. 136) was selected. Some of the pregnant adolescents lacked knowledge of family planning, childbirth and parenting, and self-care during pregnancy. (See again Table 7-3 regarding education needs for birth control and childbirth/parenting information.) Although we recognized that there are multiple reasons for adolescent pregnancy, lack of knowledge was a significant problem identified in our survey and verified in our contacts with individual pregnant adolescents.

Data are used to formulate nursing diagnosis of community client (pregnant adolescents).

There are various reasons for lack of information. Our needs assessment revealed gaps in community resources providing educational services related to adolescent pregnancy. After considering all the preceding information, our nursing diagnosis for the population of pregnant adolescents was "Knowledge Deficit (family planning; childbirth, and parenting education; self-care during pregnancy) related to inadequate community resources."

Nursing diagnosis is specified.

Planning

When planning a program for adolescent pregnancy, we selected as a priority improving educational preventive and support services for the adolescents, because of the negative impact of adolescent pregnancy on the population, coupled with data obtained in the assessment phase. Another reason for selecting teenage pregnancy was our desire to successfully establish a Maternal Health and Family Planning Program. We identified factors that could contribute to success of the program. The factors included expertise in maternal health and family planning, access to pregnant adolescents through the WIC program, and resources to target a pregnant adolescent population of 99. We lacked staff resources to serve the total maternal health population of 600.

Target population identified for health program is pregnant adolescents.

Resource identification is a crucial part of determining problem priority in the planning process.

Our next task was to design a service plan that would meet health department program certification requirements and the needs of pregnant adolescents within existing constraints. The state requires a written service plan for each health program based on assessed needs and problem priority. Required components of the plan include quantitative objectives and time frames; a description of activities and methods, including services provided by other agencies (intervention strategies); limiting factors (constraints) in achieving objectives and plans to overcome the constraints; and evaluation criteria (*Illinois Department of Public Health: Standards for Local Health Departments in Illinois*, 1981).

Health program plan is based on assessment of needs and is designed to meet health department program certificate requirements.

Our program plan contained the sociodemographic data and results of the adolescent pregnancy needs survey presented earlier. We used the state's objective for the Maternal Health and Family Planning Program as our long-term goal. The objective states "To assure women of child-bearing age the optimum chance for: (1) wanted pregnancies, (2) successful pregnancy outcomes, (3) adequate preparation for the motherhood role" (*Illinois Department of Public Health: Standards for Local Health Departments in Illinois*, 1981, p. 17). Our short-term goals were specific to adolescent pregnancy. For example, our quantified goal for case finding was "to identify at least 50 percent of the 99 pregnant teens."

Program goals relate to nursing diagnosis: "knowledge deficits in areas of family planning, childbirth, parenting education, and self-care during pregnancy."

(continued)

Case Example 7-1   *(continued)*

The methods and activities in our plan included directives for our work with clients and coordination with other agencies. For example, strategies for family planning were to offer family planning information on all postpartum home visits and to investigate the content of school health education curricula and the inclusion of sex education.

A primary concern in service design is client utilization. Factors influencing utilization range from transportation to cultural beliefs and values. Client utilization potential was evaluated for our own direct care activities and the services provided by outside agencies. For example, we advocated one agency's service delivery in the county because their program provided transportation and a pregnant adolescent support group. The support group would use peer input, an important influence in the adolescent culture.

Group dynamics or group process are incorporated in planning.

Our plan for the Maternal Health and Family Planning Program was approved because it was creditable and presented in a manner that acknowledged the values of the health board. For example, we did not propose family planning as a health department service at this time, but we emphasized the economic wisdom of family planning and endorsed health department support of the existing public family planning agency. (The agency later received health department funds for transportation, but the health board made sure the money did not finance contraception.) A local newspaper editorial dramatized the community's antifamily planning sentiment for teens. "Parents, do you like the fact that kids are encouraged to experiment sexually because they know good old planned parenthood is right there with the Pill or a quick D & C? Do you like the rewards we have reaped in our wonderful permissive society? Let's do anything we can to forever eliminate places like Planned Parenthood by cutting off its life-line, the federal government" (Editorial, 1982).

Program plans are presented in a manner accepted by the community.

Local newspapers provide insights about community values.

Implementation

There were about two years between the approval of the Maternal Health and Family Planning program and the termination of our work in the county. During the first year of program implementation, we developed the caseload and gave direct care to pregnant adolescents. Direct care included supportive counseling, anticipatory guidance, problem solving, and consultation and referral. These services to pregnant and postpartal teens were provided on home visits and at the WIC Clinic.

Coordination of multiple services to pregnant adolescents became one of our priorities. We called a series of meetings of agency representatives to continue building rapport and networking activities to avoid service duplication, facilitate information exchange, and enhance client use of appropriate services. Meeting participants agreed on geographic service boundaries, validated the role of the health department as a legitimate service coordinator, and developed a Release of Information form that all agencies could use to exchange client information.

Coordination of services and interagency collaboration are part of the implementation phase.

Evaluation

The major focus of our work in the county was service development. Since much of our work was developmental, an appropriate evaluation criterion is service establishment. Ten health department programs were certified by the state including the Maternal Health and Family Planning Program serving pregnant adolescents. Although state certification does not ensure desirable client outcomes, the certification process is a form of quality control.

Program certification achieved.

Improved client health status is the ultimate criterion for evaluating service success. Determining service outcomes of community clients requires aggregate outcome data. Examples of outcome criteria we could have used were a decrease in an adolescent pregnancy birth rate, increased numbers of pregnant adolescents attending the public family planning clinic, increased numbers of pregnant adolescents in the WIC program, and increased numbers of pregnant adolescents attending prenatal classes. Mechanisms for monitoring these variables needed further development.

About six months before we left the county, block grant funds obtained by the county health department were used to hire a baccalaureate-prepared community health nurse for the county. One of us gave the new nurse a comprehensive orientation to the health department. This nurse has continued the work we initiated with pregnant adolescents.

New funding is a measure of the community health nurse's effectiveness.

Summary

In summary, the nursing process has been presented as a desirable method of nursing clients at all levels because it provides a systematic approach for community health nursing. The nursing process also provides a general framework for the application of theory to specific client situations.

The components of the nursing process are interdependent and cyclical. Problem resolution depends on accurate problem identification. Problems are accurately identified when sufficient, relevant data are collected and the nurse interprets the data correctly. Planning is based on client-validated problems. Clients validate problems they consider important and amenable to significant change with a reasonable expenditure of resources. Planning provides the road map for change by specifying the destination for change and the route and resources for the journey. Evaluation involves determining whether the destination (goal) was reached and the efficacy of the plan and the interventions. The case example of Weca County illustrated how this process was put into practice in a real community.

Topics for Nursing Research

• What is the nature and characteristics of client autonomy in a community health center, and how is this autonomy manifested at the various levels of the nursing process?

• Design a program to evaluate the differences in treatment outcomes in a community crippled children's clinic where: (1) contingency contracts are instituted, (2) noncontingency contracts are instituted, and (3) no contracts are instituted during the planning stage of the nursing process.

Study Questions

1. The relationship between the nursing process and the application of theory to practice is:
   a. The nursing process is a method for theory application
   b. The nursing process validates theory application
   c. The nursing process substitutes for theory application
   d. The nursing process defines theory application

2. The similarity of data collection across all client levels is most significant because:
   a. Data similarity permits interchangeable data collection across client levels
   b. Data similarity enhances recognition of interrelationships between client levels
   c. Data similarity restricts theory application across client levels
   d. Data similarity reduces assessment time for any client level

3. The primary function of nursing diagnosis is to:
   a. Delineate the scope of interdependent nursing practice
   b. Decrease the necessity for interprofessional collaboration
   c. Enhance the status of nursing as a profession
   d. Provide a sound basis for nursing intervention

4. The most important reason *noncontingency* contracts are used in community health is to:
   a. Reward desired client behavior changes
   b. Require client participation in care delivery
   c. Schedule future nurse-client interaction
   d. Negotiate a working agreement for care delivery

5. Evaluating the outcomes of a stress management program would involve:
   a. Validating client need for a stress management seminar
   b. Determining whether relevant content is presented to clients
   c. Verifying the use of appropriate nursing and nonnursing theories
   d. Judging whether clients improved their stress management abilities

References

American Nurses' Association: *Nursing: A Social Policy Statement*. Kansas City, Mo.: American Nurses' Association, 1980, p. 32.

American Nurses' Association: *Standards: Community Health Nursing Practice*. Kansas City, Mo.: American Nurses' Association, 1973.

Bailon SG, Maglaya AS: Tools and guidelines for nursing care at the family level, Part I. A typology of nursing problems in family care practice. *The ANPHI Papers* (January–March) 1977; 12: 13–21.

Blair KK: It's the patient's problem—and decision. *Nurs Outlook* 1971; 19: 587–589.

Braden CJ, Herban NL: *Community Health: A Systems Approach*. New York: Appleton-Century-Crofts, 1976.

Choi T, Josten L, Christensen ML: Health-specific family coping index for noninstitutional care. *Am J Public Health* 1983; 73 (11): 1275–1277.

Cianfrani KL: The influence of amounts and relevance of data on identifying health problems. In: Kim MJ, McFarland GK, McLane AM (editors), *Classification of Nursing Diagnosis Proceedings of the Fifth National Conference*. St. Louis: Mosby, 1984.

Dyer WG: Working with groups. In: Reinhardt AM, Quinn MD (editors), *Family-Centered Community Nursing: A Sociocultural Framework*. St. Louis: Mosby, 1973.

Editorial. *Oregon Reporter* (September 25) 1982.

Friedman MM: *Family Nursing Theory and Assessment*. New York: Appleton-Century-Crofts, 1981.

Gordon M, Sweeney MA, McKeehan K: Nursing diagnosis looking at its use in the clinical area. *Am J Nurs* 1980; 80: 672–674.

Gordon M: *Nursing Diagnosis Process and Application*. New York: McGraw-Hill, 1982.

Green LW, Anderson CL: *Community Health*. St. Louis: Mosby, 1982.

Griffith JW, Christensen PJ: *Nursing Process Application of Theories, Frameworks, and Models*. St. Louis: Mosby, 1982.

Hamilton P: Community nursing diagnosis. *Adv Nurs Sci* 1983; 5 (3): 21–36.

Hanlon JJ: *Public Health Administration and Practice*. St. Louis: Mosby, 1974.

Helvie, CO, Hill AE, Bambino CF: The setting and nursing practice. *Nurs Outlook* 1968; 16: 27–29.

Helvie CO: *Community Health Nursing Theory and Process*. Philadelphia: Harper & Row, 1981.

Illinois Caucus on Teenage Pregnancy: *County Profiles/ 1980*. (Available from the Illinois Caucus on Teenage Pregnancy, 160 N. LaSalle Street, Room 300, Chicago, Ill 60601).

Illinois Department of Public Health: *Standards for Local Health Departments in Illinois.* Springfield, Ill: Author, 1981.

International Council of Nurses, 1981: *Am J Nurs* 1981; 81 (9): 1664–1671.

Johnson W, Hardin C: *Content and Dynamics of Home Visits of Public Health Nurses: Part I.* New York: American Nurses Foundation, 1962.

Lunney M: A framework to analyze a taxonomy of nursing diagnosis. In Kim MJ, McFarland GR, McLane AM (editors), *Classification of Nursing Diagnosis Proceedings of the Fifth National Conference.* St. Louis: Mosby, 1984.

Mallick MJ: Nursing diagnosis and the novice student. *Nursing and Health Care* 1983; 4 (8): 455–459.

Martin K: A client classification system adaptable for computerization. *Nurs Outlook* 1982; 30 (9): 515–517.

Pender NJ: *Health Promotion in Nursing Practice.* Norwalk, Conn.: Appleton-Century-Crofts, 1982.

Perry K: *The Nursing Care Plan as Contract: The Process, Purposes and Outcomes.* Chicago: Unpublished Manuscript, Rush University College of Nursing (August 6) 1974.

Simmons DA: *A Classification Scheme for Client Problems in Community Health Nursing.* DHHS Publication No. HRA 80-16. National Technical Information Service, 1980.

Sloan MR, Schommer BT: The process of contracting in community health nursing. In: Spradley B (editor), *Contemporary Community Nursing.* Boston: Little, Brown, 1975.

Steckel SB, Swain MA: Contracting with patients to improve compliance. *Hospitals* 1977; 51: 81–84.

Steckel SB: Contracting with patient-selected reinforcers. *Am J Nurs* 1980; 80: 1596–1599.

Swain MA, Steckel SB: Influencing adherence among hypertensives. *Res Nurs Health* 1981; 4: 213–222.

University of Illinois College of Nursing: *Agreement for Personal Health Services.* Service contract (June 6) 1983.

Visiting Nurse Association of Omaha Defined Data Base. Unpublished (The VNA of Omaha, 4500 Ames Ave., Omaha, NB 68104).

Werner JR: Effective community health nursing: A framework for actualizing standards of practice. *Nurs Forum* 1976; 15 (3): 265–377.

Chapter 8

Family Assessment

Linda Lee Daniel

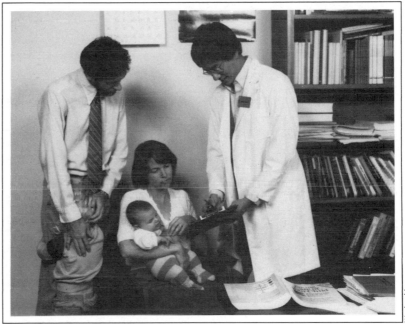

Assessing both the health status of each family member and the level of functioning for the family as a whole is a key phase in the community health nursing process.

Chapter Objectives

After completing this chapter, the reader will be able to:

- Identify the components of family assessment
- Describe three specific areas for assessment of each component
- Describe sources of data for family assessment
- Describe tools the community health nurse can use for family assessment

Family-centered care based on a family assessment is a key concept in community health nursing practice. Friedman (1981) further identifies the importance of working with the total family since any dysfunction or problem that affects one or more family members will affect the total family unit. "One can achieve a clear perspective of the individual and his or her functioning, only when the person's family is also assessed" (p. 5).

The assessment is the basis for nursing care and the yardstick against which both the nurse and the family can measure family progress. The family assessment is more than the sum of the assessments of the individual family members. A family assessment includes:

- Each family member's health status
- Family member's relationship to the other family members
- Family's functioning
- Strengths and weaknesses of the family unit
- Relationship of the family to the larger community
- Influence of the larger community upon that family

Just as each family member is a part of the larger family, each family is a member of a larger community. As the family influences the individual member, the community also influences the family.

Purpose of Family Assessment

The purpose of the family assessment is to determine the quality of family functioning, the strengths and weaknesses of the family unit and each individual member, and the health and well-being of the family and each family member. An area that is frequently missed in the area of family assessment is the identification of family strengths. In nursing there is a tendency to concentrate on needs and problems. Families are often able to identify their problems and needs, but are unable to identify their own strengths. Families must be helped to identify their strengths, because the utilization of family strengths is an important strategy for helping families overcome problems. Spradley (1981) cited the importance of emphasizing family strengths as a way of helping families have a more positive concept of themselves.

Family Strengths

The nurse may identify strengths that the family can't recognize without some assistance. When identifying family strengths, it is important to start at a very basic level. If the family is together and functioning, this is a strength that can be built upon. Otto (1973), a pioneer in the area of family strengths, developed a framework of thirteen areas for assessment. These thirteen areas are not independent variables but are interrelated and dynamic (p. 91):

1. Ability to provide for the physical, emotional, and spiritual needs of the family
2. Ability of the family to respect each other's views and decisions on child-rearing practices

3. Ability to communicate with each family member

4. Ability to provide support, security, and encouragement

5. Ability to foster ongoing growth within the family

6. Ability to assume responsible community relationships

7. Ability to grow with and through the children

8. Ability to help themselves and accept help from others

9. Ability to assume different family functions and roles as needed

10. Ability to provide mutual respect for individuality

11. Ability to utilize crisis experiences as a means of growth

12. Concern for family unity, loyalty, and intra-family cooperation

13. Flexibility of family strengths

If the nurse begins the family assessment by concentrating on the family's strengths, those involved will have a more positive feeling toward the total assessment process.

A family need is any problem, concern, limitation, or weakness that causes difficulty to the family unit or an individual family member. The family unit will be affected by needs of the individual family member, just as the individual family member will be affected by needs of the family. Nursing or other professional intervention is not always needed, as many needs can be dealt with effectively by the family.

Family Priorities

The importance the family places on the need or the strength must be assessed. This is no simple task, since what may be very important to one family may not be considered important to another family. An example might be the birth of a low birthweight infant. One family may identify this as a very significant problem, foreseeing potential difficulties for the child in future years. The family, or the mother, may see in the small size an indication that the mother is unable to produce a full-term infant. Another family experiencing the birth of the same weight infant may see it as a positive event and have no real concern since the infant is alive and expected to live. Thus, though the families experience the same event, their interpretations of its significance are very different. The community health nurse may be able to pick up clues by observing the family, but it is important to discuss the event with the family, allowing them adequate time to verbalize their concerns and questions.

An important part of the family assessment is the identification of areas where the community health nurse may not be able to intervene or to provide assistance in helping the family obtain the services of other health and social professionals through the referral process. Although several areas may be identified as needs in the assessment, each of these needs must be further assessed to determine the family's desire for intervention and the type of intervention most appropriate. A rank-ordering of family needs is a part of the assessment.

All families have areas where some work or intervention would be appropriate. However, no family can work on a multitude of areas at one time. The priority of needs may be influenced by such things as the severity of the problem, how recently the problem occurred, the relationship of that need or problem to other concerns of the family, and the family's previous experience in dealing with similar needs. The process of prioritizing needs during the assessment provides the family unit with the opportunity to determine the importance of each need, concern, or problem.

[handwritten annotations in top margin: Physical, Psychosocial, Diet, Sociocultural, Environmental]

Components of a Family Assessment

The family assessment consists of five components: physical, psychosocial, sociocultural, nutritional, and environmental. Each component is interrelated but has specific areas that must be assessed when completing a family assessment.

Physical Assessment

In community health nursing practice the physical assessment of the family may not receive as much attention as other parts of the assessment. If, for example, the major purpose of the nursing visit is for psychosocial concerns, the physical assessment may be deemphasized. However, a basic physical assessment of the family members is important to the total family assessment, because without these data, it is impossible to determine the individual members' health status.

Health Status   Basic data needed for each family member include age, sex, height and weight, blood pressure, current medication, current health status, and the individuals' perception of their own health. Although a complete physical assessment of each family member would yield useful data, it is often not possible to obtain. The emphasis is usually placed on obtaining the family members' perceptions of their own health and their perceptions of the other family members' health. These data give the community health nurse insight into the family's health status and its view of health and illness. It is important to determine what a family considers illness. How does the family describe the terms *sick, ill, well,* and *healthy?* Much of this basic information can be obtained from a health history completed by the nurse on a visit to one or more of the family members.

Ideally, the health assessment should be completed during face-to-face contact with each family member, but the limitation of the nursing service and the family schedule may prevent this. However, an in-depth physical assessment should be completed for any family member experiencing a specific health problem such as coping with the birth of a new child. The community health nurse would need to assess the mother's health status in relation to pregnancy, delivery, and lactation; her postpartum course; condition of her breasts; problems with elimination; and her adjustment to parenting. The physical assessment of the infant would concentrate on weight, sleeping, eating, and elimination. Future visits to the family would require continued assessment in the area of infant growth, progress toward developmental milestones, sleep, and physical activities, along with the psychosocial assessment. For visits to an elderly family, the emphasis might be on determining the ability of each family member to carry out the activities of daily living. The individual's hearing, vision, gait, and ability to ambulate are areas in need of in-depth assessment. The physical assessment should then be comprehensive, but at the same time related to the health needs and health status of the individual family member.

Health Promotion   An assessment of the family's activities related to self-help and optimal healthful living need to be determined. One might ask: Do the adult females in the home practice breast self-examination? Do they know how to do breast self-examination? Do they understand its importance? Does the family know the status of immunizations? Does the family practice oral hygiene with regular visits to the dentist for cleaning and prophylactic treatment? Does the family have regular vision examinations? A family's answers to these questions will indicate its interest and knowledge of preventive health practices.

Skill in assessing health promotion activities is important in obtaining a complete family assessment.

Routine Health Care   The importance of assessing routine health maintenance cannot be overemphasized. With young infants and school-age children, routine health examinations, immunizations, and measures of growth and development are an intrinsic part of normal health care practices. For the adult female in our society, routine health care is usually related to obtaining and using birth control. Adult males, unfortunately, utilize very little routine health assessment or health care. Although young males have a low incidence of illness, they are often developing a life-style that can increase the risks of heart disease and stroke, leading killers in this country. Greater emphasis should be placed on the assessment of young adult males, both in community health nursing practice and in medical practice.

The cost of routine health care for the family can drain their financial resources. The emphasis placed on prevention and health promotion can be influenced by the cost of the care.

It is important to assess the family's utilization of health care services. At what point does the family seek medical care? What are the factors that influence when care will be sought? These factors may include the family's perception of health and illness, as well as the inability to work or perform usual activities. One way to determine a family's rationale for obtaining health care can be to ask the family members why they went to the physician or clinic the last time. The number of visits to the physician or clinic in the last month or the last six months will also give clues to the frequency of health care. An exploration of why the visits were made provides an indication of the type of health concerns for which the family seeks professional intervention.

Emergency Health Care   A plan for emergency health care is frequently neglected until an emergency exists. The community health nurse should elicit the family's plan for emergency care and determine with the family the appropriateness of the source of care for both acute emergencies and minor illnesses. For families in need of care but unfamiliar with or unaware of other less expensive resources, an emergency room is both a costly and inefficient choice. The new medical walk-in clinics, open in the evening and on weekends, pro-

vide an alternative to the emergency room for less acute illnesses or injuries. It is important that the family plan for emergency care before a crisis occurs. Not only is the source of emergency care important, but the transportation the family will use to reach the emergency care needs to be planned for in advance. Emergency health care should be viewed as an adjunct to routine health maintenance, not a substitute for routine health care.

Psychosocial Assessment

Family communication patterns and styles are as varied as other aspects of family life. Communication patterns are developed early in childhood. A family with an open system of communication has greater exchange of information with the external environment, whereas a family with a closed system of communication is more mutually interdependent and does not reach out into the larger community. Friedman (1981) states that the family can handle only a limited amount of information, and the family that is indiscriminately open to information becomes chaotic and disorganized. On the other hand, closed family systems can be dysfunctional. For example, Friedman (1981), further states, "the abused child is frequently found in families that are isolated and have closed boundaries with society" (p. 112). The degree of communication within the family and between the family members can best be determined through observation of the interaction when all family members are present.

Since it is not always possible to visit the family when all family members are present, assessment of the communication patterns may have to be accomplished through communication with an adult family member. The communication between the parent and child must be assessed. How do the parents or adults in the home respond to the children's requests? Does the adult caregiver or parent berate the child, or speak to the child with a loving voice? Are the children included as part of the conversation? Are they sent away as soon as the nurse enters the home? Communication patterns identified with the children may be typical of communication patterns with other family members. The emotional tones or feelings that accompany verbal expression give an indication of the family's affection for one another in the family unit.

Family communication is often influenced by such factors as the family's ethnic background, social class, norms, and the position of individual family members. Thus, family communication must be assessed in terms of these factors (Miller & Janosik, 1980). Some families encourage the utilization of friends and coworkers as a support system for sharing family concerns and family problems. Other families view this sharing as a violation of confidentiality. Asking the family whom they see as a support system can provide vital data about the family and the family's source of support. The family that does not share concerns or crises may not accept referrals to community agencies.

The use of community resources is determined partly by the family's need, but to an even larger extent by the family's receptivity to outside assistance. Most families accept the placement of their children in public schools and the use of water and sewage in the community; however, families believing in self-sufficiency may not accept food stamps or financial assistance from the department of social services. Some families may view community services as a means of meeting their social and emotional needs, whereas other families reject the idea of any outside assistance. Asking the family whom they would first tell the good news that they are expecting a baby or news of a death in the family and how widely they would share the information can give some clues as to the tightness of the family's boundaries. Case Example 8-1 illustrates a beginning assessment of a nuclear family.

Role of the Family Members   The role each family member plays within the family is dictated in part by society and in part by the family's own social system. Every family member has many roles that are played out at various times. In community health nursing it is important not to limit the expected roles of individuals in other families to those roles that were assumed in one's own family.

First, the nurse must determine what role each family member plays within the family constellation. The next step is to determine the family member's satisfaction with that current role. Much family conflict comes about when family members are in roles in which they are not interested, for which they are unsuited, or that they are unable to fulfill. An example is the young woman assuming the role of mother with her first child. If she has been a career woman for the past few years, she may have difficulty feeling fulfilled and occupied as a full-time mother. Another example is the father who was previously the breadwinner and the head of the family but is suddenly unemployed. If he feels he has lost some of his authority and status, he may be not only uninterested but unable to fulfill his current role as husband.

Dissatisfaction with a family role may be rooted in external forces, such as being unemployed, or it may come from within the family—an expectation that certain family members will fulfill a role that they do not wish to assume. According to Miller and Janosik (1980), there can be a discrepancy between what is being done in the family and what should be done in that role as far as the family is concerned. It is important to determine the roles that exist in a family, how specific family members function in these roles, and the family's role expectations. "A viable role system depends upon consensus, role reciprocity, functional role enactment, and a normative system which is stable yet flexible" (Miller & Janosik, 1980, p. 138). All these considerations are important in assessing the nature of family functioning.

One aspect of family life concerning roles is that of role sharing. As more and more women return to the work force, the housekeeping and child-rearing role that the mother has historically assumed is now often being shared by the mother and father. In many homes sharing roles can be accepted and performed by both parents. In other homes it may present difficulties, especially if the mother had assumed the role of housekeeper and homemaker previously and has recently entered the work force. Her husband may expect her to assume a different role as well as maintain her role of wife and mother.

Case Example 8-1: A Nuclear Family With Two Children

The family consists of Brian, Mary, and their two children. Brian attended the local schools and graduated from a nearby college with a degree in journalism. He has been employed for the last two years in an advertising firm writing brochures and developing a client group. Mary is from a very small rural community. She completed only one year of college but is now an accomplished child photographer and supplements the family income.

Family has lived in the community for many years.

Differences exist in background and education between husband and wife.

The two children, ages ten and seven, attend public schools. The older child, a son, is very active in the Boy Scouts and a computer programming club through the elementary school. The daughter is interested in ballet and the arts, having her mother's artistic flair. The only major illness the family has experienced was Reyes Syndrome after the son had chicken pox last spring. He has some residual effects with slight weakness on the left side of his body. The family and physician expect a full recovery in time. The health insurance was adequate to meet the financial cost of the medical crisis, but the long recovery period have been a drain on the family income. Most of the family's savings have been spent on the son's health care.

Family has experienced major illness in one family member.

The family eats together on Saturday mornings and at least one other meal sometime during the weekend. Sunday dinner is eaten with the grandparents and is considered a time to get together and share with the larger extended family. Evening meals are eaten together at times, but because of Mary's photography schedule, fast foods are an increasing alternative to family dinners.

Family arranges for regular meals together.

The family income is adequate for their needs at this time. The husband likes his job but sees little potential for advancement. He is contemplating additional schooling and perhaps a career in computer programming. Mary is very content with her role and wants to continue to expand her creative talents.

Family income is adequate.

Husband is dissatisfied with his employment.

Family Unity Many years ago in rural America the family unit was of utmost importance. The interdependence of the family members was great, and members relied upon each other for social outlets, socialization, and support. Today the family unit is faced with many external factors influencing the interrelationship of the family and its relationship to the larger community. Children are involved in Girl Scouts, Cub Scouts, church activities, social clubs, and social activities, just as the parents are involved in social clubs, social activities, and professional organizations. The family must identify their values in relation to the family unit: How close and how circumscribed do they want the family to be? If the family is living in a very transient community, there may be less interrelationship with the community than if it were a more homogeneous or stable community. The family must determine what they view as an acceptable level of togetherness. In American society today it is not always acceptable to admit that family members are more involved with outside forces and with outside members than they are with other family members. However, the family can be a close-knit unit and can be supportive of each other, even though members do not spend a great deal of time together.

Family Stress   It is also important to identify stress, which can come both from within the family unit and outside the family. Unemployment is an example of a stress factor from the outside, whereas illness of a family member produces an internal stress. Again the importance and the value the family place on the event are indicators of how much stress the event causes a particular family. The Social Readjustment Rating Scale, developed by Holmes and Rahe (1967), attempts to measure the impact of stressors on daily living. Holmes and Rahe were among the first to recognize that any change results in stress. Change, both positive and negative, affects one's life (Table 8-1). What may be a major stress to one family may not be important to another family. The purchase of a home is an example. Though any move can be seen as stressful, a family that moves regularly, perhaps once every two years, may not see the move as threatening. However, the family that is making their first move after twenty years of living in a community may find the move very upsetting both to parents and children. The first family is accustomed to making new friends and is well acquainted with what they will face in a new community, whereas the second family may not know what to expect or how to make new friends.

When psychosocial problems or needs are identified, the next step for the nurse is to identify those family strengths that can counteract or reduce them. In today's rapidly changing society almost every family faces a multitude of psychosocial stressors. Communication patterns and roles are constantly changing. The need for support systems is increasing with the decrease in closeness of the extended family. At one time the extended family was the major support system for the young family, but today the extended family often lives thousands of miles away and only sees the younger family on holidays or special occasions (see Case Example 8-2). An important role of community health nurses is to assess the implication of these changes to specific

families. Since psychosocial assessment deals with very intimate aspects of a family's life, sensitivity to the family and a nonjudgmental attitude on the nurse's part are essential for a comprehensive assessment.

Sociocultural Assessment

The sociocultural assessment encompasses the family's cultural background and religious orientation, its place in the community, and its goals and values. Social class, which is usually associated with the occupation or employment of family members as well as with their income and education, is also important. Although some people might deny the stratification of the American society into social classes, social class does exist. Family members whose professions provide for autonomy and power are viewed as members of higher social classes. Friedman (1981) states, "Family life style, structural and functional characteristics, and associations with the external environment of home, neighborhood, and community vary tremendously from social class to social class" (p. 95). Hence, the social class factor can provide an indication of the family's life-style. Assessment of a family's social class may be difficult because multiple factors such as education, income, and occupation of household members are used to determine whether the appropriate designation is low, middle, or upper class. The employment or the occupation of the extended family is a consideration. What position did the wife's parents or the husband's parents hold in their community? Many conflicts in families arise as a result of husbands and wives coming from different social classes. Problems arise because of differences in family values, in the importance placed upon certain events, and in the value of education or travel.

Assessment of the family's income includes how the income level has changed over the last five or ten years and what future prospects are. If the income is very low, what is the reason? Is it a result of unemployment? A young family whose members are spending long years in schooling or training

Table 8-1 Social Readjustment Rating Scale

Rank	Life Event	Mean Value
1	Death of spouse	100
2	Divorce	73
3	Marital separation	65
4	Jail term	63
5	Death of close family member	63
6	Personal injury or illness	53
7	Marriage	50
8	Fired at work	47
9	Marital reconciliation	45
10	Retirement	45
11	Change in health of family member	44
12	Pregnancy	40
13	Sex difficulties	39
14	Gain of new family member	39
15	Business readjustment	39
16	Change in financial state	38
17	Death of close friend	37
18	Change to different line of work	36
19	Change in number of arguments with spouse	35
20	Mortgage over $10,000	31
21	Foreclosure of mortgage or loan	30
22	Change in responsibilities at work	29
23	Son or daughter leaving home	29
24	Trouble with in-laws	29
25	Outstanding personal achievement	28
26	Wife begin or stop work	26
27	Begin or end school	26
28	Change in living conditions	25
29	Revision of personal habits	24
30	Trouble with boss	23
31	Change in work hours or conditions	20
32	Change in residence	20
33	Change in schools	20
34	Change in recreation	19
35	Change in church activities	19
36	Change in social activities	18
37	Mortgage or loan less than $10,000	17
38	Change in sleeping habits	16
39	Change in number of family get-togethers	15
40	Change in eating habits	15
41	Vacation	13
42	Christmas	12
43	Minor violations of the law	11

SOURCE:
"The Social Readjustment Rating Scale" by T. H. Holmes, R. H. Rahe. Journal of Psychosomatic Research 1967, 11. 213–218. Copyright © 1967 Pergamon Press, Inc.

Case Example 8-2: Older Couple With Grown Children

The Miller family moved to the community forty years ago when Mr. Miller came to work in a local Chrysler automobile plant. Both Mr. and Mrs. Miller are from Tennessee. They are in their seventies, and Mr. Miller has been retired for almost fifteen years. At the time of his retirement the family's income was adequate, but in the fifteen years since, his pension has not kept up with the cost of living. Mrs. Miller never worked because her husband was able to make an above average income as a tool and die maker at the local plant. In the last few years they have not been able to afford anything above the food, clothing, and taxes on their house. Their nutrition is adequate, and they have enjoyed meals together all through their marriage. They have two daughters, one in Boston and one in Houston. The daughter living in Boston has a college degree and has worked as a schoolteacher. She is married with three children and is very involved with her own family. She talks to her parents each week but only visits once a year. The daughter in Houston lost her job two years ago and has been unable to find a new job at close to her previous salary. She is in her own crisis and is unwilling and unable to support her parents at this time.

Mr. Miller suffered a stroke five weeks ago. He was hospitalized at the local community hospital for three weeks and has been discharged for two weeks. A community health nurse now comes to their home each day. He is beginning to feed himself again and can dress with much assistance. There is a good chance he will be able to resume all of his previous activities within another five or six months.

Mrs. Miller is very frustrated and very alone at this point. Mr. Miller was the stronger of the two and made all the decisions. Mrs. Miller does not have the cash for the hospital bills. Mr. Miller was covered by Medicare, but the hospital bill for his share of the cost is greater than their savings. Mrs. Miller has lost fifteen pounds in the last few weeks. She does not drive and feels very trapped in the house. Mr. Miller does not want her to leave the house, and she is afraid to leave him alone.

Income is inadequate.

Children do not live in the area. They are not a source of support to aging parents.

Wife is unable to cope with husband's illness and added responsibility.

---

may also have an income barely adequate to meet their basic needs, but within five years, they will earn a much higher income and progress to positions of power and authority in the community.

Cultural Influence on the Family Unit Because culture is the blueprint for forming a family's values, attitudes, philosophies, and way of living, cultural and ethnic backgrounds are determined as part of the family assessment. The importance the family assigns to its heritage and the degree to which cul-

tural practices are adhered to are essential information. However, the community health nurse avoids cultural stereotyping, because what may be true for one group of people may not be true for another group of the same ethnic or cultural background. The assessment identifies a family's differences from, as well as its similarities to, an ethnic or cultural group (see Chapter 5).

For example, the family's cultural background can influence the importance of children to the family. In some cultures children are allowed to develop as individuals and are seen as individuals very early. In other cultures children are viewed more as pawns, belonging to the parents. These parents see the child not as an individual, but as an extension of themselves.

Cultural patterns define for the family what is normal and abnormal behavior. Because of the different cultural backgrounds, what may be acceptable for one family may not be acceptable for another—or for the nurse. By identifying the strengths of the cultural identification and practice for a family, the nurse gains insight into the importance of its cultural heritage. A few years ago conformity was the rule in American society, and families that had ethnic or cultural backgrounds different from the majority were looked down upon rather than identified as unique. Today families are becoming more involved with their cultural heritage and are viewing their cultural backgrounds with a sense of pride.

Congruence of the Family with the Community   A very important aspect of the psychosocial assessment is determining the congruence, or "fit," of this family with the immediate neighborhood, the larger community. An example of incongruence is the family living in a very rundown home with broken windows and littered yard in the midst of a middle-class neighborhood of manicured lawns and flower gardens. When this occurs, the family is often ostracized and the children have no friends. Another example of incongruence with a community would be the Jewish family living in a very protestant religious community in the Bible Belt. It is important to evaluate the congruence of the family with the immediate neighborhood, but it is also important to relate the family to the larger community. The low-income family with limited schooling may feel uncomfortable in a college town. Likewise, residents in the college town may feel uncomfortable having low-income residents as neighbors. It is important to ascertain the family's opinion and the family's view of its congruence with the larger community and with the neighborhood. Asking the family how they feel about living in the neighborhood, how many

friends they have, how many people in the community they talk to, and who their children play with would give some beginning assessment data on the fit of this family with the community.

Goals of Family for Each Member   It is important to identify the family's goals—the goals not only of each adult member, but also of the children as well. Families may not realize that they have goals, but all families have goals whether or not they identify them as such. Goals are frequently viewed in terms of family roles. If a mother views her role as a mother rather than a wife, her goals will revolve around child-rearing or the development of her family. If a young wife sees herself as a career person and wants to become a trust officer in a local bank rather than a mother, the family may or may not accept this goal as appropriate to her role. Conflict can result if the goals of the individual family member are different from the goals of the family unit. For example, if a woman enters school after her children are grown and away from home, she might complete her education and develop career goals that the family may consider unacceptable.

Individual family members may also have conflicting goals. For example, the husband might have the goal of an adequate bank account, whereas the wife has a goal of home ownership. Children's goals are often more oriented to the present than their parents' goals; the grandparents and the extended family may have even more future-oriented goals.

Parents' goals for their children may differ from the children's own goals. The parents may have a goal of college education for a child who has no such desire. When the child's goals and the parents' goals conflict, it can be difficult for the parents and the child to arrive at a compromise and even more difficult for children or parents to give up their goals completely. Even young children can respond to the question What do you want to be when you grow up? Deciding what you want to do when you grow up is beginning to formulate goals. Asking this question of the child in front of the parents often gives information on the parents' perception of what the child wants to do. Not infrequently

Case Example 8-3: Emerging Family

The Smith family moved to the community about six months ago. Kathy is from a small town in Utah, and Dave is from Dallas. They were married three years ago when Kathy was seventeen and Dave eighteen. Dave's father worked in a gasoline station for thirty years, and Kathy's father was a schoolteacher. They met four years ago when the two families were on a vacation in Florida. They moved to Michigan to get away from both sets of parents: Kathy has an uncle in the state. Dave is working as a mechanic at a car dealership, and Kathy will finish beautician school in another month. She is already earning some money cutting hair at home. They have postponed childbearing until they have saved enough money to buy a small house. Both Kathy and Dave would like to attend the community college to earn a degree. Kathy would like a family now, but Dave is adamant that they cannot start a family until they have a house and are able to afford a child.

Couple is from different backgrounds and has been married three years.

Their future orientation is toward more schooling, a home, and a family.

Conflict has arisen between husband and wife regarding timing of childbearing.

Kathy's mother died six months ago, and Kathy and Dave plan to raise her younger brother who is twelve. He is somewhat immature and has had a very hard time accepting his mother's death. Both Kathy and Dave have recognized the drain the brother will cause on family finances. Dave does not resent her brother, but uses him to discourage any possibility of having a child in the near future.

Couple has the added responsibility of raising the wife's brother.

---

the child has said all his life that he wants to be a police officer, but his father who wants the child to become a lawyer like himself, does not hear what the child is saying. Children need to be encouraged to develop and share their goals. This communication can bring the family together and open new areas of understanding.

This part of the assessment involves first obtaining information from all family members and then putting together as consistent a picture of family goals as possible. The community health nurse can help the family identify and verbalize their goals. He or she can also help the family determine if their goals are feasible and achievable as well as what the outcome would be if the family achieved their goals. Since goals are fluid and constantly changing, it is also important for the nurse to review periodically the goals a family has identified (see Case Example 8-3).

The Family's Values The family's values are most readily apparent in relation to their views of

recreation, education, and health. How a family uses leisure time indicates what its priorities and values are regarding recreation. Does family recreation involve the total family unit, or is it recreation for each individual family member, such as a son's playing touch football? Do the adult family members attend children's sports activities but not participate in sports themselves? Asking a family what they do for recreation helps a family to focus on how they use leisure time and what is important to them. At times a family can be so involved with survival that they do not see the importance of recreation and leisure time.

How parents view the school system and teachers and how they value the total educational process greatly influences how their children will view education. If parents themselves felt threatened by the teachers, threatened by the principal, and less than successful in the educational system, they often convey this to their children and the children assume the same attitude and devalue education. If parents view education as exciting and important, they will share these values with their children. How authority is viewed and accepted may also depend on people's experiences. For some families the teacher is very much an authority figure, whereas in other families the teacher is more a friend. Families that are future-oriented usually plan for college or other postsecondary education for their children. Children whose parents are college-educated have a greater tendency to attend college and graduate from college than do children of parents who did not attend college.

Almost every individual and every family says that health is an important value—that having good health permits one to accomplish what one wants to accomplish and to enjoy life to the fullest. However, what people say about health is less important than what they do. How much money is a family willing to invest in health care? How much time and effort are put into being healthy? What self-care practices are employed? How much emphasis is put on preventive medicine? How much time is devoted to health screening, breast self-examination, diet, or exercise? If the family has a choice of spending money for a physical exam or a new stereo, which would they choose? Whether health maintenance and preventive health services are values is usually more indicative of the family's view of health than is crisis care. All families view health care positively when there is a crisis or an acute illness, but the value placed on prevention is another issue. The importance the family places on preventive care, exercise, and proper nutrition indicates the family's values concerning health.

Nutritional Assessment

Nutrition is a very intimate part of a family's lifestyle and an area most families believe they understand at least somewhat. Most everyone has learned, usually in school, about proteins, carbohydrates, and fats. However, the adequacy of many family diets in America today is in question because of the increase in snacking and the consumption of large numbers of empty calories.

Diet Recall The nutritional assessment begins with a twenty-four-hour recall of the typical diet for each family member. There are various ways of obtaining this recall. One way is to ask all family members to record everything they ate and drank for twenty-four hours. The difficulty with this approach is the amount of time it takes to write everything down. For example, if a mother has several young children, she may not have time to complete the diet history for each one of the children. A faster way to obtain the information is simply to ask family members what they had to eat yesterday, what they plan to eat today, and if this daily food intake is fairly typical. This way the data can be gathered during the home visit. The typical diet is needed for each family member; however, if some of them are not present, the information can usually be obtained from the mother or the father. A dietary record for a period of several days gives even more data and may be needed if problems are identified. The difficulty of keeping a diet record for several days must be weighed against the usefulness of a complete diet recall.

Along with the dietary recall, important information can be obtained by asking the family to name their favorite foods and the foods they eat most frequently. Then the community health nurse can ask *why* these foods are their favorite foods. After obtaining a diet history, the next step is to analyze the diet in relation to the basic food groups, inclusion of vitamins and minerals, and the ratio of fat, protein, and carbohydrates. All these are related to the caloric needs of the individual family member. A diet that is adequate for one family member may not be adequate for another. For example, children and pregnant mothers have widely differing requirements.

Influences on Family Diet Though economic status has an influence on what a family eats, large expenditures on food do not guarantee an adequate diet. Much money might be invested in convenience foods and snacks that have limited nutritional value.

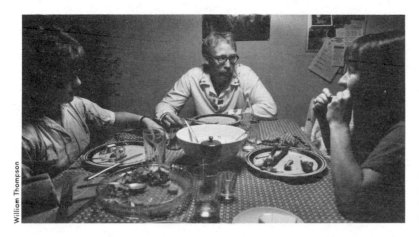

William Thompson

Patterns of family eating can reveal information about family values and relationships as well as nutrition and health status.

Food stamps and the Women, Infant, and Children (WIC) food programs have increased the availability of nutritional foods to low income families; however, the use of food stamps does not guarantee an adequate, well-balanced diet. Some segments of the population are moving toward nutritious foods, reducing the number of preservatives and the amount of fats and animal proteins they consume. However, Americans still consume a large portion of their calories from animal protein, and for many families the amount of meat and sweets they are able to purchase is a source of pride. We are all subject to a barrage of advertising that constantly encourages the American family to purchase more cupcakes, processed meats, and snack foods. And, unfortunately, although Americans today are much more sedentary than they were a few years ago, eating patterns have remained much the same as if the population were involved in hard manual labor.

Another important area to assess is who purchases the food? Is this a joint venture that includes the mother and children, or do the adults go shopping together? Is grocery shopping seen as a pleasurable outing, or is it drudgery after a long day at work? The frequency of shopping also indicates whether or not meal planning is long-range or is done at the last minute during frequent trips to the grocery store. It is also important to assess the ade-

quacy of food storage. Convenience foods and modern equipment permit the family to reduce time on food preparation, but the length of time food is stored has increased. Foods should be labeled, and the length of storage should be determined in advance. Who usually does the food preparation in the home? Is it always done by one person? If several persons are cooking, labeling is even more important. Care, management, and adequate preparation of foods directly relate to family's health and are consequently of concern to community health nurses.

Patterns of Family Eating   Patterns of family eating are as varied as any other aspect of family living. Is mealtime seen as a time for the family to eat their daily portion of calories, or is it a time to share ideas, joys, and sadness with the family unit? It is important to determine the pattern of family eating. Does the family eat together several times a week, only on weekends, or very rarely altogether? Meal patterns provide insight not only to a family's food habits, but also to the value they place on the family unit.

Another aspect to be assessed is the pattern of eating outside the home. Are fast food restaurants commonly frequented? Are they a regular substitute for meals at home, or are fast food restaurants seen as a convenience during times of crisis or extremely busy times? The nutritional quality of many fast foods is adequate, though some are over-supplied with fat and carbohydrates. Awareness of the nutritional content of foods served in fast foods and other eating facilities will help families to make informed choices about where to eat outside of their homes.

Friedman (1981) states, "It is within the context of family that faulty dietary habits are learned, involving familial behavior patterns which are central to daily life" (p. 20). The assessment of family nutrition is an essential part of the family assessment, but it is also a sensitive area that is very personal and value-laden. It is important to help the family understand that the assessment is a way to identify not just problems, but also positive aspects of their nutrition.

Environmental Assessment

The environmental assessment begins on the way to the family's home. What is the neighborhood like? Who is living in the neighborhood? Is the neighborhood in a state of transition, or is it a stable community? How close is the family's home to major shopping centers? How close is it to community activities? Are there playgrounds in the area? How close are these to the family's home? How far are the elementary schools and the high schools? How far away are the police and fire departments? What is the age of the neighborhood? Is this a rural area, an urban area, or suburban area? What is the appearance of the home from the outside? Is there a play area safe for young children? Does the area appear to be cared for, or does it appear to be in a state of neglect? How long has the family lived here? How safe is the area? Is crime increasing or decreasing in the area? The answers to these questions will form the basis for the environmental assessment.

Housing   How similar or dissimilar is the family's home to other homes in the block and in the surrounding area? The house or apartment is assessed first in terms of adequacy to meet the basic needs

of shelter; however, for a family to grow and develop, all members need some space to call their own. The provision of privacy is an important aspect of the housing. Do children have their own bedrooms, or how many children must share a bedroom? Do the parents and children share sleeping areas? Housing codes often limit the number of individuals that can live in a home, but large families may be unable to find or afford adequate living space. It may be difficult for individual family members to have adequate private space for their own needs when many people are living in one small confined house or apartment.

Sanitation and Safety   The sanitary and safety conditions of the family in its home environment are focal areas for assessment. The frequency of trash pickup or other methods of solid waste disposal should be determined for adequacy to meet the needs of this family. Home safety for all members is an important consideration. If young children live in the home, their safety and protection from dangerous objects, poisons, and burns must be assessed. If there are elderly family members who have physical limitations, the entry and exit from the home should be barrier free, the house interior should be arranged to prevent falls, and there should be adequate space to move through the home. Families often overlook safety hazards because of their familiarity with the environment. The assessment can be utilized to discuss safety hazards with the family, because awareness is the first step toward providing a safe environment.

Aesthetics   The aesthetics of the home influences the family's view of it. It is very difficult for a family to keep a house clean and neat if the structure is in very poor condition. The care and state of repair of the house may also give clues to the value the family places on their home. Do they see their home as merely a shelter to protect them from the elements, or does it provide a secure environment where they can share and grow? Is there agreement or conflict among family members on the housing arrangements? Is the housing temporary or permanent? All these issues influence the way family members view their home.

Access to Community Resources Another aspect to consider is accessibility of community resources. This is true in both rural and urban areas. How close is the home to a bus line or other types of transportation? How far is the nearest grocery store and how expensive is that grocery store? If the family does not have a washer and dryer, how far away is the nearest laundromat? Where is the family's church? How far away is medical care, both the hospital or the clinic and physicians' offices? The availability of health care—that is, the ability to reach the health care provider—may influence whether care is sought.

The physical environment is an important area for assessment because this is the place the family spends much of their time, and the quality of the environment can have a positive or negative effect on the total family unit. Much of the environmental assessment can be completed by observation and brief discussion during other parts of the family assessment.

Sources of Relevant Data

Data collection for the nursing assessment is usually accomplished by the nurse on a home visit. The approach is usually an unstructured, free-flowing exchange of information between the nurse and the family. Community health nurses often provide teaching or counseling simultaneously with the ongoing nursing assessment. If the assessment is not completed during the first or second visit, it may be spread over several visits. It is important for the community health nurse to continually point out the relevance of the assessment to the family.

Assessment as Part of Nursing Intervention

Families often question the benefit to them of the nursing assessment. By helping families understand the role of the assessment, ensuring that they participate fully in it and develop family-centered goals as a result of the assessment, the nurse aids the family in understanding the importance of the assessment. When this approach is used, the family does not feel they have been giving the nurse information without any direct benefit for themselves. Another way of involving the family in the assessment process is the continuous identification of family strengths. The identification and sharing of these strengths with the family increases their interest in the assessment process and encourages their active participation.

Timing of Assessment

Visiting the family at different times during the day and on different days of the week increases the opportunity to see the family in different situations. For example, if the family has school-aged children, and the visits are always made at ten o'clock in the morning, the community health nurse has no opportunity to assess the interaction of the children with their parents or the interaction of the children among themselves. The timing of the nursing visit is extremely important. If the nurse is trying to obtain information on the mother's approach to toilet training, visiting when the child is awake is crucial if the nurse is to observe the mother-and-child interaction. Additional insight can be obtained through the observation of family members in a clinic setting. This is often possible if the health department runs immunization, well-child, or family planning type clinics. Seeing the family in their own environment and again in a different, perhaps threatening, environment provides information on how the families respond to threatening events. Visiting around mealtime allows the nurse to obtain objective data on the family's nutrition at that meal. If the mother is having difficulty putting her two-year-old to bed for a nap, then it is important for the nurse to visit during this period of time. However, it is difficult for a mother with several small children to be attentive to and involved in teaching or counseling by the community health nurse if all the children are present. At least one visit should be made to a family when all members are present.

Written Record

The family assessment should begin with the review of the written record. If another nurse has visited this family previously, an analysis of previous nursing care should be completed before the first home visit. If the family has just been referred to the agency, some information can be obtained about the family from the referral, which may include information about the family situation by the social worker, nurse, or other health care provider. Some hospitals send copies of the nursing care plans for individual family members to the community health nurse as part of the referral. Although the nurse may wish to validate the data on the record or on the referral, he or she can use these data as a baseline for the assessment.

Before a visit the community health nurse should obtain the family name, address, telephone number, and a synopsis of the reason for the referral or the reason for community health nursing intervention. The family assessment builds on previous data and utilizes current data for a comprehensive family assessment.

Recording of Data

The recording of data is an essential part of the nursing assessment. Although the recording of observation and the written presentation of the family assessment can be a very time-consuming process, it is essential to the overall nursing intervention. Data that may not now seem important may at some later date be very critical to the nurse working with the family. The accurate recording of the complete assessment is imperative in working with the family. Although community health nursing has not yet identified a perfect recording system, the following formats are samples of commonly used recording methods.

Narrative Format

In the narrative format the community health nurse records a summary of the visit to the family. Some agencies require the recording to be broken down into subjective and objective areas of data collection. Other agencies provide blank sheets of paper for ongoing running commentary on the family, the assessment, and the nursing intervention. Figure 8-1 is an example of a narrative recording form for the family assessment, utilizing the assessment areas identified in this chapter.

Checklist Format

Some agencies have adopted a checklist format that is designed to reduce the amount of time spent doing paperwork. Another advantage of the checklist format is that information is consistently recorded in certain areas of continuing concern to the patient's welfare. The checklist or fill-in-the-blank type of assessment format not only saves time but also gives some clues to the nurse for areas that need to be assessed and increases the accessibility of information to all nurses working with the family. Figure 8-2 is an example of this format.

Summary Recording

The third type of presentation format for the family assessment is the brief summary recording (Figure 8-3). In this type the family assessment is broken into assessment areas with key words included for each section. The community health nurse writes a summary of observations and data regarding the family in relation to each applicable area. This format is a kind of compromise between the narrative and the checklist format with the advantage that it allows some flexibility for the nurse in recording the family assessment.

Each one of the formats has advantages and disadvantages. Some nurses will find one format easier to use than another. It is the quality of nursing assessment that is the important consideration. The format is an adjunct to the assessment, but the form is only a form, and no form can make a limited family assessment comprehensive.

FAMILY ASSESSMENT

Family Name_____   _____

Family Address_____   _____ Phone_____

Family Assessment (Include the family constellation, family strengths, and family needs. Consider the physical, psychological, social, and environmental areas for assessment.)

Family Health Goals (Include family priorities.)

Identify Family Needs That Require Nursing Intervention

Figure 8-1 Narrative form for family assessment.

Assessment Tools for Community Health Nurses

Several tools have been developed to assist the nurse with the assessment process. One of the major advantages of assessment tools is that they can increase the objectivity of the assessment by validating the nurse's professional judgment. However, the value of assessment tools can also be overemphasized (Spradley, 1981). In this section we'll look at three examples of assessment tools that community health nurses can use.

Family Coping Estimate

One of the first tools utilized by the community health nurse was a Family Coping Estimate (Freeman, 1970), developed jointly by the Richmond Visiting Nurse Association and the Johns Hopkins School of Hygiene and Public Health in 1964. Still in use in agencies today, the coping estimate allows the nurse to identify the family's initial level of coping in ten areas and allows for estimate of change over time (Figure 8-4).

Home Observation for Measurement of the Environment

Although questionnaires are infrequently used in community health nursing, they are tools that

FAMILY ASSESSMENT		
Family Name: _____		

DATE	CHECK (✓) APPROPRIATE COLUMN	Problem	NAP
	I. ENVIRONMENTAL		
	A. Housing		
	1. Size and adequacy for family.		
	2. Condition of physical plant of dwelling.		
	3. Adequacy & condition of furnishings.		
	4. Sanitation. a. Cleanliness of environment.		
	b. Water supply: municipal; well.		
	c. Condition of plumbing.		
	d. Sewage disposal: municipal; septic.		
	B. Safety of Environment		
	1. House, yard, & immediate environment.		
	2. Neighborhood.		
	II. FAMILY LIVING PATTERNS		
	A. Availability & use of support systems.		
	B. Decision-making patterns.		
	C. Health promotion & maintenance activities.		
	D. Family relationships & communication patterns.		
	E. Coping mechanisms.		
	F. Goal-setting patterns.		
	G. Child-rearing patterns.		
	H. Independence of family.		
	III. OTHER		
	A. Transportation.		
	B. Nutrition.		
	C. Knowledge of health condition.		
	D. General hygiene.		
	E. Financial.		
	F. Social behavior.		
	G. Attitude of family toward services.		

Figure 8-2 Family assessment, checklist format. (Adapted from Washtenaw County Health Department: *Pituch/Stanford Home Health Record.* July 1981 [revised].)

DATE	
	PLAN FOR MEDICAL EMERGENCY Medical Source: Transportation: Contact Person (address, phone):
	RECORDS AVAILABLE (Other Volumes or Sources):
	OCCUPATION & EMPLOYER:
	MEDICAL & DENTAL CARE:
	SOCIAL AGENCIES:
	FINANCIAL:
	SPECIAL CONSIDERATIONS WHEN WORKING WITH THE FAMILY
	OTHER (Include Family Concerns):

Signature _____ Date _____

Figure 8-2 *(continued)*

FAMILY ASSESSMENT

Family Name _____

Family Address _____   Telephone Number _____

FAMILY CONSTELLATION   Length of time at this address _____

Name	Date of Birth	Relationship to Head of Household	Education	Health Status

EMPLOYMENT OF FAMILY MEMBERS _____

FAMILY INSURANCE _____

SOURCES OF FAMILY HEALTH CARE _____

PHYSICAL ASSESSMENT

Family Member Name	Height	Weight	BP	Major Physical Health Problems	Current Health Status

SUMMARY OF FAMILY'S PHYSICAL HEALTH STATUS _____

ENVIRONMENTAL ASSESSMENT (include family strengths and needs) _____

PSYCHOSOCIAL ASSESSMENT (include family strengths and needs) _____

SOCIOCULTURAL ASSESSMENT (include family strengths and needs) _____

NUTRITIONAL ASSESSMENT (include family strengths and needs) _____

SUMMARY OF PREVENTIVE HEALTH PRACTICES UTILIZED BY THE FAMILY _____

SUMMARY OF FAMILY STRENGTHS _____

SUMMARY OF FAMILY NEEDS _____

Figure 8-3 Family assessment, summary format recording.

FAMILY COPING ESTIMATE

Family ——————————— Nurse ——————————— Date ————

Initial ————————————— Periodic ————————— Discharge ———

Coping Area	Rating x-status 0-est. change Poor. . . . . Exc.	Justification
Physical Independence	1 2 3 4 5 Not Applicable ☐	
Therapeutic Independence	1 2 3 4 5 Not Applicable ☐	
Knowledge of Condition	1 2 3 4 5 Not Applicable ☐	
Application of Principles of Personal Hygiene	1 2 3 4 5 Not Applicable ☐	
Attitude Toward Health Care	1 2 3 4 5 Not Applicable ☐	
Emotional Competence	1 2 3 4 5 Not Applicable ☐	
Family Living Patterns	1 2 3 4 5 Not Applicable ☐	
Physical Environment	1 2 3 4 5 Not Applicable ☐	
Use of Community Resources	1 2 3 4 5 Not Applicable ☐	

Comments

Figure 8-4 Family Coping Estimate. (Developed jointly by the Richmond IVNA City Nursing Service and the Johns Hopkins School of Hygiene and Public Health, 1964. From Freeman RB: *Community Health Nursing Practice*. Philadelphia: Saunders, 1970.)

I. Responsivity of the Mother
II. Avoidance of Restriction and Punishment
III. Organization of the Environment
IV. Appropriate Play Materials
V. Maternal Involvement
VI. Variety in Daily Stimulation

Figure 8-5 Home Environment Subscales. (From Caldwell B: Home observation for measurement of the environment. In: Humenick S (editor), *Analysis of Current Assessment Strategies in Health Care of Young Children and Childbearing Families.* New York: Appleton-Century-Crofts, 1980.

needs further exploration and greater utilization by community health nurses. One example of a questionnaire is the Home Observation for Measurement of the Environment (HOME), developed by Betty Caldwell (Caldwell, 1982). This tool attempts to assess the relationship of the home environment to the development of the infant or child. When using a tool such as the HOME, the community health nurse focuses on one particular aspect of the family (Figure 8-5).

Family Apgar

The Family Apgar developed by Smilkstein (1980) is a tool to assist health professionals in evaluation of the family. The individual family member's response indicates that person's satisfaction in the five areas of adaptation, partnership, growth, affection, and resolve (APGAR). The Family Apgar was designed not as a diagnostic tool, but rather to assist physicians in the assessment of a family's functioning in relation to a child's perception. The Family Apgar provides five close-ended questions that could apply to any family. This tool could provide initial information about these five areas of family functioning, and the area that appeared to present difficulty could be further assessed by the nurse (Figure 8-6).

Family APGAR Questionnaire

	Almost always	Some of the time	Hardly ever
I am satisfied that I can turn to my family when something is troubling me.	___	___	___
I am satisfied with the way my family talks over things with me and shares problems with me.	___	___	___
I am satisfied that my family accepts and supports my wishes to take on new activities or directions.	___	___	___
I am satisfied with the way my family expresses affection and responds to my emotions, such as anger, sorrow, and love.	___	___	___
I am satisfied with the way my family and I share time together.	___	___	___

Scoring: The patient checks one of three choices which are scored as follows: "Almost always" (2 points), "Some of the time" (1 point), or "Hardly ever" (0). The scores for each of the five questions are then totaled. A score of 7 to 10 suggests a highly functional family. A score of 4 to 6 suggests a moderately dysfunctional family. A score of 0 to 3 suggests a severely dysfunctional family.

**The Five Components of
Family Function (Family APGAR)**

1. **Adaptation:** the utilization of intra- and extra-familial resources for problem-solving in times of crisis.
2. **Partnership:** the sharing of decision-making and nurturing responsibilities by family members.
3. **Growth:** the physical and emotional maturation and self-fulfillment that is achieved by family members through mutual support and guidance.
4. **Affection:** the caring or loving relationship that exists among family members.
5. **Resolve:** the commitment to devote time to other members of the family for physical and emotional nurturing; involving a decision to share wealth and space.

Figure 8-6 Family APGAR questionnaire. (From Smilkstein G: The Family APGAR. A proposal for a family function test and its use by physicians. *J. Fam. Pract.* 1978; (6):1231–1239.)

Formulation of Nursing Diagnosis of the Family

The final step in the assessment process is the formulation of nursing diagnoses. The diagnosis is an analysis of the assessment. All data must be considered in terms of their relevance to the family unit and to each individual family member. Although some needs and concerns would appear important to the community health nurse, they may or may not be considered relevant to the family. While the data may substantiate a need for obtaining dental care for a ten-year-old child, the family may see this as a very low priority compared to obtaining birth control for the mother and obtaining eyeglasses for the husband so he can continue with his employment. The diagnosis is a concise summary of the analysis of the family assessment, including a comprehensive analysis of family strengths and family needs.

After the family's needs and strengths have been identified and the importance of these to the family have been determined, the next step is prioritizing the family needs. Priorities are fluid and change frequently as a result of new concerns and resolution of previous needs. It is important that both the family and the nurse understand the importance of flexibility in priority determination. At times, families may place a high priority on one specific need but may be unable to follow through with intervention to answer this need. If such a need can't be addressed, other needs take priority.

The priorities can now be translated into family goals. The family goals are those areas toward which both the family and the nurse will direct their effort. Family goals established must be achievable and measurable. In this way the family and nurse can determine when goals are accomplished and can measure progress toward the accomplishment of these goals.

Additional areas may be identified by the nurse as potential areas that may need nursing intervention. Although the nurse may identify an area of need, the family may not have the interest or energy to work in this area at this time. Goals must be established with the family. Establishment of family goals is a way of addressing those areas that have been identified as needs for the family. Assessment of family strengths and needs can be used again later to help the family identify additional goals.

Summary

The family assessment is an essential component of family-centered community health nursing practice. The assessment focuses on family strengths and needs, the interrelationship of all family members, and the relationship of the family with the community. The health of the family influences each individual family member, and the health of the individual affects the family. The nurse must be sensitive to the overt as well as covert needs of the family.

The most frequent data-gathering tools used by community health nurses are their own observational and communication skills. A sensitive, positive assessment that includes the family in the assessment process provides the basis for nursing intervention and evaluation. Although the assessment is the basis of practice, the assessment is also an ongoing, continuous process. The results of nursing interventions and family response must be a part of the ongoing family assessment.

Topics for Nursing Research

• What health promotion activities are performed by families in middle socioeconomic groups as compared to those in lower socioeconomic groups?

• Determine the relationship between nutrition and health by conducting a participant observation study of the practices of a family who places a high value on health compared to families who place a low value on health.

• Select a family assessment tool and determine the tool's usefulness in collecting clinical data as compared to research data.

Study Questions

1. A family assessment includes which of the following elements:
   (1) Family members' health status
   (2) Strengths and weaknesses of the family unit
   (3) Relationship of the family to the larger community
   (4) Family members' functions
   a. 1 only
   b. 1 and 4 only
   c. 2 only
   d. All of the above
   e. 1, 3, and 4

2. Which of the following statements concerning family strengths is most useful to the nurse in conducting a family assessment?
   a. Determining family strengths is time consuming and may be unnecessary.
   b. Focusing on family strengths can result in family members having more positive feelings about the assessment.
   c. Assessing family strengths is of little value to the nurse unless the family already knows how to use their strengths to improve their health status.
   d. Determining family strengths is the beginning stage of the family assessment process.

3. Which of the following questions are relevant in assessing a family's health promotion activities?

   (1) Do the females in the home practice breast self-examination?
   (2) Is the family aware of immunization schedules of the children?
   (3) Does the family have regular vision examinations?
   (4) Does the family practice oral hygiene with regular visits to the dentist?
   a. All of the above
   b. None of the above
   c. 1 and 2 only
   d. 3 and 4 only

4. Which of the following responses is the best way to determine a family's values with respect to health?
   a. Ask them how they feel about being healthy.
   b. Have them to develop a profile of a healthy life-style.
   c. Observe what self-care and preventive health practices they employ.
   d. Ask them how much they pay for health insurance.

References

Caldwell B: Home observation for measurement of the environment. In: Humenick S (editor), *Analysis of Current Assessment Strategies in Health Care of Young Children and Childbearing Families.* New York: Appleton-Century-Crofts, 1982.

Freeman R B: *Community Health Nursing Practice.* Philadelphia: Saunders, 1970.

Friedman MM: *Family Nursing: Theory and Assessment.* New York: Appleton-Century-Crofts, 1981.

Holmes TH, Rahe RH: The social readjustment rating scale. *Psychosom Res* 1967; 11: 213–218.

Miller JR, Janosik EH: *Family Focused Care.* New York: McGraw-Hill, 1980.

Otto HA: A framework for assessing family strengths. In: Reinhardt A, Quinn M (editors), *Family-Centered Community Nursing: A Sociocultural Framework.* St. Louis: Mosby, 1973.

Smilkstein G: Assessment of family function. In: Rosen G, Geyman J, Layton R (editors), *Behavioral Science in Family Practice.* New York: Appleton-Century-Crofts, 1980.

Spradley BW: *Community Health Nursing, Concepts and Practice.* Boston: Little, Brown, 1981.

Chapter 9

Community Health Assessment

Cecilia E. Dawkins

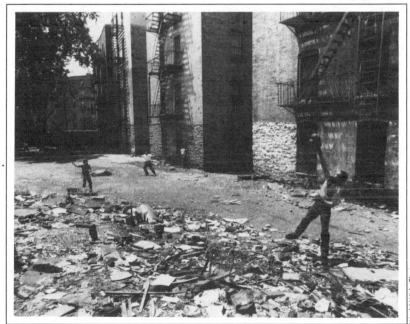

Assessing the health status and needs of a community as a whole is a special challenge to nurses, who learn to identify which factors may indicate that community residents are at risk of disease, neglect, and violence.

Chapter Outline

Definition and Purposes of Community Health Assessment

The Community as Client

Approaches for Conducting a Community Health Assessment

    Windshield Survey

    Social Survey

Participant Observation

Key Informants

Social Indicators

Nominal Group Process

Summary

Topics for Nursing Research

Study Questions

References

Chapter Objectives

After completing this chapter, the reader will be able to:

- Define and discuss the purposes of a community assessment
- Conduct an assessment of a community
- Compare and contrast the following methods as to their advantages and disadvantages for collecting data for a community health assessment: windshield survey, social survey, participant observation, key informants, social indicators, and nominal group process

As discussed in Chapter 7, assessment is the first phase of the nursing process. This phase provides the foundation for the activities that take place during the nursing process. A needs assessment of the community can enable the community health nurse to obtain information and discover resources crucial to the delivery of quality health services to the individuals, families, and groups in the community. In order to achieve this, community health nurses have to be thoroughly familiar with the community. This chapter describes the purposes of community health assessment and the methods used to conduct the assessment.

Definition and Purposes of Community Health Assessment

Assessment can be defined as the planning to determine a need. The assessment process has three phases: data collection, data analysis and presentation, and a statement of conclusions (Braden & Herban, 1976).

Accordingly, community health assessment is a process of collecting data about the community; analyzing these data; and finally arriving at the health status and needs of the community based on these investigative activities. The summary statement of conclusions derived from the data-gathering and analysis phases can be called a diagnosis. An in-depth discussion of diagnosis as a stage in the nursing process is presented in Chapter 10.

A community may be assessed for any number of reasons: to identify its needs; to know the health status of the residents; to identify high-risk groups; to identify needs of ethnic or minority subgroups in the population; to accomplish health planning and facilitate policymaking; to identify and allocate resources; to determine the need for community health nursing services; to identify the strengths and weaknesses of the community; and to know the people's attitudes toward health. This is not an exhaustive list nor is it ranked in terms of priority. However, it does demonstrate the various purposes for which the assessment may be done.

The Community as Client

The concept of the community as the client emphasizes the focus of community health nurses to define problems and provide health services at the aggregate and group levels. Accordingly, Muecke (1984) notes the following:

Community health nursing integrates the epidemiologic approach with the nursing process to make fundamental decisions about care at the level of the population as a whole. This means that the unit of concern includes not only those who seek care, as is the case in clinical nurs-ing, but those who do not. The segment of the population that has not received care is included to establish how common or rare are the health problems or needs of the care receivers, to determine if the nonreceivers need or want care and the reasons they have not obtained it, and to provide for health maintenance among the whole population (p. 27).

While the community health nurse with graduate education will be best prepared to conduct an assessment with the focus on the community as the client, the baccalaureate-prepared nurse is usually prepared to assess individuals and families in the community. This is important to note because of the increasing complexity of assessment approaches and methods as one goes from the assessment of individuals and families within a community to the assessment of a community or several communities

(see, for example, Flynn, 1984; McCarthy & Daly, 1984). The baccalaureate-prepared nurse is able to participate in the conduct of the assessment, especially if there has been a good basic preparation in epidemiology. See Chapter 6 for an in-depth presentation of epidemiology and its relationship to assessment.

Approaches for Conducting a Community Health Assessment

Various methods can be used to assess a community. This may be upsetting to someone who would prefer one procedure to accomplish the process. However, a general approach would aim to collect objective and subjective data using more than one method. Objective data are often referred to as hard data and subjective data as soft data. This is because objective data are usually quantifiable and thought to be more reliable than subjective data. For example, objective data may have been obtained from statistical reports of health records of clients who utilize the services of community agencies and hospitals, and from surveys of the characteristics and health trends of different communities or the nation as a whole. On the other hand, subjective data are observations made using the five senses: sight, sound, smell, taste, and touch.

Since both types of data should be collected in an assessment of the community, various approaches are necessary. The following six approaches are common in needs assessment activities and are especially appropriate in community health nursing practice: (1) windshield survey; (2) social survey; (3) participant observation; (4) key informant; (5) social indicator; and (6) nominal group process. Several of the approaches are also methods used to collect data in the research process, especially social survey and participant observation methods. Therefore, the student who desires more detail is referred to basic texts on research methodology.

The Windshield Survey

The community health nurse will find it beneficial and economical to begin the assessment with what is commonly called a *windshield survey*. The windshield survey is a composite of subjective data that the community health nurse collects through personal observations about the people and their lifestyles, and the environment in which they live and may work in the community. The windshield survey allows the community health nurse to use the five senses while driving as well as walking around the community. See Table 9-1 for examples of the kinds of subjective data that can be collected during a windshield survey. Case Example 9-1 describes a typical windshield survey.

The Social Survey

The *social survey* is a method to collect data on a sample of persons in a population regarding their views on diverse issues. It can be very valuable in the assessment process. Using this approach, one can determine the needs of a population at risk. In other words, information can be obtained on those individuals, families, and groups who may or may not be in the health care system, but in whom there is potential interest in serving.

The social survey is especially effective in providing information about consumers' attitudes and

Table 9-1   Examples of Subjective Data to Be Collected in a Windshield Survey

Subjective Data	Observations
Sight	What do you see as you walk or drive through the community? Are natural or artificial boundaries evident? What are the boundaries—rivers, major thoroughfares, or parks? What kinds of architecture are observable? What style and size of housing are in the community? Are the houses multiple- or single-dwelling structures? What is observable in regard to the environment? Are houses in good repair, or are there many houses in a state of disrepair? What is the appearance of yards? Do street names and buildings reveal any unique characteristics? What service facilities are seen in the area? Are there social service agencies, grocery stores, pharmacies, health care providers, schools, and churches? What modes of transportation are available to the residents? What recreational facilities are available in the community? Are there swimming pools, tennis courts, and ball fields, or are children in the streets or in vacant lots? Whom do you see on the streets? Are there women with small children? Are there teens or older adults? How are they dressed? Are they black, white, and Asian, or are some other ethnic groups present? Are there ethnic neighborhoods? What animals do you see? Are there dogs? Are they on leashes or running loose? Can rats or other rodents be seen running around? What evidence of politics is visible? Are there campaign posters? Is there a party headquarters? Is there evidence of a predominant party affiliation? What protective services are seen in the community? Are there fire stations, police stations, and ambulances or other emergency vehicles?
Hearing	What can you hear where you drive or walk through the community? Is the area quiet? Can you hear birds singing and children playing, or are there loud industrial noises, traffic sounds, loud music, and airplanes?
Taste	Use the sense of taste to assess the flavor of the community. What kinds and numbers of food establishments are in the neighborhoods? Greek, Mexican, or other specialty restaurants? Are there many fast-food stores? Or are food services old, traditional, family-operated establishments?
Smell	How does the community smell (a paper mill smells much different from a bakery)? Are there noxious industrial emissions? Or are there pleasant odors of flowering trees and honeysuckle?
Touch	Use touch to understand how it feels to be there. Is the area surrounded by a barbed wire fence, or are there open fields of wildflowers? Do you feel uncomfortable? Do residents seem friendly? Are they willing to stop and chat, or do they ignore you and hurry on their way?

SOURCE:
Taken from portions of Table 6-3, Sommerville BL: Nursing assessment: Data collection of the community client. In: Griffith J, Christensen P (editors), *Nursing Process: Application of Theories, Frameworks, and Models*. St. Louis: Mosby, 1982, pp. 74–76. Used with permission.

Case Example 9-1: Use of the Windshield Survey

Mrs. Jones, a community health nursing instructor, requires her baccalaureate nursing students to conduct a windshield survey as their initial assignment when they first come to a department of health clinic for their clinical experience in community health nursing. Although the students are based at the clinic, participation in the survey increases their understanding of the community at large. In addition to recording their observations and organizing them according to the subjective categories of the survey, they discuss their feelings about doing the survey and about the community with their instructor in their clinical supervision group. Each of the six students in the clinical rotation assesses a section (subarea) of the community. By sharing their knowledge of their subareas, they gain an understanding of the entire community.

Baccalaureate students use the windshield survey to begin a community health assessment.

thoughts about their health care. The thoughts of consumers about their needs and the ability of the health care system to meet those needs are of interest as part of any thorough community health assessment process. This information is useful in providing health services responsive to the needs and desires of consumers.

This method can also be used to enable the community health nurse to reconstruct the patterns that individuals, families, and groups have in their encounters with the health care system. For example, the nurse may raise questions about the kinds of experiences that took place surrounding an episode of illness. Additionally, the community health nurse may want to have information such as: What is the clients' usual source of care? Was there easy access to a source of care? How many return visits were made to the physician or nurse because of this episode of illness? How satisfied were the clients with the services that were received? Were the clients able to assume their normal activities such as attending school or going to work, or was it necessary to stay in bed? These are examples of the kind of information that the community health nurse can obtain when he or she is trying to determine the "paths" that people take in the health care system. Equally important, the community health nurse can determine if different subgroups of a population such as ethnic minorities

differ in how they seek care and their experiences with a health care system once they are in it.

In addition the social survey method allows estimates to be made for the population as a whole. The community health nurse collects data from a limited number of people in a community about their health status and use of health services, and then he or she projects what these attributes would be for that community as a whole. This technique, the use of a small number of observations to represent many, is called *sampling* (Aday, 1984).

Samples can be random, stratified, or purposive. In *random sampling* each case has an equal probability of being selected. For example, a community health nurse wishing to conduct a survey might take a neighborhood and decide to interview every fifth household in each block of the neighborhood. On the other hand, the community health nurse might decide to use a random numbers table after numbering every unit in the universe. (Every unit in the universe means that we know the population of eligible persons from which a sample can be obtained.) Lists for selecting a sample include such examples as the voter registration lists, lists of numbers from the telephone book, or lists from community organizations. When all the units in your universe are identified, then random sampling is an appropriate and useful procedure.

A *stratified sample* is useful when an attempt is

being made to reach a group with selected characteristics, such as a particular income group or a particular ethnic group. Both time and money may be saved by utilizing stratified sampling. This technique involves dividing the universe into strata or groups of individuals and obtaining samples within each group.

Finally, in _purposive sampling_ the researcher uses a nonrandom approach to select persons for the sample. Suppose the community health nurse decides to go into one clinic today and ask the clients present just on that one day about their opinions about the health care delivery system. Obviously, no systematization of the selection process is made. However, if the interest of the community health nurse is limited to getting a rough impression of a particular situation on a selected topic, then purposive sampling is an excellent technique.

In a social survey, data may be collected by a mailed questionnaire, a telephone interview, or a personal interview. There are advantages and disadvantages to each of these methods. Advantages in using mailed questionnaires in conducting a community assessment include the absence of an interviewer bias and its rather low cost when compared to personal or face-to-face interviews.

However, mailed questionnaires present disadvantages if the community health nurse has a need to ask complex questions requiring quite a bit of information. Additionally, there is no support present to encourage the individual to respond. In fact, since those who respond may be individuals who are interested in the topic or issue or those with similar characteristics, the result may be a biased sample.

The telephone interview is another economical way to conduct a social survey. It also has lower sampling and interviewing costs as compared with the personal interview. Drawbacks to this method include the fact that not all persons who should be represented in the sample will have a telephone. This is especially the case in some low income communities. Another potential problem is that fewer questions can usually be asked. Typically the time should not exceed thirty minutes for a telephone survey.

In the personal interview the researcher can usually cover a broad range of questions. An advantage of this technique is the higher levels of completion, since the interviewer's presence can encourage the respondent to finish the interview. While this is a potential attribute of the process, it can also be a disadvantage because of interviewer bias. Additionally, this is an expensive method as compared to the mailed questionnaire and the telephone interview. Finally, if the proposed site for the interviews is the homes of residents in the community, the sample may be limited if residents refuse to allow access to their homes to conduct the interview.

In summary, the social survey can provide quality information as compared to other available methods. Whether the mailed questionnaire, the telephone interview, or personal interview is utilized during the assessment depends on the relative advantages of each method given the desired outcome.

Participant Observation

Participant observation is the data collection method wherein the data collector is directly or indirectly a part of an ongoing social setting to observe and analyze what takes place in the setting (Lofland, 1971). This method is used to gain insight and information that probably would be otherwise unattainable.

The sampling is nonrandom. An example might be a _snowball sample_, whereby an individual who has the attributes that are sought for the study is selected and this individual provides another person with similar attributes. The sample size is usually small. A study may be limited to only people in a particular social setting or organization in the community rather than the entire community.

The methods for collecting data include interviewing people. However, the use of a structured questionnaire or interview schedule as in the social survey method is less likely in this approach.

Types of data collection may involve the examination of records by an organization; the direct observation of and/or the direct participation in the entire events as they take place. However, it must be stressed that data gatherers must impose many more controls on their own perceptions of behavior to guard against recording their influence on the behavior and responses of the people they are studying.

The participant observer must have a defined system for remembering the context in which observations were made. Even more importantly, there must be a systematic approach to retrieving notes and analyzing them. The data results are usually written up and reported in a narrative format rather than reported in tables and graphs as in the case of quantitative data. Summaries are usually made during the data collecting period. The common forms of recording in participant observation are field notes and log or personal notes. The log or personal note is a daily account of events and conversations while field notes are more in-depth accounts of observations with analytical interpretations. The participant observation method's success depends on accuracy and completeness of logs and field records.

Three categories have been suggested by Wilson (1985) as formats and approaches for organizing and recording field notes: observational notes, theoretical notes, and methodological notes. We'll present a brief definition and illustration of these categories next:

Observational Notes *Observational notes* are descriptions of events obtained by answering the questions who, what, when, where, and how. This information is obtained by listening and watching. It is imperative in recording these types of notes to limit personal interpretation. The following elements would be key factors that should be observed and noted:

- "Actors" or subjects—roles of the subjects, their characteristics, and interrelationships
- Setting—structure, atmosphere, and appearance
- Timing of events—time of day, season, weather, and other environmental factors
- Purpose of the event

- Behavior and activities of actors or subjects
- Pertinent points in the conversations, movements, and evidence of behavior manifesting nonverbal communication
- Frequency and duration of events and behavior

An example of an observational note of a prenatal class follows:

The purpose of the prenatal class is to provide couples with the Lamaze preparation. The site of the prenatal class is the community room of the local church in a suburban community. The thermostat is at 68 degrees on this spring afternoon. The room is carpeted; there are no chairs and only one table is at the front of the class. The table contains an anatomical model of a fetus and pamphlets and flyers about hospitals, nurse midwives, and home deliveries. There are flip charts near the table that contain graphic presentations of the stages of pregnancy and delivery. In the room are five couples, each sitting on the floor with two pillows. The ratio of nursing staff to couples is one to five. The nurse conducting the program is doing so as a structured class but with ample demonstration of the Lamaze techniques. The friendly, orderly atmosphere fosters frequent conversation between the couples and the nurses regarding the stages of pregnancy and birth.

Theoretical Notes The second category of recording field notes is the *theoretical note*. Theoretical notes are purposeful and directed attempts to derive meaning from observations. The objective is to apply an interpretation to the observation. An illustration of a theoretical note follows:

Three principles are essential to successful completion of the techniques described in this prenatal class. The participants must understand what is to take place during the delivery process; breathing and relaxation techniques are key to reduced pain; and support by the significant other must exist. The participant observer observed in the class distinctive elements that seemed to support each of these principles. The atmosphere and supportive material in the room were selected to complement this learning objective. The variety and comprehensiveness of the information seemed to be designed to facilitate learning, regardless of educational background or level of the couples. Key principles regarding breathing were reduced to easily memorable exercises. This technique will facilitate retention at the time of delivery when greater stress is bound to exist. And, finally, the role of the significant other was demonstrated and stressed. This is an attempt to inculcate the principles of the class and have individuals behave during the delivery exactly as taught as if the behavior was second nature.

Methodological Notes The final category for field notes is the *methodological note*. These notes serve as instructions and reminders to oneself about the methodological approach that is to be employed in the analysis of the data. An example of the methodological note might be:

In an attempt to determine differences in approaches to teaching prenatal classes, I made prior arrangements with three instructors. Each instructor was asked to identify participants who had experienced at least one prior delivery but were using the Lamaze technique for the first time. I decided to look for instances where the nurse instructors sought specific anecdotal comments from these participants to illustrate comparative advantages of the Lamaze technique. I was also interested in the degree to which these participants' knowledge was sought by other class participants or otherwise given the status as informal leaders because of their prior experiences at childbirth.

Logs or Personal Notes In addition to field notes, one other prominent form for recording participant observation is the *log* or *personal notes*. Logs or personal notes are the participant observer's reactions and reflections about the observed events. A final example from the prenatal class demonstrates the use of a log:

Tonight is the night we hear from a couple that "graduated" from the prenatal class. The couple brought their one-month-old son. They were given ten minutes to recount highlights of their experiences in the delivery and to give pointers to the class. Although our child was born at home and was attended by a nurse midwife, the "graduates" had a hospital delivery with a physician in attendance. The nurse instructor had a delivery at a hospital with a nurse midwife in attendance. I was struck by the commonality of the experience. I recalled the last session of the class I attended and the morning of my delivery. I felt a common bond with the "graduates," not

only because we had similar experiences, but also because it seemed that at one month our sons had the same repertoire of behaviors. One of the benefits of using the participant observation approach among this group is the knowledge that in addition to obtaining skills in the use of the approach, the class offers a basis for personal memories of a significant event.

There are disadvantages as well as advantages of the participant observation method. The disadvantages include: (1) the study is usually limited to a rather circumscribed group or social setting; (2) unlike probabilistic social survey sampling, no statistically determined error estimates are available on the results from samples studied from participant observation; and (3) the results are not generalizable and are limited to the sample that was studied. Ethical issues may arise as one attempts to disguise participants in the study during the writeup of the report. If one studied a small organization or group, this can be problematic in terms of maintaining confidentiality and anonymity of the subjects.

On the other hand, participant observation is a very good method of obtaining descriptive material about a social phenomenon. Second, the descriptive information obtained from this method can generate theories and hypotheses for further studies. Finally, this can be an inexpensive form of research that may be done by an individual working alone.

Key Informants

Key informants are people who know their community and will talk to an outsider about it (Green, 1982). The key informant may be a community resident or a nonresident who works in the community and has become knowledgeable about it. Health providers, social workers, law officers, hairdressers, and schoolteachers are examples of potential key informants.

In an unfamiliar community a good key informant can be a cultural guide to the community health nurse. The individual can help the community health nurse begin to understand the sub-

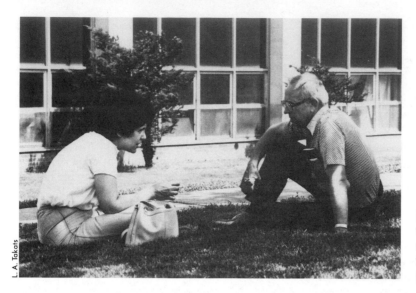

Key informants, such as social workers or school teachers, can provide helpful information while acting as a cultural guide for the nurse.

tleties and complexities of a particular community. Key informants acting as cultural guides may not be willing initially to discuss sensitive areas with an outsider, especially if the individual is from an ethnic group or profession that the community holds in low esteem. However, as rapport is established with the key informant over a period of time, the areas of mistrust can be overcome.

Finally, the community health nurse should be aware of the fact that it may be necessary to strike up a "bargain" with the key informant (Green, 1982). The key informant is giving up time and energy to help with the community health nurse's work. There may be implicit or explicit expectations of a return of the favor. Maybe the key informant would want a sympathetic ear to listen to and pass on criticism about a particular service. Maybe the community health nurse would be expected to hold a health workshop on an issue of importance to the individual and the community. The community health nurse needs to have in mind what can be offered to key informants in exchange for their confidence.

It is quite easy to fall into a practice of relying only on the opinions of others who have

worked in the community for many years, especially if they are members of the nurse's own racial or ethnic group. There are two poignant reasons for avoiding this:

First: Just because people have long familiarity with a community does not mean that they know and understand it well. Individuals can and do spend years working among persons they little understand, and their longevity is sometimes used as justification for flawed judgements. Second: Reliance upon a senior worker or others in an agency for information about the community being served deprives the worker of the direct encounters outside the relatively safe world of the agency that are essential for learning about and appreciating cultural distinctiveness (Green, 1982, p. 63).

Hence, it is important for the community health nurse to make direct contacts with people in the community and avoid an overdependency on key informants for information about the community. The key informant may be able to introduce the community health nurse to people who may provide different viewpoints about the community. Some people refer to key informants as "gatekeepers" because of their ability to grant access to key community people and organizations. Views from more than one informant can enrich an understanding of the community. It is important to note that key informants will provide perceptions, experiences, and knowledge from their individual perspectives. In itself this is a limited presentation, which may well be one-sided.

One major limitation of this method of assessment is that usually the data are not quantifiable. There has been limited use of the key informant method in quantitative research; therefore, few discussions about its reliability and validity are available (Warheit, Buhl, & Bell, 1978). When Warheit and his associates (1978) completed their pilot study to determine the practicality and utility of the social survey analysis and the key informant survey as needs assessment methods, they found the key informant survey was less useful as a needs assessment tool when compared with social survey analysis. On the other hand, Schwab (1983) noted that key informants may be better able to provide information about different kinds of programs needed in the community rather than identifying how many persons need care.

An advantage of using key informants as a needs assessment method is that key informants can provide the kinds of qualitative data that statistics hide or are incapable of revealing. For example, it may be known from the statistical tables how many families live in a particular community. However, the community health nurse would find it difficult to know from those same statistics the subtle details of family life affecting the families' health utilization and propensity to use or not use the services of community health nurses.

Social Indicators

A *social indicator* is a statistic that helps to make a comprehensive judgment about the condition of a society in a particular area (U.S. Department of Health, Education and Welfare, 1969). It is a mea-sure of the presence or absence of a social problem (Bloom, 1983). A social indicator is sometimes used as a measure of the quality of life for a community or country. For example, an inner-city community may have an infant mortality rate of 33 deaths per 1000 live births; the same rate may be 10 in the suburban community. One inference from this statistic is that the quality of life for the residents in that inner-city community is lower than the quality of life of the counterparts in that suburban community. The assumption with the social indicators method is that an estimate can be made of human service needs of persons in a community based on geographic, ecological, social, economic, and demographic characteristics of the area (Warheit, Buhl, & Bell, 1978).

Commonly used indicators include (Smith, 1979, p. 290):

Clinical

- Spatial arrangements of the community's people and institutions
- Descriptive epidemiological parameters of the population, such as age, sex, socioeconomics
- Social behavior—particularly crime, substance abuse, family patterns, and morbidity and mortality rates
- General quality of living—for example, substandard housing, overcrowding, accessibility to services, and economic conditions

Once the community health nurse has decided the objectives of the assessment, he or she can determine the data most appropriate as indicators of need. Examples of indicators whose results can point to need in a community include the following (Smith, 1979, p. 290):

- Population characteristics: density, race, ethnicity, national origin, marital status, age, sex, and family status
- Housing characteristics: type of structure, owner- or renter-occupied dwellings, persons per dwelling, and substandard indices

- Mortality and morbidity rates: tuberculosis, infant mortality, venereal disease, or suicide
- Crime patterns and arrest records: those dealing with substance or personal abuses (driving while intoxicated or assaults)
- Education

Multiple factors of need, rather than one or two, are usually used although sometimes a measure of poverty may be based on family income and family size. On the other hand, when multiple indicators are used, the result is an index. For example, an index for family stability could be divorce, separation, percentage of mother-child households, and similar factors (Warheit, Buhl, & Bell, 1978).

An advantage of this method is that it can be inexpensive because the data have already been collected and are usually available. Second, there is strong evidence that the social indicators approach is a practical and valid means for assessing human service needs.

The data for use of the social indicators approach may be obtained from local public and private sectors such as health departments, health systems agencies, private health providers, community health nursing agencies as well as the U.S. Department of Commerce, Bureau of the Census. For example, Table 9-2 provides examples of governmental data sources produced at the national level. These publications provide statistical information on vital statistics (e.g., rates for births, deaths, marriage and divorce) and data on the incidence, prevalence, and mortality rates of disease. These publications are routinely housed in many public and university libraries. In Chapter 6, Ray provides a discussion of sources of health data for the epidemiological study of a community. The reader is referred there for additional sources at the national, state, and local levels.

Nominal Group Process

The reader can find the general dynamics of groups discussed in Chapter 12, but the nominal group process is introduced here because it is a valuable method in the assessment of health needs in the community. There are times when the community health nurse wants to find out how providers, clients, or potential clients feel about their own health or their health services. These data are not always readily available or, more importantly, the data may not reflect the current feelings of community residents. One method to obtain this information is through the technique called the *nominal group process.*

The nominal group process is "a structured meeting which seeks to provide an orderly procedure for obtaining qualitative information from target groups who are most closely associated with a problem area" (Van de Ven, Delbecq, 1972, p. 338). This method of needs assessment can be utilized in diverse settings such as human service organizations, businesses, and educational institutions (Gilmore, 1977). For example, Casbergue (1975) demonstrated its use in nursing education as an effective tool for nursing faculty to identify subjective and objective problems, issues, and critical ideas in any selected area.

The key features of the nominal group process (Francis & Browdy, 1977, pp. 246–247) are as follows:

- Stimulates creative tension
- Avoids evaluation or elaborating comments while problem dimensions are being generated
- Provides participants an opportunity to engage in reflection
- Forces participants to record their thoughts
- Avoids the dominance of a group by strong personality types
- Encourages the generation of minority opinions and ideas
- Alleviates "hidden agendas"
- Prevents premature closure of problem dimension identification
- Imposes a burden upon all participants to work and produce their share of the necessary task
- Focuses on problem identification rather than problem solution

Table 9-2 Selected Governmental Publications Produced at the National Level

Governmental Publication	Description
Materials to access the data	
American Statistics Index	Comprehensive guide to statistical publications of the three branches of federal government. Indexes by subject and names, categories, titles, report numbers.
Catalog of Publications of the National Center for Health Statistics (NCHS)	Part one is a chronological listing by series and publication number. Part two indexes broad topics such as arthritis or divorce compared against factors such as income, employment, or residence size.
Facts at Your Fingertips	Topical index to statistical publications on a variety of health topics; some general nonstatistical data provided.
Data Series	
Advancedata	Issued irregularly—intended as a means of early release of selected findings from NCHS surveys.
Vital and Health Statistics Series	Covers data from surveys conducted by the National Center for Health Statistics. Publications grouped by subseries such as methodology, health, or vital statistics.
Morbidity and Mortality Weekly Report	Provisional information on selected notifiable diseases in the U.S. and deaths in selected cities; annual summary published.
Monthly Vital Statistics Report	Provisional vital statistics by geographic subdivisions; some rates and subdivisions time lag: thirteen weeks for death data and eight weeks for other information.
Vital Statistics of the U.S.	Volume One covers natality. Volume Two covers mortality. Volume Three covers marriage and divorce. Wealth of information in types of breakdown of materials. Life tables included.
Statistical Notes for Health Planners	Issued irregularly as a guide to health planners in the use of methodology.

SOURCES: E. Joseph, Librarian, University of Illinois at Chicago, January 1984, Chicago, Illinois.

Table 9-3 Cycle of the Nominal Group Process

Steps	Explanation
Step 1 Silent genera-tion of ideas in writing	Each group member works silently and independently to write down results of the silent generation of ideas.
Step 2 Round-robin recording of ideas on a flip chart	Serially, each group member presents one of his or her ideas in brief. Ideas are recorded on a flip chart, visible for all to read.
Step 3 Serial discus-sion for clarification	Serially, each recorded idea is discussed to clarify the meaning of items.
Step 4 Preliminary vote on item importance	Group members work silently and independently from the list of recorded ideas to select a specific number of ideas considered to be priority items. Each member does a rank-ordering of the selected priority items on cards. Cards are collected, votes tallied, and results recorded on the flip chart.
Step 5 Discussion of preliminary vote	This is done for clarification, not for pressure toward artificial consensus. The intent is to ensure that "spread" votes really reflect differences in judg-ment, not unequal information or misunderstanding.
Step 6 Final vote	The procedures for Step 4 are used.

SOURCE:
Adapted from Delbecq AL, Van de Ven A, Gustafson DH: *Group Techniques for Program Planning: A Guide to Nominal Group and Delphi Processes.* Glenview, Ill.: Scott, Fores-man, 1975.

The nominal group process can be conducted with a large number of people. However, they have to be divided into small groups of from six to ten individuals with a qualified group facilitator or leader. The question to pose to the group should have been carefully formulated prior to the meeting. The question formation is crucial to the success of the results of the nominal group process. It should be easily understood. Questions that require answers to hard facts or data should be avoided. The process should be designed to assess the perceptions, atti-tudes, and feelings of the participants rather than "test" participants about a particular subject. For example, one nominal group process session with community residents asked, "What do you feel is the major health problem in your community?"

A cycle for completion of a nominal group process is summarized in six steps in Table 9-3. The steps are as follows:

Step 1: Silent generation of ideas
Step 2: Round-robin recording of ideas on a flip chart
Step 3: Serial discussion for clarification
Step 4: Preliminary vote on item's importance
Step 5: Discussion of the preliminary vote
Step 6: Final vote

A guide for conducting a nominal group process session and a sample script that can be used in the classroom as well as with actual consumer groups or target groups are available (see source note for Table 9-3). It is recommended that the group leader read from a script and avoid extemporaneous explanations during the procedure. The adherence to a script serves to maintain the structure of the nominal group process. It also provides for a degree of uniformity when several groups are simultane-ously conducted to assess one question.

Case Example 9-2: Community Assessment Using Several Methods

The Suburban Cook County-Dupage County Health Systems Agency (HSA) was required by PL 91-643 to have a five-year health plan and an annual implementation plan for its service area. This health planning agency made the decision to conduct a health assessment of the residents in the communities in the two counties service area.

The general purpose of the assessment was for health planning by a government agency.

The major data collection methods included a social survey and a series of nominal group process sessions in the communities.

Several data collection methods were used in the assessment.

The social survey was done to obtain information that was not available on the current health status of residents. The purpose of the survey was also to examine the residents' use of the health care delivery system and their attitudes toward that system. Data on the environmental health of the communities were obtained.

Other goals of the assessment survey were knowledge of residents' health status, health attitudes, and use of the health system.

The Consumers' Health Survey instrument is an example of a community health assessment tool. (See Appendix 2 for the tool.) The sources used to construct the tool included the HSA's objectives and informational needs and other consumer-oriented health surveys. The survey was mailed to a probability sample of noninstitutionalized residents.

A series of nominal group process sessions were held in the various communities in the two counties to identify the health concerns and perceptions of the residents in each community.

Residents had the opportunity to make their concerns known via these gatherings.

It was possible to summarize all of the groups' concerns in a master listing of perceived health problems. It was also possible to identify a specific community's health problems as perceived by the residents who attended these nominal group process sessions.

The advantages of the nominal group process include its low cost as a needs assessment method. It can provide qualitative data about the current perceptions and attitudes of a group with data that have been collected in a structured, but democratic way. It provides a means to aggregate individual judgments. Finally, it may be used as a pilot research technique to generate hypotheses from information on a selected issue. Case Example 9-2 illustrates how a variety of assessment methods can be used together.

However, the written requirements may provide some difficulty for persons with a limited ability to read and write or for those who have difficulty writing because of advanced age or illness. The author of this chapter has participated in the nominal group process with persons who had one or more of these difficulties and found this not enough of a problem to discard using the method. What happened was that during the silent period of listing ideas on paper, those persons listed their ideas mentally. They just proceeded to verbally call out their ideas in turn during the round-robin process of listing ideas. Using this method, they were able to participate in the remainder of the meeting without difficulty.

Summary

This chapter defined and presented purposes for a community health assessment. Six approaches for conducting an assessment were discussed: windshield survey, social survey, participant observation, key informant, social indicators, and nominal group process. The community health nurse with graduate education would be involved in a leadership capacity to conduct an assessment with the focus of the community as a client. The baccalaureate-prepared community health nurse can participate in this process and is usually prepared to conduct an assessment on a group of individuals or families in a community. More than one approach should be used in the assessment process. The choices of approaches can be based on the purposes for the assessment and available resources such as money, time, manpower, technical assistance, and community input.

Study Questions

1. When doing an assessment, the community health nurse plans to interview the presidents of two community organizations with large resident memberships. This approach can be most appropriately labeled as:
   a. Social survey
   b. Key informant
   c. Nominal group process
   d. Social indicator approach
2. During the community health assessment the community health nurse reviews census data and the morbidity and mortality statistics of the community. These data are examples of:
   a. Subjective data
   b. Objective data
   c. None of them
   d. Both of them
3. The element(s) of a community health assessment consist(s) of:
   a. Data collection
   b. Analysis and presentation of data
   c. Conclusions
   d. All of the above

Topics for Nursing Research

• Evaluate the usefulness of the kinds of data that are received from key informants as part of a community health assessment.

• As a community health nurse, you have been asked to develop a program to provide services to a population of black and Hispanic residents who are primarily young women with preschool children. What specific types of data would you want to have about the community *before* planning your program, and which of the community health assessment methods will supply such data?

References

Aday L: Studying health and the utilization of medical care via the social survey method. Lecture presentation, University of Illinois at Chicago, Department of Public Health Nursing, Winter 1984, pp. 1–17.

Aday L, Sellers C, Andersen R: Potentials of local health surveys: A state-of-the-art summary. *Am J Public Health* 1981; 71: 835–840.

Bloom BL: The use of social indicators in the estimation of health needs. In: Bell R et al (editors), *Assessing Health and Human Service Needs.* New York: Human Sciences Press, 1983, pp. 147–162.

Braden CJ, Herban NL: *Community Health: A System Approach.* New York: Appleton-Century-Crofts, 1976.

Casbergue JP: The nominal group process: An effective tool in nursing education and the management of change. Presentation to the National League of Nursing, Operation Update, New Orleans, La., May 20, 1975.

Delbecq AL, Van de Ven A, Gustafson D: *Group Techniques for Program Planning: A Guide to Nominal Group and Delphi Processes.* Glenview, Ill.: Scott, Foresman, 1975.

Dever GEA: *Community Health Analysis: A Holistic Approach.* Germantown, Md.: Aspen Systems Corporation, 1980.

Flynn B: Public health nursing education for primary health care. *Public Health Nurs* 1984; 1 (1): 36–44.

Francis PR: The nominal group process. Continuing education workshop presentation, University of Illinois, College of Dentistry, 1977.

Francis PR, Browdy M: Issues and problems regarding continuing education of dental professionals in Illinois. *Illinois Dental Journal* (May) 1977: 246–252.

Freeman R, Heinrick J: *Community Health Nursing Practice.* Philadelphia: Saunders, 1981.

Gilmore G: Needs assessment processes for community health education. *Int J Health Educ* 1977; 20: 164–173.

Green JW: *Cultural Awareness in the Human Services.* Englewood Cliffs, N.J.: Prentice-Hall, 1982.

Hamilton P: Community nursing diagnosis. *Adv Nurs Sci* 1983; 5 (3): 21–36.

Joseph E: Community health data sources. Lecture presentation, University of Illinois at Chicago, Department of Public Health Nursing, Winter 1984.

Lofland J: *Analyzing Social Settings: A Guide to Qualitative Observation and Analysis.* Belmont, Calif. Wadsworth, 1971.

McCarthy N, Daly EA: Community assessment: A risk factor analysis. *J Nurs Ed* 1984; 23 (9): 398–401.

Muecke M: Community health diagnosis in nursing. *Public Health Nurs* 1984; 1 (1): 23–35.

Schwab JJ: Identifying and assessing needs: A synergism of social forces. In: Bell R et al (editors), *Assessing Health and Human Service Needs.* New York: Human Sciences Press, 1983, pp. 31–39.

Smith BC: *Community Health: An Epidemiological Approach.* New York: Macmillan, 1979.

Sommerville B: Nursing assessment: Data collection of the community client. In: Griffith JW, Christensen PJ (editors), *Nursing Process: Application of Theories, Frameworks and Models.* St. Louis: Mosby, 1982.

Stewart C: Community health assessment: A systematic approach. *Nursing Papers* 1981; 14 (1): 30–46.

Suburban Cook County-Dupage County Health Systems Agency: *The Consumers Health Survey: A Survey of Health and Health Care Needs.* Oak Park, Ill.: Author, 1977.

US Department of Health, Education and Welfare: *Toward a Social Report.* Washington, D.C.: US Government Printing Office, 1969.

Van de Ven AH, Delbecq AL: The nominal group as a research instrument for exploratory health studies. *Am J Public Health* 1972; 62 (3): 337–342.

Warheit G, Buhl J, Bell R: A critique of social indicators analysis and key informants surveys as needs assessment methods. *Evaluation and Program Planning* 1978; 1: 239–247.

Wilson, H. Research in Nursing. Menlo Park, Calif. Addison-Wesley, 1985.

Chapter 10

Nursing Diagnosis with the Family and Community

Wealtha M. Alex

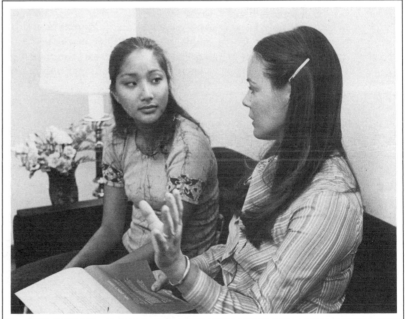

George Fry

One purpose of nursing diagnosis is facilitating communication among nurses; client involvement in the nursing diagnosis also helps achieve a second purpose, which is ensuring client participation in the plan of care.

Chapter Outline

Chapter Objectives

After completing this chapter, the reader will be able to:

- State rationale for using nursing diagnosis in community health nursing practice
- Apply the clinical judgment model of the diagnostic process in community health nursing practice
- Use nursing diagnoses contained in three classification systems
- Describe the development and major features of three nursing diagnosis classification systems
- Discuss issues relating to nursing diagnosis within the context of community health nursing

There are many important reasons for using nursing diagnosis: to improve nursing practice, to facilitate communication, to define the area of health care provided by nurses, to meet legal and political needs, and to advance nursing science (Kim, McFarland, & McLane, 1984).

This chapter describes the application of nursing diagnosis to community health nursing practice. The subject is important because diagnosis is a component of the nursing process and because studies and observation show that nursing students and practicing nurses have difficulty using nursing diagnosis.

Shoemaker (1984) decided to develop a research-based definition of nursing diagnosis when she observed that graduate students did not state a nursing diagnosis when using the nursing process and that her colleagues disagreed about the nature of a nursing diagnosis. Shoemaker's (1984, p. 109) definition of nursing diagnosis states, "A nursing diagnosis is a clinical judgment about an individual, family, or community that is derived through a deliberate, systematic process of data collection and analysis. It provides the basis for prescriptions for definitive therapy for which the nurse is accountable. It is expressed concisely and includes the etiology of the condition when known." Although the definition is long, it deserves scrutiny because it reflects the consensus of 102 nurses with identifiable expertise in nursing diagnosis. Essentially, Shoemaker's definition says that a nursing diagnosis is a clinical judgment derived from a process of data collection and analysis. The clinical judgment guides nursing therapy—nursing care planning, intervention, and evaluation. Thus, nursing diagnosis is both a process and a product; the diagnostic process yields a nursing diagnosis label (Gordon, 1982b).

Work on label development stimulated a closer look at how nurses reach conclusions about client health states. There is general agreement about the need to improve nurses' clinical judgments, but the use of nursing diagnostic labels is controversial. This chapter will briefly summarize selected points of controversy.

Defining the Diagnostic Process

We need to begin with a definition of nursing diagnosis, as it applies to nursing practice in general.

All registered nurses in all clinical settings need to make and write nursing diagnoses. The nurse's part in the diagnosis varies with the nature of the client's health state. The roles of the nurse are sometimes defined as independent, interdependent, and dependent. The independent role encompasses conditions nurses are capable and licensed to treat by themselves such as those in the area of health promotion. The interdependent role involves consultation and coordination with other health team members and might involve, for example, recognition and treatment of an ineffective breathing pattern. The dependent role is implementing another's orders as in administering medications. Some nurses believe that nursing diagnosis should be limited to health conditions nurses treat independently. Thus, nursing diagnosis does not include all areas of nursing practice (Gordon, 1982b).

According to Gordon (1982b), there are four areas of nursing practice requiring nursing clinical judgment. Nursing judgments are made when actual or potential problems: (1) relate to clients' health perceptions and health management practices; (2) occur secondary to illness, therapy, developmental changes, and life situations; (3) require referral; and (4) are treated under protocols or medical supervision. The first two practice areas require nursing diagnosis because actual and potential problems are treatable by a nurse. Since the latter two practice areas relate to interdependent or dependent nursing functions, they do not require a nursing diagnosis. That is, a nursing diagnosis is not indicated because nurses do not plan treatment.

Nurses are interested in how people respond to actual or potential health problems (American Nurses' Association, 1980). People develop typical ways or patterns of caring for themselves and dealing with health problems. Gordon (1982b) identified eleven functional health patterns and arranged them in the Functional Health Patterns Typology described in Chapter 7. (See especially Table 7-2.)

Nurses use knowledge of the universal (or general) to understand a particular client. Without knowledge of the general, nursing practice would be completely intuitive, and no nurse would have any idea of what interventions to use for a particular diagnosis (Webster, 1984). For example, community health nurses identify safety hazards in the home. Before hazards can be recognized in a particular client's house, the nurse must have a general knowledge of home safety hazards. Action to increase home safety with a given client stems from knowing how safety hazards are usually eradicated. The essential value of a nursing diagnosis is its ability to communicate the universals of nursing practice (Webster, 1984). For example, the nursing diagnosis "Potential for injury" (Kim, McFarland, & McLane, 1984, p. 470) helps the nurse recognize home safety hazards by defining and listing signs and symptoms of safety hazards in general. Nurses have always applied their knowledge of the universal into caring for particular clients. What is relatively new is the attempt to name the kinds of phenomena nurses diagnose and treat.

There are several ways to describe the thought processes used to reach conclusions about client health states. For example, the diagnostic process was presented in Chapter 7 as a process of matching client data with a published nursing diagnosis.

This chapter looks more closely at the diagnostic process using Gordon's (1982b) clinical judgment model. The model is introduced here because it describes mental operations needed to use existing and formulate new nursing diagnoses. (See Gordon's textbook for a more detailed description of the process.) The model is applicable to all nursing specialties.

"The diagnostic process is a cycle of certain perceptual and cognitive activities" (Gordon, 1982b, p. 13). The four activities of the diagnostic process are (1) information collection, (2) information interpretation, (3) information clustering (that is, grouping data), and (4) cluster naming. Although the activities are discussed sequentially, they are intertwined. Case Example 10-1 illustrates the process.

A diagnostic strategy (Gordon, 1982b) guides the activities of the diagnostic process. A diagnostic strategy is a set of decisions about what information to collect, in what sequence to collect it, and how to use the information. Though assessment guides direct the collection of basic or minimum information, nurses need to collect more information when health problems are suspected. A diagnostic strategy helps the nurse go beyond the assessment guide.

Suspected problems are identified by interpreting client cues (Gordon, 1982b). Interpretation involves using clinical knowledge and reasoning to infer possible explanations, or hypotheses, for problems suggested by client cues. The key to being a good diagnostician is the ability to generate alternative hypotheses. One suggestion is to try to think of an explanation for client cues from several areas of knowledge, such as physical or psychosocial. For example, a crying child with bruises may have fallen off a tricycle, may have been abused, or may be suffering from a bleeding disorder.

After several possible explanations have been generated, testing is required to confirm or disprove each hypothesis. Initially, testing may be done for the presence of several problems at the same time. This is called *multiple-hypothesis testing*. Such testing is done by checking for the presence of cues common to several problems. For example, a client reports that she is having trouble sleeping. The diagnostic hypotheses generated are (1) sleep onset disturbance, (2) sleep pattern disturbance—early awakening, (3) sleep pattern interruption, and (4) sleep pattern reversal. The nurse asks the client to describe her sleep pattern. Her answers provide information to test for all four sleep problems (Gordon, 1982b).

Case Example 10-1: The Diagnostic Process

Catherine Felton, a community health nurse, was referred to the Jones family by the pediatric nurse practitioner at the community well child clinic. Ryan Jones, three years old, and his mother had gone to the clinic for advice on his feeding habits. Because the Jones family had just moved to the area, the PNP sensed that there could be other family concerns that a home visit might uncover.

During the interview the mother states that she is lonely, having made *information collection* no new friends in the neighborhood. She also misses her extended family. Catherine notices that the mother seems tired and discouraged. Ryan's *information interpretation* father regularly stays late at the office and has increased his overnight *information collection* travel, while Ryan's older sisters are busily engaged with school activities and new friends. Ryan, on the other hand, stays at home with his mother and has developed no new friends. Catherine notices that Ryan clings to his mother during the interview and demands her attention at regular intervals while she is talking. The aftereffects of the recent move are a *information clustering* clear theme in the mother's remarks. Catherine decides that a possible *naming the cluster* nursing diagnosis is "ineffective family coping related to relocation."

When all but one or two hypothetical problems have been eliminated, the nurse can switch to *single-hypothesis testing*. Single-hypothesis testing is confirming or disproving problems one at a time. It is done by checking for the presence of each cue that reliably indicates the presence of the problem. Such reliable cues are called "defining characteristics" by the NANDA (North American Nursing Diagnosis Association). For example, defining characteristics of the NANDA nursing diagnosis "Coping, ineffective family: Disabling" include abandonment and intolerance (Gordon, 1982a).

Cues are *clustered*, or grouped into patterns associated with the health problems being investigated. Clustering is done by resolving inconsistencies among cues and weighing their importance relative to the hypothesis being tested (Gordon, 1982b). (See Case Example 10-2.)

After the problem or concern has been diagnosed, the nurse needs to identify the etiology, or the contributing factors. Finding the etiology is similar to problem identification—that is, alternative explanations are generated and tested to determine the reason(s) for the client's problem.

Naming the cluster involves labeling the problem that was formulated during the diagnostic pro-

cess. Mundinger and Jauron (1975) divide a nursing diagnosis into two parts: (1) statement of the unhealthful response, and (2) statement of factors that are maintaining the undesirable response and preventing the desired change. The first part of the diagnostic statement is useful for client goal-setting, and the second clause guides nursing intervention. Table 10-1 summarizes the diagnostic process.

The diagnostic component of the nursing process is not complete until nursing diagnoses are validated with clients. Validation means discussing the nursing diagnosis with clients and determining their acceptance or rejection of the nursing diagnoses. Clients have their own ideas about their health and welfare. Insight into client response to nursing diagnosis can be obtained by exploring the client's diagnostic process—identifying what they did or did not perceive about their situation, and how they interpreted their perceptions.

Knowing the client's perspective helps the nurse act effectively. Nursing diagnoses accepted by the client become the focus for nursing intervention when clients accept continued nursing service. Clients may accept the nursing diagnosis but refuse further nursing care for various reasons such as cost. In such situations, the nurse can offer other resources

Case Example 10-2: Clustering in the Diagnostic Process

Jenny Valentine, a nurse, is making a home visit to Mr. Andrews, an elderly client recently discharged from the hospital. Mr. Andrews has undergone surgery that has left him in considerable pain, for which the physician prescribed medication. Mr. Andrews lives alone, although a neighbor stops in to see him periodically.

Jenny notices that Mr. Andrews is tense, sweating, and moves gingerly. She asks him whether he feels any pain, to which he replies, "My pain isn't too bad. I haven't taken any pain medication for six hours. I'm afraid if I take the pills too often, they won't work when I really need them." After leaving Mr. Andrews, Jenny asks the neighbor her opinion of his condition. "He's not doing too good," says the neighbor. Jenny arrives at a diagnostic hypothesis of "pain self-management deficit" (Gordon, 1982a, p. 134).

Verbal report of pain severity inconsistent with nurse's observations and neighbor's report. Nurse weighs her observations and client's fear of inadequate pain control more heavily than Mr. Andrews's description of pain severity or the time interval since his last pain pill.

and/or invite clients to call if they decide later to use nursing service. A nursing diagnosis rejected by the client should be closely scrutinized to determine its accuracy. If the nurse continues to believe in its accuracy in spite of its rejection by the client, the nurse should record the diagnosis as inactive.

Clinical information used in the diagnostic process is probabilistic or uncertain. Uncertainty exists because diagnosticians may lack access to, miss, or wrongly interpret signs and symptoms of existing problems. Accurate diagnoses are made when problems exist in reality rather than in the nurse's imagination. Careful attention to each activity of the diagnostic process, retrospective review of the relationship between client cues and identified problems, and validation with clients increase diagnostic accuracy. Another factor that influences diagnostic accuracy is the clinical knowledge base and the clinical reasoning ability of the diagnostician (Gordon, 1982b).

Nursing Diagnoses within the Community Health Setting

Although the same diagnostic process is used to process individual, family, and community client data, implementing the process is different. Major differences relate to the nature of the assessment data, the theory used to interpret, cluster, and name nursing diagnoses, and the kinds of diagnostic functions performed by community health nurses.

Data of interest to community nurses vary widely in source, scope, content, reliability, and format. Sources of data range from nurse observations to the 1980 census data. The scope of the data may relate to individuals or aggregates. Data content may be about health or disease. Reliability ranges from neighborhood gossip to official reports. Data format can be verbal or statistical. These characteristics of community data affect data processing.

Each nursing speciality uses nursing and non-nursing theories and models to reach conclusions about client data. In community health, theories about individuals, families, and communities are all used to process data. Examples of nursing theories useful in processing individual or family client data are Sister Callista Roy's model and Orem's

Table 10-1   The Nursing Diagnostic Process

Activity	Purpose	Description
1. Collecting the information	To gather data about the health status of individuals, families and communities	Client cues are the "building blocks" or "raw data" (Gordon, 1982b, p. 126) from which diagnoses are formulated. Client cues indicative of possible health problems are investigated using a diagnostic strategy. A diagnostic strategy is a set of decisions about what information to collect, in what sequence to collect it, and how to use the information. A diagnostic strategy helps the diagnostician collect data beyond the minimum data requested in an assessment guide. Additional data collection is required to clarify and verify suspected problems or concerns.
2. Interpreting the information	To explain client cues relevant to health status	Clinical knowledge and clinical reasoning enable the nurse to infer possible explanations for client cues. These possible explanations or diagnostic hypothesis are tested by checking that predicted cues (i.e., defining characteristics) of nursing diagnosis are present.
3. Clustering the information	To combine client cues in patterns associated with health status concerns	Information clustering is done by resolving inconsistencies among cues and by weighing them according to their importance relative to the diagnostic hypothesis being tested. Cues are added, rearranged, or discarded.
4. Naming the cluster	To attach a label that communicates the nature of the client's health status	When the cluster is an actual or potential health problem or concern amenable to nursing intervention, it is labeled a nursing diagnosis. Persons using diagnostic labels are responsible for using them correctly—by applying the label only when client cues warrant the label.

SOURCE:
Based on Gordon's clinical judgment model. From *Nursing Diagnosis Process and Application* by M. Gordon. Copyright © 1982 by McGraw-Hill, Inc. Used with permission.

model (Griffith & Christensen, 1982). Roy's model guides nursing assessment of the family's environment and adaptation. Orem's model helps the nurse enhance a family's self-care abilities.

Hamilton (1983, p. 31) states, "nursing theory has not developed sufficiently to guide community health nurses in assessment, diagnosis, intervention, and evaluation of ways community systems influence health." She reached this conclusion after analyzing several nursing theories based on systems theory, actual community health nursing practice, and the ideal of community as client. Lack of nursing theories to guide care of the community client impedes the identification of nursing diagnoses relating to the community client. Since nursing theories and nursing diagnosis are relatively new to the profession, community health nurses can anticipate exciting developments in theory and diagnosis.

Nonnursing theories are also useful to community nurses during the diagnosis phase of the nursing process. An example of a nonnursing theory used for individual or family clients is Otto's framework of family strengths (Griffith & Christensen, 1982). Theories that can be used to process community data include the epidemiological, interactional, structural-functional, and systems approaches (Griffith & Christensen, 1982).

Theories must be selected appropriately if they are to be useful. Selection of a theory, model, or framework is based on the following considerations:

- Which theory deals most adequately with the variables of concern to the health professional? For example, Griffith and Christensen (1982, p. 8) state that a crisis theory is probably appropriate for a family whose teenage daughter has committed suicide.
- Which variables or concepts of the theory can be altered or modified to improve the client's health status and situation? For example, Erickson's developmental model is useful with children exhibiting psychosocial or behavioral problems, since the concepts address these behaviors.
- Does the theory support the main focus of change and direct the course of nursing strategies? Systems theory can be used to implement change

Table 10-2 Diagnostic Functions in Community Health Nursing

Family	Community
Assesses health-related learning needs of the family	Assesses health-related learning needs of population
Includes members of the family as partners in the assessment process	Includes members of the community as partners in the assessment process
Determines the unique combination of biological, psychosocial, developmental, and environmental factors impacting on a specific family unit	Aids in community health surveys
Uses a family theory, such as structural-functional, to guide data collection	Uses basic statistics and demographic methods to collect health data
Consults with other health and welfare agencies regarding the family	Consults with community leaders to describe the community
Analyzes data for relationships and clues to the family's health	Analyzes data for relationships and clues to the community's health
Includes members of the family in analyzing assessment data and validating nursing diagnoses	Includes members of the community in analyzing assessment data
Applies relevant theories, models, frameworks, norms, and standards to family data	Applies selected epidemiologic concepts in analyzing assessment data (population-at-risk, incidence, prevalence)
Forms ideas and hypotheses concerning data gathered in family assessment to derive inferences for nursing intervention	Forms ideas and hypotheses concerning data gathered in community assessment to derive inferences for nursing programs
	Describes present community health problems in the perspective of time (recognizes trends)

in a community (Griffith & Christensen, 1982, pp. 8–9).

Diagnostic functions performed by community health nurses while caring for family and community clients are listed in Table 10-2. These functions were derived from the literature and are presented to illustrate the diagnostic activities and conclusions encountered in the community setting.

Functions relating to the diagnostic process include analyzing data for relationships, clustering data to show relationships, deriving inferences, applying epidemiologic concepts, and applying theory. See Table 10-1 for a review of the nursing diagnostic process.

Community health nurses reach conclusions about family and community health problems or concerns and their health-related responses. Examples of the kinds of *family* problems or concerns community nurses identify are health deficits, health threats, and foreseeable crises (that is, stress points and difficulties families face in managing their health). Family responses to actual or potential health problems relate to their health capacity. Community nurses reach conclusions about a family's health capacity by evaluating their resources in relation to the estimated impact of a health problem.

Community nurses also identify the health problems or concerns and the health capacity of

Table 10-2 *(continued)*

Family	Community
Identifies health deficits, health threats, and foreseeable crises or stress points	Identifies the health status of the community including levels of vulnerability
Identifies actual or potential family health problems or concerns	Identifies common and recurrent health problems that have potential for illness consequences
Identifies possible etiology and factors contributing to family problems or concerns	Identifies forces in the larger environment that might significantly impact the community's health
Delineates the specific difficulties families face in managing their health	Identifies strengths and deficiencies in relation to preventive health practices
Identifies family resources (strengths, coping ability) to meet family health needs	Describes and analyzes resources available including patterns of utilization
Estimates health capacity of family in achieving the level of health possible for them	Describes health capability of community based on assessment
Identifies family and individual health problems	Identifies health needs of help-seeking and non-seeking populations

SOURCES:
Selected ideas from Clemen SA, Eigsti DG, McGuire SL: *Comprehensive Family and Community Health Nursing.* New York: McGraw-Hill, 1981.

Community Functions adapted from Anderson ET: Community focus in public health nursing: Whose responsibility? *Nurs Outlook* 1983; 31 (1): 46. Copyright by American Journal of Nursing Company. Reprinted by permission.

Selected ideas from Bailon SG, Maglaya AS: *Family Health Nursing—The Process.* Quezon City: University of the Philippines in Manila. 1978. p. 37–41.

the *community client*. These concerns may be common and recurrent health problems, health needs, or a vulnerable health status. To judge a community's response to health, the nurse may examine the use of health resources and identify strengths and deficiencies in relation to preventive health practices. The next section of this chapter presents three systems of nursing diagnosis labels.

Systems of Nursing Diagnoses

We'll look at three systems of nursing diagnosis: (1) the list of the North American Nursing Diagnosis Association (NANDA); (2) Classification Scheme of Client Problems in Community Health Nursing; and (3) Typology of Nursing Problems in Family Health Care. These systems were selected for discussion because they are well known or specifically relevant to community health nursing.

The North American Nursing Diagnosis Association's List

The reader may already be familiar with NANDA, so this discussion will be brief. NANDA, formerly the National Group for the Classification of Nursing Diagnoses, began in 1973. Since then, six national conferences have been held, and some of the conference proceedings have been published. The work of NANDA has spawned research and numerous publications, and NANDA's list of nursing diagnoses has been introduced into many nursing education and practice settings. For the list of accepted nursing diagnoses from NANDA, the reader is referred to Kim, McFarland, and McLane (1984). Examples of family nursing diagnoses from the list include "Coping, family: potential for growth" (see Table 10-3). Inclusion of a nursing diagnosis on the NANDA list means that the diagnosis has been accepted for clinical testing, but research is needed to validate that the condition described by the label exists in practice and is appropriately labeled.

The work of NANDA will be ongoing. Nursing diagnosis research, "especially diagnostic validation studies and inquiries into the diagnostic process"

Table 10-3 Examples of Family Nursing Diagnoses

Source	Diagnosis
North American Nursing Diagnosis Association (NANDA)	Coping, ineffective family: compromised Compromised, disabling Coping, family: potential for growth Parenting, alternation in: actual potential
Visiting Nurse Association of Omaha (VNA)	Parenting: Impairment Neglect: Child/Adult Abuse: Child/Adult

SOURCES:
Kim MJ, McFarland GK, McLane AM: *Classification of Nursing Diagnoses: Proceedings of the Fifth National Conference.* St. Louis, Mosby, 1984.
Simmons DA: *A Classification Scheme for Client Problems in Community Health Nursing.* DHHS Publication No. HRA 80-16. National Technical Information Services, 1980. (NTIS No. 14)

are priorities for the 1980s (Kim, McFarland, & McLane, 1984, p. 537). Any nurse may contribute to the work of NANDA. Gordon (1982b) describes when and how to identify nursing diagnoses in practice. Appendix D in her book tells how to submit diagnoses to NANDA. Nurses may also join NANDA, which publishes a newsletter. The address is the North American Nursing Diagnosis Association, St. Louis University School of Nursing, 3525 Caroline Street, St. Louis, MO 63104.

A Classification Scheme of Client Problems in Community Health Nursing

A classification scheme of client problems in community health nursing was developed by the Visiting Nurses' Association (VNA) of Omaha, Nebraska from 1975–1980 under a government contract. The classification "is an orderly arrangement of a nonexhaustive list of client *problems* diagnosed by nurses in a community health setting. It is subdivided into four major domains, each including the names of problems identified in each domain, *modifiers* of these problems, and *signs or symptoms* of the problems" (Simmons, 1980, p. 6). The four domains are environment, psychological, physiological, and health behaviors.

Nurses at the VNA recognized the need for a uniform nomenclature for client problems in their efforts to develop a family problem-oriented record for community health nursing. Client problems were identified inductively by community health nurses in the agency from their clinical practice. Examples of nursing diagnoses from the VNA's classification scheme include "Parenting: Impairment" and "Neglect: Child/Adult." The classification scheme underwent several cycles of testing, revision, and retesting by the VNA of Omaha and several other community health agencies. The VNA of Omaha plans to build upon this problem classification scheme by developing expected outcome and criterion measures associated with each problem label. The reader is referred to Simmons (1980) for the complete classification scheme.

Nurses using this classification scheme have reported the following advantages: increased ease in sorting significant from extraneous data, increased ability to perceive client needs in multiproblem situations, improved care planning, improved ability to evaluate problem resolution, and improved ability to interpret community health nursing services.

Simmons does not discuss the relationship of nursing theory to the classification scheme, although the references include works of several well-known nurse theorists. Perhaps the lack of a clearer relationship between the classification scheme and community health nursing theory contributed to some of the observations cited by Gordon. She states, "no evidence of problems in family coping or family dynamics were evident in Simmons' classification. Although a focus on the family and community is a stated philosophy of community health nursing, the majority of diagnoses nurses identified pertain to individuals. Perhaps most interventions are directed toward individuals in a family context rather than toward families per se" (1982b, p. 318). Freeman and Heinrich (1981, p. 557) state, "In public health nursing the family cannot be seen only as a factor to be taken into account in caring for the individual patient—the family is the patient." These two quotes point out the need for developing means, such as the classification schemes of nursing diagnosis, to help operationalize community health nursing philosophy in practice. That is, nursing diagnoses pertaining to family or community can systematically facilitate the development of interventions directed toward families or communities.

Typology of Nursing Problems in Family Health Care

The Typology of Nursing Problems in Family Health Care (Bailon & Maglaya, 1977) is a systematic arrangement of six categories of family nursing diagnoses. The typology is constructed in several levels according to the degree of generality or specificity. The inability of the family to perform one of the six health tasks is the general or main problem category under which are found the specific cues or contributory problems. Diagnoses are formulated by combining the main problem with a specific contributing problem. These diagnoses are consistent with widely accepted ideas for nursing diagnosis construction.

Freeman's (1981) family health tasks provide the organizing principle of the typology and its theoretical framework. The health tasks are:

1. recognizing interruptions of health development
2. making decisions about seeking health care
3. dealing effectively with health and non-health crises
4. providing nursing care to the sick, disabled, and/or dependent members of the family
5. maintaining a home environment conducive to health maintenance and personal development
6. maintaining a reciprocal relationship with the community and its health institutions (Bailon & Maglaya, 1977, p. 17)

Bailon and Maglaya used the health tasks in their typology because the primary function of the nurse in a community setting is to develop or strengthen the family's ability to perform health tasks.

The typology was developed and field-tested by nurse educators, practitioners, and students in the Philippines in the mid-1970s. The method of construction was inductive analysis of community health nursing with families. A review of the typology suggests that the diagnoses are treatable by nursing intervention. Potential problems are identified as "health threats," such as accident hazards, and "Stress Points/Foreseeable Crisis Situations," such as the death of a family member.

Feedback from students and faculty using the typology indicates that the typology increased cue recognition, helped implement the concept of family-centered care, improved family care planning, and defined family problems so they seemed more manageable to the nurse and the family. The reader is referred to Bailon and Maglaya (1977) for a copy of the typology.

A comparison of the three nursing diagnosis systems is found in Table 10-4. The table compares the way the systems were developed and their content.

Notable similarities among the systems are commonalities between the diagnoses, development rationale, inductive development, lack of community client diagnoses, incompleteness, and the need for widespread testing and research in practice. Parenting provides an example of a nursing diagnosis included in all three systems:

1. *NANDA*—"Alteration in Parenting due to knowledge or skill deficit" (Gordon, 1982a, p. 186)
2. *VNA*—"Parenting Impairment" (Simmons, 1980, p. 23). (Although the VNA scheme does not specify etiology, "conveys expectations incongruent with child's level of growth and development" is listed as a sign or symptom of the diagnosis.)
3. *Typology*—"Inability to care for dependent family member due to ignorance of child development and child care" (Bailon & Maglaya, 1977).

Significant differences between the classification systems are the number of nurses involved in the development, the use of nursing theory as an organizing principle, and the inclusion of etiology in the diagnostic label.

Community health nurses may choose to work with one or all of these classification systems. References (Bailon & Maglaya, 1977; Gordon, 1982a; Kim, McFarland, & McLane, 1984; Simmons, 1980) contain definitions, signs and symptoms, etiologies, examples, guidelines, case studies, and diagnostic exercises.

The presence of multiple classification systems can be viewed as a negative or a positive situation. On the negative side, multiple systems could increase the complexity of using diagnoses, may divide the profession along specialty lines, and fragment effort. On the other hand, it is reassuring to find similarities emerging from diverse efforts.

Table 10-4   A Comparison of Nursing Diagnosis Classification Systems

	North American Nursing Diagnosis Association	A Classification Scheme of Client Problems in Community Health Nursing	Typology of Nursing Problems in Family Health Care
A. Development 1. Rationale	Begun in 1973 when Gebbie and Lavin called the first national conference because they viewed nursing diagnosis as a concept critical to nursing. They asserted that the classification of nursing diagnoses represented "nothing less than the systematic description of the entire domain of nursing" (Kim, McFarland, & McLane, 1984, p. 528).	Created to provide a uniform method for documenting client needs and the services provided to meet those needs.	Developed to identify the kinds of family problems nurses deal with in family nursing practice.
2. Participants	Nurses from the United States and Canada attending six national conferences since 1973.	Community health nurses employed by VNA of Omaha. Scheme tested by community health nurses employed in three other agencies.	Nurse educators, practitioners, and students in the Philippines.
3. Method	Primarily developed inductively by nurses from all specialties of practice. Formation of nurse-theorist group to develop a theory of unitary (holistic) man which can be used to generate diagnoses deductively.	Developed inductively from the active practice of community health nurses.	Created by inductive analysis of community health nursing with families. Built on Freeman's six family health tasks. Used Roy's requirements and criteria for a taxonomy of nursing diagnosis. Developed to coincide with data base for family nursing also developed by these nurses.

(continued)

Table 10-4   *(continued)*

	North American Nursing Diagnosis Association	A Classification Scheme of Client Problems in Community Health Nursing	Typology of Nursing Problems in Family Health Care
4. Field-testing	Amount and results of field testing difficult to determine. Twenty-one research papers published in the *Proceedings of the Fifth National Conference.* Publications referring to the work of NANDA increased dramatically over the past decade.	Tested on a representative sample of ninety-nine families in agency, revised, then tested and retested by three other community health agencies. Nurses using the system reported numerous benefits.	Tested two months by faculty and undergraduate nursing students. Testing showed the typology helped nurses implement the concept of family-centered care, define family problems so they seemed more manageable, and improve family care planning.
B. Description of Classification System			
1. Inclusion of individual, family, and community nursing diagnosis[a]	Contains forty-four individual, seven family, and no community nursing diagnoses.	Contains forty-two individual, three family, and no community nursing diagnoses.	Contains six categories of family, no individual, and no community nursing diagnoses (see Appendix 3).
2. Structure of nursing diagnosis	Diagnosis written with two clauses. First clause describes the client problem. Second clause identifies the probable factors causing or maintaining the problem. Many problem labels contain a modifier, such as a deficit.	Diagnosis consists of a problem label and a modifier. Etiology is not written.	Nursing diagnosis is a two-part clause. First clause describes family's inability to perform health tasks. Second clause describes factors that contribute to the performance problem.
3. Domain of nursing practice	List intended by some to be confined to conditions that can be alleviated by nurse actions. Limiting the list to independent nursing functions is controversial among NANDA leaders.	List contains diagnoses treatable by nursing intervention and others requiring physician referral.	List composed almost entirely of diagnoses treatable by nursing expertise.

Table 10-4   *(continued)*

	North American Nursing Diagnosis Association	A Classification Scheme of Client Problems in Community Health Nursing	Typology of Nursing Problems in Family Health Care
4. Presence of potential problem diagnoses	Any nursing diagnosis may be a potential problem. Six diagnoses are labeled as potential problems on the Fifth National Conference list.	Any nursing diagnosis may be a potential problem. No diagnoses labeled as potential problems.	Potential problems are called "health threats" and "stress points/foreseeable crises situations."
5. Organization of list	Diagnoses are listed alphabetically by problem label.	Diagnoses are categorized under one of four domains: environment, psychosocial, physiological, and health behaviors.	Diagnoses organized according to Freeman's six family health tasks.
6. Completeness of Classification System	Work on the list is ongoing. Published mechanism for any nurse to participate in development.	Scheme is a "nonexhaustive" list of client problems. No published mechanism for contributing to development and refinement of system.	Presented for "peer evaluation and trial." Request feedback from nurses using the system.

SOURCES:

NANDA: From Kim MJ, McFarland GK, McLane AM: *Classification of Nursing Diagnoses: Proceedings of the Fifth National Conference.* St. Louis, 1984, The C.V. Mosby Co.

VNA: Simmons DA: *A Classification Scheme for Client Problems in Community Health Nursing.* DHHS Publication No. HRA 80-16. National Technical Information Service, 1980. (NTIS No. 14)

Typology: Bailon SG, Maglaya AS: *Family Health Nursing—The Process.* Quezon City: University of the Philippines in Manila. 1978. p. 37–41.

[a] For this count, a nursing diagnosis was not considered a family diagnosis unless the diagnosis referred to problems in family coping, family dynamics, or parenting. Any individual problem or concern could be problematic to other family members. Environmental concerns (for example, housing) could be individual or family problems.

Issues in Nursing Diagnosis

Two issues to be discussed are (1) Is it necessary to use published nursing diagnoses, such as labels developed by NANDA? and (2) What is the domain of nursing diagnosis? A discussion of these issues can help the community health nurse use nursing diagnosis more wisely.

Necessity

Williams (1980, p. 359) asks, "To do nursing, do nurses need a special nursing taxonomy of patient problems, a unique nursing language, a classification scheme?" (Williams was referring to the work of NANDA.) Shamansky and Yanni (1983) also question whether the development of nursing diagnoses and a taxonomy of nursing diagnoses are necessary for nursing practice. They are concerned that nursing diagnoses impede nursing by unnecessarily complicating practice, undermining clinical reasoning, and discouraging interdisciplinary collaboration.

Shamansky and Yanni (1983) observe that community health nursing students could collect data and articulate real and potential nursing problems but had trouble stating their nursing diagnosis using the NANDA list of diagnoses. Using nursing diagnosis was problematic because (1) many clinical situations were not described by accepted diagnostic labels; (2) it was hard to decide which label best fit a clinical situation; and (3) labels were "clumsy" and "ponderous." They believe that conclusions written by the nurse involved in the clinical situation are better than "predigested labels" because the nurse's conclusion is more precise.

Shamansky and Yanni (1983) are also concerned that nursing diagnoses may impede practice by interfering with clinical reasoning. Such interference occurs by preventing intuitive thought (quick and ready insight) and discouraging inferential thought (conjecture beyond the information given). Intuition may be stifled because it is not an acceptable method of reaching clinical conclusions. The authors argue that nurses need intuition to cope in many nursing situations. They also believe that published nursing diagnoses limit the number of alternative explanations the nurse might generate to explain client data. This limitation will occur because the lists are incomplete and nurses will use only nursing diagnoses on the list to explain clinical data. Published nursing diagnoses may also limit the number of alternative explanations nurses generate because it encourages premature labeling of clinical impressions.

According to Shamansky and Yanni (1983), published nursing diagnoses are verbose, unclear, and foreign to all health care workers including most nurses. Its use would impede interdisciplinary communication. They also believe that nursing diagnoses are designed to lay claim to an exclusive area of health care. Such a claim is inappropriate and will exacerbate turf battles among health care professionals. In their view it is no longer the prerogative of one health care discipline to claim exclusiveness in care, because the practice boundaries are overlapping at an increasing rate, especially in primary care.

Williams's question could be rephrased to ask, "Is it possible to practice nursing without using published nursing diagnoses?" The answer is obviously yes, since nursing has been practiced for years without such diagnoses. The alternative to published nursing diagnoses is a label generated by the individual nurse for specific client situations. Once a decision is made about the value of published diagnoses, concerns about usage, such as the impact on interprofessional collaboration, can be more adequately evaluated. Published and individual nurse labels could be compared in terms of their utility in practice and their potential for improving practice.

Comparison of the practical utility of individual nurse and published labels in community health nursing must specify which nursing diagnosis system is being considered. Graduate and student community health nurses were able to use the VNA of Omaha scheme and Bailon and Maglaya's typology. A more definitive evaluation of the utility of these systems awaits further field testing.

Little information about the use of NANDA labels by community health nurses is available. Shamansky and Yanni's (1983) observations of community health nursing students' difficulties in using NANDA labels relate to the list's incompleteness and need for refinement. The best way to improve the NANDA list is for community health nurses to contribute to its development.

Shamansky and Yanni (1983) believe that individual nurse labels are better than published labels because individual nurse labels are more precise. Precision relates to the specificity of the label. Any nursing diagnosis must be specific enough to permit determination of a plan of intervention (Kim, McFarland, & McLane, 1984). The NANDA list contains labels at different levels of abstraction (i.e., high abstraction diagnoses like "alteration in family process" and diagnoses at lower levels of abstraction such as "ineffective airway clearance") (Kim, McFarland, & McLane, 1984). Diagnoses at high levels of abstraction in any system of diagnosis require that the nurse generate a more precise label. Ideally these more precise labels will be fed back into the system of diagnoses to improve the system.

The major disadvantage of individual nurse labels is that they do not contribute to identifying the universal phenomena of nursing practice. Such identification is important for improving nursing practice. Identified phenomena are named so they can be communicated to others; we all know what to visualize when someone says "chair," because we know the object (thus the concept) and its label. The intent of nursing diagnosis is to name phenomena that nurses identify and treat. Such naming will improve our ability to think and talk as well as do nursing. Precise thinking and talking in the nursing field are important ingredients in research and theory development. Research and theory building can improve nursing practice.

Some evaluation data on the use of nursing diagnoses in clinical settings indicate that nursing practice improved when nursing diagnoses were used (Kim, McFarland, & McLane, 1984). Although community nurses using the VNA classification scheme and Bailon and Maglaya's typology reported numerous benefits in using nursing diagnoses, research on practice impact is needed.

One approach to responding to concerns about the impact of using published labels on clinical reasoning is to identify errors to avoid during the diagnostic process. Such errors include: (1) premature closure—insufficient data collection and/or analysis to support conclusions; (2) incorrect clustering such as labeling a chair a table; (3) lack of closure—not combining cues (Gordon, 1982b). Nursing research is needed to compare the incidence and nature of diagnostic errors related to the use of official or individual nurse labels.

Concerns about the impact of using published labels on interdisciplinary collaboration are important to community nurses. A language is always foreign until it is learned. As nurses use nursing diagnoses, the diagnoses will become familiar to nurses, other health professionals, and the general public. It is not the intent, however, to rename conditions that already have acceptable names. For example, medical diagnoses are used when making a medical diagnosis under protocol or standing orders.

Of equal importance is intraprofessional communication between community nurses themselves and nurses in other specialties. One concern about the development of systems of nursing diagnoses specific to community nursing is that such systems may divide nurses by specialty.

Domain

The second issue is the domain or scope of nursing diagnosis. Three areas of concern for community nurses are inclusion of health promotion diagnoses, inclusion of community client diagnoses, and inclusion of diagnoses requiring collaborative or interdependent nursing interventions. It is necessary to differentiate between health promotion and disease prevention before discussing the inclusion of health promotion nursing diagnoses. Pender (1982, p. 42) stated that health promotion includes "activities directed toward *sustaining* or *increasing* the level of well being, self actualization and personal fulfillment of a given individual or group. Primary prevention (encompasses) activities directed toward *decreasing* the possibility of encountering illness, including active protection of the body against unnecessary stressors."

Potential problem diagnoses include primary prevention, but they do not accommodate health promotion, because health promotion is not problem related. Although NANDA includes the health-promoting diagnosis "family coping: potential for growth," there are complex conceptual issues related to including health promotion nursing diagnosis in a nursing taxonomy (Kim, McFarland, & McLane, 1984). In the meantime nurses are invited to submit health promotion nursing diagnoses to NANDA and join a group of nurses in NANDA who are developing wellness-oriented nursing diagnoses.

Shoemaker's (1984) definition of a nursing diagnosis included the community, but there are no community diagnoses in any of the three systems of nursing diagnoses presented. The reason(s) for the lack of such diagnoses is unknown, but nurses engaged in nursing the community client have begun developing nursing diagnoses for the community client.

For example, Muecke (1984) devised a structure for stating a nursing diagnosis for a community client. It incorporates the expanded epidemiologic triangle, which consists of the health-illness problem, population characteristics and environmental characteristics, and the nursing diagnosis format of (problem) related to (etiologic factors) as manifested in (signs and symptoms). Muecke's (1984, p. 28) format for a community health diagnosis is "Risk of _____ Among _____ (community) Related to _____ (associated characteristics of the community and its environment) as demonstrated in _____ (health indications)." Her article contains an analysis of the concept of community health diagnosis, a description of the diagnostic process used to formulate a nursing diagnosis of the community client, and a case study.

At the beginning of this chapter several reasons for using nursing diagnosis were presented. Nurses active in NANDA disagree about the kinds of nursing diagnoses to include in the list. The disagreement centers around the amount of interprofessional collaboration that may be required to resolve the health condition. One group of nurses believe that NANDA's list should only contain names of health conditions nurses diagnose and treat independently. Another group of nurses believe that the list should include names of health conditions nurses diagnose and treat jointly with other professionals.

The controversy arises from differing views of how nursing diagnosis can best serve the profession and society. For example, Kim (1985) and Kritek (1985) are both concerned about defining the area of health care provided by nurses. Kim's approach is to include physiologic malfunction diagnoses such as "ineffective airway clearance," because modern health care practice necessitates collaboration and a large portion of nursing practice is interdependent. Excluding physiologic diagnoses would present a restricted picture of the domain of nursing practice. Kritek believes that interprofessional collaboration is facilitated by clearly identifying nurses' contribution to care. She advocates limiting NANDA's list to diagnoses nurses' treat independently as a means of "highlighting" the boundary between nursing and medicine.

Resolution of health problems with families, aggregates, and communities require more than independent nurse action. A recent study by Kim (1985, p. 284) demonstrates the variability of collaboration needed to resolve nursing diagnoses on NANDA's current list. Kim found that on the average 56 percent of the diagnoses required independent, 35 percent interdependent, and 9 percent dependent nursing actions. Two family diagnoses were among the eleven diagnoses requiring more than 40 percent interdependent nursing actions. Limiting the NANDA's list to health conditions nurses treat independently would exclude many family and client diagnoses.

Summary

Nursing diagnosis is a significant and important component of the nursing process. However, as the area of nursing diagnosis has developed, it has generated some controversy among nurses as well as among some professionals outside of nursing. Much of the controversy centers around the questions of whether nursing diagnosis is really needed and whether it serves to impede communication between nurses and other professionals. Despite the controversy, the diagnosis of patients' health problems will continue to be part of nursing functions as nurses continue to define and specify nursing.

Topics for Nursing Research

• Identify and validate nursing diagnosis appropriate for the community as client.
• Select existing diagnoses labels from the published lists and test their application to actual client problems (complaints and symptoms).
• Develop individual nursing diagnoses that are applicable to health promotion, and describe a method for testing the accuracy of these diagnoses.
• Design a method to seek client validation of nursing diagnoses in follow-up home visits of families with infants.

1. Identify and select published official diagnoses that would apply to this situation.
2. Identify potential individual nurse diagnoses that would apply to this situation.
3. Design a system for client validation of both types of diagnoses (1 and 2).
4. Compare the differences in diagnostic errors related to the use of both 1 and 2.

Study Questions

1. Which client situation is most likely to be resolved by independent nurse actions?
   a. Two family members have had positive stool cultures for salmonella.
   b. A high-risk resident is sequestered in her room threatening suicide.
   c. A family member asks for help to stop smoking.
   d. A client's prescription for medication has expired.
2. Which of the following is a true statement about the use of nursing theory in community health nursing?
   a. A nursing theory or model can be used only with an individual *or* a family client.
   b. A nursing theory or model has been developed for nursing the community client.
   c. A nursing theory or model *may be* appropriate for use with an individual or a family client.
   d. Any nonnursing theory could be used to care for all family clients in a caseload.
3. Acceptance of a nursing diagnosis by the North American Nursing Diagnosis Association (NANDA) means that the nursing diagnosis:
   a. Has been validated in practice
   b. Has been verified through research
   c. Has been accepted for clinical testing
   d. Has been accepted by organized nursing—that is, the ANA
4. The following is the *most* appropriate response to the state of the art of nursing diagnosis:
   a. Provide health promotion services but disregard diagnosis.
   b. Wait to use nursing diagnosis until granted agency approval.
   c. Select only the best nursing diagnoses for clinical use.
   d. Contribute your ideas to nursing diagnosis development.

References

American Nurses' Association: *Nursing: A Social Policy Statement*. Kansas City, Mo.: American Nurses' Association, 1980.

Anderson ET: Community focus in public health nursing. *Nurs Outlook* 1983; 31 (1): 44–48.

Bailon SG, Maglaya AS: Tools and guidelines for nursing care at the family level, Pt. I: A typology of nursing problems in family care practice. *The ANPHI Papers* (January–March) 1977; 12: 13–21.

Clemen SA, Eigsti DG, McGuire SL: *Comprehensive Family and Community Health Nursing*. New York: McGraw-Hill, 1981.

Freeman RB, Heinrich J: *Community Health Nursing Practice*, 2nd ed. Philadelphia: Saunders, 1981.

Gordon M: *Manual of Nursing Diagnosis*. New York: McGraw-Hill, 1982a.

Gordon M: *Nursing Diagnosis Process and Application*. New York: McGraw-Hill, 1982b.

Griffith JW, Christensen PJ: *Nursing Process Application of Theories, Frameworks, and Models*. St. Louis: Mosby, 1982.

Hamilton P: Community nursing diagnosis. *Adv Nurs Sci* 1983; 5: 21–36.

Kim MJ: Without collaboration, what's left? *Am J Nurs* 1985; 85 (3): 281–284.

Kim MJ, McFarland GK, McLane AM: *Classification of Nursing Diagnoses: Proceedings of the Fifth National Conference*. St. Louis: Mosby, 1984.

Kim MJ, McFarland GK, McLane AM: *Pocket Guide to Nursing Diagnoses*. St. Louis: Mosby, 1984.

Kim MJ, Moritz DA: *Classification of Nursing Diagnoses: Proceesings of the Third and Fourth National Conferences*. New York: McGraw-Hill, 1982.

Kritek PB: Nursing diagnosis in perspective: Response to a critique. *Image: The Journal of Nursing Scholarship* 1985; 17 (1): 3–8.

Muecke MA: Community health diagnosis in nursing. *Public Health Nursing*. 1984; 1 (1): 23–25.

Mundinger MD, Jauron GD: Developing a nursing diagnosis. *Nurs Outlook* 1975; 23 (2): 94–98.

Pender NJ: *Health Promotion in Nursing Practice*. New York: Appleton-Century-Crofts, 1982.

Shamansky SL, Yanni CR: Apposition to nursing diagnosis: A minority opinion. *Image: The Journal of Nursing Scholarship* 1983; 15 (2): 47–50.

Shoemaker JK: Essential features of a nursing diagnosis. In: Kim MJ, McFarland GK, McLane AM (editors), *Classification of Nursing Diagnoses: Proceedings of the Fifth National Conference*. St. Louis: Mosby, 1984.

Simmons DA: *A Classification Scheme for Client Problems in Community Health Nursing*. DHHS Publication No. HRA 80-16. National Technical Information Services, 1980. (NTIS No. 14)

Webster GA: Nomenclature and classification system development. In: Kim MJ, McFarland GK, McLane AM (editors), *Classification of Nursing Diagnoses: Proceedings of the Fifth National Conference*. St. Louis: Mosby, 1984.

Williams AB: Rethinking nursing diagnosis. *Nurs Forum* 1980; 19 (4): 357–363.

Chapter 11

Planning with the Family and Community

June Crayton and Beatrice L. Gilmore

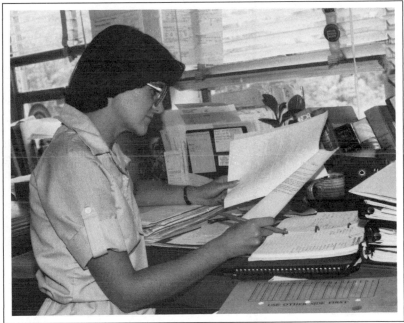

Planning is a process of setting goals for future levels of health and determining the means for attaining those goals. It must consider feelings, values, habits, traditions, as well as scientific data.

Chapter Outline

Chapter Objectives

After completing this chapter, the reader will be able to:

- Describe the relationship between planning and rational decision making
- Name factors that impact on planning at the family, community, and policy-making levels
- Describe the impacts of purpose, resources, values, and setting on planning with the family, community, and policy-making entities
- Describe the planning sequence as proposed in this chapter
- Develop a family or community health plan to address actual problems or needs in their clinical practice
- Discuss family and community health planning as discussed in this chapter in terms of their relevance to actual practice
- Describe a major health planning law enacted in 1974

This chapter explores the theoretical concept of planning and its application in community health nursing. The concept of planning is based on the belief that planning is a process that enables us to progress from where we are to where we want to be. We explain the importance of planning in this respect and describe the planning sequence. Case examples also illustrate the planning sequence and the process of family and community planning.

Theoretical Perspectives of Planning

One model for community health nursing outlined seven dimensions of the practice: service delivery; provider outreach; family as unit of concern; community-oriented population base; multidisciplinary resources; constant surveillance; and primary, secondary, and tertiary prevention and control (Chavigny & Knoske, 1983). Planning is a basic component of each of these dimensions. Traditionally, nurses have been involved in health planning with individuals and families. However, nurses also have a significant role to play in planning at the community and policy-making levels.

Planning is a corrective element in service delivery systems (Lauffer, 1979). It assumes inadequacies in existing service systems or in the connections between relevant community groups. Lacking the mandate or resources to influence basic changes in the social structure, planners examine existing services or connections and provide new, extended, more appropriate, or effective ones.

Perspectives of planning can be approached through a technomethodological process and a sociopolitical process (Gilbert & Specht, 1979). Technomethodological approaches emphasize analytical tasks such as data analysis, priority ranking, goal setting, and program designation. Sociopolitical perspectives focus on tasks such as network building, communication, and collaboration. The two perspectives are actually just two sides of the same coin, since both sets of tasks are equally essential to fruitful planning. Lauffer (1979) substituted the terms "analytical activities" for technomethodological tasks and "interactional activities" for sociopolitical tasks, and demonstrated how both sets of activities should be integrated throughout the planning process.

Planning is a process of establishing future levels of health and deciding means of attaining the desired levels (McLemore, 1982). It is a rational selection of a course of action, a process through which society makes its decisions (Kalisch & Kalisch, 1977). As a rational process, planning involves the use of analytical and interactional skills to optimize outcomes and achieve the greatest return for expended efforts (Lauffer, 1979). Common to each of these descriptions is the idea that planning is a rational, goal-directed, decision-making process.

Planning as a Rational Decision-Making Process

Generally decision making involves the following steps: (1) analyzing and prioritizing the problem in terms of the decision-maker's goals and concerns; (2) establishing goals and criteria by which a solution will be judged; (3) formulating alternative solutions by applying previous experience and systematic testing to weigh the consequences of each alternative; and (4) selecting the solution deemed best to solve the problem (Yura & Walsh, 1978). This process is used by individuals, families, or groups when confronted with problems requiring rational choices.

Feelings, values, habits, traditions, and special interests often influence rational decision making. Consequently, policies and authority relationships are often enacted to facilitate rational choices.

However, feelings, values, and traditions can impede rational decision making, especially in the absence of common goals, values, or interests among decision makers. Hence, there is a need for effective sociopolitical and interactional skills.

Planning is a conscious and deliberate process. It is the art of formulating in advance a detailed strategy for accomplishing goals—that is, the design and management of change. Planning is intended to improve performance, enabling persons or groups to anticipate and predict their future and prevent or minimize undesired change. These functions of planning are more compatible with technomethodological or analytical activities.

Factors Impacting on Planning

Bower (1977) identified three factors that impact on decision making: (1) the purpose of the decision; (2) the context in which the decision is to be made; and (3) the values, attitudes, and motives of the decision makers. Note the similarity between these factors and Ruybal's (1972) list of factors that are essential for health planning: (1) a community or social structure; (2) a cultural belief system; and (3) a process of rational action. Both sets of factors can be influencers of health planning. Consequently, factors impacting on health planning are: (1) the purpose of the planning; (2) the context or structural environment in which the planning is to be conducted; and (3) the values, cultural beliefs, attitudes, and motives of the decision makers; and (4) the planning process utilized.

The purpose of health planning may center on improved crisis management, disease prevention, health maintenance, or health promotion. These purposes may direct the selection of strategies or plans. For example, if the purpose of a diabetic client's decision to follow a prescribed diet is health maintenance, when confronted with alternative foods from which to select, the client will choose foods allowed for normal blood sugar maintenance. On the other hand, when experiencing hypoglycemia, the client's purpose is crisis intervention.

This client selects foods that will alleviate his or her crisis. Sometimes clients or consumers must be informed of the purposes to which health planning decisions are directed. Community health nurses are often in the best position to inform families of these purposes. Through their data gathering and expertise about the community's health status, nurses are also equipped to contribute to the clarification of health-planning purposes at the community or policy levels. Nurses can provide community or policy level planners information about the community's health status that is drawn from their direct observations and experiences with families. Such information can help shape the purpose of planning.

The context in which planning is conducted includes factors of the external environment, which vary with the setting. If the setting is an institution or agency, the external environment includes political, economic, social, and administrative parameters as well as regulations and policies that affect the institution or agency. In a family setting the external environment includes family structure and organization, economical resources, education, and degree of interaction with others outside the family. In a community setting the external environment includes community sociopolitical structures, biological and geographical factors, community resources, codes and regulations, and interest groups such as consumers and providers. In a policy-making setting the environment is composed of the political structure of the policy-making entity, revenues, citizens, interest groups, and educational, religious, and economic institutions.

Values, traditions, and motives of decision-makers influence the decision-making process. Values are the standards that determine how we act and what we want. A value system is a set of beliefs and ideas held by individuals and society about the relative worth of goods or actions. The value systems of policymakers and citizens determine social choices regarding the allocation of resources and the priorities placed on health relative to other goods.

The values and interests of those for whom decisions are being made also influence planning. For instance, planning has sometimes been justified on the basis that its goals serve the common good of the public. However, individuals' notions of what constitutes the common good differ. Three competing values that continually impact on social planning in the United States include (1) participative involvement of citizens in decision making in order to protect their interests and affect binding choices; (2) bureaucratic leadership to expediently and equitably mitigate conflict and competition in a complex, heterogeneous society; and (3) technocratic expertise or professionalism that is free of personal interests and geared toward merit, rationality, and objectivity. These values defy discrete distinction, often overlapping or operating inconsistently among groups or individuals (Gilbert & Specht, 1979). Therefore, effective planning requires integration and application of these values as each situation dictates. As planners, nurses, too, must consider the values, motives, and interests of themselves, consumers, and other decision makers in order to achieve effective health planning.

Sequence of Planning

Planning is often described in terms of various steps and phases. Emphasizing both technomethodological and sociopolitical tasks (or, in Lauffer's terminology, analytical and interactional activities), Kalisch and Kalisch (1977) identified six steps in the planning process. Step one, awareness and initiation, involves the redefinition of identified problems in terms of the planners' domain of control or concern. Step two, estimation, specifies the merits of alternative solutions, clarifies objectives, and analyzes resources and constraints. Step three, selection, involves identifying and testing one or more designs or alternatives, collaboration among decision makers, and the collective choice of a preferred plan. Steps four and five include implementation and evaluation of the chosen plan. Finally, in step six, termination, evaluational feedback is reviewed so that policies and programs can

be reconciled to facilitate the plan. Implementation and evaluation are discussed more fully in Chapters 12–15.

Looking specifically at nursing care planning, two other authors identified a four-phased process: (1) prioritizing the diagnosed problems; (2) differentiating those amenable to nursing interventions from those requiring other interventions; (3) designating specific actions, goals or outcomes; and (4) writing or communicating the plan to relevant parties (Yura & Walsh, 1973). Again, both analytical and interactional perspectives were reflected in this description. The planning process was analyzed within a framework of integrated systems, decision-making, perception, information, and communication theories. Consequently, analytical activities were emphasized in the planning phases, and interactional tasks were apparent in assumptions underlying their theoretical framework.

Other authors have identified activities in the planning phases such as problem definition, network construction, goal selection, collaboration, and systems adjustment (Gilbert & Specht, 1979). From these sources, decision-making theory, and the experiences of the writers, we extrapolated four major phases of planning for purposes of this chapter: (1) prioritization and goal setting, (2) selection and analysis of alternatives, (3) analysis of resources and constraints, and (4) selection and development of a plan.

Problem Prioritization and Goal Setting In this first phase of planning, health planners collaborate with consumers and other interest groups to prioritize problems on the basis of values, interests, severity of the problem, efficacy, and domain of the consumers and planners. Priorities assigned to various health problems are also determined by knowledge and other resources. Prioritization requires analysis of the domain of the planners, resources available to them, and the relative importance of the problem for the family or community. It is important, therefore, that planners permit and consider channels of input from all interested parties.

Goal setting also requires client participation. Goals are generalized statements of an aspiration or desired state of affairs. Although often used interchangeably, goals differ from objectives. Objectives are specific end-points or targets; achieving these targets brings about the reality of goals (Fox & Fox, 1983). Because objectives are measurable and are specific indicators or criteria of desired goals, they must be stated in the plan.

Objectives can be stated in terms of process criteria—what the consumers or other actors will do to alleviate the problem, improve health, or maintain wellness—or outcome criteria—expected changes in status after the plan has been implemented. Goals and objectives may suggest clues to plausible alternatives.

Selection and Analysis of Alternatives　In this second phase of planning, there are three guidelines for selecting alternatives: choosing alternatives that lead to as many desirable consequences as possible; choosing alternatives that best meet the intent while minimizing risks to those involved; or, when faced with an alternative that presents risks, choosing alternatives that yield the greatest benefits and the least danger for the greatest number at risk (Bower, 1977). The planner weighs each alternative's capacity to solve the problem and tries to foresee other consequences of the alternative. The planner is assumed to have knowledge and expertise in order to predict the probable success of alternative solutions. However, the values, goals, and resources of the planners, consumers, and other interest groups obviously influence this phase of planning.

Analysis of Resources and Constraints　Once alternatives have been selected, the planners enter the third phase of planning when they can analyze appropriate resources that might impact on the success of each alternative. These resources for analysis include the facilities, funds, networks, manpower, expertise, and other inputs needed to achieve desired outcomes. The planners can identify resources through a review and analysis of family conferences, community forums, legislative hearings, or an exchange among resource providers. For example, couples unfamiliar with family planning may want to know more about it. They may explore such resources as literature on the topic or education from private physicians, nurse practitioners, or community family planning clinics.

It is important to note that consideration of resources may sometimes precede the weighing of alternatives. The sequence of planning is not always chronological and undirectional, but rather must sometimes occur simultaneously.

Constraints within the environment can influence the probable success of alternatives at the family community and policy level. Factors such as limited knowledge or finances, inadequate transportation, and language or other cultural barriers can affect the feasibility of alternatives.

Selection and Development of a Plan　In the last phase the planners make a collective choice of a preferred plan. By now they have presumably deliberated over the probable success of alternatives, the availability of resources, the correct order of priorities. They can now select a specific course of action and allocate the resources. They can also define responsibilities for implementing various aspects of the plan, draw up time frames for accomplishment, and specify the evaluation criteria. These criteria are the basis for careful monitoring of the plan's progress. Based on this feedback, the plan may require continued alteration until desired outcomes are achieved.

These four major phases of planning should be based on accurate analysis of available data from the assessment phase of the nursing process, effective application of communicative skills, and appropriate procedural structures, which facilitate needed interaction, collaboration, or compromise among participants. Case Example 11-1 illustrates the planning sequence.

Case Example 11-1: The Planning Sequence

Mary Smith is a community health nurse directing the Child Health Services of Alp County Health Department. From a community assessment she observed that the southern end of the county needed increased services due to an increased preschool population.

Mary contacted the directors of school services in the county's southern end to verify the increase in service demand. She reviewed the area's demographic statistics and the service capacity of each clinic and discovered that the population growth and other health indices exceeded levels that the clinics could serve.

During the assessment phase Mary used key informants and demographic statistics.

Mary initiated the planning process by meeting with community leaders and consumers to determine their perception of and prioritization of their problems. Through this process the community discovered that many of the children were behind in their immunizations, and that parents lacked pertinent information regarding the services provided by the clinics.

Mary helped the community identify and prioritize problems.

With Mary's assistance the community addressed each problem in relation to its importance or urgency, and they set forth goals for alleviating the problems.

Mary assisted the community in goal setting.

Mary collaborated with the consumers and health department professionals to identify and explore some plausible solutions. However, most of the alternatives required more resources than the health department could allocate.

Mary helped to identify and analyze alternatives, resources, and constraints.

The goals and objectives of the community were reexamined. After a number of meetings with the health department officials and community residents, it was determined that the parents could be taught to provide some of the services provided by the professionals. Parents were willing to volunteer time working in the clinics if clinic hours could be arranged to accommodate their participation.

The community discovered new resources.

This solution was acceptable to the parents and professionals of the area. Mary wrote the plan of implementation, which included the goals, objectives, and interventions needed to solve the problem. The plan included specifications for quarterly evaluations of the outcome of the plan.

The community selected a plan for implementation.

Planning with the Family

Precepts for Planning

The family as the unit of service is a well-known precept in community nursing practice. However, family-centered nursing is a two-level process because its focus includes the whole family and individual family members (Friedman, 1981). In order to understand the individual client, it is necessary to analyze the client in a family context; to understand the family, it is important to learn about its individual members. This two-level approach to planning with families is a broader conceptualization of the unit of service precept. The community health nurse is guided by seven such precepts when planning at the family level.

1. Clients must be viewed in relation to their family's interactions and influences on their development and health status.
2. The family and its individual members are recognized as the unit of service.
3. Health education, counseling, and service coordination for the family and its individual members are integral parts of community health nursing.
4. The family and its members participate in various ways in all decision making regarding health attainment and maintenance of goals.
5. Community health nursing services are provided for individuals and their families regardless of their racial or ethnic origin, cultural background, social circumstance, or economic level.
6. Community health nursing services are provided by professionally prepared nurses who function as members of the health team and serve individuals, families, and population aggregates.
7. The community health nurse utilizes the nursing process to provide nursing care and coordinate health services ordered by the physician and other team members.

These precepts help clarify the purposes of planning in what Friedman (1981) referred to as the "family nursing process" (pp. 32, 34–35). The ultimate purpose of planning with the family is to select the most appropriate preventive or corrective course of action given the family's priorities, goals, resources, and values. Contingent upon the family's structural and functional context, planning also enables the family and individual members to participate in the planning sequence.

Frequently, nurses plan health care with families with special needs. These needs may arise from conditions such as deafness, blindness, musculoskeletal problems, and neurological or endocrine disorders. The aim of planning with these families is to strengthen individual and family capacity to cope with the situation and sustain optimum well-being.

Planning and Family Settings

The family and its members experience greater decision-making autonomy in the family setting than they would in an institutional setting. Therefore, the structure, function, values, and resources of the family setting provide guidelines for planning. For example, methods of decision making within families can differ according to family structure and function. Family structure and function may, in turn, be influenced by ethnic heritage or socioeconomic status. Consequently, as Miller and Janosik (1980) reported, in traditional Mexican American, Puerto Rican, or Italian American families, decisions are made by authority rule. The authority figure, usually the father or highest ranking male sibling, may make decisions that affect the health of other family members. Such decision making requires little involvement of other family members in the planning process. Other families reach decisions by consensus. To the nurse the latter arrangement might appear to be the more effective decision-making method. However, within many ethnic groups, traditional customs serve to maintain identity and ethnic solidarity, which may be important to the family's integrity and stability in the face of a strange, new environment. Therefore, nurses must resist imposing their own decision-making values on the family, but work within the family's own structural context.

The nature of the problem—whether it is acute or chronic—might influence the family's perception of it as a family or individual problem. Acute problems might be perceived to have more family implications than chronic problems to which the family might have developed homeostatic balance (Miller & Janosik, 1980). In this case the community health nurse must be skillful in recognizing ways in which health problems affect other members of the family. Certainly an individual whose goal is to control hypertension could benefit from

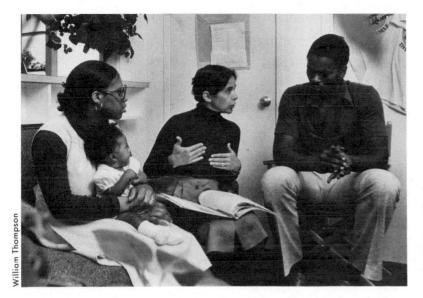

William Thompson

When planning care with a family, the community health nurse is sensitive to the family's structure, values, and traditions and makes sure the plan of care is acceptable to the family.

a family commitment to change the sodium content in its diet and adopt certain life-style changes.

The availability of resources is another component of the family's setting that affects planning. The creative nurse must frequently assist family members in utilizing resources in ways that they might not previously have known. A system of classifying resources—such as formal or informal—might provide a useful framework for identifying resources. Some formal resources are institutions such as the American Red Cross, American Can-

cer Society, local health departments, community health centers, and so on. Informal resources include key people such as politicians, local clergy, neighbors, relatives, or friends.

Family Health Service Plan

Case Example 11-2 illustrates the decision-making and problem-solving aspects of the planning sequence with the family (pp. 256–257).

Planning with the Community

The purposes of community health planning include the provision of services to meet the community's health needs, resources development, and continuity of services. Preventive services may be emphasized as an integral part of the plan in one community. Depending on community health status, resources, structure, priorities, or values, health

planners in another community might emphasize early detection services. Such differences in purpose have direct implications for the planning sequence. For example, a community whose purpose is to increase health promotional services would probably assign a low priority to a problem such as noncompliance among diabetics with treatment

Case Example 11-2: Planning with the Family

Lori Brown is a twenty-six-year-old single mother of three: Charlene, six; Mary Ann, four; and Benjamin, three months. Lori and the children live in a three-bedroom apartment in a housing project for low income families. Because Benjamin was born at the County Hospital and has no other source of health services, he was referred to the Coors County Well-Child Clinic.

Joan White, a community health nurse who works for Coors County Department of Health Services, coordinates the services of the Well-Child Clinic for the geographic area where Lori Brown lives.

After talking with Lori by telephone Joan decided that a home visit prior to Benjamin's clinic visit would provide additional assessment data on the family and their environment and enhance the planning of their health care.

Initial assessment

Upon visiting the family Joan compiled a health history, wrote a health profile of the family, and conducted a survey of the physical environment. She also completed physical assessments on Benjamin and Mary Ann. She learned from Lori while developing the health profiles that Lori and Charlene's health care evaluations were current. All data were compiled to form the family data base, and this was written on structured forms provided by the department of health.

Joan reviewed the data. She found that various family stressors were present. Lori's income was insufficient to meet more than the survival needs of the family. She depended on her parents for assistance with recreational needs of the children. She had problems forecasting income to cover the entire month. She frequently "ran out" of money by the last week of the month. Lori felt that her parents expected her to devote much more attention to the children than she was physically able. She experienced constant confrontations with her parents about childrearing.

---

regimens. Consequently, an alternative to improve patient compliance would not be selected as a high priority by this community.

Health Planning in the Community Context

Health planning often involves the allocation of scarce resources and results in controversy regarding the relative merit of goals and alternatives. Community health planning is planning with the community so that citizens determine their own goals and health plan. Collaboration among con-sumers, providers, and economic and political institutions is essential to effective planning. Community health nurses must prepare themselves to participate in community planning processes. They should know how to assess the community's health status (see Chapter 9) and pinpoint relevant needs. They should acquaint themselves with influential community activities, know where and when planning meetings are held, and be familiar with their agendas and participants. It is also important that community nurses take positions on the relevant health issues and develop alliances with supporting consumer and provider groups. They should identify supporters or resisters to their position prior to

Benjamin needed to be evaluated by a pediatrician. He had not been examined since his four weeks evaluation. Mary Ann was developing normally but had not been evaluated by a pediatrician for two years. She had never been seen by a dentist.

Lori frequently yelled at the children and spanked them. She sent them outdoors to play on sunny days to "get them out of her hair."

Joan reviewed with Lori her ideals for her family. Lori had higher standards set for her family than what she felt she was achieving. She was concerned that her children develop normally. She was concerned that they "would not become ill and would eat properly."

Lori and Joan identified and prioritized four nursing diagnoses as follows: (1) Potential deficit in health maintenance related to insufficient health evaluations and follow-up. (2) Deficit in parenting skills related to lack of knowledge. (3) Deficit in financial resources related to poor management. (4) Hostile communication with parents related to different notions of childrearing. *Identification and prioritization of family nursing diagnoses*

Joan discussed goals and objectives with Lori. They agreed on objectives related to each of the nursing diagnoses and on interventions to effectively eliminate or decrease the problems. They also analyzed and selected alternatives based on the perceived probable success of each alternative. *Goal setting*

Selection and analysis of alternatives

Joan explored resources and related constraints with Lori. She explained other options that could be considered. Together they chose resources and interventions that each felt could best meet the goals and objectives of the plan. *Identification of resources and constraints*

Joan wrote the plan and Lori agreed on the monitoring criteria as specified in the evaluation column. It was agreed that the implementation plan would begin the following day when Lori made an appointment with the clinic. *Collaboration to select a plan for implementation*

Specification of the plan for implementation

meetings through early consultation and collaboration. Crucial aspects of collaboration include having a give-and-take attitude as opposed to a win-lose stance, knowing which points of a position are negotiable, and identifying other programs that one is willing to support in exchange for support of one's own programs (McLemore, 1982).

The success of community health planning also requires the use of the community structure to facilitate planning. Community health nurses should be currently informed of relevant political, legislative, or professional activity regarding the community's health. They should know the local health ordinances, the community health service plan, and appropriate community resources. Resources such as home health agencies, community health centers, local health departments, public or private health providers, or ratios of health professionals to population are also important to know.

Community health nurses should also be familiar with the community's health status and, consequently, the community's needs and goals. For example, a rural community with an inadequate supply of physicians might experience gaps in its diagnostic and treatment services. Such a community might plan to provide these services through the use of family nurse practitioners or school health detection programs.

Community Beliefs and Values

Consumer characteristics are other indices of how the context of the community can influence the purposes and goals of planning. An example may be demonstrated by contrasting a suburban community consisting largely of young, middle-class working adults against an urban population consisting of a large percentage of elderly, poverty level or other high risk groups. The suburban community would be less likely than the urban community to experience health problems such as malnutrition, lead poisoning, hypertension, or diabetes. Therefore, the suburban community might prioritize programs having wellness or health promotional purposes. On the other hand, the urban community might preferably allocate resources to programs related to specific disease prevention, early detection, and treatment.

Community priorities are determined not only by the perceived seriousness or urgency of problems, but also by the values, customs, and motives of citizens. Our example of the suburban and urban communities will also serve to illustrate this relationship. It was assumed that the suburban community with its larger percentage of middle-class working adults might value healthier life-styles than their urban counterparts, and value health promotional programs more highly than the higher

risk urban groups. However, given a conservative political system, highly influential physicians on planning boards, and a highly saturated physician market, the same suburban community might choose to promote programs that serve the interest of the medical profession—treatment oriented medical programs.

Patterns and channels for communication among consumers, planners, and interested groups are other factors in community settings that affect planning. Nurses' knowledge of the community setting enables them to anticipate the values and interests of relevant community groups.

When planning for communities, community health nurses may develop plans for specific community groups. However, these plans must fit within the context of the community setting, its goals, and the agreed-upon plan.

Sequence of Community Health Planning

With the increased complexity of the health care system, community health planning has grown more complex. Case Example 11-3 illustrates the nurse's involvement in community health planning and the complexity of the process (pp. 260–261).

Health Policy Planning

Although plans for improved coordination and delivery of health services were previously recommended, the first comprehensive, nationally supported health planning policy was P.L. 79-725, the Hospital Survey and Construction Act of 1946—better known as the Hill-Burton Act. The Hill-Burton Act provided funds for hospital construction based on statewide priorities and standards of need (Phillips, 1983). More significant health planning initiatives occurred during the 1960s when "Great Society" policies, such as Section 202 of

P.L. 89-4, the Appalachian Region Act of 1965; P.L. 89-239, the Heart Disease, Cancer and Stroke Amendments of 1965; and P.L. 89-749, the Comprehensive Health Planning and Public Health Service Amendments of 1966, authorized federal funds to states, regions, or communities to plan coordinated resources development and improve health services utilization (Kalisch & Kalisch, 1977). The Hill-Burton Act was criticized for stimulating the construction of too many unneeded facilities (Phillips, 1983). Although $163 million were spent from 1967 to 1974, the Comprehensive Health Planning Act failed to achieve its goals because of language that minimized its ability to influence private medical practices and organizational arrangements that limited public scrutiny, consumer input, or enforcement of its responsibilities. At the local level health providers exerted disproportionate influence on decision making. Because consumers lacked the necessary technical knowledge to exercise meaningful impact, the local agencies were often dominated by local hospitals or medical associations (Kalisch & Kalisch, 1977).

Emphasis on national health planning peaked in the mid-1970s after passage of the National Health Planning and Resources Development Act of 1974, P.L. 93-641, which repealed functions of the existing Hill-Burton Act, Regional Medical Programs Act, and Comprehensive Health Planning Act. The National Health Planning and Resources Development Act created a new network of planning and regulatory agencies including Health Systems Agencies (HSA), State Health Planning and Development Agencies (SHPDA), and Statewide Health Coordinating Councils (SHCC). HSAs were required to develop long-range health plans and annual implementation plans for their respective communities. SHCCs were responsible for reviewing and approving health plans for compliance with federal funding statutes. In contrast to the Comprehensive Health Planning Act, the National Health Planning and Resources Development Act was strengthened by its requirement that HSAs consist of a consumer majority, hold public meetings, provide technical assistance to its members, and remain financially independent of special interest groups.

Purposes of Health Policy Planning

Effective planning rests on collectively understood and accepted purposes. Health planning policies were directed toward improved access and utilization of services, consumer involvement, cost containment, health promotion, and disease preven-

tion. Unfortunately, the purposes of major United States planning programs such as P.L. 93-641, the National Health Planning and Development Act of 1974, were understood differently by federal, state, and local governments; providers; consumers; and other interest groups. Some thought the purpose was cost containment. Others suspected a congressional aim to centralize resources allocation and give the federal government greater control. Uncertainty about the purposes of policy planning led to continual resistance from interest groups, inadequate funding of planning efforts, compromised congressional support, and its eventual demise during the Reagan administration.

Health planning at the policy level declined after the mid-1970s. By the 1980s health planning programs, like many other social programs of the previous two decades, were virtually phased out. Some attributed the demise of health planning at this level to numerous unresolved controversial issues raised by P.L. 93-641. Resistance arose from local and state governments, who felt they had been bypassed by the law that gave regulatory powers to HSAs, voluntary agencies, that had no public accountability. Resistance also arose from physicians and hospitals who were subject to the regulatory statutes of P.L. 93-641 (Phillips, 1983).

Unresolved questions regarding the feasibility and desirability of health policy planning remain. As a democratic process leading to consensus on acceptable services, health planning policies were considered to have merit. However, as a rational, economic decision-making process, health policy planning may seem impractical in the face of current emphasis on competition and free choice as better means of cost containment and resource allocation (Phillips, 1983).

Planning in Policy-Making Settings

In contrast to community health planning—which is often initiated by community providers, institutions or networks—health planning policies such

Case Example 11-3: Planning with the Community

Brighten, Illinois, is a suburban community of culturally diverse, largely middle-class residents. Fifteen percent of the community's residents are teenagers. A 1982 community health assessment indicated that Brighten was experiencing high pregnancy and birth rates among its teenage females coupled with high infant mortality rates among teen births—17 infant deaths per 1,000 live teen births compared to 9 infant deaths per 1,000 live births to adult females. Additionally, pregnancy accounted for sixty-five percent of all female high school dropouts. A community task force was convened to develop a plan to address this problem.

Barbara Clark, a community health nurse for the Brighten City Health Department, was appointed by the Public Health Director to serve on the task force. Other representatives to the task force included the Director and Psychologist of Teen Surrogates, a community counselling and referral center for teenagers; a pediatrician and director of pediatric clinics in the local community hospital; a social worker from a private, community social service organization; a school health nurse; two teenagers; two community parents; and a local alderman. The planning sequence proceeded as follows:

The Director for Teen Surrogates, the community-based teen center, made personal contacts with heads of each community agency serving teenagers to elicit their participation in a community task force forum on teen pregnancy.

Interactional or sociopolitical activity facilitates communication and collaboration among interest groups.

During this forum members formulated the purpose of the task force—that is, to develop plans to improve the quality of life among teenagers by preventing unwanted pregnancies, improving pregnancy outcomes for pregnant teenagers, and promoting healthy life chances for infants of teen mothers. Barbara Clark shared data regarding the extensiveness of the teen pregnancy problem and its consequences for the community.

Barbara contributes to the task force's definition of the problem.

A number of problems were identified throughout the discussion. However, based on observations and experiences contributed by Ms. Clark, the Teen Surrogates' representative, and the school health nurse, two problems were deemed most amenable to the task force's purpose and scope: (1) inadequate sex education and pregnancy preventive services accessible to teenagers and (2) inadequate coordinated, com-

Problem is prioritized based on the scope of the task force and the expertise of its members.

as P.L. 93-641 were initiated by the federal government or government-appointed commissions. Consequently, the strength, integrity, and effectiveness of these policies were contingent upon the political attitudes of government officials, voters, or organized pressure groups. The availability of resources and the competing demands for those resources exerted influence on the structure, process, and outcomes of planning policies. For example,

at the height of its funding, health planning consumed only 75 cents per capita. However, the delivery of health services consumed approximately 1,000 dollars per capita. In other words, the planning expenditures were less than 0.1 percent of the expenditures for services delivery (Phillips, 1983). It is doubtful that such a lack of enthusiasm for planning would occur in rational commercial industries.

munity support services available to pregnant teenagers or infants of teenagers.

The views and recommendations of representatives were heard and information was shared regarding each agency's services.

Resource analysis takes place early.

Two goals for community action were developed by the task force: (1) educate sexually active teenagers about pregnancy prevention and family planning and (2) provide coordinated counselling, referral, and prenatal and support services for teen mothers and their infants from early pregnancy to three years after delivery.

Community goals and objectives consensually established by task force members.

During the course of this and other forums held by the task force, a number of approaches to goal attainment were explored and negotiated. Considered more desirable were comprehensive approaches that spread the costs of services among community agencies while minimizing gaps and duplication. Progressive values influenced a proposal involving sex education in the high school, the provision of family planning clinics in the Teen Surrogate Center and the implementation of a continuing education program in the high school for pregnant teenagers. However, conservative influences dictated that family planning services through the Teen Surrogate Center be provided very confidentially; the continuing education program for pregnant teenagers be removed from the high school to an off-site community location; and that no sex education would be provided in the elementary and middle schools.

Alternatives are identified.

Values impact on planning.

Any increase in services required additional funding, or that community services providers absorb the additional cost. The Director of the Teen Surrogate Center informed the task force members of federal funds for comprehensive teen family planning and health care services, and suggested that a grant application be submitted based on a comprehensive interagency community plan. The Teen Center would prepare the grant application, receive the funds, purchase services from other community health care providers and coordinate the program. Other alternatives were also considered and weighed in terms of their cost effectiveness, likelihood of success, and acceptability to all interest groups. However, the federally funded, comprehensive approach was selected. Ms. Clark communicated the task force's plan to the Public Health Director and secured the health department's commitment to provide its share of the planned services.

Resources and constraints are identified and analyzed.

Plan is selected for implementation.

Barbara coordinates the health department's input to the plan.

Summary

Planning is a rational decision-making process whereby community health nurses in collaboration with their clients, families and communities, determine how to attain desired levels of health. The concept of planning is based on the belief that the plan of care should be based on specific principles and research and should outline specific realistic goals to be accomplished. Planning is an important step in the nursing process. Its success depends on successful accomplishment of the previous steps (assessment and diagnosis); equally, the success of the steps following planning (implementation and evaluation) is dependent upon a well-developed plan of action. Community health nurses participate in planning at individual, family, community, and policy levels. Regardless of the level at which planning takes place, the goal is the same—better implementation of health services for clients.

Topics for Nursing Research

- Design health services plans for the family and the community and include evaluation procedures for measuring the effectiveness of each plan.
- Explore the relationship between family structure, function, cultural values, and family involvement in the planning process.
- How is consumer involvement in planning of health services operationalized and implemented in a high income community compared with a low income community?

Study Questions

1. The major differences between the sociopolitical and the technomethodological approaches to planning are:
   a. Technomethodological approaches emphasize communication networks, computerized planning activities, and objective techniques, while sociopolitical approaches emphasize involvement of politicians and members of grassroots organizations in the planning process.
   b. Technomethodological approaches emphasize tasks such as data analysis, priority making, goal setting, and program designation, while sociopolitical approaches emphasize tasks such as network building, communication, and collaboration.
   c. Technomethodological approaches to planning emphasize the nursing process

while sociopolitical approaches emphasize social systems concepts.
   d. There are no major differences between the sociopolitical and the technomethodological approaches to planning.

A community health nurse was asked to plan health service for a community whose residents consist of predominantly single-parent mothers and young children. A community assessment determined health care needs of the community to be family planning, immunization and follow-up care for young children, and routine health examinations for the women. Questions 2 and 3 relate to this situation.

2. As the community health nurse develops a health services plan for the community, which of the following actions is most likely to result in increased utilization of the health services by the community residents?
   a. An efficient plan developed and presented to the community by the community health nurse.
   b. An efficient plan developed by the community health nurse but presented to the community by their local council representatives.
   c. The incorporation of community residents and community leaders in the development of the plan.
   d. The incorporation of health promotion provisions in the plan.

3. Which of the following factors are most important for the community health nurse to consider in the planning process?
   (1) The social structure of the community
   (2) Values and cultural beliefs of community residents
   (3) Community decision-makers
   (4) Power-structure of the community
   (5) Existing health services
      a. 4 and 5
      b. 1, 2, and 3
      c. 5 only
      d. 1 only
      e. All of the above

4. Which of the following are part of the planning sequence?
   (1) Prioritization and goal setting
   (2) Selection and analysis of alternatives

(3) Analysis of resources and constraints
(4) Selection and development of a plan
   a. None of the above
   b. All of the above
   c. 1 only
   d. 1 and 4 only

References

Aguilera DC: Coping with life stressors: A life-cycle approach. *Family and Community Health* 1980; 2 (4): 61–70.

Becker MH: *The Health Belief Model and Personal Health Behavior.* Thorofare, N.J.: Charles B. Clask, 1974.

Beckhart R, Harris RT: *Organizational Transitions: Managing Complex Change.* Menlo Park, Calif. Addison-Wesley, 1977.

Bennis WG et al: *The Planning of Change,* 3rd ed. New York: Holt, Rinehart and Winston, 1976.

Benson E, McDevitt J: *Community Health Nursing Practice.* Englewood Cliffs, N.J.: Prentice-Hall, 1976.

Bower LF: *The Process of Planning Nursing Care: A Model for Practice.* St. Louis: Mosby, 1977.

Carpenito LJ: *Nursing Diagnosis Application to Clinical Practice.* Philadelphia: Lippincott, 1983.

Chavigny KH, Kroske M: Public health nursing in crisis. *Nurs Outlook* 1983; 31 (6): 312–316.

Clemen SA et al: *Comprehensive Family and Community Health Nursing.* New York: McGraw-Hill, 1981.

Cordes SM: Assessing health care needs: Elements and processes. *Family and Community Health* 1978; 1 (2): 1–16.

Crawford CO, Leadley SM: Interagency collaboration for planning and delivery of health care. *Family and Community Health.* 1978; 1 (2): 35–46.

Dalis GT, Strasser BB: Decision making and health education. *Teaching Strategies for Values, Awareness and Decision Making in Health Education.* Charles B. Slack, 1977.

Elkins CO: *Community Health Nursing Skills and Strategies.* Bowie, Md.: Robert J. Brady, 1984.

Fox DH, Fox RT: Strategic planning for nursing. *The J Nurs Adm,* 1983; 8(5): 11–17.

French WL, Bell CH: *Organizational Development.* Englewood Cliffs, N.J.: Prentice-Hall, 1978.

Friedman MM: *Family Nursing Theory and Assessment.* New York: Appleton-Century-Crofts, 1981.

Gilbert N, Specht H: Who plans. In: Cox F M et al (editors), *Strategies of Community Organization.* Itasca, Ill.: F. E. Peacock Publishers, Inc., 1979.

Goodall B, Kirby A: *Resources and Planning.* New York: Pergamon Press, 1979.

Griffith JW, Christensen PJ: *Nursing Process Application of Theories, Frameworks, and Models.* St. Louis: Mosby, 1982.

Hanlon JJ, Pickett GE: *Public Health Administration and Practice.* St. Louis: Times Mirror/Mosby College Publishing, 1984.

Hersey P, Blanchard KH: *Management of Organizational Behavior: Utilizing Human Resources.* Englewood Cliffs, N.J.: Prentice-Hall, 1977.

Kalisch PA, Kalisch BJ: *Nursing Involvement in the Health Planning Process.* HHS Publication No. (HRA) 78-25. US Department of Health and Human Services, 1977.

Lauffer A: Social planning in the United States: An overview and some predictions. In: Cox FM et al (editors), *Strategies of Community Organization.* Itasca, Ill.: F. E. Peacock Publishers, Inc., 1979.

Lee C: *Models in Planning.* New York: Pergamon Press, 1973.

McLemore MM: Nurses as health planners. In: Spradley BW (editor), *Readings in Community Health Nursing.* Boston: Little, Brown, 1982.

Miller JR, Janosik EH: *Family Focused Care.* New York: McGraw-Hill, 1980.

Mott BJT: The new health planning system. In: Levine A (editor), *Health Services: The Local Perspective.* New York: Academy of Political Science, 1977.

Phillips HT: The role of health planning in the delivery of personal health services. In: Jain SC, Paul JE (editors), *Policy Issues in Personal Health Services.* Rockville, Md.: Aspen Systems Corporation, 1983.

Reinhart AM, Chatlin ED: Assessment of health needs in a community: The basis for program planning. In: Reinhart AM, Quinn MD (editors), *Current Practice in Family-Centered Community Nursing,* St. Louis: Mosby, 1977.

Ruybal SE: Community health planning. *Family and Community Health* 1978; 1 (1): 9–18.

Schelling TC: Government and health. In Lindsay CM (editor), *New Directions in Public Health Care: A Prescription for the 1980's.* San Francisco: Institute for Contemporary Studies, 1980.

Spiegel AD, Hyman HH: *Basic Health Planning Methods.* Rockville, Md.: Aspen Systems Corporation, 1978.

Spradley BW: *Contemporary Community Health.* Boston: Little, Brown, 1975.

Stanhope M, Lancaster J: *Community Health Nursing Process and Practice.* St. Louis: Mosby, 1984.

Yura H, Walsh MB: *The Nursing Process: Assessing, Planning, Implementation, Evaluation.* Washington, D.C.: Meredith Corporation, 1973.

Chapter 12

Group Process:
Implementing Strategies

Barbara L. Dancy

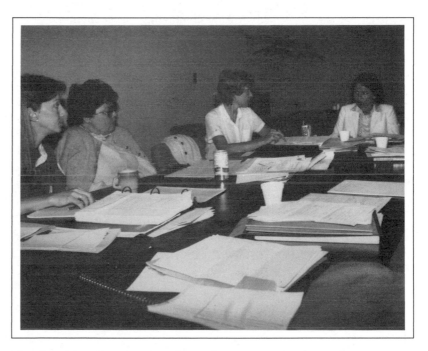

The dynamics of group process are important to implementing care for families and communities. Effective use of group process is also a necessary skill for nurses to evaluate and plan community health programs. (Linda Daniel/courtesy of Washtenaw County Health Department and the Huron Valley VNA)

Chapter Outline

Definition and Characteristics
    Types of Groups
    Group Membership and Size
    Formal and Informal Groups
    Advantages and Disadvantages of Groups
Elements of Group Process
    Norms
    Cohesiveness
    Roles
    Leadership
    Power

Stages of Group Development
    Initiation Phase
    Working Phase
    Termination Phase
Evaluation of Group Process
Summary
Topics for Nursing Research
Study Questions
References

Chapter Objectives

After completing this chapter, the reader will be able to:

- Describe the five types of groups that community health nurses encounter in their practice
- Compare and contrast formal and informal groups
- Examine the advantages and disadvantages of group process
- Analyze group process in terms of group membership, size, norms, cohesiveness, roles, leadership style, and power
- Discuss the stages of group development
- Determine the effectiveness of groups by evaluating group process and the degree of goal attainment

Community health nurses work primarily with communities and families and, consequently, conduct much of their practice in group settings. These groups may include teenage mothers unfamiliar with the role of parenting, community action groups composed of tenement dwellers demanding adequate and safe housing, an interdisciplinary outreach group assisting the homeless in finding shelter, a nursing peer support group coordinating referral sources for nurses abusing drugs, a family consisting of delinquent children, and a city-sponsored committee studying a particular health problem such as the outbreak of hepatitis in the public school system.

Community health nurses assume a variety of roles when they participate in different kinds of groups. Some of these roles are health educator, consumer advocate, change agent, liaison, planner, facilitator, consultant, and researcher. By understanding the interpersonal dynamics underlying these roles, and aspects of group process such as leadership style, cohesiveness, power, and conflict, community health nurses can become more effective in fulfilling their roles. Then they will make their maximal contribution to the group's success in accomplishing its goal. Community health nurses know that their effectiveness and efficiency are contingent upon their ability to identify the needs of the group members and to help their constituents solve problems. They not only function within a particular group setting but also become members of those groups.

This chapter, therefore, presents the basic concepts of group dynamics in order to foster an understanding of the essential characteristics of groups. Among the topics considered are types of groups, group membership and size, formal and informal groups, advantages and disadvantages of groups, group process, norms, cohesiveness, roles, leadership, power, stages of group development, and evaluation of group process.

Definition and Characteristics

A group can be defined as three or more individuals who interact together and, as such, are interdependent. The relationship existing among group members is one in which each member, by his or her nonverbal and verbal behavior and by his or her perceptions and beliefs, is influenced by and influences every other member (Cartwright & Zander, 1968; Sampson & Marthas, 1981; Van Servellen, 1984). Groups, therefore, can be viewed as social systems with distinct boundaries that delineate the group members from nongroup members. The boundaries also distinguish the membership in terms of the various roles each member plays within the group (Berne, 1963; Stuart & Sundeen, 1983).

Types of Groups

In their service to the community, community health nurses can become involved in the following types of groups: teaching-learning groups, task-directed/planning groups, support groups, socialization-centered groups, and self-help groups. These groups focus on the here-and-now, not the past, and, therefore, emphasis is on the present task to be completed, the current learning needs of the group, or the incorporation of more adaptive ways of increasing or maintaining current levels of functioning. They do not focus on the redevelopment or reconstruction of group members' personalities.

Teaching-learning Group The major emphasis of the teaching-learning group is to use the group process to disseminate information and/or to teach techniques and skills to individuals who need knowledge and skills related to certain health issues. For instance, individuals who are diagnosed as having hypertension, diabetes, or leukemia, or who require a colostomy, have special learning needs pertaining to diet, medication, skin care, and other

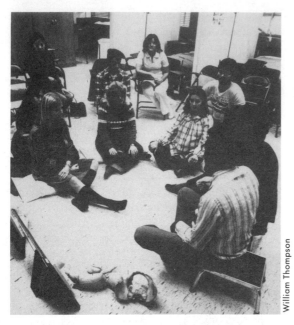

A prenatal exercise and education class is an example of a teaching-learning group.

areas. Also, postpartum mothers need to learn about the care of the newborn, child development, and family planning.

The facilitator uses the group process to advance learning from the acquisition of facts on the part of the group members to an actual incorporation of these facts in the group members' everyday lives. Group members demonstrate their learning behaviorally in their personal lives. Whether community health nurses function as leaders-facilitators or consultants, they use simple words and audiovisual aids when presenting information and allow enough time to ensure that group members will have a chance to ask questions about the information presented and to practice the skills and techniques demonstrated. Adequate time is also needed to allow the facilitators to assess each group member's learning and to encourage the expression of feelings and thoughts about the incorporation of the information and skills into group members' lives.

Task-directed/Planning Group   The focus of the task-directed/planning group is the completion

of the establised task; emphasis is primarily on the job to be done and the establishment of a strategic plan to fulfill the group's goals. Individuals in a community may organize a group for the purpose of reducing crime in their neighborhood. This group will consist of those individuals who are interested in accomplishing the goal of crime reduction. Group members will work diligently in planning and implementing specific strategies designed to lower the crime rate in their neighborhood. When the task has been successfully achieved or it becomes evident that the task is unachievable, the group disbands. Community health nurses may initiate and lead task-directed/planning groups after making astute assessments of the community's needs, strengths, and weaknesses. They may also be invited or volunteer to participate in already existing task-directed/planning groups. Their participation would then most likely be as group members. Regardless of whether community health nurses function as leaders-facilitators or members in these groups, their role is to ensure that the group membership is representative of the community residents who have vested interests in the task and of professional and political individuals who may be able to assist the residents in their endeavor. In addition, community health nurses can assist the group toward the successful completion of its task.

Support Group   The purpose of a support group is to support its members through a crisis situation. Generally, the group members are psychologically healthy individuals who are experiencing a crisis in their lives. Loss of employment, divorce, death of a child, and sexual assault are types of crises that may be experienced. These individuals need emotional support to work through the crisis and either to maintain or advance their current level of coping. Members are encouraged to practice adaptive coping strategies to facilitate crisis resolution. Community health nurses serve as leaders-facilitators who create a caring, nonjudgmental, and accepting environment conducive to support.

Socialization - centered Group   Community health nurses generally function as the leaders-facilitators of socialization-centered groups. These groups consist of members who either do not know, or know but are unable to behaviorally display, social skills acceptable to the dominant culture. Oftentimes, those individuals, who may be chronic mentally ill outpatients, prisoners, or senior citizens, are rejected by society. The socialization-centered group is, therefore, designed to assist members to develop more adaptive and appropriate social skills that will facilitate not only their integration into the dominant culture, but also their ability to function and interact effectively within the dominant culture.

Sometimes, however, the leader-facilitator will need to motivate members to want to become more involved, interested, and active in their community. On these occasions the leader-facilitator may use various kinds of activities to stimulate interest and facilitate group interaction. For example, the group may attend a play, go to a dance, or prepare a picnic. During the activities the leader-facilitator encourages social interaction. As members become comfortable with each other and with the leader-facilitator, who models an accepting and nonjudgmental attitude, they are encouraged to share their experiences. Members are urged to practice more appropriate social skills in this caring, supportive, nonthreatening atmosphere and, finally, to practice their skills in the community. Members should acquire positive views of themselves and a willingness to become reinvolved in the community.

Self-help Group Self-help groups emerging over the years have as their primary purpose the provision of emotional support and constructive assistance to their members. Members are individuals who have similar social, emotional, and physical problems. They have organized to meet common needs that they feel have not been addressed by professionals and the larger society. Generally, professionals are not included in the membership but instead function as consultants and/or referral sources (Van Servellen, 1984). Perhaps the oldest self-help group is Alcoholics Anonymous. Recently self-help groups have been established by and for professionals who have common problems, such as nurses who abuse drugs.

All self-help groups strive to create an atmosphere where solutions to problems can be discussed, where suggestions can be made, and where group support is offered to encourage group members to implement the suggestions. Group members serving as role models are an important feature because their coping effectively with their problems can serve as a motivator for other members to make behavioral changes (Van Servellen, 1984).

Community health nurses may find that the groups they encounter in the community can be a mixture of any of the five types. Any given group can have both primary and secondary purposes. For example, self-help groups can have a socialization, task-directed, and/or teaching-learning purpose. In some self-help groups—for example, Herpes Resource Center and Alcoholics Anonymous— members are encouraged to acquire and practice more adaptive social skills and to learn factual information about their disease. Sometimes self-help groups actively strive to effect political and legal changes. Both Remove Intoxicated Drivers and Mothers Against Drunk Drivers not only provide members with emotional support but also have as a task the promotion of laws regulating intoxicated drivers. In addition, inherent in all groups is the element of emotional support. See Table 12-1 for a brief overview of the purposes and some examples of the five types of groups.

Group Membership and Size

Group membership is determined by the group's purpose. Membership consists of individuals who are most likely to accomplish the group's purpose and who are highly motivated and committed to the purpose. The group's purpose also dictates the demographic characteristics, the medical and social conditions, and the skills and knowledge base of the group's membership. If the purpose of the group is to provide support to recently divorced fathers, membership consists of divorced adult men who are parents. For this group, the criteria for membership is a function of age, sex, and marital status. Likewise, if the purpose of the group is to teach adolescents with a diagnosis of diabetes about their

Table 12-1   Purposes and Examples of Types of Groups

Types of Groups	Purpose	Examples
Teaching-learning	Disseminate information and/or teach techniques and skills	1. Prenatal classes for adolescent girls 2. Teen Outreach focusing on issues of adolescent sexuality 3. Hypertensive group for young Afro-American men 4. Herpes Resource Center 5. Alcoholics Anonymous, Alateen, and Alanon 6. Lamaze classes
Task-directed/planning	Get the job done	1. Various community task force and planning groups: Neighborhood Watch groups, political groups, task force to pass school bond, community action groups 2. Educational Advisory Board 3. Mothers Against Alcoholic Drivers 4. Remove Intoxicated Drivers 5. Gray Panthers 6. Task force of professional nurses to establish peer assistant programs

disease, the membership's age and medical condition are specified as selection criteria for membership. Task-directed/planning groups generally specify the skills and expertise of its membership.

Whether the group consists of homogeneous or heterogeneous membership is also determined by the group's purpose. Heterogeneous membership tends to be best for task-directed groups because individuals with different academic backgrounds and skill levels bring a variety of ideas to the group and thus foster problem-solving. Groups in which the membership is homogeneous tend to be more supportive and accepting of each other and create a comfortable, secure group atmosphere. These groups, however, often discuss topics on a more superficial level than heterogeneous groups (Lubin, 1976; Van Servellen, 1984).

When considering membership, community health nurses need to be aware of the cultural and ethnic backgrounds of potential members. Culture, ethnicity, and economics shape individuals' values, beliefs, perceptions, health orientation, social ties, and religious and political affiliations. (Leininger, 1982). Community health nurses need information regarding individuals' cultural values specifically in relationship to groups. If a sense of privacy is important in a particular culture, it may be difficult for members to establish an effective

Table 12-1 *(continued)*

Types of Groups	Purpose	Examples
Support	Promote adaptation during and after crisis	1. Support groups for victims of floods, tornados, and mud slides 2. Support groups for survivors of rape 3. Support groups for recently divorced parents 4. Support groups for families surviving suicide 5. Support groups for children of incest
Socialization-centered	Encourage the acquisition of adaptive and appropriate social skills	1. Groups for recently discharged schizophrenics 2. Remotivation groups for senior citizens 3. Socialization groups for the borderline retarded 4. Socialization groups for Vietnam veterans
Self-help	Provide emotional support and strategies to cope with problems	1. Alcoholics Anonymous, Alanon, and Alateen 2. Remove Intoxicated Drivers 3. Mothers Against Alcoholic Drivers 4. Fathers United for Equal Rights 5. Gray Panthers 6. Bulimia/anorexia self-help

group because they will be reluctant to discuss issues related to them in this setting.

Group size also helps to determine the effectiveness of the group. Yalom (1975) suggests that group size should range from five to ten members with the ideal size being seven. When group size is smaller than five, interaction among group members is adversely affected: group members are more likely to interact with the leader-facilitator on a one-to-one basis as opposed to interacting with the other group members. When the group size is larger than ten members, the individual efforts of the group members tend to drop: group members discuss topics on a superficial level, feel less responsible, participate less due to time constraints, are dissatisfied, and tend to form subgroups. In addition, group members need more time to make decisions, and individual members have increased difficulty relating to each other as unique individuals (Berkowitz, 1980; Sampson & Marthas, 1981).

However, in certain situations large groups can be effective because increasing the size of the membership also increases the possibility that the membership will be heterogeneous and that members will have a variety of talents and resources. This variety is especially helpful for task-directed/planning groups. In addition, the formation of subgroups can be a positive factor if the subgroups' purposes are consistent with the larger group's purposes. Subgroups can be considered a means of dividing labor.

Formal and Informal Groups

Groups may be classified as informal or formal based on their structure. Informal groups have a loose structure, whereas formal groups have a rigid, well-defined structure. Members interact differently depending on the group's structure. In informal groups members tend to be more intimate and friendly toward each other. Their interactions are spontaneous, open, supportive, and noncompetitive; sharing is encouraged. The success of an individual member is viewed as success for the group. There is a strong attraction to the group, and the group is highly valued by its members. Rules and regulations are generally unwritten and emerge from the group process through the nonverbal interactions of the group members and the leader-facilitator. Leadership is flexible and may be assumed by different members depending on the members' skills and expertise and the group's needs.

On the other hand, interactions among the members in formal groups are usually competitive, more limited, less personal, and maybe less satisfying. Expectations, norms, rules, and regulations are more formalized; these are dictated from an authorized body and are in writing. Leaders are also officially appointed by an authorized body and have well-delineated roles, a title, and official power. The roles of the leader-facilitator and members, and the type or relationships existing among them, are explicitly defined (Sampson & Marthas, 1981).

Informal groups are generally smaller than formal groups. In fact, as the membership increases, the group tends to become more formal. Generally, however, within the formal group, informal subgroups emerge. These subgroups tend to be smaller and, consequently, reduce some of the negative qualities of the formal group. The formation of subgroups, however, has certain disadvantages. Sometimes subgroups develop purposes and norms that are incompatible with the purposes and norms of the larger group. Loyalty to the subgroup may overshadow loyalty to the larger group, leading to deterioration and destruction of the larger group (Olson, 1979; Yalom, 1975).

The primary purpose of the formal group is similar to that of the task-directed/planning group—that is, to get the job done. Even though some members may be selected, others can and do volunteer. The primary purpose of the informal group, on the other hand, is to meet its members' social and emotional needs. The informal group may also have a protective function; members band together against perceived or actual threat. Examples of formal groups include a health advisory board, a hospital's board of directors, a community health planning board, a legislative health task force, and a neighborhood block association. Examples of informal groups include social and hobby groups such as dance groups, photography groups, and friendship groups.

Advantages and Disadvantages of Groups

Groups have some definite advantages over one-to-one interaction. The obvious advantage is that the leader-facilitator is able to assist, support, and promote the growth of several individuals in the group setting. In the group, members are more likely to realize that their problems are similar to the problems of others. They begin to perceive themselves as individuals who are not alienated from the rest of the world because others too have similar concerns, needs, and feelings. Groups also provide their members the opportunity to interact with others and to use problem-solving skills in the resolution of their own and other members' problems. Group members begin to understand that they can be of assistance and provide support to others. Consequently, the feelings of belonging, security, and self-esteem, as well as interpersonal and problem-solving skills, are greatly enhanced by the group process. Groups are, therefore, influential in shaping behavior, feelings, and thinking. Lastly, groups are advantageous when complex decisions requiring a wide range of talents and skills are to be made (Eaton, Peterson, & Davis, 1981; Van Servellen, 1984).

A disadvantage of groups is that individual members must share the leader-facilitator and, consequently, receive less attention. When certain individuals require the leader-facilitator's undivided attention, they are not ready for the group. These individuals may not have either the minimal communication skills needed for group interaction or the motivation to participate in the group. Another disadvantage of groups concerns confidentiality. Even after explaining to group members that everything stated in the group should stay in the group, community health nurses cannot vouch for the confidentiality of the group members (Eaton, Peterson, & Davis, 1981).

Elements of Group Process

Through the social interaction occurring among the members of the group, the group process or group dynamics evolve. Social interaction exists on a verbal level and a nonverbal level. Any interaction on a verbal level is defined as the group content. The *group content* is simply what is said or written and can be concrete or symbolic. The group content carries minimal significance when delineating the true essence or nuance of the group. To discern what is really occurring in the group, one needs to look at the group process, which addresses the types of relationships existing within the group and between group members and the group leader-facilitator (Yalom, 1975).

The *group process* consists of all nonverbal communication occurring within the group and includes how group members relate to each other and their group leader-facilitator. The nonverbal messages given and the nonverbal feedback received can be determined by an astute examination of the overt behavior of the group members and the group leader-facilitator. What body language are members displaying toward each other and toward the leader? Where do members seat themselves? Do group members tend to have seating arrangements that isolate any particular group member? Do certain group members always sit in close proximity to each other? Do certain group members always sit either close or far away from the group leader-facilitator? Who speaks to whom? Do group members address themselves only to the group leader-facilitator and seldom to each other? Are certain group members given little opportunity to express their opinions and feelings? Is there a member who talks all the time and monopolizes the group's time? What tone of voice is used by group members when they address each other and when they address the group leader-facilitator? What types of gestures do group members use? Do group members tend to smile, frown, grimace, or look uninterested? Are group members casually dressed? Is the style of dress consistent among group members? In what type of setting does the group generally meet? (Yalom, 1975).

The answers to these questions provide a foundation for determining the group process—that is, how group members are relating to one another and to their group leader-facilitator. In Case Example 12-1 a community health nurse observes the group process of a self-help group that has been in existence for some time.

Norms

Norms, which are rules defining the behavior of the group members, can be either implicit or explicitly verbalized. Norms establish standards of behavior that are acceptable by the group. These behavioral standards are helpful because they lend a certain degree of predictability to the members' relationships with each other. Members know what types of behavior to expect from others, as well as

Case Example 12-1: Group Process in a Self-Help Group

While visiting a family in the community, Mrs. Jones, a community health nurse, was asked if she would attend a meeting that would be held that evening. When Mrs. Jones inquired about the meeting, she found that ten mothers had been meeting biweekly in the church basement for the past two months to talk about effective ways of handling their children's behavioral problems in the home and at school. Mrs. Jones was told that these parents wanted to talk to a nurse about child development, specifically behavioral problems.

Self-help group is formed.

Mrs. Jones decided to attend this meeting in order to decide in what ways she could be of assistance to these parents. Upon arrival Mrs. Jones noticed that these mothers were seated in a circle. One woman, who was talking incessantly, was seated somewhat outside the circle. This parent continued in a lengthy monologue about her problems, not only with her children but also with her husband and job. Oftentimes, she disclosed very personal information about her relationship with her husband.

Group members are seated in a circle. One member, who is seated somewhat outside the circle, is monopolizing the group.

The other parents seemed inattentive and withdrawn. They looked bored, and occasionally Mrs. Jones observed them passing irritated glances among themselves. Three parents were talking softly among themselves. From her observation of the group process, Mrs. Jones concluded that the group members were permitting one of its members to dominate the group. There was an obvious behavioral problem that no one was addressing. It was not apparent that any member wanted to assume the role of group leader-facilitator. The monopolizer was isolated from the other group members as evidenced by her sitting outside the circle and by the unresponsiveness of the other members to her verbal outpouring. No one talked to her or appeared to be listening to her. In addition, no one attempted to place limits on her behavior. Three group members were talking to each other as a means of coping with the monopolizer. The group appeared to be individual people with minimal relationship among themselves and no direction. The group was not cohesive.

Nonverbal communication among group members includes inattentiveness, unresponsiveness to monopolizer, irritated glances, monopolizer seated outside of circle, and withdrawn behavior—failure to listen to or communicate with the monopolizer. Verbal communication includes three members talking among themselves and incessant monologue.

Unproductive norm: group members allow one member to monopolize while constructive feedback on the group process is not permitted.

Subgroup—the three members talking among themselves—has formed.

Mrs. Jones decided to intervene. She briefly summarized the concerns expressed by the monopolizer and asked if the other mothers had similar concerns. She stated that it would be helpful for the group to hear from everyone. She encouraged the others to express their concerns.

Mrs. Jones assumes the function of leader-facilitator.

what behaviors are expected of them. All group norms are based on group consensus and are adhered to by the group members. However, those norms that are most important to the group's purpose are the ones most strictly adhered to by group members. Consequently, there may be a hierarchy of norms based on the importance of the norm in the group process. If a member's behavior fails to meet the standard dictated by the norm, that member will receive some form of reprimand by the group (Sampson & Marthas, 1981; Thibaut & Kelly, 1959). For example, a member whose behavior does not conform to the group's norm may be the target of the group's criticism, ridicule, and ostracism. Various types of subtle pressure are often exercised by the group to ensure that this member will change the nonconforming behavior. If, however, the member is persistent in exhibiting this nonconforming behavior, his or her membership in the group is terminated.

Norms can be categorized as either productive or unproductive. Not only are productive norms characteristic of groups that are cohesive, but they also play an important part in developing that cohesiveness. The following are examples of productive norms:

- All members have the right to express their ideas and feelings.
- All members are important, and their ideas and feelings are respected.
- All ideas and feelings, however diverse, are allowed.
- Feedback on group content, group process, group goals, and group norms is encouraged.
- Feedback is constructive and designed to promote the growth and development of the group as well as of the individual members of the group. Constructive feedback is objective and focuses on the behavior of group members. It is delivered in a supportive, caring atmosphere.

Unproductive norms are the opposite of productive norms. They do not lead to cohesive groups. Examples of unproductive norms are:

- Only members of certain rank or status are allowed to speak in the group.
- Diverse ideas and feelings are not sanctioned.
- Feedback is not encouraged.

Cohesiveness

The likelihood of group purpose being achieved is directly related to how cohesive a group is. Groups that are cohesive have a greater potential for accomplishing their purpose than groups that are not (Sampson & Marthas, 1981; Thibaut & Kelly, 1959). Consequently, cohesiveness is very important to group functioning.

Cohesiveness refers to individual group members' desire to be a part of the group. An individual member's desire to be in a particular group is determined by several factors. One factor is the perceived similarity among group members. Do individual members perceive themselves to be similar to the other members in demographic characteristics and in values and attitudes? A second factor determining desire to be in a group is the degree to which an individual member feels accepted and understood by the other group members and by the group leader-facilitator. Does the behavior of the other group members communicate to particular members that they are viable members of the group whose contributions are valued and respected? How attractive the individual member perceives the group and the group members to be is the third factor determining the desirability of a group. In other words, what are the perceived benefits to be derived from being a member of a particular group? A fourth determining factor is the attractiveness of the group purposes to the members. Are the group purposes consistent with the individual member's values and needs? Are the group purposes and tasks relevant to the individual member's mode of operating? Do the group purposes concur with the individual member's goals? The fifth factor determining desirability is the attractiveness of the leadership style characteristic of a particular group to the member (Bednar & Kaul, 1978; Berkowitz, 1980; Cartwright, 1968; Thibaut & Kelly, 1959; Yalom, 1975).

Members of groups with a high degree of cohesiveness experience a sense of loyalty to the group; have a higher level of involvement and participation in the group; demonstrate a desire to share and explore ideas, thoughts, and feelings in a nonjudgmental fashion; and are more inclined to accept, support, and enforce group norms. Members in cohesive groups also tend to give feedback that focuses on overt behavior and does not put value judgments on behavior or make assumptions about the reason for the behavior. In addition, in cohesive groups, members have more influence over each other and can tolerate conflict and disagreement. In cohesive groups the group members are more inclined to attend the group meetings on a regular basis and less inclined to discontinue their membership (Cartwright, 1968; Yalom, 1975).

Case Example 12-2 describes a cohesive task-directed/planning group. The group members are working cooperatively to resolve a common problem. The purpose and goals of the group have been agreed upon by the group members, and constructive norms are being established.

Cohesiveness is sometimes confused with total conformity. This interpretation, however, is erroneous. Cohesive groups are not afraid of disagreement; they actively encourage members to present even divergent viewpoints. Cohesive groups work on the principle that only after all viewpoints have been discussed can realistic resolutions evolve. Total

Case Example 12-2: Cohesiveness in a Task-directed/Planning Group

By observation Mrs. Hayes, a community health nurse in a small urban community characterized by high unemployment, determined that there was a lack of recreational facilities for the children in the neighborhood. After talking to several community residents who had voiced their concerns about this problem, Mrs. Hayes decided to organize a task-directed-planning group to address this problem. She invited all interested residents; twenty parents attended the first meeting.

During the first meeting there was a spontaneous discussion among the parents about the lack of recreational facilities and about their concerns that the streets were their children's playground. Mrs. Hayes noted that everyone wanted to talk during the discussion. A tall, distinctive middle-aged man, Mr. Jacks, made sure that everyone had an opportunity to speak by establishing a time limit. He also made sure that the group members did not stray from the topic. Several times during the discussion, Mrs. Hayes asked for clarification. Generally, Mrs. Smith, who not only was born and raised in the community, but had raised her children and now her grandchildren there, made clarifications and answered questions. Mr. Camp, who was characteristically quiet, spoke up several times to encourage people to present their viewpoint. He said that he thought this project was a worthwhile endeavor and that he was very pleased that people were talking about this problem in a constructive manner.

After the problem had been defined and discussed to everyone's satisfaction, Mrs. Hayes stated that it was now appropriate to entertain

Open discussion occurs.

Mr. Jacks ensures input from everyone.

Mr. Camp encourages people to talk and comments on group process.

conformity, on the other hand, leads group members blindly to accept issues and positions without questioning them; no dissension is tolerated. This type of situation has been described as *groupthink* by Janis (1971).

In groupthink situations, pressure is placed on any member who does not conform or who dares to express opinions, thoughts, and feelings contrary to the established opinions, thoughts, and feelings of the group. Critical thinking and critical analysis of a problem are unacceptable. Only those facts that support the position of the group are presented. Other information is either ignored, discounted, or distorted. As a result, decision making is generally ineffective (Janis, 1971).

Groupthink situations are common in juvenile gangs and social elite groups. The norm in these groups does not allow dissension. These groups tend to be closed and inflexible. They screen input from the outside world, admitting only input consistent with their philosophy. In addition, group members, according to Janis, tend to be arrogant and cruel to nonmembers. Their cruelty can take the form of either physical or verbal abuse.

A group leader-facilitator can avoid the development of groupthink by facilitating the development of norms that encourage group members to respect all feelings and opinions expressed and to examine all issues thoroughly and critically. Also, group members should be encouraged to perceive

---

possible solutions to the problem. Mr. Camp said that maybe Mrs. Hayes could tell them what to do since she was a nurse. Mrs. Hayes, however, felt that if she assumed this role it would be detrimental to the development of the group. Mrs. Hayes instead facilitated the discussion regarding possible solutions by encouraging the group members to present what they felt were feasible solutions. Even though many solutions were presented, the group repeatedly verbalized that they needed more concrete facts about the children's needs. Mrs. Hayes summarized where the group was at this point by enumerating all the solutions that had been suggested and by stating that the group felt that they needed more facts before a feasible solution could be obtained.

The group members, however, could not think of any ways to obtain the necessary facts. Mrs. Hayes suggested a needs assessment that would emphasize the specific needs of the children within the community. Mrs. Hayes knew that she would not be able to do the needs assessment, since she did not have the educational background or experience to be a researcher. She felt, however, she could function as a research assistant. The group discussion now focused on who could do this type of research. The parents had no money to pay a researcher's fee and would thus need to find a researcher willing to volunteer his or her time and expertise. The group members also felt that they would like to participate as research assistants in this research endeavor, because they wanted to be involved in every facet of resolving their problem. After more discussion the group members decided that one of the community health nursing faculty at the university might serve as their research consultant. An ad hoc committee consisting of Mr. Jacks, Mr. Camp, and Mrs. Smith was formed to further explore this idea.

Mrs. Hayes encourages discussion of possible solutions and, thus, fosters the norm that group members work together in problem solving.

Mrs. Hayes summarizes to help group members stay focused on the task.

Members are committed to group purpose.

Ad hoc committee (a subgroup) is formed as instructed by the larger group with a specific goal—to explore the possibility of eliciting the services of a research consultant.

critical assessment and evaluation as constructive components of effective problem solving.

Roles

Roles are closely related to norms and evolve from the group process. *Roles* reflect the group's norms and as such define a person's behavior and function within the group—that is, how that group member is to behave in relationship to other group members (Smith, 1982; Thibaut & Kelly, 1959).

Many roles develop within the group context. Benne and Sheats (1948) have described three categories of roles that can be assumed by group members. The first two categories, group task roles and group maintenance roles, are considered to be group-centered roles, because their major function is the development and maintenance of an effective group. The third category of roles, on the other hand, is individual or self-centered.

The role assumed by a particular member of a group depends on the dynamic interplay between the individual's needs and the needs of the group. The individual's need for achievement, recognition, and acceptance and his or her wants and desires play an important part in determining the type of role a person will assume. Equally important is the need of the group in terms of its structure. Whether a group is formal or informal will determine the types of roles that emerge within it. Formal groups tend to have a larger number of task roles than informal groups, which are typically characterized by a larger number of maintenance roles.

Group Task Roles　The first category is the group task roles (Benne & Sheats, 1948), which are concerned with the accomplishment of group purpose. Individuals who are task oriented and, thus, function in the group task roles facilitate the group in defining and analyzing its common problems and in selecting the most appropriate strategy for solving the problem. Here are some examples of group task roles:

- *Initiator*—group member who suggests innova-

tive ideas and who offers a different perspective to group problems
- *Information seeker*—group member who elicits facts and requests clarification of ideas
- *Information giver*—group member who gives factual information to the group
- *Opinion seeker*—group member who focuses on values
- *Coordinator*—group member who coordinates activities and integrates ideas

Group task roles are described in Case Example 12-2. Mr. Jacks, Mrs. Hayes, and Mrs. Smith functioned in the group task roles. Mr. Jacks assumed the functions of coordinator. This role was shared with Mrs. Hayes, who also functioned in the role of information seeker at the beginning of the group and as information giver toward the end of the group. The role of information giver was also filled by Mrs. Smith.

Group Maintenance Roles　The second category described by Benne and Sheats is group building and maintenance roles. These roles specifically focus on the relationship component among group members and function to sustain and retain individual members within the group. Some examples are:

- *Encourager*—Group member who facilitates group involvement by praising and accepting group participation
- *Harmonizer*—Group member who attempts to maintain peace among group members by acting as mediator
- *Gatekeeper*—Group member whose major responsibility is to keep the lines of communication open
- *Commentator*—Group member who comments on the group process

The group maintenance roles depicted in Case Example 12-2 are encourager and commentator, both of which were filled by Mr. Camp.

Individual Roles The third category of roles discussed by Benne and Sheats is individual roles. These roles meet the idiosyncratic needs of the individual group member and are not conducive to the development of group task or group maintenance roles. The probability of individual roles developing is low when the group purposes are well defined and appropriate for the group level of functioning. The following are examples of individual roles:

- *Blocker*—group member who is negativistic in approach
- *Recognition seeker*—group member who uses the group as a forum to self-aggrandize
- *Help seeker*—group member who elicits sympathy from other members
- *Self-confessor*—group member who discloses inappropriate personal information; the self-disclosure is too personal

Case Example 12-1 provides an excellent example of group members who have assumed individual roles. The group member who was talking incessantly about her personal problems has taken the role of a self-confessor. Since she also monopolized the group's time, she had the additional role of monopolizer, an individual who dominates a disproportionate amount of group time on issues irrelevant to the group purpose and goals. A monopolizer can preoccupy the group with any irrelevant issues, not necessarily personal issues. The other group members have assumed the role of the passive aggressors. This role, like the monopolizer, is an example of individual roles. These passive aggressive group members were passively acting out their hostility as a means of coping with their frustration. They remained silent, established a subgroup, and isolated the verbose member.

In Case Example 12-3 the group includes persons in all three role categories. Note that the same group members can assume different roles.

Rank and Status Rank and status are closely related to roles. The members *rank* a group according to their roles relative to each other. *Status* is the prestige attributed to a particular role (Smith, 1982). Every role assumed by a group member has attributed to it a particular rank and status. Generally, roles with high rank also have high status within the group. The leader-facilitator of a particular group usually has considerable prestige within the group; that task role is considered very important relative to other roles. Group maintenance roles may also have relatively high rank and status. In groups where the atmosphere is tense, the group member who functions as harmonizer and gatekeeper is perceived as a valuable member to the group, and has high status and high rank within the group. On the other hand, group members who assume individual-centered roles will generally find that their roles carry little prestige and relatively low rank.

In addition, if group members can work together to achieve the group purpose, the status of the group as a whole will be likely to rise. When the group acquires status, the status of individual members is also positively influenced (Thibaut & Kelly, 1959).

Leadership

Leadership encompasses the dynamic relationship among group members and exists within the relationship, not just within the individual identified as the leader. In this relationship both leader and members are interdependent and, as such, influence each other. The success of the group is contingent upon the type of relationship emerging between leader and group members. All members have responsibility to work effectively and cooperatively for the purpose of establishing and maintaining a group that is functioning at its maximal capacity. The leader shares that responsibility and also assists group members to fulfill their responsibility to the group and to maximize their own growth. The group is more successful in accomplishing its purpose when leadership functions are shared among members. Since group members ordinarily have different skills and strengths, drawing from each member's assets would be beneficial

Case Example 12-3: Roles in a Task-directed/ Planning Group

Susan Smith, Roberta Jones, James Cook, Sally Parks, Mary Sams, Ann West, and Tim Blank are community health nurses at one of the local city health clinics. They have agreed to meet once weekly for seventy-five minutes for the purpose of resolving professional and personal issues existing among them. In their first meeting, Roberta suggested that the group start with relatively simple problems because the more emotionally loaded problems would surely bog the group down and nothing would ever be accomplished.

Roberta assumes the role of initiator.

After no response for several minutes, Mary asked her colleagues if anyone else had other suggestions or ideas. The silence continued. Roberta said that she would appreciate receiving some feedback on her suggestion. At this point, Ann stated that she was not sure what simple problems the group would initially discuss because from her perspective all of their current problems were emotionally loaded.

Mary and Roberta assume the role of information seeker.

Ann functions in the role of blocker.

Tim agreed but added that maybe the group could list all their current problems and select from the list the problem most conducive to problem-resolution. Mary thought his suggestion was excellent and stated that she felt that the group could work through their problems.

Tim acts as coordinator and Mary as encourager.

Susan stated that she didn't think what Tim said was any different from what Roberta had said earlier. Tim asked Susan if she was implying that he was parroting Roberta. Tim emphasized that he had a mind of his own and could think quite well without assistance from anyone. For the next five minutes, he talked about all of his professional accomplishments.

Susan comments on group process.

Tim seeks recognition.

Mary interjected that Susan was not making any negative implications but was simply pointing out the consistencies of the two suggestions and that Tim had expanded on an idea. The group members nodded in agreement. Mary described what had happened up to this point and asked the group for its opinion. Members nodded.

Mary assumes the role of harmonizer, commentator, and opinion seeker.

After a few seconds, Ann stated that she thought this idea of meeting was a waste of precious time. She had more important things to do. Susan, who had not said anything since her last statement, now spoke in a whining voice. She thought the group was a good idea but was having problems concentrating because she was so preoccupied with her own personal problem. She requested that the group understand and be patient with her.

Ann continues to act as blocker.

Susan seeks consolation and sympathy.

Roberta stated that maybe the group members should begin to formulate a list of their problems. Members agreed. Ann, however, said, "Okay, but don't say I didn't warn you. There is nothing this group can do to solve anything."

Roberta functions as coordinator.

Ann continues to act as blocker.

to both the group and the individual member's development (Benne & Sheats, 1948; Berkowitz, 1980; Heimann, 1976; Sampson & Marthas, 1981).

Function of Leader-Facilitator Whether appointed by an official body or selected by the group members, the leader-facilitator assumes group task or group maintenance roles. When fulfilling these roles, leader-facilitators must be able to adequately assess the group process and intervene when necessary to ensure that their own behavior and that of the other group members do not adversely affect the group's achieving its purpose. Group leader-facilitators also foster cohesiveness and ensure that the group process has positive outcomes on its members. Therefore, they encourage openness to all ideas and suggestions, facilitate discussion and participation, coordinate activities and tasks, allocate adequate time for discussion, assign tasks and responsibilities, assist in problem solving and decision making, eliminate unnecessary stress and anxiety, assist in the establishment of goals and the evaluation of progress, facilitate learning by focusing on both positive and negative accomplishments, and foster the growth of both individual members and the group. To foster individual members' growth, the leader-facilitator assists them to recognize their strengths and to use their talents and assets effectively in the achievement of the group purpose. The group task and group maintenance roles, as well as the functions just discussed, can be assumed by other members besides the designated leader. They are, however, more consistently performed by the leader-facilitator (Sampson & Marthas, 1981; Van Servellen, 1984).

Leadership Styles Three types of leadership styles—authoritarian-autocratic, democratic, and laissez-faire—have been described by White and Lippitt (1968) and Heimann (1976). Not only may groups prefer different leadership styles, but also within the life span of a particular group, different leadership styles may be required.

The *authoritarian-autocratic* leader has complete control over the group. This leader dominates the group by establishing group policies and goals, for-

mulating strategies for implementing the designated goals, and deciding when the goals have been achieved. There is very little sharing of information with group members, and questioning is discouraged. All decision-making activities are accomplished without any input from the group members. The authoritarian-autocratic leader is primarily concerned with getting the task done and is very active in directing group members toward completion of the task (Heimann, 1976; Sampson & Marthas, 1977; White & Lippitt, 1968).

Group members function as followers and perceive their authoritarian-autocratic leader as giving them orders that they must obey. Almost all communication is directed toward the leader, who does not encourage communication among group members. Interpersonal contact among members is minimal. In addition, all evaluations come directly from the authoritarian-autocratic leader. These evaluations, however, are not usually based on the indivdual's performance but rather on the individual's personal attributes (Heimann, 1976; Sampson & Marthas, 1981; White & Lippitt, 1968).

Consequently, group members are oftentimes fearful of, or angry with, the authoritarian-autocratic leader, who will not allow them the opportunity to participate actively in the group and to share in the decision-making activities. An atmosphere of intense frustration among group members evolves. This frustration is displayed in the form of hostility and aggressiveness, which is generally not expressed directly to the leader. Instead group members may displace their hostility and negative thoughts and feelings onto another group member, and the stage is set for scapegoating. Also, group members may act out in passive-aggressive ways as a means of expressing their hostility—i.e., being tardy or not participating at their potential (Heimann, 1976; Sampson & Marthas, 1981; White & Lippitt, 1968).

The *democratic* leadership style is characterized by group involvement and group cohesiveness, as well as independent and interdependent functioning. The democratic leader's most salient function is to serve as a facilitator who actively fosters the development of norms that lay the foundation for a cohesive group. These leaders encourage group members to function independently of the leader and to work interdependently, cooperatively, and collaboratively with each other. The democratic leader facilitates maximal group involvement in decision-making activities. Through group discussions the democratic group leader, in conjunction with the group members, decides the group policies and goals, the strategies for implementing the group goals, and the criteria for goal achievement. In addition, the democratic leader not only permits but promotes group interaction, and, consequently, communication flows between and among group members. Members feel secure and are able to discuss their views, ideas, and concerns without feeling threatened (Heimann, 1976; Sampson & Marthas, 1981; White & Lippitt, 1968).

The group and its functioning as an efficient and cohesive unit are more important to the democratic leader than maintaining power and/or being the leader. In the group led by a democratic leader, the growth of the group is directly correlated to the growth of the individual group members. As the group grows, so do the individual group members and vice versa. Neither the growth of the group nor the growth of individual group members is jeopardized. In contrast, authoritarian-autocratic leaders place more emphasis on their position as leader than on the development of a cohesive group (Heimann, 1976; White & Lippitt, 1968).

The third leadership style is the *laissez-faire* leader. These leaders emphasize neither their own power role nor the development of a cohesive group but rather the growth of individual group members. They function primarily as consultants or resource persons who interact with individual group members only upon request. As such, they may appear aloof and minimally involved with the activities of the members of the group. When their services are requested, these leaders cordially respond to the specific needs of individual members. The laissez-faire leader, however, does not exert any control over group members, who can accept or reject any recommendations. Direction is minimal. The laissez-faire leader's goal is to improve the individual's

effectiveness by encouraging the growth and development of individual members (Heimann, 1976; White & Lippitt, 1968).

Group members in a laissez-faire group, like group members in an authoritarian-autocratic group, often experience frustration. Their frustration, however, is due to lack of direction—goals are unclear, decisions are not made, and evaluations are not done. Group members in the laissez-faire group generally manifest their frustration by scapegoating, and the group becomes confused and disorganized, all of which adversely affect the level of productivity. In addition, members become apathetic and withdrawn from active participation within the group. (Heimann, 1976; Sampson & Marthas, 1981; White & Lippitt, 1968).

Table 12-2 presents strengths and limitations of the three leadership styles.

Power

Leadership implies *power*, the ability to influence and to produce changes. Power and leadership coexist and, therefore, like leadership, power takes place within interpersonal relationships. These relationships are interdependent and are characterized by cooperation, collaboration, and the sharing of power for the purpose of promoting the growth of the group and of the individual group members. Consequently, power does not necessarily imply control, complete domination, and manipulation, nor does power reside solely in the identified leader (Claus & Bailey, 1977; Olson, 1979; Welch, 1979).

Claus & Bailey (1977) view power as the interplay among three factors: strength, energy, and action. Strength denotes the person's ability, skill, competency, talent, and aptitude in a specified area, whereas energy implies the person's readiness and eagerness to become involved and to take risks. The person's action or performance, which results from that strength and energy, leads to observable changes. One uses strength, energy, and action to increase a power base and, subsequently, to be influential.

Those individuals with authority have the official right to use power and, as such, to be the leaders. Authority can be assigned on a formal basis, as when an organization designates a person to an official position with a title and written regulations defining that authority. On the other hand, a person can gain authority on an informal basis when the group grants that person the authority of leader. This authority would be based on that individual's personal actions resulting from the maximal use of his or her strength and energy (Claus & Bailey, 1977).

Community health nurses wishing to maximize their power when working with groups can do so by (Claus & Bailey, 1977; McCurdy, 1982; Morrison, 1982; Olson, 1979; Welch, 1979):

- Developing creative solutions to problems
- Becoming visible by joining committees in health agencies and the community
- Cultivating assertive behavior—maintaining eye contact, speaking clearly and distinctly, standing erect, etc.
- Including others in the establishment of goals, decision making, and the resolution of problems
- Acquiring knowledge about the process of change and problem solving
- Interacting effectively with people on an individual and group level for the purpose of impacting upon their behavior, feelings, and attitude
- Being competent in a given theoretical or technical area
- Appraising realistically their strengths and weaknesses
- Knowing when to be persistent and when to be flexible in their approach
- Being objective—giving feedback based on objective data
- Being aware of the types of power and how to use them

Types of Power Five types of power have been described by Wilson and Kneisl (1983):

1. *Reward and coercive power* exists when the leader gives positive rewards and negative sanctions,

respectively, to group members. The amount of influence a leader has would be a function of the leader's ability to control the rewards delivered to group members.
2. *Referent power* exists when the group members identify and internalize the leader's values. Charismatic leaders generally have referent power.
3. *Expert power* occurs when the leader is viewed as having a special body of technical knowledge and experience.
4. *Informational power* exists when the group members perceive the leader to have information that is not available to the group.
5. *Legitimate power* is synonymous with authority, which is the official right to govern the group members.

All five types of power can be used by community health nurses, whether they are the designated leaders or group members. In addition, a person can use more than one type of power. Community health nurses who have expert power may also have referent power. For example, their expert power, which may be child development, can be enhanced by the group members' desire to incorporate the community health nurses' values regarding child care. Community health nurses can also have legitimate power; they can either be assigned by their supervisor to lead an interdisciplinary task force or can be elected by group members to be the leader based on their expert, referent, and information power. Reward power occurs when the community health nurse praises and compliments group members' effort. Strange as it may seem, community health nurses, even though they are generally nonmembers, can exert reward power when they praise self-help groups and make appropriate referrals.

Community health nurses most often, however, use expert power; they share their expertise in child care, prenatal and postnatal care, family planning, child development, and immunization. In Case Example 12-4, Mrs. Doe exhibits expert power.

Informational power is also used by community health nurses. In Case Example 12-5, Mrs. Dew uses informational power.

Table 12-2 Strengths and Limitations of Leadership Styles

Leadership Styles	Strengths	Limitations
Authoritarian-Autocratic	1. More conducive to larger groups and formal groups 2. More beneficial when decisions have to be made quickly	1. Impersonal relationships 2. Lack of cohesiveness 3. Highly competitive 4. Passive aggressive behavior, hostility, and scapegoating 5. Level of productivity is a function of leader's presence 6. Preponderance of individual roles 7. Low group morale 8. Members are dependent on leader 9. Formation of subgroups that have purposes inconsistent with the larger group purpose
Democratic	1. High group involvement 2. High interpersonal interaction among members 3. High group cohesiveness 4. Consistent level of productivity 5. Group members function interdependently	1. Takes time to develop cohesiveness and to make decisions

Case Example 12-4: Using Expert Power

Mrs. Doe, a community health nurse, scheduled weekly meetings for teenage mothers for the purpose of teaching infant care. She organized her teaching to complement the educational and maturity level of these mothers. To ensure that the information was being perceived correctly, she encouraged members to discuss the content and to indicate in what ways this information could be used by them. Time was allocated for demonstration of skills learned. In subsequent meetings, members agreed to share with the group the ways they actually used the information and skills in their everyday lives.

Mrs. Doe organizes teaching-learning group in which she uses expert power.

Table 12-2   *(continued)*

Leadership Styles	Strengths	Limitations
	6. Commitment of group members to the group purpose 7. Useful for group dealing with feelings and values 8. Valuable when groups have to handle complex problems	
Laissez-Faire	1. Leader acts as a consultant	1. Members function independently 2. Level of productivity is usually low. Quality of work is usually poor 3. Preponderance of individual roles 4. Lack group cohesiveness 5. High confusion 6. Scapegoating exists 7. Formation of subgroups that have purposes inconsistent with the larger group

SOURCES:
Benne KD, Sheats P: Functional roles of group members. *Journal of Social Issues* 1948; 4 (2): 41–49.

Heimann CG: Four theories of leadership. *J Nurs Adm* 1976; 6 (5): 18–24.

Sampson EE, Marthas M: *Group Process for the Health Professions.* New York: Wiley, 1981, pp. 27–47, 261–304.

White R, Lippitt R: Leader behavior and member reaction in three social climates. In: Cartwright D, Zander A (editors), *Group Dynamics: Research and Theory.* New York: Harper & Row, 1968, pp. 318–335.

Stages of Group Development

Before the first meeting of the group the leader-facilitator performs preliminary functions to ensure that the group achieves its purpose. These are preliminary functions:

1. Performing a needs assessment to determine if a need that is common to a number of individuals actually exists
2. Determining, by considering the advantages and disadvantages of a group, if a group format is the most effective means of meeting this need
3. Formulating an overall purpose based on the need, and deciding which of the five types of groups would best meet the purpose
4. Establishing criteria for membership and determining the size of the group based on the purpose
5. Contacting and interviewing potential mem-

Case Example 12-5: Using Informational Power

In community Y, five school children have been sexually assaulted in the past four weeks. A task force was formed by Mrs. Blanket, the school nurse, for the purpose of determining in what ways they could address the needs of the community. Members of the task force consisted of Miss Dew, a community health nurse; Mrs. Seems, a community resident; Mrs. Jones, social worker from the Division of Family and Children's Services; Dr. Banks, a pediatrician; Dr. Keith, a community psychologist; Mrs. Sights, an emergency room nurse; and Sergeant Davis from the Sexual Assault Control Unit.

Task-directed/planning group is organized.

Mrs. Blanket introduced everyone and started by stating that the recent incidents of sexual assaults were affecting the entire community. Parents were escorting their children to and from school. Teachers were noticing that children were not attentive in the classroom and had questions that the teachers did not always feel comfortable in addressing.

Mrs. Blanket has legitimate power.

Mrs. Blanket asked those members who had information about the community's reactions to sexual assault to share it with the group. Mrs. Seems and Miss Dew had specific information about the community's reactions. From Miss Dew's community assessment, it was revealed that parents in the community were requesting information on how to protect their children. In addition, it was revealed that everyone in the community was expressing concern and fear and was angry and frustrated with the police department because of its failure to arrest the assailant. Mrs. Seems concurred and added that parents of children victimized were concerned about their children's nightmares and reluctance to be alone. According to Mrs. Seems, these parents were seeing their children change from active to fearful young people who had periods of unpredictable crying. Mrs. Seems ended by saying that both the parents and the children needed assistance during this stressful period.

Miss Dew and Mrs. Seems have informational power.

bers to determine if they satisfy the criteria for membership and to determine their commitment to the group purpose

6. Selecting a meeting place and time conducive to members assembling. The meeting place should be consistent throughout the groups' existence and in a safe, quiet, and convenient location. There should be enough space to accommodate the group and to permit a circular seating arrangement.

Groups evolve through three phases: initiation phase, working phase, and termination phase. Throughout these phases the leader-facilitator of the group, in conjunction with group members,

must be cognizant of promoting an environment to enhance the development of a cohesive group. He or she must guide the group in the direction of establishing norms that encourage total member involvement in the formation of goals, in decision making, and in conflict resolution. These three phases may overlap, and only the first and last phases are seen in all groups (Yalom, 1975).

Initiation Phase

The first phase is called the initial phase (Yalom, 1975) or the *initiation phase*. During this phase the members are meeting together for the first time in

Dr. Keith had talked to some concerned residents, but had not seen any of the victims or their parents. Mrs. Seems and Miss Dew both stated that parents were reluctant to bring their children to the local mental health clinic for fear that the community might label them "crazy."

Dr. Banks and Mrs. Sights had treated these children in the emergency room but have had little contact with them since then. Both thought that these children were in a state of shock and very frightened when seen in the emergency room.

Mrs. Blanket asked if other members had comments they would like to make. Sergeant Davis said that his staff was pursuing all clues. There were very few clues, however, and most of them were not substantial. He could understand the community's frustration and was eager to participate in whatever way he could to make this task force a success. Other members also expressed their commitment to the group.

Sergeant Davis expresses his commitment to the group and other members concur.

Mrs. Blanket thanked everyone for their commitment. She said that valuable information had been presented and maybe the group could talk about specific things it could do to assist the community. Based on the information given, the task force decided by group consensus to prepare a ninety-minute presentation in which all interested and concerned community residents would be invited. The purpose of the presentation would be to present some factual information about sexual assaults—i.e., typical reactions of the victims, their families, friends, and the community, and common myths about sexual assaults. Also to be included in this presentation would be a discussion on safety tips. The presentation for the community would be given three times weekly at different days and times during the week. For school children, the presentation would be given during the school hours several times a week.

Mrs. Blanket ensures that everyone has an opportunity to participate.

The task force also felt that a support group for victims and a support group for their families should be organized. The group decided to discuss this possibility at their next scheduled meeting.

this group context. Generally, but not always, the members are strangers. Whether some members know each other prior to their group membership does not diminish the fact that members must become acquainted with each other in this particular context. Members are asking themselves what to expect from each other and from the leader-facilitator and what each person's role will be in this particular group. The trust level is not high, and testing between and among members occurs. Through the interaction developing during this phase the foundation for group norms is laid. This foundation determines how cohesive the group will become (Yalom, 1975).

The group develops specific goals to achieve the group purpose. These goals should have group consensus and should be defined explicitly to eliminate confusion and to ensure goal achievement. All members must be involved. If members are not encouraged to participate in goal formation, they may not share the same goals and, consequently, may have different expectations. The strategies of intervention for the achievement of these goals should also have group consensus. When there is group consensus regarding the purpose, goals, and strategies for goal achievement, the probability of resistance occurring within the group is minimal (Thibaut & Kelly, 1959; Yalom, 1975).

Contracting, an agreement between leader-facilitator and group members, is useful during this phase. The group leader-facilitator and members come to a mutual understanding about the group purpose, goals, and strategies, as well as what everyone has to offer the group, and what everyone is expected to do. The contract also provides an estimation of when the goals are to be completed and the method of evaluation (Sampson & Marthas, 1977; Sloan & Schommer, 1982). Contracts can either be in writing or verbal but are always clear and explicitly stated. They are dynamic and renegotiable.

Since this phase is characterized by some degree of uncertainty—roles, norms, and goals are evolving—the leader-facilitator must ensure the emergence of appropriate roles, norms, and goals consistent with the group purpose. The leader-facilitator, therefore, should clarify information about the group purpose, encourage discussion, comment on and summarize essential points as a means of informing the group of its progress, make and elicit suggestions, and create an atmosphere in which members can feel comfortable.

Working Phase

During the second phase, the *working phase*, the group develops into a cohesive unit and begins to function as a team in its attempts to accomplish its goals. However, this cohesive entity emerges as a result of the group's ability to resolve conflict (Yalom, 1975).

Resolving Conflict Conflict, which normally occurs during the working phase, is the tension that results from disagreements or differences (Kramer & Schmalenberg, 1976). Conflict may arise from four sources:

1. Frustration due to a sense of helplessness in accomplishing a difficult task
2. Disagreement related to personal power struggles existing among members who are attempt-

ing to maximize their status and rank within the group
3. Disagreement among group members about strategies, techniques, and priorities
4. Disagreements resulting from members having loyalties to other groups

The first two sources can lead to unproductive or destructive conflict, whereas the last two have the potential to lead to productive or constructive conflict (Sampson & Marthas, 1981).

Constructive conflict results in the group's accomplishing its purpose—members are receptive to the discussion of all issues and the unfolding of disagreements and to the rational resolution of problems. Members are willing to compromise. Destructive conflict, on the other hand, results in chaos; members are not receptive to input from other members, are confused and uncertain about the group purpose, are critical and refuse to compromise, and wish to dominate the group. The group purpose is not accomplished, and issues recur because no solutions are ever reached (Sampson & Marthas, 1981).

Conflict can be manifested in the form of resistance. Resistance can either be passive or active. Members who actively resist may discontinue their membership, scapegoat other members, or form subgroups with purposes inconsistent with the group purpose. Members who passively resist may withhold information, participate minimally, withdraw from the group discussion and problem solving, or sabotage the agreed-upon plan by forgetting to fulfill their responsibilities and by being marginally committed to the group purpose (Olson, 1979; Yalom, 1975).

The role of the leader-facilitator in conflict resolution is to recognize that a conflict exists and to label the situation accordingly. The leader-facilitator then assists group members to recognize and not be frightened by the conflict. When assisting group members to recognize the conflict, the leader-facilitator describes the behavior that is occurring in the group and what feelings this behavior evokes in him or her. Then he or she states that disagreements are natural and inevitable and provide the group the opportunity to utilize their problem-solving skills. The leader-facilitator and members explore the basis for the conflict and the meaning the conflict has for the group. In the final step the leader-facilitator encourages members to recognize commonalities, to discuss possible resolutions, and to negotiate a mutually agreeable solution for the members (Sampson & Marthas, 1981).

It is, however, important that conflict be resolved as soon as it becomes evident. Failure to do so only prolongs the conflict and may inadvertently communicate to the group members that conflicts are to be feared and avoided. The group may feel helpless and demoralized; they may feel that conflicts are unmanageable. When conflict is successfully resolved, group members will be better equipped to cope with future conflict—they will accept disagreements as nonthreatening and as a potential growth experience (Sampson & Marthas, 1981).

Solving Problems and Making Changes
Rodgers (1973) has delineated the following five steps in problem solving:

1. *Problem Identification:* The problem is stated.
2. *Assessment of Problem:* Data are collected and from the data base the problem is diagnosed. When collecting data, the group looks at all facets of the problem. What are the advantages and disadvantages of resolving or not resolving the problem? Who would or would not benefit from problem resolution? What are the strengths and weaknesses of the group? What are the forces encouraging and hindering changes? As the facilitator, what are the reasons for initiating or facilitating change?
3. *Intervention Planning:* Components of the contract that were established in the initiation phase are reexamined and are defined more explicitly. Clear, concise strategies, alternatives, and criteria for evaluation are formulated. Who will do what in a specified time frame is spelled out, and commitments are reconfirmed.
4. *Intervention.* Implementation takes place.

5. *Evaluation:* Appraisal is done on criteria established.

Inherent in problem solving is change. Lewin's theory of change describes this process. This theory consists of three stages: unfreezing, moving, and refreezing. In the unfreezing stage, there is a growing awareness that a problem exists. This problem disturbs the group because the group's stability or equilibrium is upset. The group is highly motivated to restore its equilibrium and attempts to diagnose the problem, explore various solutions to the problem, and select the most appropriate means of combating the problem. At this point, the group enters the second stage, moving. Here the group plans in detail its strategy of action and the implementation of this strategy. To encourage and maintain planning and implementation of plans, the group needs to be rewarded for its efforts. During the first two stages there are driving forces that make change easier and restraining forces that hinder or impede the process of change. The leader-facilitator must be alert to both forces and assist group members in developing an awareness so as to build upon the driving forces while minimizing, modifying, or avoiding the restraining forces. The last stage, refreezing, occurs when the changes are integrated into the value system of the group. The group members incorporate the change into their everyday function, and equilibrium is restored. During all three stages feedback and constructive criticism are helpful to ensure successful progress (Olson, 1979; Rodgers, 1973; Welch, 1979).

Problem solving and Lewin's theory of change are similar in that the first two steps of problem solving are synonymous with Lewin's unfreezing stage and the last three steps are consistent with Lewin's stage of moving. To be effective, the process of change and problem solving must be shared by all group members. In addition, group consensus must be sought during each of the steps. Group consensus occurs when there is mutual acceptance among group members of whatever issue is currently being discussed. No group members feel that they have lost, and, consequently, commitment from all members is likely to occur (Smith, 1982; Wilson & Kneisl, 1983).

Making Decisions Decisions are part of the problem-solving process. Four types of decisions are:

1. Decisions made by the leader-facilitator with or without the benefit of group discussion
2. Decisions made by a subgroup
3. Decisions made by majority vote
4. Decisions made by group consensus

Decision by group consensus, the last type, generally takes a long time to evolve.

It is important that groups make decisions that are realistic, sound, and acceptable to the group members. These decisions occur when all ideas are taken into consideration, when the assets and talents of all members are used, when the group spends its time focusing on the task, and when the group members are committed to the decision and are actively involved in implementation. When decisions are realistic, sound, and effective, group members feel pleased with their problem-solving abilities.

Termination Phase

The contract established by the group prescribes when the group will be terminating. The group members and leader-facilitator decide whether termination will occur after a certain number of meetings or on a specified date, or whether termination will occur after goals have been achieved. If termination is stated in terms of time, the goals may or may not be accomplished. In those cases where goals have not been accomplished, group members determine if the goals were realistic and whether more time is needed. If group members decide more time is needed, they renegotiate a new contract that will either extend the time to another target date or extend the existence of the group indefinitely until goals are achieved.

When the group reaches the termination phase, group members may experience a multitude of feelings and thoughts. Common feelings are joy, happiness, sadness, anger, fear, relief, a sense of belonging, and grief. Typical thoughts focus on the quality of one's performance in the group and the quality of the group itself. These strongly influence whether people want to have similar experiences again, whether they feel successful or not, and whether they wish to maintain contact with other group members after termination. These feelings and thoughts are closely related to each group member's self-concept and sense of loss (Sampson & Marthas, 1981).

In those groups where there is a high degree of cohesiveness and where goals have been accomplished, the group members feel successful and experience an elevated status and a positive view of group work. However, in those groups where cohesiveness does not evolve and the group functions in a state of turmoil, either individual members will discontinue membership, or the group itself will dissolve (Yalom, 1975).

Some groups are terminated prematurely, and individuals also leave groups before the termination date. For example, Bednar and Kaul (1978) comment on the case when individuals leave the group during its working phase. They leave the group because they perceive the group to be unresponsive to their needs, because they have unrealistic expectations of the group, or because their goals are inconsistent with the group goal. Regardless of the reason, loss of group members may have an ominous effect upon those who remain; their morale is lowered. If the group terminates prematurely, the group members may feel frustrated and experience a sense of failure and reduced self-esteem. Sometimes, however, these members may feel a sense of relief that they are no longer involved in an unproductive group (Sampson & Marthas, 1981; Yalom, 1975).

Often members are unaware that the feelings and thoughts they are experiencing are related to termination, or they are reluctant to confront the issues of termination. They deny feelings, avoid the topic, refuse to recognize the significance of the group, and disengage from the group through tardiness, absenteeism, emotional separation, and limited and superficial involvement. The leader-facilitator must assist group members to recognize that their feelings and behavior are closely related to an imminent termination. Adequate time should be allocated for discussion. Approximately three weeks prior to the last meeting the leader-facilitator initiates discussion by acknowledging that the group members may be experiencing feelings and thoughts related to termination. Members are asked to summarize the experiences that have occurred in the group. When doing so, the group members analyze and evaluate the progress the group has made as well as examine the effect of the group process on themselves. Group members are encouraged to review their successes and failures and to learn from them. By sharing personal feelings and thoughts about the group process and progress, the leader-facilitator assists members to become more aware of the issues of termination, more ready to share their perceptions, and to begin to cope with termination. Members who have needs that have been unmet by the group should be referred to the appropriate resources (Sampson & Marthas, 1981; Van Servellen, 1984).

Evaluation of Group Process

Group members and leader-facilitators evaluate the group not only in terms of the degree to which goals are achieved but also in terms of the process of goal achievement. To determine the degree of goal achievement, it is imperative that the group purpose and goals have been clearly stated.

Evaluating the process of goal achievement is done on an ongoing basis at the end of each group meeting. Group members examine their behavior as it affects group cohesiveness, motivation, problem solving, and decision making. Group members are encouraged to express their feelings and thoughts about the meeting and attempt to minimize those that are not conducive to the group process.

For example, after one group meeting, members thought that the meeting was a waste of time and, consequently, felt angry. Group members were encouraged to examine their thoughts and feelings and concluded that their thoughts and feelings stemmed from the fact that no relevant issues were discussed during the meeting. The leader-facilitator assisted the group in focusing on factors that might have been operating in the group causing it to deal only with irrelevant issues. The group members were then able to decide what the group could do to alter its present course.

Sometimes, however, it is helpful to have an objective nonmember observe and evaluate a group meeting. This is especially true when the group members are engaged in unproductive conflict. Regardless of whether group members or an objective observer evaluates the group process, it is important that members realize that the productivity of each group meeting influences whether the group purpose and goals are achieved. It is highly unlikely that the group goals will be achieved if the process evaluations of the majority of the group meetings are poor.

According to Berkowitz (1980), Sampson and Marthas (1981), and Wilson and Kneisl (1983), effective groups are able to:

1. Develop and maintain cohesiveness but are not controlled by cohesiveness to the point that the group will not be able to tolerate any disagreements or dissensions. Disagreements are not viewed as threatening to the group's existence but instead provide the group the oppor-

tunity to resolve conflict in a constructive manner. The ability to solve problems is a high priority for the effective group.

2. Encourage and facilitate maximal participation of its members. The effective group creates an atmosphere in which all members feel free to express their feelings and thoughts about the group process. Through group discussions, group goals and strategies are determined, clarified, and modified as a means of achieving group consensus. Members are encouraged to generate many possible solutions to the group's problems in order to facilitate making the best decision. Flexibility and creativity are paramount for effective decision making.

3. Share the leadership role among its members based on the individual group members' expertise and the group needs. The primary concern is goal achievement rather than control.

4. Establish and utilize criteria to evaluate the degree to which the goals are or are not accomplished.

5. Terminate with a sense that the group members have learned from their successes and failures and have a positive view about the group process.

Summary

In group settings community health nurses work collaboratively and interdependently to ensure that the group purpose and goals are achieved. They promote group cohesiveness, the development of productive norms, and the emergence of group task and maintenance roles. They are alert to behavior occurring in the group and work to maximize behavior that positively impacts upon the group process. Conflict is perceived as an opportunity to grow and, as such, to advance the group to a higher level of functioning. An awareness that leadership and power go hand-in-hand and are a function of the group relationship assists the community health nurse to serve the group more effectively.

Promotion of the health and welfare of the community, which is the task of community health nurses, takes place when they work with groups within the community. Moreover, their time and expertise are enhanced when they are actively involved in groups. Their involvement includes working in planning groups and health education groups and providing support, recognition, encouragement and assistance to aggregates of residents. Emphasis is placed on primary prevention, which is facilitated by the group process.

As members of interdisciplinary and intradisciplinary groups, community health nurses can assist in the formulation of health policies, legal regulations, and ethical principles. Likewise, community health nurses are involved in the political arena, oftentimes a group setting. Their ability to understand group process, decision making, power, and leadership enhances their capacity to serve as advocates for the community and for their profession.

Study Questions

Mary Dans, a community health nurse, established and led a group whose purpose was to provide assistance to parents who had recently lost their infants from Sudden Infant Death Syndrome. An understanding, supportive nurse, Miss Dans facilitated the sharing of feelings and thoughts among parents.

Mrs. Silvers, a soft-spoken parent, talked about the shock and guilt she experienced. She was receptive to other members and praised them for their ability to share their experiences and feelings with the group. Mr. Thomas was not as receptive and requested a lot of group attention.

Questions 1 through 6 refer to this vignette.

1. Mary Dans has established a
   a. Socialization-centered group
   b. Support group
   c. Task-directed/planning group
   d. Self-help group
2. Mrs. Silver is functioning in the role of
   a. Monopolizer
   b. Coordinator
   c. Help-seeker
   d. Encourager
3. To be effective, Miss Dans realizes that
   a. The membership should consist of at least twenty parents, some of whom have not experienced Sudden Infant Death Syndrome
   b. She must focus exclusively on what is said in the group
   c. Each member must feel understood and accepted by the group
   d. Norms that foster restrictive communication among group members must be established
4. The type of power that Miss Dans uses is most likely
   a. Referent power
   b. Coercive power
   c. Informational power
   d. Both *a* and *b*
5. If Miss Dans chose to function as a laissez-faire leader-facilitator, you would predict that
   a. The group would dissolve because of limited group interaction and frustration
   b. The group would maintain its membership because group interaction is maximized
   c. Miss Dans would shift to an authoritarian-autocratic leadership style to encourage group interaction
   d. Miss Dans would shift to a democratic leadership style to increase her control over the group
6. Evaluation of the group
   a. Should be done by Miss Dans two weeks after the group has terminated
   b. Is more effective when it is done by Miss Dans on a regular basis without input from the group members
   c. Will most likely be positive if group members work cooperatively to achieve the group purpose
   d. Is based entirely on whether the group achieves its goal

References

Bednar RL, Kaul TJ: Experiential group research: Current perspectives. In: Garfield GL, Bergin AE (editors), *Handbook of Psychotherapy and Behavior Change: An*

An Empirical Analysis. New York: Wiley, 1978, pp. 769–815.

Benne KD, Sheats P: Functional roles of group members. *Journal of Social Issues* 1948; 4 (2): 41–49.

Berkowitz L: *A Survey of Social Psychology.* New York: Holt, Rinehart, & Winston, 1980, pp. 418–437.

Berne E: *The Structure and Dynamics of Organization and Groups.* Philadelphia: Lippincott, 1963, pp. 54–59.

Cartwright D: The nature of group cohesiveness. In: Cartwright D, Zander A (editors), *Group Dynamics: Research and Theory.* New York: Harper & Row, 1968, pp. 91–109.

Cartwright D, Zander A: Groups and group membership: Introduction. In: Cartwright D, Zander A, (editors), *Group Dynamics: Research and Theory.* New York: Harper & Row, 1968, pp. 45–62.

Claus KE, Bailey JT: *Power and Influence in Health Care: A New Approach to Leadership.* St. Louis: Mosby, 1977, pp. 16–27.

Clemen SA, Eigsti DG, McGuire SL: *Comprehensive Family and Community Health Nursing.* New York: McGraw-Hill, 1981, pp. 535–547, 195–234.

Eaton MT, Peterson MH, Davis JA: *Psychiatry: Medical Outline Series.* New York: Medical Examination Publishing, 1981, pp. 403–445.

Freeman RB: *Public Health Nursing Practice.* Philadelphia: Saunders, 1963, Chapter 13.

Heimann CG: Four theories of leadership. *J Nurs Adm,* 1976; 6 (5): 18–24.

Janis J: Groupthink. *Psychology Today* (November) 1971; 5 (6): 43–46.

Kozier B, Erb G: *Fundamentals of Nursing: Concepts and Procedure,* 2nd ed. Menlo Park, Calif.: Addison-Wesley, 1983, pp. 389–409.

Kramer M, Schmalenberg CE: Conflict: The cutting edge of growth. *J Nurs Adm* 1976; 6 (8): 19–25.

Leininger M: The cultural context of behavior: Spanish-Americans and nursing care. In: Spradley BW (editor), *Readings in Community Health Nursing.* Boston: Little, Brown, 1982, pp. 351–363.

Lewin K: Frontiers in group dynamics: Concept, method, and reality in social science. *Human Relations* 1947; 1 (1): 5–41.

Lewis JH: Conflict management. *J Nurs Adm* 1976; 6 (10): 18–22.

Lubin B: Group therapy. In: Weiner IB (editor), *Clinical Methods in Psychology.* New York: Wiley, 1976, pp. 393–450.

McCurdy JF: Power is a nursing issue. In: Muff J (editor), *Socialization, Sexism, and Stereotyping.* St. Louis: Mosby, 1982, pp. 359–365.

Morrison EG: Power and nonverbal behavior: Indicators and alternatives. In: Muff J (editor), *Socialization, Sexism, and Stereotyping.* St. Louis: Mosby, 1982, pp. 366–377.

Olson EM: Strategies and techniques for the nurse change agent. *Nurs Clinics of North America* 1979; 14 (2): 323–336.

Rodgers JA: Theoretical considerations involved in the process of change. *Nurs Forum* 1973; 12 (2): 160–172.

Sampson EE, Marthas M: *Group Process for the Health Professions.* New York: Wiley, 1981, pp. 27–47, 261–304.

Sloan MR, Schommer BF: The process of contracting in community health nursing. In: Spradley BW (editor), *Readings in Community Health Nursing.* Boston: Little, Brown, 1982, pp. 197–204.

Smith M: Group and organizational theory. In: Haber J et al (editors), *Comprehensive Psychiatric Nursing.* New York: McGraw-Hill, 1982, pp. 341–364.

Spradley BW: *Community Health Nursing: Concepts and Practice,* 2nd ed. Boston: Little, Brown, 1985, pp. 224–265, 553–585.

Stanhope M, Lancaster J: *Community Health Nursing: Process and Practice for Promoting Health.* St. Louis: Mosby, 1984, pp. 361–378.

Stuart GW, Sundeen SJ: *Principles and Practice of Psychiatric Nursing,* 2nd ed. St. Louis: Mosby, 1983, pp. 701–724.

Thibaut JW, Kelly HH: *The Social Psychology of Groups.* New York: Wiley, 1959, pp. 100–125, 126–148, 239–255.

Van Servellen GM: *Group and Family Therapy: A Model for Psychotherapeutic Nursing Practice.* St. Louis: Mosby, 1984, pp. 44–64, 67–96, 113–130, 131–159.

Welch LB: Planned change in nursing: The theory. *Nurs Clinics of North America* 1979; 14 (2): 307–321.

White R, Lippitt R: Leader behavior and member reaction in three social climates. In: Cartwright D, Zander A (editors), *Group Dynamics: Research and Theory.* New York: Harper & Row, 1968, pp. 318–335.

Wilson HS, Kneisl CR: *Psychiatric Nursing,* 2nd ed. Menlo Park, Calif. Addison-Wesley, 1983, pp. 214–235.

Yalom ID: *The Theory and Practice of Group Psychotherapy.* New York: Basic Books, 1975, pp. 45–69, 105–168, 276–300, 301–330.

Chapter 13

Health Promotion: Implementing Strategies

Nola Pender

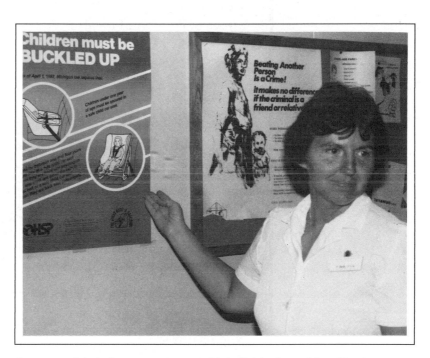

Because of their frequent contact with individuals and families in their own environments, community health nurses can be especially effective in implementing health promotion strategies. (Linda Daniel/courtesy of Washtenaw County Health Department and the Huron Valley VNA)

Chapter Outline

Chapter Objectives

After completing this chapter, the reader will be able to:

- Analyze the similarities and differences between health promotion, health protection, and illness prevention
- Examine the multidimensional role of the community health nurse in promoting health among families, communities, and society
- Discuss the benefits of school and worksite health promotion programs
- Compare and contrast information dissemination, appraisal and assessment, life-style modification, environmental restructuring, and building social-cultural support as strategies for the promotion of health in aggregates
- Critique values clarification, life-style review, and health promotion and protection planning as approaches to enhancing the health of families
- Examine strategies that community health nurses can use to influence health policy

The idea of health promotion is not new. It has been a fundamental concept in public health for decades. What is new is the focal position of health promotion in evolving national health policy and the increasing interest and activity generated by health promotion within society. Today few Americans, including health professionals, would disagree philosophically with any of the following statements:

- Living longer and enjoying life more are goals likely to be attained best by a healthy life-style rather than through destructive personal habits (Polakoff, 1982).
- Promoting health, and preventing illness when possible, are more desirable approaches to health care than curing illness.
- Educating people to stay healthy will cost less than treating them after they become sick.

In fact, a National Survey of Personal Health Practices and Health Consequences conducted by the federal government (Harris, 1981) indicated that 92 percent of the people surveyed agreed that eating more nutritious food, smoking less, maintaining proper weight, and exercising regularly would do more to improve the health of Americans than anything physicians could do.

While health-promoting life-styles have considerable potential for increasing longevity, improving the quality of life, and reducing health care costs (Niblett, 1975), many questions have also been raised concerning health-promoting care. Critical questions for community health nurses to address include: What are the responsibilities of individuals, families, groups and communities in promoting health? What role should health professionals, in particular nurses, play in the redirection of society toward healthier life-styles? What is the role of social and health policy in supporting healthful life patterns? These questions will be considered in this chapter and alternative solutions offered for consideration.

As a context for the discussion of strategies for health promotion, we need to take a brief look at recent evolutionary changes in the focus of national health policy. In 1979, the Surgeon General of the United States, Julius B. Richmond, issued a landmark document entitled *Healthy People,* which clearly set forth national policy for the prevention of illness and the promotion of health among Americans (*Healthy People,* 1979). It was the premise of the document that if progress were made in the target areas identified, significant improvement in the health of Americans would result. In 1980, a related government report entitled *Promoting Health/ Preventing Disease: Objectives for the Nation* was issued (*Promoting Health,* 1980). This document set forth specific objectives in fifteen areas, which were organized into the categories of preventive health services, health protection, and health promotion as shown in Table 13-1. The objectives set forth for the nation are primarily preventive in orientation, since they are based on evidence that certain behaviors increase mortality and morbidity from specific diseases (Green, 1984b). While health promotion is addressed, it receives less attention than prevention. However, for the first time in many years, prevention and health promotion came to the forefront as equally deserving of attention in national health policy, along with treatment of disease and rehabilitation.

Specific areas of health promotion targeted in the objectives for increased effort on the part of health professionals and laypersons are nutrition, physical fitness and exercise, control of stress and violent behavior, smoking, and misuse of alcohol and drugs. All of these areas can be characterized as behavioral—that is, an acquired part of life-style—and thus amenable to change.

The objectives are intended to provide guidelines not only for the federal government but also for states and the private sector. As federal spending on health decreases, states will assume increased responsibility for the health of their people. In addition, the private sector will also shoulder more of the responsibility for health initiatives.

Formation in 1984 of the U.S. Task Force on Prevention is still another indication of the increasing national emphasis on proactive (illness prevention) as opposed to retroactive (treatment of disease) policy in health care. The charge of the

Table 13-1   Fifteen Areas Targeted for Action in *Promoting Health/Preventing Disease: Objectives for the Nation*

Preventive health services
    High blood pressure control
    Family planning
    Pregnancy and infant health
    Immunization
    Control of sexually transmitted diseases

Health protection
    Toxic agent and radiation control
    Occupational safety and health
    Accident prevention and injury control
    Fluoridation and dental health
    Surveillance and control of infectious diseases

Health promotion
    Smoking and health
    Prevention of misuse of alcohol and drugs
    Improved nutrition
    Physical fitness and exercise
    Control of stress and violent behavior

SOURCE:
Promoting Health/Preventing Disease: Objectives for the Nation. US Department of Health and Human Services, US Public Health Service, 1980.

Task Force is to develop recommendations for the appropriate delivery of preventive services in clinical settings. Prevention as well as health promotion will become more salient aspects of health care in the next decade.

While emergence of illness prevention and health promotion as major tenets of health policy within the United States represents one of the most exciting and challenging trends in health care during recent decades, actual health expenditures by the federal government have not followed policy. It has been estimated that only 2.5 percent of the total national health budget is spent on disease preven-

tion and a miniscule 0.5 percent on health promotion. This means that 97 cents of every health care dollar is still spent on treatment of disease (Polakoff, 1982). Organized pressure by the public and concerned health professionals will be critical during the coming years to ensure that promotion of health becomes the dominant focus for health care expenditures in the twenty-first century. Major emphasis on health promotion will mean fostering health-enhancing life-styles, self-responsibility as opposed to passive reliance on health professionals, societal norms supportive of health, and social policy that provides incentives for wellness.

Key Concepts in Health Promotion

Before health promotion strategies can be discussed, several key concepts must be defined: health; health behavior; health promotion; health protection, or illness prevention; health education; and change.

Health

The concept of health is complex and multidimensional. In Chapter 1, Barkauskas described Smith's (1981) four models of health and in Chapter 4, Crayton mentioned ecological and sociological definitions of health.

With respect to Smith's (1981) models of health, to be considered healthy, not only must individuals be free from the signs and symptoms of disease and able to perform satisfactorily in social roles, but they must adjust to the ever-changing conditions of the environment with a minimum of negative stress and strain. In addition, according to the eudaimonistic or most comprehensive definition proposed, health is creative self-fulfillment, actualization of inherent and acquired potential, and exuberant and zestful well-being (Smith, 1983). With the increasing emphasis on health promotion in our society, the adaptation and eudaimonistic definitions of health are becoming the norm. Based on Smith's work, Laffrey (1982) has developed the Health Conception Scale to measure the definition of health to which individuals subscribe.

An early advocate of a eudaimonistic definition of health was Halbert Dunn (1959) who defined health or wellness as: "An integrated method of functioning which is oriented toward maximizing the potential of which the individual is capable. It requires that the individual maintain a continuum of balance and purposeful direction within the environment where he is functioning" (p. 449). The World Health Organization's definition of health as "a state of complete physical, mental and social well-being and not merely the absence of disease and infirmity," which has been mentioned in pre-vious chapters, is also eudaimonistic (Temkin, 1953:21). Definitions of health that have appeared in the nursing literature have been primarily adaptive (Hadley, 1974; Murray & Zentner, 1975), eudaimonistic (Bermosk & Porter, 1979; Hanchett, 1979), or a combination of both adaptive and eudaimonistic (King, 1971; Pender, 1982; Wu, 1973).

The eudaimonistic or actualizing definition of health will be used as a basis for the discussion of strategies for health promotion in this chapter. The terms *health* and *wellness* will be used interchangeably, since the author views optimum health and high-level wellness as synonymous concepts.

Health Behavior

In 1966, Kasl and Cobb published a typology of health-related behaviors, which identified the following three types:

1. *Health behavior*—Any behavior undertaken for the purpose of preventing disease or detecting disease in an asymptomatic state
2. *Illness behavior*—Any activity undertaken by people who feel ill, for the purpose of defining the state of their health and discovering suitable remedy
3. *Sick-role behavior*—Any activity undertaken by people who consider themselves sick, for the purpose of getting well

As conceptualized by these authors, health behavior includes aspects of both primary prevention (specific protection against disease) and secondary prevention (early or presymptomatic diagnosis), not health promotion. However, the work of Kasl and Cobb clearly identified a category of legitimate health-related behaviors that could occur in the absence of disease. This was an important theoretical contribution to the field of behavioral health.

Health Promotion, Health Protection, and Illness Prevention

In *Healthy People* (1979) the Surgeon General differentiated between health promotion, health protection, and preventive health services in the following way:

- *Health promotion*—individual and community activities to promote healthful life-styles
- *Health protection*—actions of government and industry to minimize environmental threats
- *Preventive health services*—actions of health care providers to prevent health problems

In 1979, Harris and Guten (1979) used the term *health protective behavior* for *any* behaviors in which individuals engage with the intent of protecting their health, whether these behaviors are medically approved or not and whether they are objectively effective or not. In their description of health protective behavior, Harris and Guten included a broad range of behaviors viewed by individuals as preserving or conserving personal health. They combined health promotion and prevention behaviors in their definition. Primary, secondary, and tertiary prevention have been defined in Chapter 1, and the concept of health has been introduced as well. However, considerable differences exist in the literature regarding the use of the terms *health promotion, health protection,* and *prevention*. In previous work the author has suggested that health promotion should be a category separate from primary prevention (Pender, 1982a). Health promotion as a separate category could be defined in the following way:

— Health promotion consists of activities directed toward increasing the level of well being and actualizing the potential of individuals, families, communities and society.

Primary prevention consists of activities directed toward decreasing the probability of specific illnesses or dysfunctions in individuals, families and communities, including active protection against unnecessary stressors.

Health promotion is "approach" behavior while primary prevention is "avoidance" behavior. Since prevention consists of avoiding or protecting the self against harm or the threat of disease, in this chapter, the terms *prevention* and *health protection* will be used interchangeably.

In a linguistic analysis of the use of the term *health promotion* in the literature, Brubaker (1983, p. 4) makes the following observations:

- The term *health promotion* is widely used but seldom defined.
- The term *health promotion* is sometimes used interchangeably with *disease prevention* and *health maintenance*.
- Writers frequently imply that *health promotion* and *disease prevention* are *not* the same thing.

Brubaker argues that even the dictionary definitions support the differentiation between *illness prevention* and *health promotion*. To prevent is to keep from occurring, while to promote is to help or encourage to exist or flourish. She also contrasts the definition of *promote* with that of *maintain*, which means to preserve, keep unimpaired, or continue. She concludes that the review of literature suggests that a number of authors "reject the idea that health promotion is merely preservation of stability (maintenance) or avoidance of risk factors (prevention); instead, they believe that health promotion is directed toward self-development, growth and high-level wellness" (pp. 4–5).

The question can be posed as to what makes a specific behavior or life-style health promoting. Is it the intent of the behavior, the source of motivation, the resulting direction of movement on the health continuum, the type of activities in which individuals and families engage, or the outcomes of behavior? These definitional issues will need increasing attention as our nation's energies are turned toward large-scale efforts to improve the health of Americans throughout the life continuum.

Health Education

The difference between health promotion and health education needs clarification. *Health education* is defined as: "Any combination of learning experiences designed to facilitate voluntary adaptations of behavior conducive to health" (Green, 1984, p. 186). Still another definition of *health education* is: "A process for aiding consumers in making informed decisions about their personal, family and community wellbeing" (Lancaster, McIlwain, & Lancaster, 1983, p. 42). While these definitions imply that health education is not only the dissemination of information but a planned, multifaceted educational process oriented toward positive life-style change, health education is only one of many emerging strategies for the promotion of health. Use of stress management techniques (relaxation, music therapy, biofeedback, cognitive reappraisal); exercise; massage; intensive counseling (nutrition, sexuality, assertiveness); and support system enhancement are just a few of the other strategies for the promotion of health of individuals and families. Community strategies for the promotion of health include environmental restructuring and building organizational and interorganizational networks supportive of health promotion efforts. Thus, health education is an important approach for the promotion of health but only one of a growing number of strategies for use with individuals, families, and communities.

Change

The integration of health promotion as a part of life-style and as a major component of national health policy will require change at multiple levels within society. *Change* can be defined as altering, transforming, or causing to be different. Change includes the processes of destabilization, or unfreezing, and refreezing. Groups or aggregates contemplating change generally show the following characteristics:

- Dissatisfaction with the status quo
- Motivation to search or consider alternate courses of action
- Realization that change might create more desirable conditions than currently exist
- Willingness to try new approaches on a pilot or tentative basis
- Less concern with tradition than progress

A great deal of literature has appeared in recent years concerning behavior change processes at the individual level (Kazdin, 1980; Martin & Poland, 1980; Panyan, 1980; Pender, 1985). Less literature focuses on change processes at the aggregate level, yet the success of health promotion within families, communities, and society will depend on how well nurses understand and implement group approaches for facilitating change. Despite the relative scarcity of literature focused on aggregate change, several excellent references are available on planning for change at the community and societal levels (Archer, Kelly, & Bisch, 1984; Bennis et al, 1976; Milio, 1981). The community health nurse should become familiar with the principles of change presented in these references as a basis for developing effective health promotion strategies.

Incentives for Health Promotion

Both social and economic forces mandate that scientists take a more aggressive role in researching health and in clarifying the fundamental processes underlying healthy functioning. This knowledge can serve as a basis for planning a proactive and coordinated approach to health promotion in our society. Economic incentives also must be developed for both health professionals and consumers of health care services to move in the direction of health promotion and increased consumer self-responsibility. While policy provides guidelines for implementing strategies, money and resources are essential to make implementation of health promotion programs and services possible. Community health nurses must participate in the exploration of financial incentives that can be built into the health care payment system to facilitate development of health promotion care options and to encourage healthful life-styles. Possible incentives might be:

- Third-party payment for health promotion programs and services
- Reduced insurance rates for individuals and families who engage in health-enhancing behaviors
- Paybacks by Medicare or Medicaid and private insurers for regular use of health promotion facilities such as fitness centers
- Health days paid for by employers if illness days are not used

Without a doubt, economic considerations will serve as important determinants of the rate of adoption of health-promotion life-styles.

Role of the Community Health Nurse

The community health nurse has an important role in health promotion within the evolving health care system. The United States is moving toward an era not only of health promotion but also of cost containment in health care. Health care providers will need to consider "economy of scale" in developing health promotion strategies and in implementing health promotion programs nationally and locally. Dunn (1980) identified five areas of optimum health or wellness that provide a classificatory scheme for health promotion efforts:

- Individual wellness
- Family wellness
- Community wellness
- Environmental wellness
- Societal wellness

Economy of scale suggests that family, community, environmental, and societal wellness are the levels at which the health promotion efforts of community health nurses should be focused. Over a decade ago Roberts and Freeman (1973) stressed the importance of fully developing concepts and models of population-based nursing. Williams (1981)

has commented that the primary focus of community health nursing practice is defining problems and proposing solutions at the population or aggregate level. Williams (1984) points out the importance of distinguishing between population- or aggregate-focused nursing and clinical nursing delivered in community settings. In population-based nursing, the community is the client. Community health nursing requires attention to multiple aggregates in the community (adolescents, for example, or older adults living independently), or the so-called "big picture." This orientation for community health nursing will be used throughout the chapter, and health promotion strategies for families (small aggregates), groups, communities, and society as a whole will be discussed. The nurse's role in assessment, planning, implementation, and evaluation of health promotion initiatives at micro- and macro-aggregate levels will be discussed.

The preparation needed to provide nursing care to aggregates depends on the level of education being considered. Undergraduate students need knowledge and skills in family-centered care, group dynamics, community assessment, and health education. The content areas identified by Archer (1982) as essential for the community health nurse specialist at the graduate level include: research methods and statistics, biostatistics, epidemiology, community analysis, political processes and strategies, public health issues, health promotion and prevention strategies, health education strategies, and public health administration, including health planning and field experience in agencies that provide population-based nursing.

Settings for Heath Promotion

Based on the classification scheme suggested by Dunn (1980), the critical target settings for health promotion aimed at aggregates are family, community, and environment. These settings for health promotion will be discussed in this chapter.

Family

While the traditional nuclear family (married male and female parents, and children) will undoubtedly continue to be the dominant family pattern in American society, many other variant family forms are emerging that have both similarities and differences when compared to nuclear families. Some of the variant forms are: one-parent families; extended families (nuclear plus a relative, often older); augmented families (additional members, not blood relation); blended families (parts of two preexisting families); and unmarried adult dyads (heterosexual, relational, or homosexual). See Chapters 16 and 17 for more detailed discussions of traditional and nontraditional families, respectively.

Conceptual models applicable only to traditional white, middle-class, nuclear families are of limited value as a basis for implementing health promotion interventions with families of differing structure. For instance, developmental models generally assume that families are relatively stable small groups that go through predictable stages during their family life cycle (Duvall, 1977; Thompson, 1984). Terkelson (1980) has stressed that even in developmental theories descriptive of traditional families, paranormal or unpredictable events,

such as separation, divorce, unemployment, and miscarriage, must be included, because they often alter the natural sequence of family development.

Studying fifty-nine one-parent families headed by women, Duffy (1984) noted that such families differ from other family forms. Not only are the resources of only one adult member available, but stresses in the one-parent family differ both quantitatively and qualitatively from the two-parent family. From the data it appears that early in the experience of single parenthood, parents perceive their options to be limited, use well-established habits to maintain feelings of security, are reluctant to change, and experience high levels of fatigue. After the initial period of single parenthood, parents begin to seek new options by redefining themselves as persons, risking change and garnering heightened energy levels. Finally, transcending options is the stage in which single parents are optimizing their circumstances and creating new options for themselves and their family. Approaches to promoting health in the one-parent family are illustrated in Case Example 13-1. Further qualitative studies of family form and related family lifestyles are critical to the formulation of theories helpful in understanding the milieu for the promotion of health in variant family forms.

The structural-functional model of the family described by Friedman (1981) will be presented briefly here, since it provides an excellent framework on which to base health promotion interventions. Within this framework the family is viewed as a system with the following structural and functional features: value structure, role structure, power structure, communication patterns, affective func-

Case Example 13-1: Health Promotion in a One-Parent Family

Linda M. and her two children, Michael and Jennifer, live in a small two-bedroom home in a low income neighborhood. Linda was divorced four months ago and is attempting to adjust to new living arrangements. Linda is frustrated by the overwhelming responsibility that she shoulders for the children's care and economic security. She is extremely tired at night and sometimes loses her patience with the children. Slowly, the family is beginning to adjust to their new life. Linda feels that she can relax and be herself since the divorce. Linda is exploring new life-style options and relationships. She recently joined a single-parent group. At one of the group meetings, Linda met Donna B., a community health nurse, who spoke to the group on "Your Health Investment." Linda made arrangements with Donna B. for a family visit.

Variant family form: one-parent family

Evidence of coping function problems

Step toward building social support systems

On her first visit, Donna asked Linda and the children to complete the Rokeach Value Survey, with health included, to determine the importance of health in relation to other values. In addition, Donna assessed family role structure, family strengths, communication patterns, and family coping effects. Donna explored the health care function of the family. Specifically, she asked about dietary patterns, participation in exercise, sleeping patterns, and family use of leisure time. She was particularly concerned about how the family handled stress, since she knew that everyone had to "pitch in" and help. The work that had been shared by four people had to be completed by three individuals. The family appeared affectionate toward one another, using touch frequently and talking easily.

Use of values clarification

Application of structural-functional framework to family

Use of life-style review

Evidence of adequate affective functioning

Linda, Michael, and Jennifer learned a great deal about each other during Donna's visit. They said that it had been fun exploring their family life-style. The entire family expressed excitement about Donna's next visit when they would begin to identify areas of their lives in which health-promoting changes could be made.

Development of a family health promotion and protection plan

---

tion, socialization function, health care function, and family-coping function. This approach provides a meaningful way of studying not only the internal processes of a family but also the family's linkages to other institutions within society. Internal dynamics of the family and external forces affecting it can be analyzed.

Decision-making patterns in relation to health (power structure), communication patterns, and the extent to which family members provide support and nurturance for one another (affective function) are all important indicators of family health status. The place of health in the value structure of the family and the family's perception of their health care function are important factors in the predisposition of the family to engage in health-promoting behaviors. Specific questions that can be explored in relation to family health care function include:

- What is the extent of health knowledge within the family?
- What health-promoting behaviors does the family already engage in regularly?
- Are these behaviors characteristic of all family members, or are patterns of health-promoting behavior highly variable throughout the family system?

- What are the perceived benefits of specific health-promoting behaviors?
- What are the barriers to adopting new behaviors that will enhance health?
- Is there consistency between stated family health values and health actions?

Reutter (1984) has proposed integration of family systems theory, specifically Friedman's structural-functional approach and Orem's self-care nursing framework (1985) as a basis for a theory of family health that can be applied to all family forms. Friedman's framework was selected because it views the family in the context of subsystems and suprasystems. Orem's framework was selected because it focuses on self-care actions critical to the health promotion process. According to Orem, the appropriate nursing care system to meet families' needs for health promotive care is the supportive-educative system in which families are assisted in overcoming their self-care limitations through education and supportive counseling by the nurse. Reutter's work suggests that synthesis of existing theories may be a fruitful approach for the development of new theories undergirding the promotion of health in families.

Community

Within the community, programs that reach large aggregates are the most cost-effective. The four major types of community health promotion programs that will be described briefly here include school, worksite, hospital, and communitywide programs.

School Health Promotion Programs   Multiple influences affect the acquisition of health-promoting behavior by young children: parents; other adults with whom the children come in contact; siblings; peers; television; and institutions such as preschool, school, and church. The degree of influence exerted by each depends on the child's age and the extent to which the child is responsive to significant others (Mullen, 1983). (The reader is referred to Chapter 19 for an in-depth discussion of school health.)

School-based health programs have four important roles in health promotion:

1. Presentation of fundamental health concepts early in life to a large segment of the population as a basis for developing self-care competencies and the knowledge base for informed decisions about individual and family health
2. Promotion and reinforcement of positive attitudes toward health and wellness
3. Development of complex health-enhancing skills necessary for effective functioning as a self-actualizing individual
4. Structuring of the environment and social influences to support health-promoting behaviors

School health programs that are comprehensive can provide the foundation necessary for children of all ages to understand factors affecting personal and societal health. In addition, they can assist students in acquiring the skills necessary to successfully carry out health-promoting behaviors (Kolbe, 1982).

In 1974, the President's Committee on Health Education reported that school health programs were hindered by antiquated laws, indifferent parents,[1] passive school boards, poorly prepared teachers, lack of governmental leadership, lack of funds, lack of scientifically sound knowledge on which to base programs, and lack of sound plans for evaluation.

Few studies evaluating school health programs have measured behavioral outcomes. Most have measured knowledge and attitudes. It is possible that failure to substantiate the behavioral outcomes of such programs has resulted in the current lack of support for school health endeavors. Given the nationwide reduction in support for education, existing health programs in schools are seriously threatened and the resources for augmenting school health efforts are minimal (Green, 1984).

Bartlett (1981) stresses the importance of coordinating school health programs with family and community resources to promote effectiveness and cost efficiency. Health-promoting life-styles can be achieved by a significant proportion of the school-age population only with support from families, health professionals, and the wider community. Hopp (1978) demonstrated the feasibility of joint parent-child education for achieving success in cholesterol control, weight control, and smoking cessation.

According to Bartlett (1981), successful school health programs:

- Are based on behavioral science theory
- Encourage a high level of student and family involvement
- Coordinate with and utilize community resources
- Contribute to community health promotion efforts

In 1982, Noak reported that twenty-four states required students to complete health course work in the schools. Thirty-five states had published curriculum or planning guides for school health education. Emphasizing the important role that schools play in the development of health behaviors Kolbe and Iverson (1984) commented:

Having completed their high school education, no adult should be ignorant about the consequences of individual decisions and social actions that ultimately will influence the health of their families and the communities in which their families reside. To the extent that the educational system fails to gain pace in disseminating and accumulating the complex understandings about health and human actions that influence it, we can expect that our people will be considerably less healthy than they could be (p. 1109).

Worksite Health Promotion Programs   Over the last decade, employers in the United States have accepted increasing responsibility for the health of their employees. Yearly, employers pay an increasing proportion of the cost of employee health insurance. Thus, it is not surprising that a 1978 Harris poll found a substantial shift toward prevention in the orientation of business and corporate leaders (Harris, 1978). Seventy-nine percent of business leaders and eighty-nine percent of labor leaders believed that the health care system should direct increased effort toward prevention rather than curative medicine. How many artificial hearts can the health care system afford to pay for to replace hearts damaged by reckless life-styles when the total cost may be as high as $500,000 per person? Billions of dollars could be spent each year on replacing only one body organ. Clearly, mass replacement of hearts and other organs with artificial devices is not the answer to lower medical expenditures or enhanced quality of living.

All businesses share a dependency on human resources. Especially today, when American businesses are working to improve their competitiveness in the world marketplace, a healthy and fit labor force is especially important (Gray, 1983). American corporations are supporting health promotion programs aimed at permanent changes in their employees' life-styles as a means of improving the quality of life for employees and of reducing employer health care costs. More and more employers are realizing that every dollar spent today may save $10 or $100 in the future (Gray, 1983).

O'Donnell (1984) identified the major benefits of work place health promotion programs as shown in Table 13-2. However, more evidence is needed from well-designed studies concerning the actual impact of employer-sponsored health promotion programs on employee health, quality of life, longevity, and corporate costs and profits.

Health promotion at the worksite creates a cultural milieu that rewards healthful life-styles. It restructures the social and physical environments to increase their health-enhancing potential. New health norms are developed by providing a work environment that supports healthy behaviors (Richard, 1984).

Wilbur (1983) stressed the importance of offering worksite health promotion programs and services in a variety of different ways to increase their appeal to employees of differing ages and with varying cultural backgrounds. He proposed that such programs be based on fundamental marketing principles—that is, the "product" should be well-defined

Table 13-2   Outcomes of Worksite Health Promotion Programs

Employee Benefits	Employer Benefits
Increased cardiopulmonary fitness	Decreased absenteeism
Weight control	Decreased health care costs
Increased strength and endurance	Increased productivity
Decreased stress and tension	Improved corporate image
Enjoyment	Improved employee morale

and priced to sell, immediate benefits from participation should be emphasized and barriers to participation minimized, and the program should be widely publicized and individualized for all participants.

Evaluation of the impact of corporate health promotion programs has been difficult. The reasons for this difficulty include lack of uniform methods for measuring cost savings across departments and corporations, inadequate systems to measure short-term outcomes, and insufficient time to measure long-term impact (Richard, 1984). Proposed long-range outcomes of worksite health promotion programs that need to be tested through longitudinal studies are increased employee productivity over time, decreased utilization of curative health services, and longer periods of independent living for retirees who have participated in a corporate health promotion program when compared to those who have not.

Some labor and employee groups have been concerned about the lack of attention to environmental and occupational conditions as part of comprehensive health promotion programs in industry. While promoting increased responsibility on the part of employees for their own health is desirable, many environmental and occupational conditions require changes on the part of employers. A well-planned health promotion program must take into

consideration both individual and corporate responsibility, involve top level management, and achieve collaboration between employer and employees. Case Example 13-2 illustrates the potential of a health promotion program at the worksite for increasing healthful behaviors among employees.

Hospital Health Promotion Programs   The shift to health promotion as a national policy priority has impact on hospitals nationwide. In addition, the rising cost of hospital care has far outstripped the increases in cost for ambulatory care, resulting in decreased utilization of inpatient facilities and services in most geographic areas. As never before, hospitals are looking for additional ways to generate income and to fulfill their societal mandate to enhance the health of the population that they serve.

Many hospitals began their wellness emphasis by developing programs for their employees. Given the stressful nature of work with acutely ill and sometimes terminally ill patients, emphasis on employee health was seen as a priority. Despite the responsibility that hospital personnel assume for teaching others about health and illness care, that knowledge frequently is not applied to their personal life-styles. Thus, assisting personnel in hospitals to adopt behaviors that improve their health

Case Example 13-2: Health Promotion at the Worksite

Peggy N., a nurse with a master's degree in community health nursing, is director of the Health Promotion Program at Sunshine Corporation, a midwestern firm with 375 employees. The chief executive officer of the corporation is committed to health promotion as a way of decreasing illness, increasing morale, and enhancing productivity of employees.

Work-site health promotion program
Employee and employer benefits

Since Peggy organized and publicized the health promotion program, 200 employees have joined the corporate health club. Many employees exercise in the fitness center and attend workshops on topics such as smoking cessation, stress management, and use of leisure time. Each employee who enters the program completes a life-style assessment that assists the employee in identifying health enhancing aspects of current life-style and areas for needed change. The employees can attend classes on how to use various techniques to change their life-style. In the classes they learn how to monitor their behavior, engage in self-modification, and reward themselves for positive changes. They also work on changing how they think about themselves. They learn to focus on their personal strengths and avoid engaging in "defeatist" thinking such as "I'll never lose weight," or "I don't have the discipline to exercise regularly."

Information dissemination program

Appraisal and assessment program

Life-style modification program

Use of operant conditioning principles

Use of cognitive restructuring

The health promotion program is creating an environment supportive of healthful practices among employees. The cafeteria now has a wide selection of salads, yogurts, and whole grain breads on the luncheon line. Empty calorie "pops" have been replaced in vending machines by juices and sparkling water. The employees encourage each other to exercise and attend health promotion classes. Joggers on the track around the company are a common sight early in the morning and at noon.

Environmental restructuring program

Social-cultural support

Peggy has developed an innovative and creative health promotion program for the Sunshine Corporation. She is always looking for new ways to expand the program and diversify its offerings. She encourages her staff to spend time in individual counseling sessions with employees and tailor health promotion approaches to meet the needs of employees with different cultural and ethnic backgrounds.

Role of the nurse in health promotion

Use of an individualized approach to programming

provides positive role models within the hospital setting.

Realizing that persons who have experienced a recent catastrophic illness may exhibit a high degree of readiness to learn how to prevent reoccurrence of illness and improve their health, many hospitals have incorporated health promotion concepts such as nutrition, stress management, and smoking cessation into their cardiac rehabilitation programs. Still another area in which health promotion efforts of hospitals are expanding is in community-oriented programming. Hospitals rich in resources and facilities that are sometimes underutilized are developing health promotion programs for communities. While some hospitals have mounted stellar programs in health promotion, others have utilized in-house personnel ill equipped to carry out programs focused on health promotion rather than care in illness. Quality programming characteristics of many hospitals in caring for the ill is sorely missing in health promotion efforts (Behrens et al, 1981). Hospitals that have achieved success in health promotion programming realized the importance of hiring community health nurses, nutritionists, exercise physiologists, and other health professionals with a community-wellness orientation.

Ardell (1980) identified the following benefits to hospitals from establishing health promotion programs: good public relations to increase use of inpatient and other hospital facilities, increased income from payment for programs, enhanced community service image, and enhanced patient satisfaction. Some hospitals have marketed their services to local industries and corporations where limited company resources preclude hiring full-time on-site health promotion personnel.

Cotanch (1984) expressed concern about the lack of integration of wellness services into inpatient care. It appears that many hospitals still see their wellness efforts as isolated services provided only to well people and not appropriate for the ill. Cotanch suggests that hospitals reevaluate their inpatient services and plan for integration of health promotion concepts into the ongoing care of patients in units throughout the hospital. Time in the hospital could be better utilized by familiarizing patients with the health promotion services that the hospital offers or by implementing strategies that motivate patients to examine their life-style and/or begin to make behavior changes that are health enhancing.

Community-wide Health Promotion Programs
The community-based model for health promotion potentially has at its disposal all of the resources of the community—including the health care networks and the systems of communication, transportation, education, recreation, social service, and government. Programming within this megastructure requires the selection of behavior acquisition and behavior maintenance strategies that can be used with large populations. The communitywide studies to date have focused on risk reduction for specific diseases rather than on programs that enhance the health status of large population groups. S. Weiss (1984, p. 1138) has cited a number of benefits of the community-based intervention model:

- It enhances opportunities for information exchange and social support among members of the target population.
- It allows for testing the efficacy of programs that can be generalized more widely than clinic-based trials.

- It allows for observation not only of the efficacy of public health programs but also of related outcomes that might have broader implications for public policy.
- It reduces the unit cost of interventions because large groups, rather than individuals, receive health promotion services.

Other advantages of community-wide programming include:

- It allows for use of interorganizational networks that are a part of the community system.
- It can provide a basis for changing societal norms regarding health and health behavior.
- It is a holistic rather than a piecemeal approach to promotion of health in large populations.

One of the best-known communitywide projects focused on risk factor reduction was the Stanford Three Community Survey (Stein et al, 1976) conducted between 1971 and 1977. In the study, mass media were the primary mechanisms used in one community for educational intervention. In a second community, intensive face-to-face counseling was used in addition to mass media education to lower risk factors associated with cardiovascular disease. A third community serving as a control received neither intervention.

The data from the study revealed that the health education campaign utilizing mass media resulted in a 20–40 percent decrease in cholesterol and saturated fat consumption among both men and women. Intensively instructed men tended to outperform men exposed to mass media alone, while women responded equally well to mass media and counseling approaches. Improvements in eating patterns were maintained over the two years of the study, indicating the potential of a community-based approach for significantly changing behaviors. The critical factor in the success of the program appeared to be the teaching of specific skills to facilitate use of the information presented via mass media and/or intensive counseling.

Building on the Three Community Survey, the Stanford Heart Disease Prevention Program has initiated a second trial of community-based intervention in the Five City Project (Farquhar et al, 1984). Of the five cities, two will serve as experimental sites and three as control communities. The major aim of the project is to test the hypothesis that a significant decrease in risk for the experimental communities will lead to a decline in morbidity and mortality from cardiovascular disease that is larger than the current national downward trend. A six-year education program is designed to stimulate and maintain changes in life-style. The program has three goals: (1) to achieve a transformation in knowledge and skills of individuals and in the educational practices of institutions such that risk factor reduction and decreased morbidity and mortality are achieved; (2) to carry out the community-based intervention program in a way that creates a self-sustaining health promotion structure within the organizational network of the communities; and (3) to derive a model for cost-effective community health promotion.

The Pawtucket Heart Health Project (Abrams & Elder, 1981; Elder et al, 1981) is another example of communitywide strategies for prevention. The goal of the program is to prevent cardiovascular disease by modifying life-style, thus lowering risk. Specific risk factors that are the focus of the program include: high blood pressure, smoking, high cholesterol diets, obesity, sedentary life-style, and high stress. The primary personnel delivering the program are volunteers who have been trained in behavior change techniques. Volunteers lead group programs and design strategies for achieving supportive changes at the organizational level within the community. The goal is a self-sustaining program that can run with minimal reliance on health professionals. Evaluation results from the program will be available in 1986.

Other communitywide interventions to reduce risk for cardiovascular disease include the Minnesota Heart Health Program (Blackburn et al, 1984) and the North Karelia Project in Finland (Puska et al, 1983). Early evaluation results of these programs indicate that community-based interventions can result in short-term changes in community health behavior.

While the community intervention trials thus far have been focused primarily on lowering risk for and incidence of cardiovascular disease, large-scale aggregate projects that focus on promoting health-enhancing life-styles in the community without a specific disease target are needed. Positively oriented community programs focused on enhancing the quality of life as well as extending longevity may have greater overall impact on the nation's health than more narrowly focused programs of disease prevention.

Types of Programs for the Promotion of Health

It is important that nurses be familiar with the various types of programs for the promotion of health. The typology of health promotion programs presented in Figure 13-1 provides the community health nurse with an overview of programming approaches that can be used singly or in combination. Proceeding clockwise from information dissemination to social-cultural support, the programs deal with increasingly larger aggregates and become more complex to develop and implement.

Information Dissemination

Health promotion programs focused on information dissemination represent the most fundamental type of programmatic approach to changing attitudes, beliefs, and behaviors. This approach makes extensive use of mass media, billboards, posters, brochures, health fairs, and health exhibits. The goal of such programs is to inform the citizenry about the components of a health-damaging life-style and ways of enhancing health and the quality of life.

Information dissemination raises the consciousness of individuals, families, and communities that a problem exists about which something should and can be done. Often the informational publicity about the problem or concern includes a motivational device to facilitate behavior change as well as suggesting how the target behavior is to be changed. Examples of information dissemination campaigns include smoking cessation posters and television announcements, brochures describing approaches to weight control, articles on physical fitness in the local newspaper, dental posters encouraging flossing or frequent brushing, and bumper stickers reading "Have you hugged your child today?"

Information dissemination programs build awareness and the knowledge base for use of further strategies to modify health habits and life-style. Seldom is information alone sufficient to significantly change behaviors on a large scale. Some individuals may make major changes in habits and life-style in response to information only, but these persons are probably the exception rather than the rule.

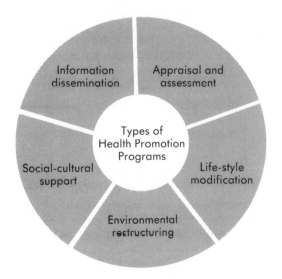

Figure 31-1 Types of health promotion programs.

Appraisal and Assessment

Appraisal and assessment programs are extremely popular as a motivational device to encourage persons to reduce risk factors for disease and adopt a healthier life-style. However, the nurse should be aware of the difference between appraising risk factors for a specific disease or diseases and assessing total life-style patterns.

Health Hazard Appraisal/Health Risk Appraisal (HHA/HRA) is a method for estimating individual risk for disease or death from a person's medical history, physical examination, physical fitness evaluation, and nutritional assessment. Risk of death from a particular illness is then estimated for the target individual using five- to ten-year probability tables of death from specific causes (LaDou, Sherwood, & Hughes, 1975).

The principle behind risk appraisal is that the health hazards of an individual can be quantified if his or her characteristics are known, based on the mortality experience of a large group of cohorts with similar characteristics. Individual data are matched to data banks of actuarial statistics from information gathered by the National Center for Health Statistics and insurance companies. The ultimate purpose of HHA/HRA is to provide individuals with a realistic evaluation of health threats to which they are particularly vulnerable prior to the development of signs and symptoms of disease.

Health Hazard Appraisal was formally introduced as an assessment and motivational tool by Robbins and Hall (1970) in their work on how to practice prospective medicine. Since that time, many risk appraisal tools have been developed. In 1981, the Public Health Service Office of Health Information, Health Promotion and Physical Fitness and Sports Medicine published *Health Risk Appraisal: An Inventory* (US Department of Health and Human Services, 1981) in which many of the HHA/HRA tools available at that time were described. S. M. Weiss (1984) presents a more recent overview of health hazard/risk appraisal tools.

Doerr and Hutchins (1981) and Goetz and McTyre (1981) present an excellent discussion of the psychometric properties of HHAs/HRAs—their limitations and need for further testing. Descriptive studies to determine the extent to which HHAs/HRAs motivate individuals to make short-term and long-term behavioral changes are critically needed. A major advantage of HHAs/HRAs is that they can be applied to large aggregates since some HHAs/HRAs are computer administered, many are computer scored, and most resultant risk profiles are computer generated. Group profiles of risk can be constructed for employees of a company or residents in a specific geographic location.

While it is generally assumed that awareness of level of risk for specific diseases is desirable, it borders on the unethical to apprise people of their risk level *without* providing supportive education to help people understand ways in which personal risk factors can be lowered. Some of the early HHA/HRA programs provided minimal feedback to the persons completing questionnaires other than probabilities of death within the next five or ten years from specific diseases and a brief list of suggestions for lowering risk. Community health nurses should be aware of their moral and professional responsibility to provide feedback to individuals or groups following appraisal, and supportive education to assist in lowering identified risk factors.

Life-style assessment and wellness inventories represent a positive approach to appraisal and assessment that is focused on enhancing wellness as opposed to identifying risk factors for specific diseases. Early pioneers in the field of life-style assessment include Dr. John Travis of Wellness Associates, Mill Valley, CA; Dr. William Hettler, Institute for Lifestyle Improvement, University of Wisconsin at Stevens Point; and Medical Datamation of Bellevue, OH.

A Health Habits and Lifestyle Assessment (HHLA) tool was developed by the author to be used by community health nurses with individual clients (Pender, 1982a). The instrument focuses on total life-style. In addition, a refined instrument, the *Health Promoting Lifestyle Profile* (HPLP) based on the HHLA has been developed and tested for reliability and validity on over 1,100 adults in communities in North Dakota and Illinois (Walker, Sechrist, & Pender, manuscript in preparation).

Doerr and Hutchins (1981) noted that HHAs/

HRAs appear to be more effective in motivating change with older rather than younger individuals. It is possible that since feelings of threat from chronic illness are minimal in younger individuals, the motivational impact is lost. Perhaps assessment tools that focus on positive aspects of life-style and "approach" rather than "avoidance" behaviors will be more effective than HHAs/HRAs in facilitating behavior change among young adults and children. Further research is needed to test this hypothesis.

Life-style Modification

Life-style modification strategies assist individuals and families to take responsibility for their own health and make appropriate changes in behavior that improve the quality of life and potentially extend longevity. This approach is more comprehensive than either of the two types of health promotion programs discussed thus far. Attempts at changing behavior are based on the acquisition of disseminated information and on appropriate appraisal and assessment. Life-style change programs generally require contact between the health professional and client over an extended period of time.

Life-style modification programs should be based on principles of social learning theory, operant conditioning, and/or cognitive psychology to maximize their probability of success. Rather than relying on the manipulation of their behavior by the health professional, individuals and families develop self-modification skills that allow them to select those behaviors they wish to change and implement self-change strategies that facilitate achievement of the goals that they have set. Factors to be considered when facilitating family changes in life-style include reasons for change, available knowledge and skills to initiate and sustain change, ratio of payoffs for present behavior versus payoffs for new behaviors, and the extent of social support for changed behavior within the social and physical environment (Kanfer & Karoly, 1972).

Discussion of the many strategies that individuals and families can use to promote positive change in life-styles is beyond the scope of this chapter.

However, the later section entitled "Developing a Family Health Promotion and Protection Plan," presents an overview of behavior change techniques appropriate for use by families in promoting healthier life-styles. Further discussion of behavior modification techniques is available in Martin and Poland (1980), Pender (1982a), and Pender (1985).

Environmental Restructuring

Restructuring the environment is an approach to health promotion that complements the previous three program types. The goals of environmental restructuring are to increase the availability of healthful options, optimize the quality of the proximal environment, and support health-promoting behaviors. The environments to be considered in health promotion include the physical, social, and economic environments of a community.

The major emphasis of environmental health programs to date has been on prevention as a reaction to the growing number of contaminants of human origin introduced into our environment within recent decades. Landrigan and Gross (1981) state that "there are already in our environment sufficient quantities of hazardous wastes to provide a legacy of disease and death to our descendants for generations to come" (p. 985). Such pollutants have contaminated our air, water, food, and land.

In a survey of 110 citizen action community organizations (Freudenberg, 1984), 153 potential dangers to environmental health were identified. The most common issues that these community action groups reported addressing were, in order of priority: (1) toxic dumps, (2) herbicide or pesticide spraying, (3) air pollution, (4) water pollution, (5) nuclear wastes, (6) nuclear power plants, and (7) mining. The major impetus for organization of the citizen groups was concern about people adversely affecting the quality of the environment and suspicion that health-damaging consequences would result.

Of the organizations studied, health fears dominated their concerns. Esthetic or economic concerns were rarely mentioned as important inducements to action. Suspected health problems were cancer, respiratory problems, birth defects, reproductive problems, and kidney-liver damage.

Press coverage of environmental health problems in communities such as Love Canal, Three Mile Island, and Times Beach has made the public increasingly aware of hazards to health posed by our industrial and technological society. New sources of pollution receiving attention are use of wood stoves and fireplaces in urban areas, use of diesel engines for transportation, and rise in carbon dioxide in the environment due to combustion of fossil fuels that can cause global temperatures to increase and ocean levels to rise.

Citizens in many communities have organized to preserve the rich resources within the environment. These organizations can become valuable allies for governmental agencies charged with environmental protection.

In addition to prevention, which has monopolized the attention of many citizen action groups during past years, health promotion through improvement of the esthetic, social, and economic dimensions of the environment is beginning to receive more attention. Health promotion concerns go beyond toxic waste, air pollution, and water pollution to considerations of the esthetics or attractiveness of the environment, mental health or social wellness of the population, and the quality of school and work environments.

Taylor (1984) views the environment as a health-strengthening field. He describes health promotion in the environment as designing surroundings to positively influence populations so that individuals and groups can maximize their potential. Taylor emphasizes the need for research in architectural psychology and related fields to determine the environmental variables that promote human motivation, creativity, and self-fulfillment. His premise is that environments should be adjusted to the needs of people rather than people having to adjust to undesirable or uncomfortable environments. For instance, creating buildings for visual release—that is, allowing long distance views of beauty—can relax eye muscles that are tense from hours of close work. Also, the positive psychological impact of sunlight should be optimized. Persons who must work in surroundings without win-

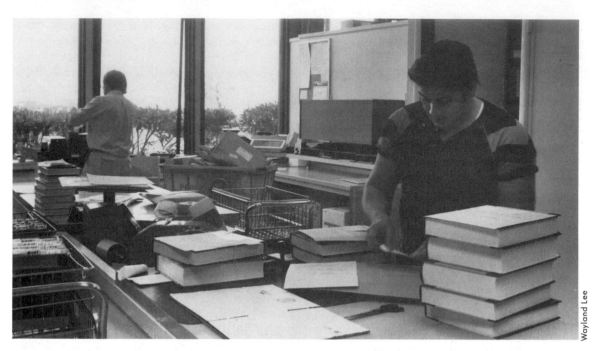

Wayland Lee

A workplace that provides ample sunlight, with the view, ventilation, and warmth windows provide, can ease stress and job-related tension.

dows or the visual or warming effects of sunlight may perform at less than their optimum. The esthetics of the environment can determine the level of tension under which people work and the extent to which they can actualize their creative powers and talents.

The social environment or the cohesiveness of aggregates is another critical aspect of a health-promoting environment. Assisting groups to develop social support systems that foster feelings of concern and belonging enhances the social climate in which group members live, work, and grow. Social support systems can establish health-promoting behaviors as the norm and can facilitate efforts of families and groups to sustain healthful life-styles.

The economic dimensions of the environment must also be considered. Health-promoting life-styles require a minimum level of economic security and comfort. High rates of unemployment have been shown to adversely affect the mental health status of families and populations. Establishing

effective mechanisms for ensuring that the economic needs of families and groups are met adequately is an important strategy for environmental health promotion.

Social-Cultural Support

An analysis of current American culture suggests that our society is more oriented to the heroics of reparative, "band-aid" medicine than to the less sensational but undoubtedly more effective health promotion services and self-care activities. Failure of insurance companies and Medicare and Medicaid to cover the cost of health promotion activities and services is diametrically opposed to the spirit and intent of the Surgeon General's 1979 report, *Healthy People.* Allocation of less than 1 percent of the national health budget for health promotion, in spite of the policy commitment, raises many questions about the power of vested interests in our society and the sincerity of the federal intent to make health promotion the backbone of the health care system.

While families and other aggregates can do much to enhance their own health, attention to policies in the wider social arena is critical to optimize the national environment for health promotion. Chin and Benne (1969) have described normative or reeducative strategies for change that take into account the social nature of human populations and their predisposition to be influenced by social mandates and social norms.

A recent Gallup poll (Harris & Gurin, 1985) found that 54 percent of the 1,019 adults surveyed reported exercising regularly. The quest for health is the primary reason that people gave for exercising. Even among nonexercisers the Gallup poll found that 35 percent of the persons interviewed in the telephone survey reported eating more fruits and vegetables than in the past. Many exercisers and nonexercisers have quit smoking, although the quit rate is higher among exercisers. In the group aged eighteen to twenty-nine, 66 percent reported aerobic workouts. Fifty-seven percent of the thirty to forty-nine-year-olds reported regular exercise while forty-one percent of persons over fifty exercise. These data suggest that the momentum for cultural and social support of health-promoting life-styles is occurring from the bottom up rather than from the top down just as Naisbitt (1982) predicted.

The public appears to be in the forefront of the health promotion revolution. Since federal, state, and local health promotion programming is implemented currently on a piecemeal basis, public pressure will need to be brought to bear to ensure an integrated approach. Lay initiatives and consumer pressure can influence policy formation, resulting in the adoption of laws and programs that support health-promoting life-styles.

Approaches to Intervention

Focus on the Family

The family is the primary social structure for health promotion within society. Within the context of the family health behaviors are learned and life-styles formed. Yet little attention has been given in previously published works to the critical role that families play in promoting healthful life-styles on the part of their members. In its commitment to the health of the total population, community health nursing has traditionally viewed the family as a major unit for intervention (Reutter, 1984). Focusing on the family as a small aggregate is important in order to see the interconnection, rather than the separateness, of family members. Health promotion within the family context presents community health nurses with the challenge of integrating principles of community health, behavioral health, family systems, and self-care theory as a basis for practice.

This section discusses such strategies as values clarification, building support systems, life-style review, and developing a family health promotion and protection plan. Prior to implementing any intervention strategy, however, assessment of the family from some theoretical perspective (see Chapter 2) is critical, and use of a particular family assessment guide (see Chapter 8) may be necessary. Assessment data related to the family's structure and function and interactional patterns provide the community health nurse and the family with valuable information on which to base health promotion interventions (Maurin, 1982).

Values Clarification Values clarification can increase a family's awareness of value priorities and the degree of consistency between values, attitudes, and behavior. Values clarification can result in reaffirming existing values, reprioritizing values, abandoning existing values, or acquiring new values (Pender, 1982b).

Values can be categorized into two types (Rokeach, 1973): (1) *terminal values* such as pleasure, self-respect, social recognition, health, and family security, which represent desired end-states of existence, and (2) *instrumental values* such as ambition, courage, responsibility, and self-control, which are desirable modes of conduct. A number of tools can be used by families to assess their value hierarchy. Such tools include the Rokeach Value Survey (Rokeach, 1973); the Survey of Interpersonal Values (Allport, Vernon, & Lindzey, 1960); and the Health Value Scale (Kaplan & Cowles, 1978). For instance, completion of the Rokeach Value Survey can be an interesting game for the entire family. The instrument has "sticky labels" that can be moved about in rank-order until the family is certain that they have identified the order of values that best represents family thinking. Even children can have fun moving the labels about and discussing what is most important to them. One word of caution about the Rokeach Value Survey: "health" is not in the set of terminal values. Thus, the nurse will have to add "health" on an identical sticker prior to administration of the instrument.

Congruent and conflicting values among family members can be identified by use of the Personal/Family Values exercise described by Pender (1982b). Families can examine how they express their values in everyday living by having the family as a unit complete the Values-Action Review (Pender, 1982b).

Many families will rank health high on their list of priorities, but there will be marked value and behavior discrepancies. These families need to be assisted in bringing their behaviors in line with their values, particularly in the area of health. In other families, a low value will be placed on health as a terminal goal. In these families the nurse should be sensitive to whether family members perceive health to be an *enabling factor*. That is, health is not valued as a goal in itself but is viewed as essential to the attainment of other desired goals. By individualizing health promotion strategies, the nurse can assist families with both value structures to achieve a healthier life-style.

The family value system provides directions or principles for action. Heightened awareness of values can assist families in systematically moving toward value-consistent behaviors. Careful analysis of values should not be overlooked as an integral part of the family health promotion process.

Building Interpersonal Relationships and Support Systems The family serves as a milieu for mutual nurturance, acquisition of appropriate communication patterns, and development of caring relationships. Family members' ability to relate to others outside the family and sustain meaningful, goal-directed relationships throughout their lifetime depends on the extent to which they have learned to function as a supportive and contributing family member. Social support can be defined as the subjective feeling of belonging or of being accepted, loved, esteemed, valued, and needed for oneself, not for what one can do for others. It also incorporates the idea of responding in kind to others (Moss, 1973).

Family members support and assist each other in many ways, such as the following (Tolsdorf, 1976, p. 408):

- *Tangible support*—money or active assistance
- *Intangible support*—encouragement, personal warmth, love, and emotional support
- *Advice*—information or guidance on how to achieve a certain goal or complete a particular task
- *Feedback*—provision of evaluative statements regarding how expectations or requirements for reaching goals are being met; provision of information on how well family members or the family as a unit is performing

The community health nurse can assist the family in strengthening its capacity as a social support system. Strategies that the nurse can help the family use for this purpose include (Pender, 1982b):

- Increasing frequency of contact among family members
- Committing to common life values
- Setting goals mutually to achieve common directions in actions and efforts
- Increasing frequency and/or intensity of expressions of encouragement, personal warmth, and love among family members
- Supporting of coping efforts in dealing with life experiences
- Enhancing self-esteem of family members
- Encouraging self-expression of family members
- Dealing constructively with conflict
- Encouraging growth, maturation, and self-actualization of family members and the family as a unit
- Promoting family identity and pride
- Encouraging use of extrafamilial support as a complement to intrafamilial support

With the importance of social support to the acquisition and maintenance of health-promoting behaviors in families, the community health nurse should place high priority on assisting families to augment their support functions. Efforts to change family health behavior are likely to be more successful than efforts to change individual health behavior in isolation, since natural social support mechanisms within the family system can be utilized.

Life-style Review *Life-style* can be defined as a way of life, mode of living, or constellation of behaviors that reflect the attitudes and values of a particular individual or group. Life-style patterns that tend to persist throughout life are developed within the family context. With a supportive family, however, it is just as easy to adopt patterns of living that are health promoting and pleasurable as to learn patterns that are health damaging.

Family life-style review is a means of exploring strengths of life-style that the family already exhibits. While a healthy life-style does not guarantee optimum well-being and freedom from illness, it does increase the probability of an illness-free and fulfilling existence.

Areas for life-style review include nutritional practices, physical and recreational activities, sleep and relaxation patterns, family sense of purpose, family relationships, and practices for actualizing family potential. These areas are best explored using interviewing techniques and open-ended questions. A short life-style review section is incorporated into the family health promotion and protection plan that appears in Figure 13-2.

Through systematic review of life-style, a family is able to identify the extent to which existing behavior patterns are supportive of family health and the health of individual family members. In families where few strengths are apparent, the family should be praised for those positive qualities that they exhibit. Even in the most disorganized families, the community health nurse can find strengths to reinforce.

Developing a Family Health Promotion and Protection Plan Following use of life-style review, the family has a great deal of information from which to make decisions about areas of behavior to strengthen or change. The community health nurse can assist the family in developing a health promotion and protection plan through which health goals can be identified and progress in behavior change monitored.

The family should prioritize those areas discussed in the life-style review that they wish to focus on in their efforts to change behavior. In some areas, the family may see their life-style as health enhancing and in need of little alteration. What the nurse must remember is that the family is in charge of making decisions about life-style change. The goal of health promotion planning is to help families assume responsibility for self-care and work out a life-style change program that meets their needs and is fun and rewarding.

An example of a health promotion goal that family members may wish to concentrate on as a group is increasing their level of physical activity. A family can plan exercise that involves all members. They may make a commitment to swim, play tennis, bike, or take a brisk walk together

Designed for (Family Name): _____
Family Form: _____
Family Members:

Name	Sex	Position in Family	Birth Date	Occupation (if employed)
_____	___	___	___	___
_____	___	___	___	___
_____	___	___	___	___

Home Address: _____
Home Telephone Number: _____
Cultural/Religious Orientation: _____
Type of Housing: _____
Major Formal Roles of Family Members: _____

Community Affiliations of Family: _____

Communication Patterns (Verbal and Nonverbal, including expression of caring/affection): _____

Family Decision-Making Patterns: _____

Family Values with Highest Rank:
1. _____
2. _____
3. _____
4. _____
5. _____
Rank-Order of Health as a Value (if not listed above):_
Value Conflicts in Family (if any): _____
Goals Important to Family: _____

Mutual goal or Specific to dyad (D) or triad (T)

Family strengths: _____
Major Sources of Stress for Family (if any) and Perceived Ability to Deal with Stressors: _____

Current or Recent Family Developmental or Situational Transitions: _____

Family Concerns or Challenges: _____

Family Self-Care Patterns
Current Health-Protecting or Preventive Behaviors (e.g., immunization, self-examination, periodic screening or examination by health professionals, avoidance of toxic exposure, use of seat belts)

Current Health-Promoting Behaviors (Life-style Review)
Nutritional Practices _____
Physical or Recreational Activities _____
Sleep or Relaxation Patterns _____
Stress Management _____
Family Sense of Purpose _____
Family Actualization Efforts _____
Relationships with Others _____
Environmental Control _____
Information-Seeking Patterns of Family in Relation to Health Promotion
Use of Health Promotion Facilities and Services by Family _____
Other Behaviors_____
Consistency Between Family Values, Goals, and Health Actions: _____

Family Health Goals

Goals	Family Priority (1 = Most Important)
_____	_____
_____	_____
_____	_____
_____	_____

Areas for Improvement in Family Health
Target Health Goal:

Specific Behavior Change	Area of Change (See Categories under Family Self-Care Patterns)	Family Priority (1 = Most Desirable)	Approaches Selected to Facilitate Family Change
___	___	___	___
___	___	___	___

Evaluation of Progress Toward Change in Family Life-style
Two weeks: _____
One month: _____
Three months: _____
Six months: _____
One year: _____

Figure 13-2 Format for a family health promotion protection plan.

two or three times a week. Such activity can improve physical fitness as well as enhance family relationships.

When joint activities are impossible, each family member should select an individualized activity that will contribute to the family goal of improved physical fitness. Families can keep a chart of the frequency of their activities from which they can determine the extent to which daily or weekly exercise goals are achieved. Family members can encourage each other and reinforce progress that they have made toward a more "active" life-style. Goal attainment can be rewarded by a trip to the theater or some other special family event. The approach to change just described is based on operant conditioning principles of learning in which reward or reinforcement for behavior plays a central role.

Change should be a slow process if the resultant behaviors are to be enduring and integrated as a permanent part of life-style. Families should set realistic goals and shape behavior over time. Too

rapid change is likely to lead to failure and abandonment of family change efforts. A suggested format for a family health promotion and protection plan appears in Figure 13-2.

Discussion of specific approaches that families can use to facilitate change is beyond the scope of this chapter. However, techniques such as associative learning, cognitive restructuring, counterconditioning, operant conditioning, self-confrontation, and stimulus control can be applied to aggregates. An overview of self-modification techniques appears in Table 13-3. For further information the reader is referred to references on self-initiated change (Bulechek & McCloskey, 1985; Martin & Poland, 1980; Pender, 1982a).

Wright and Leahey (1984, pp. 174–181) have summarized a number of concepts concerning change that the community health nurse should keep in mind when working with families:

- "Change is dependent upon context." The family must create a physical and social environment

Table 13-3   Behavior Change Strategies That Families Can Use To Modify Life-style

Strategy	Brief Description of Technique and Rationale
Associate learning	Through repeated pairing of the same context with a given behavior, the behavior becomes automatic, habitual, and an integrated part of life-style.
Cognitive restructuring	By changing the way an individual labels or evaluates a specific situation or event, the emotional reaction to the situation can be modified; positive rather than negative self-statements and self-evaluations can result.
Counter-conditioning	The aim of this approach is to break an undesirable bond between a stimulus and a maladaptive or health-damaging response and replace the bond with a more desirable or health-promoting one.
Operant conditioning	Through manipulation of outcomes or consequences, the frequency of a given behavior can be increased or decreased. New behaviors are gradually shaped by repetition and reinforcement.
Self-confrontation	Change results from the arousal of an affective state of dissatisfaction within the individual due to recognition of inconsistencies in personal values-beliefs-behavior system or between personal system and that of persons who are admired.
Stimulus control	By changing the antecedents of behavior—that is, the stimuli or events preceding behavior—it is possible to decrease or eliminate an undesirable behavior or increase the frequency of a desirable behavior. Target stimuli for change can be physical, social, or intrapersonal.

supportive of change. Attention to and manipulation of stimuli in the environment (stimulus control) can enhance the probability of successful change.

- "Change is dependent upon the perception of the problem." The family should discuss and clarify their understanding of any life-style problems that they identify as targets for change. Sharing perceptions assists all family members in arriving at a common world view as a basis for developing a health promoting family life-style.
- "Change is dependent on realistic goals." Setting short-term as well as long-term goals provides a series of realistic and achievable steps for families in their quest for permanent, health-promoting changes in life-style.
- "Understanding alone does not lead to change." Providing information to a family relevant to a problem will seldom result in resolution of the problem until the family develops skill with specific change strategies.
- "Change does not necessarily occur equally in all family members." Some family members may react more enthusiastically and energetically to change than others. The early adopters can provide motivation to other family members who are more reticent about making change.
- "Directing change is the nurse's responsibility." Part of the nurse's professional responsibility is to direct the course of change of families. This does not imply that the nurse should have preconceived ideas about how the family should change. It is more important that the family be satisfied with changes they have made in life-style than that the nurse be satisfied.
- "Change can be due to a myriad of causes." Change is affected by so many variables that it may be difficult to determine the exact causal chain for new behaviors. The nurse should credit the family for changes that they have made rather than personally taking credit for positive changes in behavior.

The readiness of the family to learn about health promotion from the community health nurse should be assessed prior to intervention. Questions to determine learning readiness include:

- Has a relationship been established by the nurse with the family?
- What experience has the family had with preventive and health-promoting behaviors?
- What knowledge and skills prerequisite to effective health-promoting behavior has the family already mastered?
- To what extent does the family view it as their responsibility to enhance the health of all family members?
- Does the family exhibit motivation to engage in learning and the life-style change process?
- Is development of a health promotion and protection plan viewed by the family as helpful and challenging?

The family that sets health goals and strives to attain them is fulfilling its function as a dynamic, evolving, and health-generating aggregate (Petze, 1984).

Focus on the Environment

This section discusses approaches for improving the environment, including such specific strategies as monitoring the quality of the environment, action groups, and participatory management.

Monitoring Activities   Monitoring the quality of the physical, interpersonal, and economic environment in which we live is everyone's business. On the other hand, it has been said that "what is everyone's business is no one's business." Organized monitoring activities are best carried out by interested aggregates. Groups established for monitoring purposes may also take action to enhance the quality of the environment.

The community health nurse should be aware of groups that have organized within the community to attend to environmental issues. These groups can be close allies of private and public health agencies concerned with environmental quality.

Freudenberg (1984) has described the formation process for environmental monitoring and action groups from a survey of 110 such groups in thirty-one states. The first stage of organization is information gathering. Survey respondents reported that the following activities were critical to their group becoming informed to deal knowledgeably with environmental issues: attending conferences or meetings dealing with environmental quality or specific toxic products, reading relevant government reports, meeting with activists from local or national environmental groups, consulting experts on specific topics, and following press coverage of environmental issues.

In the survey conducted by Freudenberg (1984), 88 percent of the groups reported that they had difficulty getting information about the particular environmental issues of concern. Almost half, 45 percent, reported that they perceived governmental agencies as obstructive rather than facilitative in their attempts to learn more about environmental health issues. All groups indicated that they eventually did obtain enough relevant information to monitor their own immediate environment and take organized action.

Lee (1984) described the formation of environmental interest groups in the work setting. He stressed the importance of educating employees regarding aspects of the work environment that pose immediate or future threats to health or that can enhance well-being. Important strategies for environmental change include:

- Worker training programs that enable knowledgeable employees to spot potential hazards and monitor safety of work procedures
- Worker training programs that focus on augmenting the esthetic and health-strengthening aspects of the environment
- Organized program for employee monitoring of work performance areas
- Inspection committees and environmental improvement committees with employee members

- Employee consultants to management on environmental issues

Lancaster and Brown (1984) also emphasized the importance of monitoring the quality of the psychosocial environment. For instance, the stress level of the work environment should be carefully evaluated. An environment in which workers are harrassed, verbally abused, and never recognized as contributors is a major threat to health and well-being. While persons are surprisingly resilient and can adapt to short periods of stress, repeated stressful experiences and conditions that create chronic stress are detrimental to physical and mental health. Work settings, where the majority of adults spend their lives, can provide social support and nurturance or cause stress. Work can be a major factor in self-actualization or a continuing threat to growth and self-esteem.

Astute employee-monitoring groups will identify work settings that are health damaging rather than health strengthening and plan action strategies that increase the interpersonal quality of the work environment. Monitoring the environment is the first step toward maintaining a health-enhancing milieu in community and organizational settings.

Action Groups Action groups have been particularly effective in dealing with environmental issues. Among their strategies are obtaining media coverage or publicity about environmental issues; distributing educational materials to inform the community of possible environmental options; speaking at community meetings; lobbying city councils, county boards, state agencies, and/or federal agencies; taking legal action; and engaging in civil disobedience.

Group spokespersons interviewed in the Freudenberg (1984) study indicated that they found obtaining media coverage, distributing educational materials, and speaking at community meetings the most effective actions for mobilizing citizens and creating pressure for action. Of those interviewed, 37 percent of the citizen action groups judged themselves to be very successful in achieving their goals; 50 percent reported elimination of the problem that was causing concern; and 35 percent reported increased community awareness concerning the environmental issue.

Discussing action strategies for maintaining a hazard-free work environment, Lee (1984) identified the following components of an effective group effort to minimize environmental threats to health:

- Require clear labeling of all industrial and office supplies as to their contents and posting of warnings concerning operation of equipment or office machines
- Promote aggressive policies that enforce compliance and sanction negligent employers and employees
- Identify alert clinicians who carefully consider environmental sources of distress and disease in their diagnostic work
- Cultivate working relationships with public health officials who take steps to monitor and enforce environmental policies that are health enhancing
- Encourage hiring of health professionals and managers who are sensitive to safe toxic exposure levels, appropriate lighting conditions, and esthetic dimensions of the environment

The community health nurse should encourage formation of citizen action groups to safeguard the environment and maximize its health-enhancing properties.

Participatory Management A positive way to deal with environmental problems, in work, school, or community settings is through participatory management. This is an administrative approach used by corporations or agencies to gain input from employees or citizens into managerial decision making. Participatory management is proactive, rather than reactive like many action groups.

Howlett and Archer (1984) discuss some of the advantages of including employee or community representatives in groups that make management decisions:

- Increased information (from differing perspectives) on which to base institutional or agency planning and decision making regarding environmental concerns
- Enhanced employer-employee communication concerning the environmental milieu
- Augmented problem-solving potential
- Increased worker or citizen health and safety
- Expanded opportunities for cooperation and collaboration among employers and employees or officials and citizens in moving toward mutually defined environmental goals

In participatory management, concerned individuals and administrators collaborate as a team to address environmental issues.

Focus on the Community

This section focuses on implementation strategies for health promotion in the community at-large. Archer, Kelly, and Bisch (1984) described the community planning process as "a collaborative, orderly, and cyclic process to attain a mutually agreed on desired future or goal" (pp. 21–22). Thus, successful community strategies for change must be characterized by collaboration, orderliness, and clearly identified goals. The community change process includes assessment of needs, and development, implementation, and evaluation of change programs.

Community Assessment Focused on Health Promotion A community assessment or analysis of health promotion concerns, practices, facilities, and resources is essential prior to identifying needed changes. Data that should be obtained include level and types of physical activity characteristic of all age groups, nutritional practices, sources of stress within the population, extent to which recreational and cultural facilities are utilized, continuing educational resources available, patterns of interaction among families within the community, patterns of interorganizational networking, and utilization of health services for cure, illness prevention, and health promotion. Schultz (1982) has identified four areas that need to be carefully assessed prior to implementing change in the community:

1. Community characteristics
2. Health status of community residents
3. Patterns of interorganizational relationships
4. Characteristics of provider organizations

Data sources for obtaining this information should include community residents of all ages, lay community health leaders, key informants from organizations that provide health or health-related services, leaders in industry and education, and personnel in local government. See Chapter 9 for more discussions of approaches for obtaining information in community assessment.

West (1984) identified the goal of community health nursing as high-level wellness for the population as a whole. She presented a community health assessment tool based on Maslow's hierarchy of needs (physiologic, safety, love, esteem and self-actualization) and a framework of unitary man. The assessment focuses on the quality of community-environment interaction. The purpose of community assessment according to West is to identify positive community attributes supportive of health. Community analysis promotes an understanding of people, the environment in which they live, and patterns of population-environment interaction.

Following assessment, a community profile can be developed to reflect prevalence of healthful lifestyles, available health promotion resources, and their level of use. Based on the needs identified, the community health nurse and community residents can establish long-term and short-term goals for increasing healthful life-styles and enhancing the health-strengthening characteristics of the environment.

Developing Communitywide Health Promotion Programs Almost all community-based intervention models tested and reported in the literature have focused on reducing risk factors for cardiovascular disease, cancer, or some other threatening ailment. The reader is referred to the section earlier in this chapter "Types of Programs for the Promotion of Health," for a brief review of some of these communitywide programs. Even health education programs conducted to enhance knowledge and change attitudes of school children have focused primarily on the reduction of risk factors for disease (Eng et al, 1979; Williams, Carter, & Eng, 1980).

Despite the disease focus of current community intervention efforts, much can be learned from these programs about implementation strategies. The following guidelines for implementing communitywide health promotion programs emerged from careful analysis of the experimental risk-reduction programs conducted to date:

- Use a population-based approach involving as many small groups, organizations, interorganizational networks and communitywide structures as possible.
- Obtain official endorsement of program from governmental agencies (mayor's office, city council, governor's office, local and state health departments).
- Base program on an aggregate or population theoretical framework.
- Focus on intensive community action with a trained and well-organized health service structure as backup.
- Ensure that the program has legitimacy by involving respected community leaders and reputable health professionals.
- Plan the time sequence of program components so that adequate time is allowed for each program phase and the overall time frame is manageable.
- Throughout the program, develop a sense of community ownership and control of the program.
- Enlist community volunteers as change agents to promote participant modeling.
- Incorporate strategies to promote both acquisition and maintenance of healthful life-styles.
- Attend to ethnic and sociocultural aspects of the community in designing the program and in tailoring health promotion strategies to subpopulations.

• Develop means for monitoring and evaluating the success of the program and for providing feedback to participating populations concerning progress in reaching program goals.

In the North Karelia (Finland) Project (Puska et al, 1983), which focused on the prevention of cardiovascular disease, strategies for promoting communitywide life-style changes included: (1) information dissemination through media; (2) persuasion techniques based on local pride, sense of contribution, and credibility image of project directors and supporting organizations; (3) training of persons in the skills needed to successfully accomplish behavior change; (4) use of natural social units such as families and small groups to accomplish and support change; (5) promotion of environmental change such as increased availability of low-fat products and fresh vegetables; and (6) establishment and maintenance of relationships with organizations and community leaders. These approaches proved to be effective in lowering the level of risk factors for cardiovascular disease among residents of North Karelia, Finland.

In Belgium, a large-scale study has been designed to investigate relationships between smoking, dietary behavior, and cancer and between the same behaviors and cardiovascular diseases (Kittel, 1984). The objectives of the health education program, which is part of the study, is to modify existing risk factors in the adult population and prevent or modify their development in adolescents. The program will involve a variety of health professionals and health-related associations. Components of the program include:

• Health education and disease prevention programs in industrial settings
• Health education and disease prevention programs oriented toward youth
• A health education program for the primary schools (ages five to twelve)
• A health education program for the general population oriented toward control of hypertension

Anticipated changes in behavior include decrease in total and saturated fats, prevention of smoking in youth, prevention or reduction in obesity, reduction of hypertension, and promotion of physical activity during leisure, work, and schooltime. The health education program will be promoted through mass media, posters, teaching materials, conferences, action projects, and face-to-face counseling. Begun in 1984, this education effort will last three years.

Another program with which the community health nurse should be familiar is the Stanford Five City Project (FCP) described by Farquhar et al (1984). Because the goals of the project were described earlier, only implementation strategies will be discussed here.

The strategies for the Five City Project are built on what the community-based intervention study team learned from the Three Community Study. The goal of the project is to lower morbidity and mortality from heart disease within the experimental cities through:

presenting a single lifestyle that is most likely to be healthy. It involves being vigorous, active, and self-confident, eating a wide variety of enjoyable foods, and not smoking. It is this basically healthy and happy image that binds together the various elements of the intervention and makes the educational programs and materials coherent and, to an extent, indivisible (Farquhar et al, 1984, 1157).

Within the FCP, a communication-behavior change conceptual framework will be used. Components of this framework are:

• Gaining the attention of the public and increasing their awareness of the problem
• Increasing the knowledge of the public about the problem
• Increasing motivation for change by providing incentives
• Providing training in skills necessary for change as a means of increasing perceived self-efficacy and developing self-management skills

- Providing cues in the environment to trigger action
- Developing an environment of social support for risk-lowering behaviors

Principles of social marketing will also be employed. Kotler (1982) identifies four aspects of social marketing to be taken into consideration: providing the right *product* backed by the right *promotion* in the right *place* at the right *price*.

In the FCP, community organizations and organizational networks are considered critical components in the initial success and durability of the program. Organizations are viewed as augmenting the effects of mass media, enhancing interpersonal influence, expanding the delivery system for educational programs, and creating a sense of community ownership for programs (Farquhar et al, 1984).

Healthstyles (Black & McDowell, 1984) is a four-year demonstration project located in Ottawa, Canada, and funded by the W. K. Kellogg Foundation. The overall objective of this unique adult health promotion program is to promote the abandonment of unhealthy habits and the adoption of health-enhancing behaviors through intensive workshops and an eighteen-month follow-up support program. In Healthstyles, specific disease agents and processes are not singled out and targeted for intervention. Instead the goal is to move people toward optimum wellness and health-promoting life-styles.

Healthstyles Basics (O'Hagan, 1984) is a two-and-a-half-day workshop that offers adults the opportunity to assess the impact of their present life-style on personal health. During the workshop, participants become aware of specific methods they can use to improve personal health. Workshops are offered on weekends for fifteen to twenty people.

The primary goal of the workshops is to assist adults in beginning the process of adopting healthy habits that will last a lifetime. The Healthstyles program focuses on four areas: nutrition, physical activity, stress management, and habits. Emphasis is placed on behavior change as central to one's purpose and meaning in life. The program also points out the need for self-responsibility in adopting and maintaining a health-promoting life-style.

The model used by Healthstyles to begin and maintain the process of change consists of the three A's—awareness, acceptance, and adjustment. Participants must be *aware* that change is needed, develop and *accept* a plan for change, and *adjust* to the demands that the life-style change requires.

Following the weekend workshops, the Healthstyles Support program (Kort, 1984) begins to provide continuing encouragement to participants working toward specific health goals. Five kinds of assistance are provided: (1) telephone support calls; (2) follow-up group sessions to facilitate peer support and exchange of ideas; (3) bimonthly health awareness sessions focused on a broad array of health topics; (4) dissemination of health information through books, articles, etc.; and (5) individual counseling sessions.

The 660 individuals participating in the program will be compared with 1320 matched controls to determine if there are differences between the groups in food choices; physical activity; stress management methods; use of tobacco, alcohol, and drugs; weight control; attitudes toward health, and exercise of self-responsibility for health. Study results will be available in 1987.

Community health nurses are in an ideal position to provide leadership in the design, development, implementation, and evaluation of health promotion programs in their own communities. Financial support for implementation and evaluation of such programs should be sought from public and private sources.

Focus on Society

Implementation strategies at the societal level focus on development of policy. Williams (1983) proposed policy formulation as one of the most crucial practice domains of community health nursing, since policy is a primary modality for influencing the health of defined populations. Population-based nursing, according to Williams, is the primary focus of community health nursing.

Health care policies in the United States are in a state of flux. Health care in our nation is intimately involved with the political process. It is the nation's politicians, and indirectly their constituents, who set health care priorities (DeLeon & Vandenbos, 1984). The federal government pays 40 percent of the nation's health bill. Thus, health policy initiatives frequently emanate from the federal level. National health policy affects health institutions, health professionals, and the public at-large.

Development of effective health policy requires assessment of health and health-related population data as a basis for informed decision making. With the technological capabilities of high-speed computers, maintaining population level data sets is becoming increasingly feasible. Not only can initial data analyses answer important questions, but secondary analyses from differing perspectives can enlighten public and private health policy. Knowing how to address meaningful questions with policy implications through secondary analyses is a critical skill for the population-focused health practitioner.

Due to decades of preoccupation with diagnosis and treatment of disease, as opposed to illness prevention and health promotion, current health policies at federal and local levels are generally illness policies. New policies are needed to implement the health mandates set forth in the Surgeon General's report, *Healthy People,* and the companion document, *Promoting Health/Preventing Disease: Objectives for the Nation.*

To put evolving health policy within the United States in appropriate historical perspective, it should be noted that Canada preceded the United States by five years in focusing on the importance of health promotion in public policy. In 1974, Marc Lalonde (1974) issued a landmark document, *New Perspective on the Health of Canadians,* that already is a classic in health policy. In the report, Lalonde pledged national attention to the environment, lifestyle, and human biology as well as to traditional health care delivery.

An Epidemiological Model for Health Policy
Dever (1980a) proposed an epidemiological model for health policy that focuses on the following elements: life-style, environment, human biology, and the system of medical care organization. He contends that this model provides a more balanced approach to policy analysis and formation than the traditional model of diagnosis, therapy, and rehabilitation, or the alternative model of public health, mental health, and clinical medicine. Dever (1980a, pp. 29–30) notes that the advantages of his model include:

- The model raises life-style, environment, and human biology to a level of categorical importance equal to that of the system of medical care organization.
- The model is comprehensive. The etiology of any health problem can be traced to one or more of the four elements.
- The model allows a system of analysis by which a disease may be examined in relationship to the four elements in order to assess their relative significance and interaction (what percent each element contributes to causation).
- The model permits further subdivision of the four major elements (e.g., life-style into leisure activity risks, consumption patterns, and employment or occupational risks; environment into the physical, social, and psychological dimensions).
- The model provides a new perspective on health that creates a recognition and exploration of previously neglected fields.

While this model is still disease-oriented, rather than illness-oriented, the position taken by Dever is a progressive one within the medical community. Application of the model would involve four steps: (1) the selection of diseases that are high risk and that contribute substantially to overall morbidity and mortality, (2) the proportionate allocation of the contributing factors of the disease to the four elements of the epidemiological model, (3) the proportionate allocation of total health expenditures to the four elements of the epidemiological model, and (4) the determination of the difference between (2) and (3). This approach to health policy would do much to redistribute the heavily concentrated expenditures on systems of medical care.

Strategies for Influencing Policy   Planning at the policy level is system changing and future creating. Systems are changed and created through policy in a variety of ways. Storfjell and Cruise (1984) conducted a survey of 166 administrators and staff nurses in community health agencies. They identified the following strategies for affecting policy:

- Testify regarding identified community health needs before policy- and law-making bodies.
- Lobby decision makers regarding health issues.
- Attend city or county board meetings and other legislative sessions to voice your perspectives and opinions.
- Use the media to educate the public regarding health concerns so that consumers can become allies for desirable policy change.
- Participate in interorganizational networks to achieve mutual policy goals that promote the public good.

Additional strategies include:

- Run for local, state, or federal public office.
- Develop positive working relationships with legislators, public health administrators, and leaders within the executive branch of government.
- Contribute to the development of policy positions within the agency in which you work.
- Seek appointment to health and health-related boards and commissions that will influence current and future health policy.
- Work with consumer groups to increase their impact on policy issues.
- Clearly articulate the policy positions of your employing agency to community organizations, the public, and mass media.
- Articulate to the media the level of public interest in health promotion (billions of dollars are spent each year on health foods, exercise equipment and facilities, vitamins, and recreational opportunities).
- Write about health policy issues in the popular press emphasizing health promotion perspectives.

DeLeon and Vandenbos (1984) report that few (1 percent) of the nation's politicians have any background in health care, yet they are the persons who ultimately make health care decisions. In the Ninety-seventh Congress (1980–1982) 45 percent of the 435 members of the House of Representatives had a background in law, while 59 percent of the Senate members were lawyers. Health staff for members of Congress have a surprisingly high turnover rate of approximately 90 percent every five years.

There is a critical need for persons knowledgeable in the area of health to fill elected offices. Many community health nurses have skills that would qualify them for such positions: appreciation of population issues, grassroots experience with the political system, good interpersonal skills, background in delivery of health care, orientation toward health promotion and illness prevention, and experience with persons of differing ethnic and sociocultural backgrounds. Case Example 13-3 illustrates the role of the community health nurse in initiating policy formation supportive of health promotion.

Because health policy formation creates a future for the public, and nursing as a profession has a commitment to create the healthiest future possible, community health nurses must play a key role in the development of health policy at the local, state, and national levels.

Case Example 13-3: Health Promotion in Society

Jim T. is a community health nurse who recently completed his baccalaureate degree and is now enrolled in a masters program focused on population-based nursing. He has become increasingly concerned about the lack of payment by third-party payors for health promotion services such as health education, life-style assessment, and life-style modification. Being aware of the importance of organizational systems in health promotion at the societal level, Jim has decided to work with the local health department and hospital in preparing a presentation on the benefits and potential cost savings from health promotion programs. He plans to present this information to a local insurance company that provides health insurance for several corporations and organizations in the area. Jim is preparing a flip chart for his marketing effort, in which he takes into consideration *product, promotion, place,* and *price* considerations for health promotion services. He wants to encourage the insurance company to pay for selected health promotion services on a trial basis. He knows that important information for his presentation can be gleaned from constructing statistical profiles from epidemiological studies of health practices among the population that is the focus for concern.

Jim just completed a course on policy formation and realizes that administrative personnel are often the primary persons responsible for policy initiatives. Therefore, he will gear his presentation to the chief executive officer and the vice presidents of the insurance company. Policy change, even on a trial basis, will be a major step forward in moving toward policy support of health-promoting services and life-styles.

Populations as critical domain for intervention by community health nurses

Organizational and interorganizational systems as the targets for change at the societal level

Use of social marketing principles

Use of secondary analysis as a source of data

Administrative initiatives in formation of policy

Goal of building support for health promotion

Issues in Health Promotion

Many health care issues face our nation in the decades ahead. The *major question* is whether health promotion, rather than treatment of disease, will indeed become the pivotal point around which health care is organized. Will a second public health revolution occur, as predicted by Michael (1982)? The potential for change exists. Long-standing health policy is being questioned. The climate is ripe for change. On the other hand, many vested interests resist change. Care in illness has been a lucrative business. Those health professionals who can best provide health promotion services are not necessarily those who are best at providing illness services.

Five major issues that will need to be addressed by decision makers in the area of health promotion will be described briefly in this section. The first issue concerns the appropriate mix of self-care and professional care for optimum and cost-effective health promotion. Related questions include: What can the public do for themselves? How much professional guidance will be needed to help the public initiate and maintain health-promoting self-care practices? Which health professionals will deliver and be reimbursed for health promotion services?

A second issue is the appropriate mix between health promotion strategies focused on the individual, the family, the community, and society as a whole. Economy of scale for health promotion interventions will be extremely important in the coming decades. Individual, aggregate, and population approaches will need to be mixed appropriately to provide quality services at acceptable cost.

Another pressing issue in health promotion is deciding who will bear the expense of health promotion services—private or public third-party payors. Unfortunately, at this point, public third-party payors appear to view health promotion as an additional expense to an already overburdened health budget. This view seems shortsighted, since paying for health promotion services now will likely diminish the amount of money paid out for illness care and disability in future years. Some private payors are experimenting with reimbursement for various health promotion services. Development of payment mechanisms and incentives for health promotion is an important area for policy formation.

A fourth issue is deciding on realistic expectations for short-term and long-term gains from family and community involvement in health promotion activities and health-promoting life-styles. Consensus conferences on current knowledge about the impact of various health practices or constellation of practices on health status should be organized. Consensus conferences held under the auspices of the National Institutes of Health would assist scientists in assessing the "state of the art" in health promotion and in identifying areas for further investigation.

A final issue is whether interdisciplinary or physician-centered care will characterize a health system focused primarily on health promotion. It is apparent that some reorganization in health care delivery systems is necessary and desirable. The nation cannot implement new health priorities with outdated delivery mechanisms.

Community health nurses must be informed about the issues surrounding health promotion and the delivery of health promotive services. Thoughtful dialogue with nurse colleagues, consumers, and other health professionals will sharpen the analytical and decision-making abilities of community health nurses, allowing them to address policy issues in an informed and articulate manner.

Summary

The shift to health promotion as a national priority presents many challenges to community health nurses. The foremost challenge is to increase the competency of community nurses in aggregate- and population-based assessment and intervention strategies. In addition, nurse scientists need to design and conduct studies of the impact of health promotion interventions on selected populations. Still another challenge for community health nurses is to increase their participation in the health policy arena. Through exercising leadership in the area of health promotion, community nurses can create a better future for the populations they serve.

Topics for Nursing Research

• What are the fundamental behavioral mechanisms underlying healthy functioning in families?
• What factors explain or predict the extent to which families engage in health-promoting life-styles?
• How can families serve as support systems for life-style change?
• How is health status measured in communities and populations?
• What community-based health promotion strategies are effective and economical?
• What are the patterns of health beliefs and health-promoting behaviors among groups with varying cultural and ethnic orientations?
• What social policies are supportive of healthy life patterns?

Study Questions

1. Approximately what percent of the total national health budget is currently spent on health promotion initiatives and programs?
   a. More than 95%
   b. 50%
   c. 15%
   d. Less than 1%
2. Which of the following programs represent an economic incentive for health-promoting life-styles?
   a. Availability of "leave days" for illness
   b. Early retirement programs
   c. Reduced insurance rates for persons who exercise regularly
   d. Comprehensive hospital care benefits
3. What type of health promotion program increases the availability of healthful options to families?
   a. Information dissemination
   b. Life-style modification
   c. Environmental restructuring
   d. Social-cultural support enhancement
4. What is the *primary* purpose for engaging in health-promoting interventions with families?
   a. Decrease the occurrence of disease
   b. Maximize the growth potential of the family
   c. Modify existing family structure
   d. Promote rehabilitation following illness
5. Data sources useful in the community assessment process include:
   a. Key informants
   b. Community residents
   c. Personnel in local government
   d. All of the above
6. The Stanford Five City Project is an example of a:
   a. Community rehabilitation project
   b. Policy formation initiative
   c. Community-based intervention trial
   d. Family-focused clinical trial
7. The major focus of community-based studies conducted to date has been:
   a. Risk reduction for specific diseases
   b. Health promotion for populations of all ages
   c. Early detection of chronic health problems
   d. Curative therapy for stress-induced diseases
8. An important strategy for answering questions relevant to population-based nursing is:
   a. Primary data collection
   b. Analysis of individual medical records
   c. Review of census collection procedures
   d. Secondary analysis of aggregate data
9. Which of the following is an important issue in the area of health promotion:
   a. Value of health promotion
   b. Mix of self-care and professional care for health promotion
   c. Right of families to health promotive care
   d. Compatibility of health promotion with illness prevention
10. The most important strategy for health promotion at the societal level is:
    a. Formation of policy
    b. Analysis of existing health legislation
    c. Enforcement of regulatory standards
    d. Evaluation of bureaucratic organizational structures

References

Abrams D, Elder J: Pawtucket Heart Health Program general theoretical model. *PHHP Technical Report.*

Pawtucket, R.I.: Pawtucket Heart Health Project, 1981.

Allport GW, Vernon PE, Lindzey G: *Study of Values,* 3rd ed. Boston: Houghton Mifflin, 1960.

Archer SE: Synthesis of public health science and nursing science. *Nurs Outlook* 1982; 30 (8): 442–446.

Archer SE, Kelly CD, Bisch SA: *Implementing Change in Communities: A Collaborative Process.* St. Louis: Mosby, 1984.

Ardell D: And what's in it for hospitals? *Promoting Health* 1980; 1: 4–6.

Bartlett EE: The contribution of school health education to community health promotion: What can we reasonably expect? *Am J Public Health* 1981; 71 (12): 1384–1391.

Behrens·R et al: Past year saw large increase in number of hospital programs. *Hospitals* 1981; 55: 105–108.

Bennis WG et al (editors): *The Planning of Change,* 3rd ed. New York: Holt, Rinehart & Winston, 1976.

Bermosk LS, Porter SE: *Women's Health and Human Wholeness.* New York: Appleton-Century-Crofts, 1979, p. 11.

Black A, McDowell I: Healthstyles: Moving beyond disease prevention. *Canadian Nurse* 1984; 80(4): 18–20.

Blackburn H et al: The Minnesota Heart Health Program: A research and demonstration project in cardiovascular disease prevention. In: Matarazzo J D et al (editors), *Behavioral Health: A Handbook of Health Enhancement and Disease Prevention.* New York: Wiley, 1984, pp. 1171–1178.

Bulechek GM, McCloskey JC: *Nursing Interventions: Treatments for Nursing Diagnoses.* Philadelphia: Saunders, 1985.

Brubaker BH: Health promotion: A linguistic analysis. *Adv Nurs Sci* 1983; 5 (3): 1–14.

Chinn R, Benne K: General strategies for effecting change in human systems. In: Bennis W, Benne K, & Chinn R (editors), *The Planning of Change,* 2nd ed. New York: Holt, Rinehart and Winston, 1969.

Cotanch PH: Health promotion in hospitals. In: Matarazzo JD et al (editors), *Behavioral Health: A Handbook of Health Enhancement and Disease Prevention.* New York: Wiley, 1984, pp. 1125–1136.

DeLeon PH, Vandenbos GR: Public health policy and behavioral health. In: Matarazzo JD et al (editors), *Behavioral Health: A Handbook of Health Enhancement and Disease Prevention.* New York: Wiley, 1984, pp. 150–163.

Dever GEA: Holistic health: An epidemiological model for policy analysis. In: *Community Health Analysis.* Germantown, Md.: Aspen, 1980a, pp. 25–40.

Dever GEA: Planning and evaluation for health. In: *Community Health Analysis.* Germantown, Md.: Aspen, 1980b, pp. 41–71.

Dishman RK: Compliance/adherence in health-related exercise. *Health Psychology* 1982; 1: 237–267.

Doerr BT, Hutchins EB: Health risk appraisal: Process, problems and prospects for nursing practice and research. *Nurs Res* 1981; 30(5): 299–306.

Duffy ME: Transcending options: Creating a milieu for practicing high level wellness. *Health Care for Women International* 1984; 5(1/3): 145–161.

Dunn HL: *High-level Wellness.* Thorofare, N.J.: Charles B. Slack, 1980.

Dunn HL: What high-level wellness means. *Can J Public Health* 1959; 50: 447–457.

Duvall EM: *Marriage and Family Development,* 5th ed. Philadelphia: Lippincott, 1977.

Elder JP et al: Social skills and health protective behaviors: Generating interpersonal support for risk factor reduction. Paper presented at the annual convention of the Association for Advancement of Behavior Therapy, Toronto, 1981.

Eng A et al: Increasing students' knowledge of cancer and cardiovascular disease prevention through a risk factor education program. *J Sch Health* 1979; 49: 505–507.

Farquhar JW et al: The Stanford Five City Project: An Overview. In: Matarazzo J D et al (editors), *Behavioral Health: A Handbook of Health Enhancement and Disease Prevention.* New York: Wiley, 1984, pp. 1137–1139.

Freudenberg N: Citizen action for environmental health: Report on a survey of community organizations. *Am J Public Health* 1984; 74(5): 444–448.

Friedman MM: *Family Nursing: Theory and Assessment.* New York: Appleton·Century·Crofts, 1981.

Goetz AA, McTyre RB: Health risk appraisal: Some methodology considerations. *Nurs Res* 1981; 30(5): 307–313.

Gray HJ: The role of business in health promotion: A brief overview. *Prev Med* 1983; 12: 654–657.

Green LW: Health education models. In: Matarazzo JD, et al (editors): *Behavioral Health: A Handbook of Health Enhancement and Disease Prevention.* New York: Wiley, 1984a, pp. 181–198.

Green LW: Health promotion and research development. *Ala J Med Sci* 1984b; 21(2): 217–219.

Hadley BJ: Current concepts of wellness and illness: Their relevance for nursing. *Image* 1974; 6: 24.

Hanchett E: *Community Health Assessment.* New York: Wiley, 1979, p. 162.

Harris DM, Guten S: Health-protective behavior: An exploratory study. *J Health Soc Behav* 1979; 20 (1): 17–29.

Harris L et al: *Health Maintenance: A Survey Conducted for Pacific Mutual Life Insurance Company.* New York: Pacific Mutual Life Insurance Co., 1978.

Harris PR: *Health United States 1980: With Prevention Profile.* DHHS Publication No. (PHS) 81-1232. Washington, D.C.: U.S. Government Printing Office, 1981.

Harris TG, Gurin J: New eighties lifestyle: Look who's getting it all together. *American Health* (March) 1985; 42–46.

Healthy People: The Surgeon General's Report on Health Promotion and Disease Prevention, U.S. Department of Health, Education, and Welfare Publication No. (PHS) 79-55071, U.S. Public Health Service, 1979.

Hopp JW: Health education program for parents and children who exhibit high risk factors of coronary heart disease. Presented at the annual meeting of the American Alliance for Health, Physical Recreation and Education, Kansas City, 1978.

Howlett M, Archer V: Worker involvement in occupational health and safety. *Family and Community Health* 1984; 7(3): 57–63.

Kaufer FH, Karoly P: Self control: A behavioral excursion into the lion's den. *Behavior Therapy* 1972; 3: 398–416.

Kaplan GW, Cowles A: Health locus of control and health value in the prediction of smoking reduction. *Health Education Monographs* 1978; 6: 129–137.

Kasl SV, Cobb S: Health behavior, illness behavior and sick role behavior. *Arch Environ Health* 1966; 12 (2): 246–266.

Kazdin AE: *Behavior Modification in Applied Settings*, 2nd ed. Homewood, Ill.: Dorsey Press, 1980.

King IM: *Toward a Theory of Nursing*. New York: Wiley, 1971, p. 24.

Kittel F: The interuniversity study on nutrition and health. In: Matarazzo JD et al (editors), Behavioral Health: A Handbook of Health Enhancement and Disease Prevention. New York: Wiley, 1984, pp. 1148–1153.

Kolbe L: What can we expect from school health education? *J Sch Health* 1982; 52 (3): 145–150.

Kolbe LJ, Iverson DC: Comprehensive school health education programs. In: Matarazzo JD et al (editors), *Behavioral Health: A Handbook of Health Enhancement and Disease Prevention*. New York: Wiley, 1984, pp. 1094–1116.

Kort M: Support: An important component of health promotion. *Canadian Nurse* (April) 1984; 80(4): 24–26.

Kotler P: Social marketing. In: Kotler P (editor), *Marketing for Non-Profit Organizations*, 2nd ed. Englewood Cliffs, N.J.: Prentice-Hall, 1982.

Kotler P, Zaltman G: Social marketing: An approach to planned change. In: Lazer W, Kelley E J (editors), *Social Marketing Perspectives and Viewpoints*. Homewood, Ill.: Richard D. Irwin, 1973.

LaDou J, Sherwood JN, Hughes L: Health hazard appraisal in patient counseling (preventive medicine). *West J Med* 1975; 122: 177–180.

Laffrey S: Health behavior choice as related to self-actualization, body weight, and health conception.

Dissertation Abstracts International, 43, 3536B (University Microfilms No. 83-06904), 1982.

Lalonde MA: *A New Perspective on the Health of Canadians: A Working Document*. Ottawa: Government of Canada, 1974.

Lancaster J, Brown V: Environmental and occupational health and safety. In: Stanhope M, Lancaster J (editors), Community Health Nursing: Process and Practice for Promoting Health. St Louis: Mosby, 1984, pp. 285–315.

Lancaster W, McIlwain T, Lancaster J: Health marketing: Implications for health promotion. *Family and Community Health* 1983; 5 (4): 41–51.

Landrigan PJ, Gross RL: Chemical wastes: Illegal hazards and legal remedies. *Am J Public Health* 1981; 71: 985–987.

Lee JS: Cadmium, mercury and lead: the heavy metal gang. *Family and Community Health* 1984; 7(3): 8–14.

Martin RA, Poland EY: *Learning to Change: A Self-Management Approach to Adjustment*. New York: McGraw-Hill, 1980.

Maurin J: Family structure model. In: Clement IW, Buchanan DM (editors), *Family Therapy: A Nursing Perspective*. New York: Wiley, 1982, pp. 59–69.

Michael JM: The second revolution in health: Health promotion and its environmental base. *Am Psychol* 1982; 37: 936–941.

Milio N: *Promoting Health through Public Policy*. Philadelphia: F. A. Davis, 1981.

Moss GE: *Immunity and Social Interaction*. New York: Wiley, 1973.

Mullen PD: Promoting child health: Channels of socialization. *Family and Community Health* 1983; 5 (4): 52–68.

Murray R, Zentner J: *Nursing Concepts for Health Promotion*. Englewood Cliffs, N.J.: Prentice-Hall, 1975, p. 7.

Naisbitt J: *Megatrends: Ten New Directions Transforming Our Lives*. New York: Warner Books, 1982.

Niblett D: Health promotion: A rediscovered social imperative. *Can J Public Health* 1975; 66: 357–358.

Noak M: *State Policy Support for School Health Education: A Review and Analysis*. Denver: Education Commission of the States, 1982.

O'Donnell MP: The corporate perspective. In: O'Donnell MP, Ainsworth T (editors), *Health Promotion in the Workplace*. New York: Wiley, 1984, pp. 10–35.

O'Hagen M: Healthstyles Basics: Lifestyle and behavior change. *Canadian Nurse* 1984; 80 (4): 21–23.

Orem DE: *Nursing: Concepts of Practice*, 3rd ed. New York: McGraw-Hill, 1985.

Panyan M: *How to Use Shaping*. Lawrence, Kans. HPH Enterprise, 1980.

Pender NJ: *Health Promotion in Nursing Practice.* Norwalk, Conn: Appleton-Century-Crofts, 1982a.

Pender NJ: Self-modification. In: Bulechek GM, McCloskey JC (editors), *Nursing Interventions: Treatment for Nursing Diagnoses.* Philadelphia: Saunders, 1985, pp. 80–91.

Pender NJ: Values clarification. In: Pender NJ (editor), *Health Promotion in Nursing Practice.* Norwalk, Conn.: Appleton-Century-Crofts, 1982b.

Petze CF: Health promotion for the well family. *Nurs Clin North America* 1984; 19 (2): 229–237.

Polakoff PL: Pathology vs. prevention: The health promotion debate. *Occup Health Saf* 1982; 51(6): 13–15.

Pratt L: *Family Structure and Effective Health Behavior.* Boston: Houghton Mifflin, 1976.

President's Committee on Health Education: *The Report of the Committee.* New York, 1974.

Promoting Health/Preventing Disease: Objectives for the Nation. US Department of Health and Human Services, US Public Health Service, 1980.

Puska P: Community-based prevention of cardiovascular disease: The North Karelia Project. In: Matarazzo JD et al (editors), *Behavioral Health: A Handbook of Health Enhancement and Disease Prevention.* New York, Wiley, 1984.

Puska P et al: Change in risk factors for coronary heart disease during 10 years of a community intervention programme (North Karelia Project). *Br Med J* 1983; 287: 1840–1844.

Reutter L: Family health assessment: An integrated approach. *Journal of Advanced Nursing* 1984; 9(4): 391–399.

Richard E: A rationale for incorporating wellness programs into existing occupational health programs. *Occupational Health Nursing* 1984; 32 (8): 412–415.

Robbins LC, Hall JH: *How to Practice Prospective Medicine.* Indianapolis: Slaymaker Enterprises, 1970.

Roberts DE, Freeman RB: *Redesigning Nursing Education for Public Health.* US Department of Health, Education and Welfare, 1973.

Rokeach M: *The Nature of Human Values.* New York: Free Press, 1973.

Schultz PR: Health planning implications of a comparative community field study. *Proceedings of University of Edinburgh, Nursing Studies Research Unit Conference,* 1982.

Shamansky SL, Clausen CL: Levels of prevention: Examination of the concept. *Nurs Outlook* 1980; 28: 104–108.

Smith JA: The idea of health: A philosophical inquiry. *Adv Nurs Sci* 1981; 3 (3): 43–50.

Smith JA: *The Idea of Health.* New York: Teachers College Press, 1983.

Stein MP et al: Results of a two-year health education campaign on dietary behavior: The Stanford Three Community Study. *Circulation* 1976; 54: 826–832.

Storfjell JL, Cruise PA: A model of community focused nursing. *Public Health Nursing* 1984; 1 (2): 85–96.

Taylor CW: Promoting health strengthening and wellness through environmental variables. In: Matarazzo JD et al (editors), *Behavioral Health: A Handbook of Health Enhancement and Disease Prevention.* New York: Wiley, 1984, pp. 130–149.

Temkin O: What is health? Looking back and ahead. In: Gladston I (editor): *Epidemiology of Health.* New York: Academy of Medicine, Health Education Council, 1953.

Terkelson K: Toward a theory of the family lifecycle. In: Carter EA, McGoldrick M (editors), *The Family Lifecycle: A Framework for Family Therapy,* New York: Gardner Press, 1980, 21–52.

Thompson MK: Family development theory. *Nurse Practitioner* 1984; 9 (6): 54–58.

Tolsdorf C: Social networks, support and coping: An exploratory study. *Family Process* 1976; 15: 407–417.

US Department of Health and Human Services. Public Health Service. Office of Disease Prevention and Health Promotion, Office of Health Information, Health Promotion and Physical Fitness and Sports Medicine. *Health Risk Appraisal: An Inventory.* PHS Publication No. 81-50163, June 1981.

Walker SN, Sechrist K, Pender NJ: *Development of the Health Enhancing Lifestyle Profile (HELP).* Unpublished manuscript.

Weiss SM: Community health promotion demonstration programs: Introduction. In: Matarazzo JD et al (editors), *Behavioral Health: A Handbook of Health Enhancement and Disease Prevention,* New York: Wiley, 1984a, pp. 1137–1139.

Weiss SM: Health hazard/health risk appraisals. In: Matarazzo JD et al (editors), *Behavioral Health: A Handbook of Health Enhancement and Disease Prevention.* New York: Wiley, 1984b, pp. 275–294.

West M: Community health assessment: The man-environment interaction. *J Community Health Nurs* 1984; 1(2): 89–97.

Wilbur CS: The Johnson and Johnson Program. *Prev Med* 1983; 12: 672–681.

Williams CA: Making things happen: Community health nursing and the policy arena. *Nurs Outlook* 1983; 31(4): 225–228.

Williams CA: Nursing leadership in community health: A neglected issue. In: McCloskey JC, Grace HK (editors), *Current Issues in Nursing.* Oxford, England: Blackwell Scientific Publications, 1981, p. 290.

Williams CA: Population: Focused practice. In: Stanhope M, Lancaster J (editors), *Community Health*

Nursing: Process and Practice for Promoting Health. St. Louis: Mosby, 1984, pp. 805–815.

Williams CL, Carter BJ, Eng A: The "Know Your Body" Program: A developmental approach to health education and disease prevention. *Prev Med* 1980; 9: 371–383.

Wright LM, Leahey M: How to intervene with families. In: Wright LM, Leahey M (editors), *Nurses and Families: A Guide to Family Assessment and Intervention.* Philadelphia: F. A. Davis, 1984.

Wu R: *Behavior and Illness.* Englewood Cliffs, N.J.: Prentice-Hall, 1973.

Chapter 14

Partnerships in the Community:
Implementing Strategies

Iris R. Shannon and Rojean Madsen

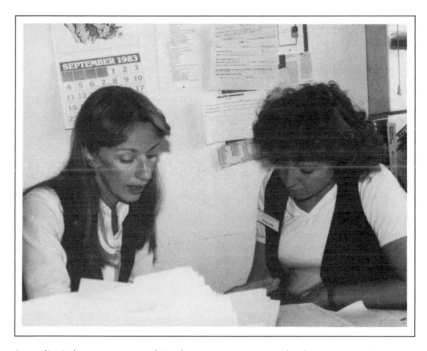

Interdisciplinary partnerships between nurses and other community-oriented professionals evolve out of a mutual commitment to improving the quality of life of the client, family, or community at large. The combined skills of these professionals often result in creative and effective strategies for care. (Linda Daniel/courtesy of Washtenaw County Health Department and the Huron Valley VNA)

Chapter Objectives

After completing this chapter, the reader will be able to:

- Identify partnerships in nursing that affect populations at greatest risk of illness, disability, and premature death
- Describe multidisciplinary collaboration in the context of community health
- State the issues that affect power in partnership relationships
- Discuss the purpose and types of community networks in nursing
- Define consumer advocacy and its uses

Public health nurses have historically considered the development of partnerships an important aspect of their practice. Partnerships are formed between people who work together to develop or achieve mutual goals. Traditional nurse-patient and nurse-family relationships can be thought of as partnerships, formed to work toward improving the health and quality of life of the patient or family or to increase the comfort and support the dignity of death.

Partnerships of nurses with community representatives, lawyers, teachers, legislators, physicians, or social workers are also familiar aspects of population-based nursing practice. Within these kinds of partnerships, nurses can play a wide variety of roles; in previous chapters, systems theory has been used to clarify the ways in which nurses may affect clients as individuals, families, and communities.

The focus of this chapter, however, will be on multidisciplinary collaboration, networks, and consumer advocacy, as specialized forms of partnership that are *uniquely* important to all nurses who work with programs committed to the improvement of the health of population groups and communities at greatest risk.

Partnerships in the Community

Partnership activities can help nurses transform their commitment to high-risk communities into a meaningful reality. Partnerships can be a means by which nurses meet their professional responsibilities to (1) identify and establish relationships with clients or potential clients; (2) collaborate with community and political leaders, consumer representatives, professionals from other fields, and other nurses and health care workers; (3) maintain networks to facilitate the exchange of information and sharing of power in the health system; and (4) be advocates for clients who are population groups within particular communities, as well as the families and individuals that make up these communities. In other words, a partnership can be seen as a strategy for the identification, implementation, and evaluation of goals identified through the nursing process.

Community as a Basis for Partnerships

As discussed in Chapter 3, the term *community* can mean a geographic place, a group of people who have some need or interest in common, or a social system. Throughout this chapter the term *community* will be used to refer to *all* types of communities. For example, nurses work with communities at greatest risk of disease disability or premature death; these communities may be specific groups of people living in one location, or they may be persons with similar needs, such as young parents and their children. Often the community at greatest risk in urban and rural areas can be most usefully defined in terms of a social system—for example, all families who have some specific type of need and who live within some specific geographic area not well served by existing health care programs and institutions.

Goals of Partnerships

A commitment to communities at greatest risk has been traditionally required in public health nursing as that specialization has been defined by the American Public Health Association. The public health nurse's commitment to communities at greatest risk implies not only feelings of concern, but also an investment of time and energy in reducing health risks for high-risk aggregate clients—

whether this means working with a few families or individuals or with the community as a whole.

Types of Partnerships

Partnerships in the community should be formed for special purposes. Depending on their level of educational preparation and experience, community health nurses may develop partnerships with powerful community leaders, clients and their representatives, or other professionals. These partnerships are developed because nurses and their partners work together in the process of reducing health problems in high-risk communities. *Multidisciplinary collaboration* is a term for cooperation and knowledge sharing that involves two or more persons with different knowledge and skills. *Networking* is a kind of partnership that primarily involves the exchange of information among or between partners. *Consumer advocacy* is a kind of partnership that occurs when professionals act to see that health care resources address highest priority client needs.

Partnerships imply shared goal-setting. The nurse most often uses the partnership to allow clients, or representatives of clients, to share in the decision making about the kinds of services needed to reduce health risks and subsequently to work with these groups to see that needed services are obtained. Most effective partnerships encompass a combination of multidisciplinary collaboration, networking, and/or consumer advocacy.

Nursing practice with a commitment to communities at greatest risk *must* be based on partnerships. Not all nurses working in programs or agencies serving communities will use all three of the forms of partnerships; however, nurses who practice in community settings can be more effective if they understand how to use partnerships to identify populations at greatest risk, develop service intervention methods, involve communities in decision making about community health risks, and engage in effective consumer advocacy when needed.

Partnerships and Power

Partnerships facilitate the development, sharing, and achievement of common objectives. Partnerships can be formal or informal; they can be long term or short term; and they can involve traditional nurse-patient and nurse-family relationships and planned interactions between the nurse and the community being served. For example, when addressing child abuse problems, the nurse's logical partners are parents, community representatives, lawyers, teachers, legislators, pediatricians and social workers. In contrast, members of the Gray Panthers, clergy, and community organizers may be partners with the nurse when addressing issues related to shelters for the homeless aged.

Within the context of systems theory (see Chapter 2), partnerships are expressions of relationships between systems and subsystems. Individuals function in subsystems (communities) of the larger society, and one of these subsystems is the health care system. Systems theory can help nurses analyze the relationship of those population groups at greatest health risk with the health care system, and in particular identify the socioeconomic, political, or organizational resources necessary to improve the groups' access and reduce their health risks.

These communities must then seek to acquire the power and resources that have been identified. The concept of power is a particularly important dimension of partnerships. Nurses possess professional knowledge and skill to deliver health services, access to the system through which services are given, and the legal authority to deliver these nursing services. In this situation, provider knowledge and skill and sometimes legal authority represent expert power. Clients negotiate with providers to use these attributes in order to attain or maintain some state of health. Clients also have some power in such negotiations, which they can exercise by refusing services. The result of non-participation could lead to a decrease in demand for nursing services, which would in turn reduce employment opportunities, or to decreased program or agency effectiveness, which might reduce funding or other support systems.

As stated earlier, partnerships help people work together to develop or achieve mutual goals. Put simply, power is the ability to implement plans to reach goals. The issue is not whether nurses must use power; the issue is *how* they can use power responsibly. Partnerships are only one way of using and influencing power, but, more than any other exercise of power, partnerships contribute specifically to the goals of nurses working with communities.

Raffaele (1974) presents an unconventional view of systems theory in which power is a central concept. He posits a conflict between, on the one hand, cultural groups who have limited power but who need service and, on the other hand, service agency professionals and managers who have power and who use their authority (power) to impose their own values on, and thereby influence the care of, relatively powerless cultural groups. Raffaele suggests that resolution of this power conflict should involve negotiation for institutional changes such as changes in the health care system itself. The types of partnerships discussed in this chapter and the power they generate can be used by nurses to promote this kind of change. Raffaele also suggests other ways of resolving conflict between those with power and client groups with limited power: the creation of opportunities for client participation in decision making through networks; and the conversion of health services management into coordination and information dissemination (such as through multidisciplinary collaboration and advocacy).

Raffaele's view of systems theory is helpful for understanding the many power issues reflected in the interactions between health care professionals and representatives of the population groups at greatest risk of disease, disability, and premature death. Issues related to the distribution of power in the delivery of community health services are often debates about the degree of client involvement that is appropriate for nursing and health services administration. Although involvement of clients in decision making is consistent with the philosophy and practice of nursing, within the professions there is disagreement about how clients should participate—i.e., as equal partners with professionals, as unequal partners, or merely as advisors to professionals who act as the major decision makers about the use of health care resources.

Examples of consumer participation in the management of their health resources were plentiful during the 1960s when "maximum" consumer participation in health and social programs was federally mandated (Sardell, 1983). Nursing and other health services associated with the War on Poverty were initially funded through the Office of Economic Opportunity (OEO) and were significantly influenced by this policy and the structures it created. (See Case Example 14-1.)

Although some power was shared with community groups at risk of poor health and many effective partnerships were formed, the actual implementation of the concept of maximum community participation created conflicts between consumers and providers of health services. For example, consumer advisory boards of OEO-funded Neighborhood Health Centers became dissatisfied over time with their limited power in decision making. In response to this dissatisfaction, advisory boards restructured themselves to become boards that could assume more authority in NHC policy and more control over NHC funds.

During succeeding political administrations in the late 1970s and 1980s, federal commitment to consumer participation as public policy has eroded from public policy, and discussions of equity in the delivery of community-based services occur less frequently than in the 1960s and early 1970s. Present federal health policy emphasizes efficiency through cost-containment measures (Sardell, 1983).

Case Example 14-1: Consumer Involvement in the Selection of Nurses

The OEO-funded Neighborhood Health Center (NHC) for which one of the authors worked required that all employees (professional and nonprofessional) be screened and approved for employment by an advisory board committee made up of neighborhood residents. Interviews were held in the community but not at the NHC site. Access to the place of the interview required the applicants to travel through the community.

Community participation in management decisions represents a partnership.

Health professional applicants, including nurses, who went before the committee were questioned about their reasons for wanting to work for the community, the type and amount of experience with similar populations (poor, predominantly black with multiple health and social problems), and their attitudes about such populations.

All applicants interviewed by the committee had already been screened by professional peers and judged qualified for employment. Some applicants and staff resented the required advisory board interview; however, the NHC advisory board held fast to its right to screen all applicants and its ability, through such interviewing, to identify those applicants with attitudes unacceptable to the community. Rarely were applicants found to have unacceptable attitudes, but when they were, the matter was referred back to the NHC director for additional inquiry and final resolution.

The terms and roles of participation must be negotiated, accepted, and clearly understood by all participants.

Multidisciplinary Collaboration

Multidisciplinary collaborations are extremely effective partnerships for identifying and assessing communities' health risks. Some multidisciplinary cooperation also involves the actual delivery of services. Often service delivery involves two or more professionals with different training working together by sharing clients, dividing up patient care tasks that will lead to a common goal, or using team management of particular clients' care. This type of collaboration among professionals is as important to nurses working with communities as it is to nurses working with families and individuals.

Multidisciplinary collaboration can facilitate many nursing functions in the community, among which are:

1. Assessment of community health needs
2. Determination of population subgroups at greatest risk of disease, disability, or premature death
3. Program planning and resource allocation
4. Identification of researchable issues

Of unique and particular importance to the practice of nursing in the community, however, is the use of multidisciplinary collaboration for identifying subgroups at greatest risk.

Complex factors, such as the incidence and effects of poverty, legal and ethical implications, cultural and spiritual needs, and public policy issues must be considered in a holistic approach to community health care. Multidisciplinary teams are often a most effective means of achieving community health goals and identifying subgroups at greatest risk. In such teams, members of different professions (as well as members of the community) bring their own special skills and understanding to the needs assessment process. Especially useful are partnerships of nurses with sociologists, clergy, psychologists, economists, planners, and other professionals who study how society is structured and how individuals and families fit into social groups. Consumers and their representatives can also contribute insight into the multiple and complex factors that influence the health status of population groups. Other clinicians such as occupational therapists, public health epidemiologists, and school social workers can provide information about unique social problems, environmental hazards, and health problems of a particular community. (See Case Example 14-2.)

For example, substantial evidence shows that poverty increases health risks (Institute of Medicine, 1981; Ryan, 1972; US DHEW, 1979, 1980; US DHHS, 1980). Groups at high risks in many communities include racial and ethnic minorities, the aged, and children. Recent social spending cuts have been associated by some with an increase in poverty (McNulty, 1985) as well with other negative consequences (Davis, 1981; Navarro, 1984). In 1971, the percentage of Americans living in poverty was reported to be 12.5 percent; in 1983, it was reported that 15.2 percent of Americans were living in poverty (Bureau of the Census, 1985). Analysis of health data such as morbidity and mortality statistics, combined with analysis of demographic and income statistics, can help the multidisciplinary team investigate and compare the effects of social policy before and after changes in policy and program funding. Thus, multidisciplinary collaboration can result in advocacy efforts on behalf of groups at high health risks.

Case Example 14-2: Multidisciplinary Research Efforts

Many types of illness are believed to be related to stress, problematic interpersonal situations, economics and the individual and family life styles of clients. In a recent study of the problems of residents of low income neighborhoods in Chicago, a multidisciplinary research team designed and analyzed a study based on personal interview data. The team included a sociologist, urban planners, a geographer, and a health services researcher. The study examined how residents were affected by a wide range of problems—housing, unemployment, hunger, crime, and illness. Many households were coping with unemployment and illness by living with relatives and sharing resources. Surprisingly, even the unemployed and uninsured had very few untreated medical problems in these neighborhoods, but two of every three households studied were found to be most in need of mental health services. A more traditional assessment of health needs in these areas would have failed to detect the extent of untreated mental health needs (Hemmens, 1984).

Investigations of the effects of social influences on health require the knowledge of several disciplines.

Goals of Multidisciplinary Collaboration

In general, the goal of multidisciplinary collaboration is to benefit from the knowledge and skills of more than one profession. These partnerships have the goal of producing better answers to complex questions. More specifically, multidisciplinary collaboration can help nurses to identify at-risk subgroups through community health assessments and to conduct research to add to the body of knowledge available to nursing. Another goal is to develop cooperation among partners to facilitate further program planning, implementation, and evaluation effectiveness.

Special Roles for Nurses

The following are roles nurses in the community can play in multidisciplinary collaboration:

- Emphasize commitment to identifying population subgroups at greatest risk—To say that an aggregate or subgroup is at greatest risk is to make a judgment based on comparisons of population groups. The multidisciplinary team should be encouraged to (1) identify the largest total population relevant to the agency or program or sponsoring group's mission, (2) consider several conceptual ways of defining subgroups of this population, and (3) identify the subgroup that seems to be at greatest risk and document the evidence that supports this conclusion. (See Case Example 14-3.)
- Assess the accuracy and relevance of community health assessments—The nurse can compare epidemiologic evidence of health risk to the knowledge of a community that he or she has gained through daily activity. Do the impressions of the nurse agree with the implications of research and epidemiological study and with the impressions of community members? If not, the multidisciplinary team may not be using a helpful conceptual scheme for identifying subgroups. Or perhaps the community does not have enough

published or formally collected information about health status and services to accurately identify subgroups at greatest risk. Or perhaps the perceptions of the nurse from individual practice are somehow biased or incomplete reflections of community needs. Nurses in the community must decide with others what is a valid determination of those "at greatest risk" and subject this to critique by other health professionals.

- Use and contribute to the nursing research literature—When involved in multidisciplinary collaboration, nurses can use nursing research literature to develop their own knowledge and skills and can bring relevant nursing literature to the attention of other partners from different backgrounds. Nurses without graduate training rarely head research efforts, but have a professional responsibility to identify researchable problems, to participate in the collection of data, and to review the results of local research efforts.

Nurses involved in multidisciplinary collaboration also bring the insights of other disciplines to the field of nursing. For example, a nurse who collaborates with transportation system planners will gain a fuller understanding of how public transportation can better meet the needs of physically handicapped clients. This nurse can share her knowledge with other nurses and inform clients of available services and/or encourage consumer advocacy to obtain improved transportation services that reduce health risks. Ideally, the nurse and her partners will also publish articles that summarize their increased knowledge from a nursing perspective and contribute to the breadth and relevance of nursing research and practice.

Preparation of health professionals for participation in multidisciplinary teams has been a concern of faculty groups for several years. As a result of research, much literature is available about group process, conflict management, leadership and communication skills. These are essential skills for nurses who work with communities, whether these skills are developed in formal coursework or through practical experience.

Case Example 14-3: Infant Mortality in Chicago, I

Infant mortality has been persistently high in the city of Chicago throughout the 1970s and the early 1980s. Concern about this problem led to the development of multidisciplinary collaboration and the formation of the Task Force on Infant Mortality. The Task Force is not an official agency; it is composed of interested professionals from several disciplines and a number of agencies and institutions in Chicago. The broad-based coalition includes representation from such groups as the American College of Nurse Midwives, Centro Latino (a consumer group), Chicago Health Systems Agency, Chicago Nurses' Association, Illinois Caucus on Teenage Pregnancy, Planned Parenthood Association of Chicago, and others.

Political action coalitions are partnerships representing organizations or individuals whose collective efforts stimulate changes in systems.

Members of the Task Force have worked together to document the fact that in certain areas of Chicago, particular age groups of mothers and some racial and ethnic minority groups are at greatest risk of high infant mortality rates in the future. These risks have been traced to poverty, inadequate access to health care, the lack of some kinds of health services, dietary patterns, and hereditary health factors. This multidisciplinary collaboration, a partnership of many different kinds of professionals, has effectively identified the subpopulations in Chicago at greatest risk and has related the health risks affecting these population subgroups to a complex set of circumstances that must be changed.

Networks

Networking refers to building and expanding partnerships of people who share information about common interests and solve problems. Members exchange ideas and resources on a continuing basis. Networks can be useful forms of partnership in almost all nursing activities, but they are particularly important for effective nursing practice in the community.

This section focuses on using networks to make nursing's contribution more effective in reducing previously identified health risks. The popular press has encouraged us to think of networking as exchanging information about job opportunities, work conditions, and training possibilities for personal career advancement and benefit. Although useful to individual nurses, this is not the use of networks discussed in this section. This chapter concentrates on networks that involve the exchange of information about client needs, effects of services, and the availability of health care resources within a community.

Goals of Networks

One basic goal of using networks for nurses working with communities is to improve the information available to people who influence community residents' behavior and people who influence the availability of health care resources. Through networks, nurses collect information about needs—why services are used, when services are perceived to be effective, and how resources for services can be obtained. The nurse also interprets health needs, explains service availability, convinces others to control health risks, and documents why more resources are needed for particular aggregates or programs. The nurse who uses networks effectively exchanges information with people who can help change situations beyond the control of the individual nurse or agency.

Nurses can use networks to reduce community heath risks, because networks facilitate the nurses' access to and acceptance within the community. Networks also help to establish the lines of communication and the patterns of cooperation that will assist the group at greatest risk. Networking can be important in developing and maintaining community cooperation for new health promotion programs that require life-style changes. Finally, networks are a means for creating and maintaining the working relationships with other professionals that facilitate multidisciplinary collaboration and consumer advocacy.

Community Access and Acceptance

Community access and acceptance are key concepts in designing programs to reduce health risk. A program with community acceptance is not a set of activities designed for community residents by "outsiders," but a program that the residents or clients feel belongs to them, that they will help support, and that they can change when and if their needs change. A network linking health professionals with community representatives can build community acceptance for new and existing programs and increase their effectiveness in reducing health risks. To develop network effectiveness, the nurse must carefully consider the kinds of community representatives needed. The interests of subgroups at greatest risk must be credibly represented by the community residents involved in planning health services.

Community Gatekeepers

Some community health workers have been concerned about how to identify these community representatives. Will and Sherrow (1977) describe *community gatekeepers* as leaders who determine the openness of the community system and who influence that system's functioning and survival. Community gatekeepers may be local residents, professionals, politicians, or religious leaders (Freeman & Heinrich, 1981). Gatekeepers can play a major role in coordinating the needs of the local community with the larger society through interpreting the needs and actions of community groups to professionals or negotiating for resources for their neighborhoods with nongovernmental and governmental agencies.

Kaufman (1977) suggests that it is important to identify gatekeepers by the amount of coordination they achieve, as opposed to their formal position or the amount of direct control they seem to hold. "Leaders most active in local programs are also most influential in the use of resources from the larger society" (Kaufman, 1977, p. 402). Gatekeepers are often either the informal or official leaders of grassroots organizations and they can discourage or encourage community residents' acceptance and cooperation with nurses and other health professionals. They can also provide information about reasons for and levels of client compliance with health programs.

Nurses may work with gatekeepers directly, but in many situations the nurse must rely on other community residents and clients to exchange information with gatekeepers. Every situation in every community will be somewhat different, and the community-based nurse must be flexible and willing to work directly or indirectly with gatekeepers to gain community acceptance for programs. Often gatekeepers can be found most easily through grassroots organizations.

Grassroots Organizations

Grassroots organizations are groups whose members (mostly unpaid volunteers) are residents of a community. These members are usually not health care professionals but rather citizens who are concerned about one or more local problems. Grassroots efforts often begin as reactions to unresponsiveness of providers to the needs of the poor and exclusion of the poor from health planning processes. Research literature suggests that grassroots organizations' efforts are sometimes ineffectual, because the groups lack experience in communicating with complex formal organizations. Also, many local groups fail to work through other, more powerful groups such as public agencies, political parties, or hospitals to achieve their goals. Nurses working with communities can include these large, powerful organizations in their network activity and help grassroots organizations work with more powerful service agencies.

Grassroots, or neighborhood, organizations, have always been part of American society. During the War on Poverty and the infusion of public monies into Community Action Programs (CAPs) during the 1960s, however, grassroots organizations became more politicized. CAPs could be funded only if they could show grassroots involvement and support for services. Competition for available government funding increased the political power of poor communities to demand the services they wanted and forced the poor's entry into health planning. Conventional provider organizations were often in competition with grassroots organizations for available funding for health services. Clients in poor communities could refuse to participate in a project and their refusal could result in the withdrawal of government funding.

As a result, in many cities and towns new health-related programs and agencies were created, and some hired and trained local residents as staff members. Often these new programs tried to adapt to the particular customs and problems of neighborhoods. Others tried to make government agencies and hospitals more responsive to the needs of the poor. Many CAP agencies were established in the 1960s and still exist. (See Case Example 14-4.)

During the 1970s most grassroot groups became less political and their programs were incorporated into the traditional health and social services system. Client participation in program planning, even when mandated by law, is now organized by agencies rather than by grassroots organizations.

It is important to understand that changes can occur in agencies, even agencies founded by grassroots organizations, when funding sources change. Gittell (1980) addresses this issue in her report of a two-year study of community organizations involved in school politics. The membership and leadership of sixteen organizations were examined and the political, economic, and social subsystems in which they function were analyzed. Findings from this study demonstrated a pervasive shift in lower-income organizations from advocacy to service functions.

The activist groups of the 1960s evolved into the service groups of the 1970s, because these groups grew dependent on outside funding for their services. Existing service programs absorb the resources of an organization and detract from the energy and commitment required for new program design and advocacy.

Continued client involvement in health planning often seems to be dependent on the viability of grassroots, or community, organizations. The nurse in the 1980s can play an important role by establishing a network that provides agencies with information about community needs as viewed by grassroots organizations. The nurse can also provide information to grassroots organizations about agency programs and opportunities for influencing health planning and program planning. Some observers of society believe that grassroots organizations have been regaining strength during the 1970s and early 1980s. Boyte (1983), in particular, has written about the activities and potential strengths of grassroots organizations of the 1980s in his book *Backyard Revolution.*

Vertical and Horizontal Community Network Links

Working with grassroots organizations, however, is only one way to use networks. Any group of influential people can be a useful "community network."

Case Example 14-4: Consumer Involvement in Neighborhood Health Centers

As mentioned earlier, public policy in the 1960s was associated with the War on Poverty and was characterized by mandated involvement of the poor in decision making about their health and welfare services, which was a shift from earlier decision making done primarily by providers. During the 1960s funding for neighborhood health centers (NHCs) to provide comprehensive continuous health care was targeted at improving the health of the poor. Consumer participation in planning was viewed by federal, state, and local governmental funding agencies as a way of building community acceptance, and as a way of involving community residents and professionals together in planned change. Federal guidelines for the establishment of NHCs required client participation in the planning and selection of types of health care services to be offered.

Effective networks that create partnerships between clients and health care providers can help improve agency effectiveness and increase utilization by community residents.

The Mile Square Health Center was one of the NHCs established in Chicago in the early 1960s. It was carefully developed through work with grassroots organizations and community gatekeepers. Community-based professionals built a network that included a major local hospital, Rush-Presbyterian-St. Luke's Hospital, and the poor, black residents of Chicago's near West Side. Utilization by community residents was an indicator of the high degree of community acceptance that this center achieved. During its first year, 1964, The Mile Square Center had over 64,000 patient visits and by 1972 this figure had risen to nearly 109,000 (Mile Square Health Center, 1974).

This health center still exists today, although grassroots participation currently consists primarily of community residents serving on the board of the center. Community health nurses can and do contribute information to the network that links local clients and potential clients to the administration and board of Mile Square Health Center.

Often nurses can become effective members of networks that already exist. Community networks are inherent parts of the community as a system. The number of people involved in a network is the simplest measure of a network's level of activity and ability to speak for or influence many community residents. Even small networks, however, may be very effective when members accurately assess and express community residents' needs and opinions. Nurses who help clients or community groups become part of large networks may influence their effectiveness in promoting improved health.

Both vertical and horizontal networks can func-

tion in a community. *Vertical* links connect community organizations to agencies or institutions with other types of power and funds (state agencies, financial institutions, hospitals, federal government, and businesses). Vertical networks, therefore, include relationships among groups with different types of power—for example, between patients and service professionals, or between administrators of provider agencies and leaders of neighborhood organizations. *Horizontal* contacts include relationships that link groups with similar kinds of power, such as relationships among different racial and ethnic consumer groups or links among local governmental agencies. Gittell (1980) reports that community organizations engaged in advocacy are often those with the highest levels of networking activity. Certainly, nurses who are part of networks with vertical and horizontal links will be exposed to new ideas for change and will be able to communicate their plans for change to both clients and persons who influence agency policies and services funding. (See Case Example 14-5.)

Barriers to Including Clients and Community Leaders in Networks

Many different groups and individuals within a community use networks to change community conditions—that is, they regularly share information and ideas about what should change and how changes can be accomplished. Nurses are among those who use health care resources to develop or improve programs that reduce health risks within a community. Networking is a type of partnership that can be particularly effective as a means of developing and gaining community cooperation with programs to reduce health risks. However, many health professionals are uncomfortable with requirements for community participation in health planning. For example, a study of twenty-seven NHCs by Sparer, Dines, and Smith (1969) reported that many professionals were unwilling to turn over professional matters to community groups, wanted to maintain control over hiring of health care professionals, and did not want community representatives involved in establishing personnel policies for the NHCs. Other studies reported similar attitudes in other NHCs (Goldberg, Trowbridge, & Buxbaum, 1969; Sheps, 1974; Zwick, 1974).

In the 1980s some health professionals continue to resist community demands for changes in health services and participation. These are the kinds of barriers to network building that nurses are expected to overcome. Because they are committed to consumer involvement in planning, nurses must overlook their own hesitations about consumer involvement, encourage other health professionals to accept consumer involvement, and encourage community residents to actively participate in the development of reasonable, effective health care agency policies and programs.

Case Example 14-5: Infant Mortality in Chicago, II

As discussed earlier, there is a citywide coalition in Chicago that is working to reduce the city's high infant mortality rate. This coalition is using network activity (in addition to the multidisciplinary collaboration mentioned earlier). The broad-based coalition of more than thirty organizations is sharing information about available services and possible coordination. Although the coalition's efforts are just beginning, it was successful in raising the issue of infant mortality for media exploration and for debate in the mayoral campaign of 1983. The organizational members of the network have also been involved directly and indirectly with Project Life, sponsored by the Executive Service Corps (retired business executives) and the State of Illinois' Parents Too Soon Initiative.

The media can be a very useful part of a network that a nurse uses to disseminate information about a community's health needs and problems.

Horizontal networks pool resources.

Vertical relationships draw support from more powerful sources.

Consumer Advocacy

The nurse with a special commitment to those population subgroups or aggregates at greatest risk brings a unique and important perspective to health planning. She or he enters consumer advocacy partnerships that work to see that subgroups at greatest risk within a community receive the resources and services they need. This kind of partnership should always involve the nurse, the client, and persons with power. The partners with power may be political leaders, other professionals, community leaders, or others.

Goals of Advocacy

Advocacy has been defined as a further attempt at problem solving when resolution of a conflict is inconsistent with the clients' interests (Grosser, 1976). Nurses are expected to be advocates, to take further action, when the needs of subgroups at greatest risk are not being addressed by the agency or program that employs the nurse or by the health care system as a whole. The nurse takes action to see that the plans made by a network of community representatives and health professionals are actually carried out in a manner that effectively results in the benefits intended. Advocacy in this sense may be action to increase funds available, to increase the professional time available to particular patients, or to change agency policy about the kinds of health professionals hired, where services are delivered, or the hours at which services are available. Client involvement should be an essential aspect of advocacy.

The Advocacy Process

A very wide range of activities have been used in advocacy, and new approaches to advocacy continue to be developed. The basic steps that nurses should follow, however, are:

1. Nurse and client or community representatives reach agreement that clearly identifies a problem that neither the nurse nor the client can solve without help from a more powerful partner.
2. Nurse and the client or community representatives decide how they will work together to address the problem—that is, they develop an advocacy strategy.
3. Participants define and jointly agree upon their advocacy roles and activities.
4. The nurse speaks on behalf of the community or client according to the advocacy strategy and the role planned for her or him.

Two types of activities of nurses involved in advocacy partnerships are most common: (1) After reaching agreement with the client, the nurse may use his or her professional status to get the attention of people with power, and he or she will try to influence these power-holders (her partners) to redirect resources to reduce previously identified health risks by supporting particular programs; or (2) the nurse may try to establish a partnership between community representatives and people with power (i.e., the nurse becomes an indirect participant in the partnership).

Planning Advocacy Strategies

Grosser (1976) suggests that advocacy should be based on careful consideration of the following issues:

1. The person(s) or institution (clients, nurse, or agency) who will be affected by the advocacy should be identified, and there should be clear foreknowledge of how they will be affected.
2. The purpose of the advocacy should be clear and carefully identified.

3. An advocacy approach should be chosen based on consideration of the resources of the nurse and the receptivity of the people with power.
4. The way in which the power-holders are contacted or affected by the advocacy should be carefully considered.
5. The results of each attempt at advocacy should be evaluated.

This list is provided to illustrate the importance of viewing advocacy as a professional skill that must be studied and practiced with care; advocacy is not merely speaking about clients' needs whenever an opportunity happens to arise. Consumer advocacy should also only be attempted with the explicit participation of the client or, if the client is a subgroup, with community representatives. Effective advocacy can, however, produce change to better meet clients' needs. Most change requires the use of power, and partnerships for advocacy can often help the client and the nurse, as partners, influence people with power. (See Case Example 14-6.)

Advocacy and Personal Values

While advocacy is considered an important activity for all nurses (Kohnke, 1982), the degree and focus of that advocacy will often depend on the nurse's individual values. White (1982) offers two "dynamics" in her conceptualization of community health nursing: the nursing process and the valuing process. Valuing processes involve moral values and judgments, which, in turn, form the basis of commitment. White (1982) offers the following comments on the importance of the nurse's value system: "Value judgements guide what we do and don't do, determine our real commitments, and serve as the bases for our advocacy and practice. But, in order to value something one must be able to conceive of it, and to relate to it on some intellectual level" (pp. 529–530). For example, if poverty increases the risk of poor health and the nurse is working with a poverty population, then the nurse's value judgments about poor people will influence his or her level of commitment and advocacy.

Case Example 14-6: Mile Square Health Center

The development of Mile Square Health Center (described briefly in Case Example 14-4) also provided opportunities for advocacy. Center personnel and the center's advisory committee (all community representatives) were careful in identifying and negotiating advocacy roles. For example, board members preferred to represent themselves in issues before the city council or other legislative bodies where distribution of resources were involved. When technical information was needed regarding the health needs of the population, the advisory committee expected the professional staff to interpret these needs, but within the broader social context of the center's program and the center's leadership and staff. Formal agreements were reached with city agencies responsible for improved nursing follow-up, case finding of maternal and child health programs, and tuberculosis follow-up. Mile Square Health Center was allowed to assume responsibility for these activities and to effectively develop better services to reduce health risks for the poor, medically underserved population subgroups the health center regarded as high risk, high priority clients.

Advocacy requires clear role identification in order to maintain or attain an effective working relationship between the professional and the community.

A nurse's value judgments concerning poor people may be based on his or her beliefs about the causes of poverty. For instance, a nurse whose values are based on conservative economic theory may look for the cause of poverty in terms of some individual characteristic over which the poor person is presumed to exercise control. The nurse's commitment and type of advocacy will reflect these beliefs. Commitment based on liberal economic theory might include advocacy that recognizes the causes of poverty to be partially societal and partially the individual's characteristics. Finally, the nurse who accepts a radical theory of poverty may believe the causes of poverty to be outside the individual's control, in economic markets and other societal institutions (Wachtel, 1974). It is essential for all nurses to understand their own value systems and how these systems influence their commitments, interactions, advocacy, and decisions about people and communities.

The nurse's level of commitment to advocacy is influenced by personal, professional and organizational values. If conflict exists among these values, it should be reconciled in favor of the client's interests. (See Case Example 14-7.)

Summary

In this chapter we have discussed only a few examples of how partnerships can be used by nurses who work with communities, and who are committed to reducing the health risks of populations at greatest risk. The opportunities for partnerships will vary from situation to situation, as will the specific goals and means used in each partnership.

Two general criteria can guide the nurse trying to identify opportunities for effective partnership:

1. When the nurse needs more resources, skills, information, or credibility to reach goals, he or she should consider establishing a partnership.

Case Example 14-7: School Health Policies: Opportunity for Advocacy

Advocacy may involve working to change the policies of institutions. A school nurse found that school system policies forced her to call for an ambulance to remove students to the hospital if they fell unconscious and could not be revived using standard first aid procedures. This policy often meant that parents had to leave their employment and also had to pay local hospital emergency room fees. In one circumstance involving a student known to have psychogenic seizures, the nurse was required to follow this policy even though it contradicted the wishes and advice of the girl's psychiatrist and mother. The school's policy and medical management were in conflict. Eventually, because of the recurring problem, the girl was excused from school attendance and her education was interrupted. Perhaps through creative advocacy by the school nurse, PTA, local medical society, school board and other interested persons, a solution could have been found that would have avoided the interruption of the student's education.

Advocacy at the system level requires communication with all persons and organizations affected and requires extensive organizing.

2. When a nurse's client (whether individual, family, or population subgroup) is not effectively being served by the existing health care system, the nurse has a responsibility to develop partnerships to change the situation.

As suggested in Figure 14-1, interaction within partnerships is always mutual, and these partnerships are always focused, explicitly or implicitly, on the reduction of health risks for those population subgroups at greatest risk of disease, disability, or premature death. The kind of partnership activity the nurse should develop may be different in each circumstance. Generally, the nurse must identify whether clients' needs are unmet and develop a partnership accordingly:

1. If needs are not well known, multidisciplinary collaboration for research may be needed, or the nurse may need to establish or join a network that includes community representatives and gatekeepers who are knowledgeable about the community.

2. If awareness of health needs and risks is contributing to a community's problems, partnerships may help the community health nurse raise levels of awareness. As a professional, the nurse may be able to involve many potential partners (funding sources, health professions, and grassroots community groups) in an information-sharing network. The use of a network may also attract attention to health risks and needs for resources.

3. If other forms of action and partnership have failed to solve a problem in a community or the problem of a particular group of clients, the nurse may want to develop a partnership for consumer advocacy (see Table 14-1).

Partnerships should always involve some type of client participation. In previous years federal policy and funding sources mandated much more client

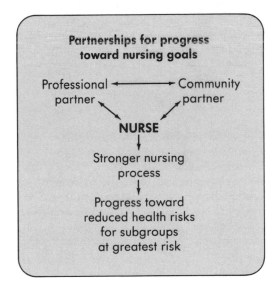

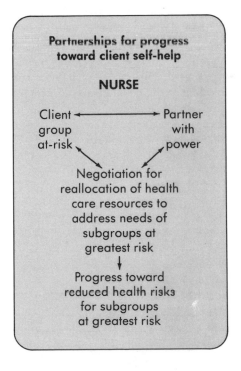

Figure 14-1 Models for using partnerships

Table 14-1   Choosing Appropriate Partnerships

Primary Obstacles to Meeting the Needs of Clients at Greatest Risk	Type of Partnership Most Likely to Be Useful
Health risks are not known to the nurse and/or the agency or program with resources.	Multidisciplinary collaboration or Network of community representatives and professionals
More awareness of and action to reduce health risks is needed.	Network of community leaders and representatives and professionals and persons with control of resources
Resources for reducing known risks are not available or particular problems have not been solved through ordinary administrative policy and action.	Advocacy with client to affect persons with power

and consumer involvement in the health care system than is the case today. For nurses, however, professional responsibility for client involvement is just as important today as ever. Although nurses must be guided by their own personal values as they identify particular opportunities for partnerships, client participation in partnerships is an important professional value they all should implement.

Working with vulnerable populations requires understanding of the communities in which these populations live. Multidisciplinary collaboration can help provide this understanding. Networks of nurses and community residents can lead to planning of services that will effectively reduce health risk. Awareness of the problems and environment of populations at greatest risk can inspire the nurse's commitment to these populations and to the process of advocacy on their behalf.

Topics for Nursing Research

Jackson Heights (population 25,000), a subdivision of a large midwestern metropolitan community, aggressively sought and received funding from a private foundation to plan a comprehensive free-standing health center. The grant to the Jackson Heights Association was based on the community's many established health needs: high infant mortality rates; high teenage pregnancy rates; increasing incidence of tuberculosis; and low levels of immunization among its children. In addition, the Heights community lacked an ambulatory facility that provided family-centered comprehensive health care. The average family income in 1980 was $12,000.

The Association's plan is to seek other funding from governmental and private sources to implement and evaluate the health center being planned. Since the Association is made up of community leaders, it plans to maintain control over the center by establishing a corporate board of its members.

• Identify and describe the nature and types of partnerships that would facilitate planning for the center.

• What system could be developed for client-input in care?

• What networks have developed between the various health agencies and professionals in Jackson Heights? How well do the networks function, and what areas exist for improvement of network function?

• Develop a viable method of collaboration between the nurse and members of grassroots organizations. Evaluate the outcomes and effectiveness of this collaborative process.

• Identify and describe the nurse's role in the Heights community.

Study Questions

1. How can public health nurses use partnerships with communities to meet their responsibilities to subgroups at high risk of poor health?
   (1) By identifying and establishing relationships within the community
   (2) By collaborating with community and political leaders
   (3) By collaborating with other nurses and health professionals
   (4) By maintaining networks to facilitate exchange of information
   Choose one answer:
   a. 1 and 4
   b. 1 and 2
   c. 2 and 4
   d. All of the above

2. When used in nursing practice in the community, what outcomes of a network relationship are *always* desired?
   (1) Frequent sharing of information
   (2) Formalization of relationships (e.g., contractual agreements)
   (3) Formation of a political coalition
   (4) Correction of a specific problem
   Choose one answer:
   a. 1 only
   b. 2 and 3
   c. 4 only
   d. 1 and 4

3. How does the concept of power influence nursing partnerships with communities at high risk of illness?
   (1) It is not an issue—nurses are always more powerful in such a relationship because of their knowledge and skill in health.
   (2) Members and groups in high-risk communities can exert their power through such activities as support, participation, and cooperation that contribute to the success or failure of a program or intervention.
   (3) Nurses can use the power they generate to promote institutional changes that will reduce the health risks to vulnerable groups in the population.
   (4) Client groups with perceived limited power must be provided the opportunity to participate in decision making about the organization and use of health resources designed to meet their needs.
   Choose one answer:
   a. 1 only
   b. 1 and 2
   c. All of the above
   d. 2, 3, and 4

4. What characteristics are important in the identification of community gatekeepers?
   (1) They must be professionals—politicians or religious leaders.
   (2) They must be able to coordinate the needs of the community with the larger society (governmental and nongovernmental).
   (3) They must be formal leaders of grassroots organizations.
   (4) They should be identified by what they achieve in the community as opposed to the amount of direct control they seem to hold.
   Choose one answer:
   a. 1 only
   b. 2 only
   c. 2, 3, and 4
   d. 2 and 4 only

5. How can one develop a network of support that will enhance continued funding and continuity for a health center?
   a. Develop vertical linkages, but only with governmental agencies
   b. Develop horizontal linkages with similar consumer groups
   c. Develop vertical and horizontal linkages in order to expose, communicate, and interpret the center's program and needs
   d. Develop vertical and horizontal linkages with interested agencies and persons who represent consumers, policymakers, and other influential persons and groups.

References

American Public Health Association: Definition and role of public health nursing in the delivery of health care. *American Journal of Public Health* 1982; 72: 210–212.

Boyte H: *The Backyard Revolution.* Philadelphia: Temple University Press, 1983.

Davis K: Reagan administration health policy. *J Public Health Policy* 1981; 2(4): 312–332.

Freeman RB, Heinrich J: *Community Health Nursing Practice.* Philadelphia: W. B. Saunders, 1981.

Gittell M: *Limits to Citizen Participation: The Decline of Community Organizations.* Beverly Hills, Calif.: Sage Publications, 1980.

Goldberg GA, Trowbridge FL, Buxbaum RC: Issues in the development of Neighborhood Health Centers. *Inquiry* 1969; 6: 37–48.

Grosser CF: *New Directions in Community Organization from Enabling to Advocacy.* New York: Praeger, 1976.

Hemmens G et al: *Household Needs and Community Response in Three Chicago Neighborhoods,* Unpublished manuscript, University of Illinois, School of Urban Planning and Policy, Chicago, 1984.

Institute of Medicine, National Academy of Sciences: *Health Care in a Context of Civil Rights.* Washington, D.C.: National Academy Press.

Kaufman H: Community influentials: Power figures or leaders? In Warren RW (editor), *New Perspectives on the American Community.* Chicago: Rand McNally, 1977.

Kohnke MS: Advocacy: What is it? *Nursing and Health Care* (June) 1982: 314–318.

Lashof J: Comments on issues in the development of Neighborhood Health Centers. *Inquiry* 1969; 6: 48–49.

Lashof J: Mile Square Neighborhood Health Center: An Overview. *Rush-Presbyterian-St. Luke's Medical Center Bulletin* 1971; 3: 81–92.

McNulty T: Lost society infects cities: Permanent underclass may be developing. *Chicago Tribune* (September 15) 1985; Section 1:1.

Mile Square Health Center: *1973 Annual Report,* Chicago, Ill.: Author, 1974.

Navarro V: Selected myths guiding the Reagan administration's health policy. *J Public Health Policy* 1984; 5(1): 65–73.

Raffaele JA: *System and Unsystem.* New York: Wiley, 1974.

Ryan W: *Blaming the Victim.* New York: Vintage Books, 1976.

Sardell A: Neighborhood Health Centers and community-based care: Federal policy from 1965 to 1982. *J Public Health Policy* 1983; 4: 485–503.

Shannon IR: Nursing service at the Mile Square Health Center of Presbyterian-St. Luke's Hospital. *Am J Public Health* 1970; 60: 1726–1732.

Sheps CG: The influence of consumer sponsorship on medical services. In: Zola IK, McKinlay JB (editors), *Organizational Issues in the Delivery of Health Services.* New York: Prodist, 1974.

Sparer G, Dines GB, Smith D: Consumer participation in OEO-assisted Neighborhood Health Centers. *Am J Public Health* 1969; 60: 1091–1102, 1969.

Styles M: Reflections on collaboration and unification. *Image: The Journal of Nursing Scholarship* 1984; 16: 21–23.

US Department of Commerce, Bureau of the Census: *Current Population Report Characteristics of the Population Below the Poverty Level: 1983.* Washington, D.C.: Government Printing Office, 1985.

US Department of Health, Education and Welfare: *Healthy People.* DHEW-PHS Publication No. 79-55071. Washington, D.C.: US Printing Office, 1979.

US Department of Health and Human Services: *Health-United States 1980.* DHHS-PHS Publication No. 81-1232. Washington, D.C.: US Printing Office, 1980.

Wachtel HM: Looking at poverty from radical, conservative, and liberal perspectives. In: Roby A (editor), *The Poverty Establishment.* Englewood Cliffs, N.J.: Prentice-Hall, 1974.

White M: Construct for public health nursing. *Nurs Outlook* 1982; 30: 527-530.

Will SJ, Sherrow V: Student analysis of clinical learning environments. In: Hall JF, Weaver BR (editors), *Distributive Nursing Practice: A Systems Approach to Community Health.* Philadelphia: Lippincott, 1977, pp. 287–297.

Zwick DI: Some accomplishments and findings of neighborhood health centers. In: Zola IK, McKinlay JB (editors), *Organizational Issues in the Delivery of Health Services.* New York: Prodist, 1974.

Chapter 15

Evaluation of Family and Community Health Nursing Practice

Naomi E. Ervin and Shu-Pi C. Chen

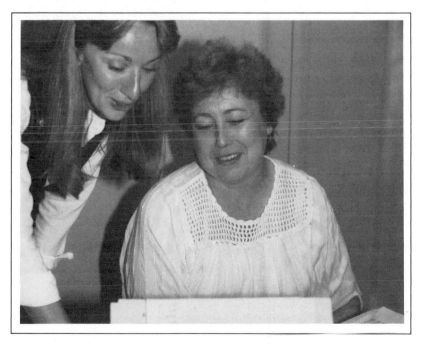

One aspect of evaluation is the appraisal a community health nurse supervisor offers to coworkers. The process of applying scientific methods in making a judgment operates as effectively for the caregiver as the care. (Linda Daniel/courtesy of Washtenaw County Health Department and the Huron Valley VNA)

**Chapter
Outline**

**Chapter
Objectives**

After completing this chapter, the reader will be able to:

- Define evaluation
- Describe the levels at which evaluation is done
- Discuss evaluation as a component of the nursing process
- List criteria for writing objectives
- Describe a method for evaluating nursing care
- Discuss the relationship of accountability to evaluation

Evaluation is the appraisal of changes that are intended as the result of an intervention. Evaluation is a process of judgment. "Evaluation is concerned with values, with measuring results against standards and coming up with a value judgement on the significance of the result" (Braden, 1984, p. 373). Although both subjective and objective information are used in making appraisals, the scientific method of evaluation emphasizes the use of objective information in making a judgment. The process of applying scientific methods in making a judgment is called the evaluation process. The evaluation process can be applied at two levels: the individual and the aggregate.

To evaluate care at the individual level, the evaluation question focuses on the extent to which the nursing care or interventions met the individual's or family's needs. To evaluate care at the aggregate level, the evaluation question focuses more broadly on aspects of the quality of care, operations, costs, and outcomes. In this chapter evaluation at aggregate levels includes evaluation of the department or division of nursing, program evaluation, quality assurance, peer review, performance evaluation, and self-evaluation. We look at evaluation at the individual level as a component of the nursing

process, which includes assessing, diagnosing, planning, implementing, and evaluating. Although the purpose of doing evaluation on any level is basically the same—to determine the worth of a program or service based on stated objectives and data—the content and focus will vary with the background of those evaluating, available time to complete the evaluation, money, and other resources available for the evaluation process.

The first section here addresses the aggregate levels of evaluation that most directly include nursing in a community health agency. Although each agency varies in the type and amount of evaluation activity undertaken, all agencies include at least some aspects of the types of evaluation discussed. The staff level professional nurse will not likely be directly involved in all areas of evaluation, but will be expected to participate in accurate data collection and some committee activities, such as quality assurance or audit. In order to be an informed, contributing member of a nursing division, the community health nurse should have a working knowledge of evaluation on several levels and awareness of how these relate to individual nursing practice.

Evaluation at Aggregate Levels

Institutional Levels

Evaluation at the institutional level may consist of evaluation within a division of nursing or of a program.

Division of Nursing Evaluation Although the separation of evaluation for the division of nursing and for program may be artificial, there are needs for doing evaluation for both areas. The division of nursing in a community health agency has objectives that differ from, but augment, those of the total agency and those of a specific program. This will be illustrated a little later in this section. The overall division of nursing objectives are usually aimed at the improvement of nursing practice within the division, resource allocation, or use and development of new nursing programs or program com-

ponents. Examples of some division of nursing objectives are shown in Case Example 15-1.

In order to evaluate whether these objectives had been met, those in charge would need data collection mechanisms. For example, they would want to keep a record of the number of staff development programs held, a count of the number of home visits made last year, and the total number of visits made each day by each nurse. Each staff community health nurse is a part of the division of nursing evaluation for some aspects of data collection. Thus, the nurse who is knowledgeable about the division of nursing evaluation will be a more competent data collector and record keeper.

Generally, a division of nursing would not undertake an evaluation of the total division each year, but may participate in an evaluation done periodically by

Case Example 15-1: Division of Nursing Objectives

To hold six staff development programs this fiscal year

Contribute to improvement of nursing practice

To increase home visit productivity by 10 percent this year

Resource allocation

To establish prenatal classes by October for pregnant adolescents in two high schools

New program component

an external agency, such as the National League for Nursing or the state health department. Such evaluations done by external accrediting or regulatory bodies are based on criteria that were established by the specific agency and are used as the basis of granting accreditation or for a license.

Program Evaluation   *Program evaluation* is defined as the measurement of success in reaching stated objectives of an organized health program (Suchman, 1967). A health program is an organized response to reduce or minimize health problems; this usually involves achieving objectives, increasing performance, and/or acquiring resources. At this aggregate level, the evaluation focuses on the health program's quality, operation, cost, and outcomes. Based on the stated objectives and data obtained, evaluators judge the worth of the health program. Table 15-1 gives an example of how agency, division of nursing, and program objectives may be stated.

As in a nursing care plan, objectives do not specify how the objectives are to be achieved. These actions are delineated as activities or action plans after objectives have been written.

Professional Levels

Quality Assurance   *Quality assurance* is the systematic evaluation of the degree of excellence of the results of care based on predetermined standards or criteria, and the systematic correction of deficiencies so as to result in a higher level of quality (Zimmer, 1974). This approach for evaluating nursing care is a

process and is often depicted as a cyclical model as illustrated in the American Nurses' Association (1975) model in Figure 15-1. Although the first two steps of the cycle (identify values and identify standards and criteria) will not necessarily be repeated at the beginning of each cycle, the other steps will need to be completed for a systematic approach and for changes in care to be realized. If only the measurements were secured and the process stopped at that point, nothing would result from the data collection phase. The American Nurses' Association quality assurance model gives direction for avoiding this pitfall.

The continuous nature of the quality assurance process provides a forum in which nurses can more objectively assess, change, and ensure the quality of nursing care to consumers as a group. Nurses have always been concerned about care that is less than optimal. The quality assurance model offers individual nurses the opportunity and responsibility to become involved in improving care for all clients, not just those to whom each nurse attends during a particular period.

Within agencies what is done in quality assurance may differ, but many agencies include some type of retrospective record audit. In this method of assessing the quality of care, the client's record is evaluated after service is discontinued or the record is closed to nursing services. The criteria used for the audit are determined by a group of professionals in the process of a quality assurance program. The retrospective record audit may be conducted by someone who is not a nurse, but is frequently done by nurses as part of their participation on an audit committee.

Criteria are predetermined elements against which quality of care is compared. Criteria are used in audits

Table 15-1   Objectives for a Community Health Agency: Division of Nursing and Specific Programs

Agency	Division of Nursing	Programs
To reduce the infant mortality rate by 10 percent in two years		*Family Planning Program*
		To provide services to fifty new clients sixteen to nineteen years of age each quarter
	To hire during this fiscal year two nurse practitioners for the women's services	
	To develop criteria in two years for evaluating the quality of nursing care provided in the women's health programs	To implement by April a follow-up system for clients who did not keep appointments
		Maternal Health Program
		To establish within six months a maternal clinic in the area of the county with the highest infant mortality
		Child Health Program
		To enroll in the child health program within the first three months of life 25 percent of all infants in the highest infant mortality area in the county
	To provide at least one home visit during this program year to every first-time mother under eighteen years of age	
To achieve an immunization level of 90 percent each year for children five to seventeen years of age		To immunize one-half of all children needing immunizations during preschool round-ups

and may be process or outcome. Process criteria are statements about the activities used by health providers in the management of a health condition. For example, the nurse obtains a blood pressure reading on each home visit to a newly diagnosed hypertensive. Outcome criteria are statements about the end-results of care (Donabedian, 1969). An example of an outcome criterion is: Client states two side effects of antihypertensive medication. Outcome criteria are always written about changes in the client's knowledge, behavior, or health status. An example of a partial audit for outcomes is shown in Case Example 15-2.

Although an agency must provide the lead for development of a quality assurance program, the indi-

vidual community health nurse should join the quality assurance committee, and thereby be involved in and contribute to the development of process and outcome criteria to be used in audits.

Peer Review   *Peer review* is the evaluation of a nurse's clinical nursing practice by associates. Peer review may be included as part of quality assurance or may be viewed as a separate process that is usually initiated by nurses on peer levels, such as community health nurses, nurse practitioners, and clinical nurse specialists. Peer review is concerned with clinical knowledge and performance. Peers judge each other on the degree to which they fulfill written, accepted, objective criteria.

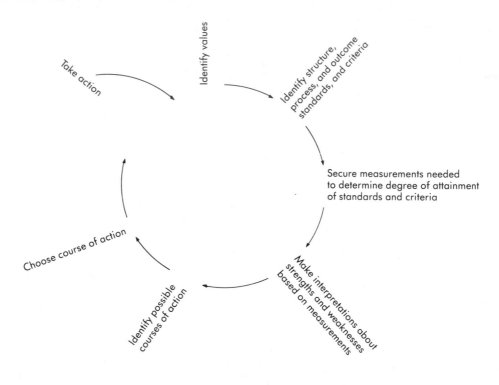

Figure 15-1 Model for Quality Assurance

SOURCE:
From *A Plan for Implementation of the Standards of Nursing Practice.* Published by the
American Nurses' Association and reprinted with permission of ANA.

Case Example 15-2: Outcome Criteria Audit for an Adult with Hypertension

Criteria	Not Met	Met	NA	
1. Client describes reason for taking medication as prescribed.				*Knowledge measurement*
2. Client loses or maintains weight.				*Behavior measurement*
3. Client lists food high in sodium.				*Knowledge measurement*

If nurses use the recommendations from the peer review process, they should experience improvements in the quality of their nursing care (Vengroski & Saarmann, 1978).

Performance Evaluation Just as peer review is part of a professional's responsibility, *performance evaluation* is an integral part of an agency's responsibility in providing safe care to clients. Performance evaluation provides an agency with a procedure for assessing the work behavior of the nursing personnel and determining where improvements are needed.

Each agency sets its own standards for staff members' performance. A new employee has the right and responsibility to become acquainted with the agency's performance evaluation process. Since new nursing employees are generally on probation for about the first six months of employment, they should be aware of what performance expectations are and how they are measured—that is, whether measurement is done with a performance evaluation tool, by observation of clinical practice with use of a tool, through self-evaluation, or with competency-based criteria. Also, the new nurse employee should know who conducts the evaluation. In most situations the immediate supervisor is responsible for conducting the evaluation interview and completing the written evaluation tool.

The evaluation process consists of a series of continuous steps. As a first step, the new nurse employee should be oriented to the specific job description and the performance evaluation tool. In some agencies, a baseline assessment is done of the new employee's skills so that orientation can be primarily directed at deficits. A second step of evaluation should involve an objective-setting conference with the employee's superior. This will provide the employee with specific direction for improvement over the next specified time frame. The third step of the process is a series of regularly scheduled conferences between nurse employee and superior. These conferences should be aimed at assisting the nurse to evaluate progress toward expectations and objectives, to develop skills and knowledge to meet job requirements, and to identify methods for acquiring the needed skills and knowledge. The fourth step is the formal evaluation itself in which the nurse and supervisor discuss the actual achievement of each point on the evaluation tool. The nurse should come to the evaluation session with a self-evaluation, either one's own or a completed copy of the agency's performance evaluation tool. Out of the formal evaluation session should come an agreed-upon written evaluation and revised objectives for the next evaluation period.

Self-Evaluation The last step of the performance evaluation process just described is an example of *self-evaluation* that need not be dependent upon a request from a supervisor for completion. The professional nurse should have a system for self-evaluation if the agency does not provide one. Even though self-evaluation is a subjective process, the nurse is challenged to keep an open mind about his or her own performance. Using an objective tool, such as the agency's performance evaluation tool, may assist the nurse to evaluate himself or herself by a consistent set of criteria. Another tool that can be used is the American Nurses' Association *Standards of Community Health Nursing Practice* (ANA, 1973) (see Chapter 1). This document contains statements that are nursing process oriented—that is, what the nurse is expected to do in giving care to individuals and families. One of the helpful features of the *Standards of Community Health Nursing Practice* is the accompanying assessment factors to be used to measure movement toward achieving the standards. For example, Standard II is: "plans for nursing service include goals derived from nursing diagnoses." One of the assessment factors is: "goals are assigned a time period for achievement."

One approach for using the standards and the assessment factors is to arrange them into an audit format and conduct self-audits on a few records each month. The value of conducting the self-audits is in the identification of patterns of practice behaviors that reveal strengths and weaknesses. For the nurse newly practicing in community health nursing, this type of consistent approach to self-evaluation is a valuable tool for developing professional accountability, which will be addressed later in this chapter. Another technique for self-evaluation is testing of one's performances against descriptions in new nursing literature that describes nursing practices (Peplau, 1971).

Evaluation as a Component of the Nursing Process

Overview of the Nursing Process

As described in Chapter 7, the nursing process consists of five components: assessing, diagnosing, planning, implementing, and evaluating. Applying each part of the nursing process is important if the outcome is to be worthwhile to the client. Since the accuracy of each component is dependent upon the preceding ones, the need for thoroughness and accuracy is obvious. Because the nursing process is primarily an intellectual activity, the nurse demonstrates the results mainly through what is written in the record. If the record is not complete or is inaccurate, the evaluation of nursing care will be incomplete and difficult to perform.

Assessing Usually the record format used by an agency has areas designated for each part of the nursing process. The record serves as a guide and sets a minimum for what information the nurse is to document. In some instances other information not specifically required, such as work hours of a husband or the name of a babysitter, will be needed on the record. The data collection part of assessing still requires that the nurse individualize what and how much data are collected in each family or community situation.

Collecting information that will not or cannot be used is unproductive. Because there is not a formula to follow in deciding what and how much data to collect, the new practicing nurse usually collects more data than are needed to provide safe and competent nursing care. With experience and careful review of the assessment content, the nurse

can limit data collection to only necessary information.

Diagnosing After data have been collected and synthesized, the nurse develops problem statements or nursing diagnoses. These will change as reassessments are done and as the family's situation changes. The list of problems or nursing diagnoses is the basis upon which the nursing care plan is developed.

Planning Developing a care plan is an ongoing process. Although the nurse commits to writing an entire care plan after one or two home or clinic visits, he or she should make changes as more data are obtained and as the client's situation changes. Often the nurse makes mental alterations in the care plan, but does not write the changes as part of the record. Not only does this lack of documentation present potential difficulties for the agency in maintaining an accurate picture of nursing care, but also leaves gaps in information for subsequent nurses and for the profession's study of effective nursing practice.

The nursing care plan for a specific client and/or family should contain objectives that are measurable, realistic, time-oriented statements that have been agreed upon by the appropriate people. The objectives may be written as patient outcomes or goals, but they should include a verb in the active voice, only one purpose or aim, specification of a single end-product or result, and specification of the expected time for achievement (Mager, 1962; Shortell & Richardson, 1978). For example, by the end of the first home visit, Mrs. Brown states three side effects of her antihypertensive medication.

Each objective is directly related to at least one problem or nursing diagnosis identified from the collection of information. For example, the problem "lack of information about infant care" requires achieving several objectives, such as the following, in order to be resolved:

- Mother demonstrates correct technique for bathing infant on first home visit.
- Mother describes by end of first home visit appropriate feeding schedule for infant.
- Mother demonstrates appropriate bottle-feeding technique during first home visit.
- Mother demonstrates correct procedure for preparation of formula on first home visit.

Because the number of objectives could be numerous for some problems, the nurse and client need to decide what are the most important objectives for each problem or diagnosis.

Another part of the care plan is nursing interventions or actions. These are specific activities that the nurse plans to perform in order to achieve the objectives. Although not every detail of the interventions must be included in the care plan, enough description must be contained in order for the nurse who wrote it or another nurse to carry out the plan. Table 15-2 is a care plan for a seventeen-year-old mother, Linda, and her week-old infant, Nicole.

Implementing If the interventions in the nursing care plan have been developed with enough detail, implementing them requires only that the nurse has the requisite knowledge and the appropriate equipment. Often during a client encounter the nurse will need to adjust the interventions to accommodate various situations that arise and additional information.

The nurse needs a variety of approaches for implementing the specific interventions, because each client is different in terms of such characteristics as learning styles, learning abilities, manual skills, motivation, and interest. Although the assessment will provide the nurse with some of the information about characteristics, not all of this will ever be known. Thus the nurse must include the client in every aspect of implementing the interventions. The last step in the nursing process, evaluating, is in practice an inseparable part of implementing.

Evaluating Evaluation, as a component of the nursing process, is not started and stopped at specified times, but is continuous and must occur simultaneously with implementation. For example, as community health nurses demonstrate the technique of taking an infant's temperature, they seek confirmation that the mother is gaining knowledge at each step. During the return demonstration, the community health nurse again evaluates the mother's grasp of the total temperature-taking technique. On a second home visit, the community health nurse may seek further confirmation of the mother's learning by requesting information about the infant's last temperature or by asking the mother to again demonstrate the temperature-taking technique or some aspect of it.

Within the nursing process, evaluation is completed for the same purpose as other types of evaluation. That is, evaluation is done to appraise changes that are intended as the result of an intervention. In the nursing process the changes that result from interventions are changes in the client's behavior, health status, or knowledge. Since nursing is purposive, the results of the nurse's interventions should be measurable and should result in improvements in the client's behavior, health status, and/or knowledge.

Unless these client changes are monitored through evaluation, the nurse does not have information to determine when to schedule the next home visit or clinic visit, what should be included in the next visit, what changes to make in the care plan, and when to terminate a client or family. The evaluation process provides the nurse with data collected systematically at appropriate intervals to make timely decisions about the care of a client and family.

However, the nurse does not make these decisions alone. The other key persons are the client and significant others. Without the involvement

Table 15-2   Nursing Care Plan

Problem or Nursing Diagnosis	Objectives	Nursing Interventions	Date Completed
1. Linda lacks information about sources of health care for Nicole.	1a. By second visit, Linda states choice for regular source of health care for Nicole.	1a. Discuss Linda's criteria for source of health care. Give list of sources that meet criteria.	
	b. On first visit Linda states reasons for need for health care for Nicole.	b. Discuss content of health care visits (e.g., physical exam, immunizations, developmental assessment). Leave pamphlet.	
2. Linda lacks information about contraceptive methods.	2a. On second visit Linda describes two types of contraception control (e.g., barrier, pill).	2a. Give information about types of contraception. Use kit to demonstrate methods.	
	b. By third visit Linda states short-term plans for additional children.	b. Discuss spacing children, plans for school or job, relationship with Nicole's father, and place of additional children in plans.	
3. Nicole wakes and cries four to five times per night.	3a. First home visit, Linda describes three techniques that may encourage Nicole to sleep for longer intervals (e.g., bath at night, holding and rocking, thorough burping).	3a. Assess current techniques. Describe and/or demonstrate others.	
	b. First home visit, Linda describes ways to facilitate rest for herself.	b. Assess current methods. Offer suggestions (e.g., nap when infant sleeps, alternate care-giving with aunt during day).	

Table 15-2   *(continued)*

Problem or Nursing Diagnosis	Objectives	Nursing Interventions	Date Completed
4. Nicole spits up formula after every feeding.	4a. On first home visit, Linda demonstrates proper bottle-feeding technique.	4a. Assess technique. Give additional information as needed.	
	b. On first home visit, Linda demonstrates proper burping technique.	b. Assess burping technique. Demonstrate proper or alternative techniques. Advise re: other actions if spitting up is excessive.	

of recipients of care, the nurse has an incomplete data base and has neglected to include those who have the most to gain or lose as a result of nursing intervention. Clients and their families should be included throughout all phases of the nursing process. If this is done, the involvement of clients in the evaluation process is facilitated. Although it is not easy to incorporate clients' involvement in appropriate phases of the nursing process, the results can be very rewarding for both clients and the nurse. Since the nurse has more knowledge than the client, the nurse's tendency is to assume that her decisions are superior to those of the client. However, professionals need to be ever mindful that decisions are made not on facts alone, but on feelings, preferences, history, and ethical concerns. All decisions are thus more complex than dealing with facts in the abstract. This consideration returns us to the original premise that evaluation is a process of judgment and is concerned with values. The client's involvement in evaluation is not only a matter of ethical "rightness" but also is one approach to securing better evaluation results and decisions.

Logically, before evaluation can be done, the criteria upon which evaluation will be based must be developed. In an effective evaluation of the care

of an individual client and family, the basis of the evaluation necessarily begins with a thorough and accurate assessment. If faulty data are used to generate a care plan, it follows that the interventions will more likely be faulty.

Methods of Evaluating

Objectives   If objectives are written according to the previously identified criteria, the evaluation of care includes deciding whether each objective has been met. The usual reasons for objectives not being met are as follows (Fromer, 1983, p. 353):

- The data base was incorrect or incomplete.
- The problem was based on faulty data.
- The client did not participate in the development of the nursing care plan.
- The objectives were unrealistic or unmeasurable.
- Nursing intervention was ineffective.
- Nursing interventions were not directed at achieving the objectives.
- The client thwarted achievement of the objectives.

Another common reason, not mentioned by Fromer, that objectives appear not to have been met is that the clients' responses, reactions, and changes in health status are not stated in the record. Without the written data, the nurse is forced to rely on memory to determine if the objectives were met. The old adage "If it isn't in the record, it wasn't done" also applies to client behaviors.

If objectives are met, the client and family can be discharged from service. Often when one set of objectives is met, families develop a totally new set of problems that continue to require the nurse's services. In these situations the community health nurse should concentrate on working with the family on problems they feel that they alone cannot manage and on areas for assisting the family to become better at seeking appropriate resources. Almost all community health nurses have experienced working with families that go from one crisis to the next. These types of families may benefit from long-term nursing intervention, but often they accept assistance and make changes only at times of crisis.

If objectives have not been met, the nurse may take one of several actions:

1. Determine with the client or family if the objective is still desirable.
   a. If yes, revise the objective based on new or additional data.
   b. If no, delete the objective.
2. Determine different nursing interventions to meet the original objective.
3. Revise the time frame for the objective.

At times nurses write objectives that are not related to or influenced by nursing interventions—for example, "Client will be free of infection in two weeks." The nurse may influence the client's behavior by offering information about taking medication or seeking medical care, but the nurse does not directly relate to the resolution of the infection by diagnosing it and prescribing medication. Another example is, "Client keeps postpartum clinic appointment." The obvious desired behavior is for the client to have her postpartum clinic visit, but the nurse does not control the patient's behavior to attend the clinic. If this objective is not met, should the nurse change it or put a new time frame on it? Perhaps the nurse's concerns should be foremost that the client is not having any abnormal symptoms, knows where care is available, has the resources to obtain care, and knows about alternate contraceptive control measures. In other situations, such as a mother not taking an ill infant for care, the nurse has the responsibility to continue to closely monitor the infant's condition and take other steps, depending upon the child's condition. Most community health nurses have experienced the need to make decisions for others who are ill and cannot make sound decisions for themselves, especially the young and the aged. In these instances the nurse would very much influence the client behavior by reporting incidence of child neglect or by having an ill, aged client transported to a hospital for admission.

As was stressed previously, clients must be included in the process of determining objectives. Since clients control their own lives, they have the right to choose what they will and will not do. Nursing care cannot be optimal if the nurse does not have cooperation of the client.

Effectiveness of Nursing Interventions
Another issue of evaluation is that all the objectives may be achieved without any real improvement in the client's health status or other indicators. This may happen for several reasons. Perhaps the objectives deal with areas that are tangential to the problems. For example, Mr. Ballard, a newly diagnosed diabetic, lacks knowledge about his disease. Many objectives can be written for this problem. Those that would be most appropriate are related to Mr. Ballard's understanding in order to gain control over his life, thus improving or maintaining his health status. Other objectives that would be ideal or would increase Mr. Ballard's knowledge may not necessarily improve his health status or self-care functioning and are, therefore, to be avoided. For instance, "Mr. Ballard describes the

function of the pancreas in the regulation of blood sugar level." The client requires basic knowledge about the action of insulin, but this need is tempered with the client's desire to know and the use that will be made of the knowledge. Knowledge that is of interest and needed by us as professionals is not always needed or wanted by clients.

Another difficulty in evaluating the effectiveness of nursing intervention is that interventions are not precise and most have not been tested to determine with whom and under what conditions they should be used. In addition to using all his or her own knowledge and skills to develop effective interventions, the community health nurse must frequently use appropriate interventions from other fields and seek consultation from nurse specialists.

For the evaluation of care for the individual client and family, much of what the community health nurse does is not readily measured because it is within the rubric of support, encouragement, and other psychosocial aspects of nursing care. This does not mean that evaluation should exclude these areas. On the contrary, efforts should be especially directed at developing methods for the accurate, if not scientific, evaluation of the psychosocial aspects of care.

In order to evaluate the effectiveness of nursing interventions and thus the achievement of objectives, the nurse should maintain adequate records of his or her actions, as well as the client's responses or outcomes. The nurse may also need to develop flow charts or other similar forms to monitor specific client parameters or behaviors. For example, the nurse might use a form such as the one in Case Example 15-3 to record smoking behaviors of a pregnant woman with whom a community health nurse is working to stop smoking.

Because nursing is a profession that applies information and findings from relevant fields, the community health nurse is always in need of sources of information to update knowledge and skills. Reading journals, attending continuing education

Case Example 15-3: Behavior Monitoring Forms

Client: Kay Pote

Date	Intervention	Number of Cigarettes		
7/15/84	Interval smoking	15		*Form in nursing*
7/18/84	Interval smoking	10		*record that shows*
7/20/84	Interval Smoking & Delayed Start	4		*progress over time.*

Time of Cigarette	Activity	Mood	Habit (H) or Emotional (E)	*Form that client*
8 a.m.	Coffee	Relaxed	H	*kept to link smoking*
9 a.m.	Phone call	Tense	E	*behavior with feelings.*
10 a.m.	Paying bills	Angry	E	

offerings, and participating in professional discussion groups are some techniques that nurses use to improve the effectiveness of nursing interventions. In addition, many areas of clinical research are needed in order to develop effective nursing interventions that contribute to the achievement of specific objectives.

Other Methods of Evaluating In addition to the forms for monitoring client parameters and behaviors, other types of data may contribute to a more thorough evaluation of the effectiveness of care. Two more commonly used pieces of data are client satisfaction and tests of client knowledge.

Client satisfaction data may be a legitimate part of evaluation if they are collected anonymously after care has been discontinued. The nurse may use a short questionnaire that the client completes and returns in a preaddressed stamped envelope. Client satisfaction should not be confused with other more objective measures of care. At times a good level of rapport in the nurse-client relationship may give the client the sense that the total nursing service was at a good level.

Pre- and post-tests may be used by the community health nurse to assist in evaluating the client's achievement in areas of knowledge. Paper and pencil tests have many drawbacks such as client dislike, appropriate reading level, and content validity, but they may be appropriate for some clients. The use of written tests should be mutually agreed upon before the client is asked to complete such an item. Tests that have been used in various content areas may be available in the literature, as well as from some voluntary agencies, such as the American Cancer Society and the American Lung Association. Some agencies have also developed their own tests for specific program areas.

Evaluation as Professional Accountability

Accountability within Nursing Practice

Definition *Accountability* means to be answerable for the responsibilities that one assumes. While *responsibility* refers to expectations of performance, *accountability* refers to the actual performance of the nurse in providing or making services available (Michigan Nurses' Association, 1980). In being accountable the nurse is liable "to be called to account," in a legal sense, for actions taken compared with expected performance. Although accountability and evaluation are not the same, they do overlap. Evaluation is concerned primarily with effectiveness, while accountability is concerned with effectiveness and efficiency (Passos, 1973).

Accountability in Practice In order to be accountable, the nurse must commit to writing the specifics of nursing care upon which his or her accountability will be judged. That is, if no one, including the nurse, knows what the nurse is projecting to accomplish, he or she cannot be held answerable for anything. Accountability for the community health nurse may be viewed as accountability to several "masters," such as supervisor, nursing director, agency administrator, agency, client, and community. Accountability is, however, foremost and most importantly to the client.

In most settings community health nurses work with individuals and families with a great deal of autonomy. This creates a mandate for the nurse to practice at a level characterized by competence in practice, efficiency and economy of services, and an effective nurse-client relationship (Michigan Nurses' Association, 1980). In addition, accountability is manifested from the legal perspective. Hence nurses are subjected to have lawsuits filed against them. Nursing's concern for accountability, though, comes not just from this legal perspective but from other factors external to nursing, such as the following:

- The rising cost of health care without an accompanying improvement in the quality of health
- The increasingly better educated public exposed to formal education as well as information about the limits of health knowledge
- The increasing governmental involvement in financing health care leading to an increased accounting to the public for health services and their costs

Factors internal to nursing have also contributed to an increased concern with accountability:

- Higher education in nursing no longer permits nurses to function routinely and primarily be directed by others. The nursing process and the problem-solving approach require analysis and thus accounting to oneself and others.
- The nursing ethic is moving more toward valuing people and an accompanying view of the client-nurse relationship as a partnership.
- The scope of responsibility in nursing has increased as a result of the expansion of the role of nursing. This has resulted in nurses having the need to share, report, be judged, and be approved (Bergman, 1981).

Accountability and Evaluation

Relationship   Evaluation can be used as a mechanism through which the individual nurse can demonstrate accountability to and for the clients with whom she works. In the process of evaluating, the community health nurse can delineate for clients and himself or herself which objectives have been achieved and how each has contributed to the outcomes. The process is not one of attaching blame, but of being answerable to the client about the nursing care delivered. This kind of nurse-client relationship is one of a professional model and assists the client in understanding what a professional nurse has contributed to an individual's health care. If this kind of professional relationship were established by all community health nurses, the public would have a better idea of what nursing is and how it may differ from medicine and other health care disciplines.

Barriers   The idea of demonstrating accountability partially through evaluation has some problems because of barriers and constraints in the nurse's practice environment. Agency policies may mitigate against the community health nurse implementing some desirable interventions, such as doing home visits in the evening and on weekends when all family members are likely to be home.

Another barrier to accountability through evaluation may be lack of autonomy for nursing in the agency. For example, all orders may need to be signed by a physician, even if the orders require only nursing care. Often this is required by third-party payor reimbursement policies. Agency practice may also create difficulty for nurses in being accountable (e.g., inadequate time for recording and assignments changed without adequate advance notification). The nurse will be unable to follow through on care plans if time and assignments are not, at the least, items that can be negotiated with the immediate supervisor.

These types of barriers to full accountability will probably always exist in some settings in which nurses practice. The nurse's responsibility is to find approaches that allow enhancement of accountability within the barriers and constraints of the specific health care agency. For example, if policy does not allow for evening and weekend home visits, a telephone call to a client's home in the evening may partially accomplish an objective of speaking with the father. Also, at times an exception to a policy may be approved if there is sufficient justification. Other approaches that have been used by community health nurses to reach working parents include a meeting at the place of the parent's employment during a lunch break, a home visit before the parent goes to work, and a meeting at the agency office or other location after working hours. Many constructive solutions to constraints to practice may be shared in case conferences and through using nurse consultants.

Summary

Evaluation is the appraisal of changes that are intended as the result of an intervention. Evaluation occurs at various aggregate and professional levels: division of nursing, program, quality assurance, peer review, performance evaluation, and self-evaluation. This chapter focused on evaluation as a component of the nursing process. Although evaluation has the same purpose at all levels, the methods and tools change, except for the common characteristics of the use of objectives.

For evaluating nursing care, objectives in measurable client-oriented terms provide the most critical tool for evaluating care to the individual and family. These types of objectives state not what the nurse does, but rather what the status of the client will be at the time specified in the objective. The nurse must also evaluate the activities or interventions that were used in implementing the plan of care. This is especially crucial if the objectives were not achieved. Since assessment data serve as the baseline against which progress toward objectives is measured, the nurse must obtain and document an adequate and accurate data base.

One key to a successful evaluation is the inclusion of the client in the process. Clients have the most to gain or lose from nursing care and have control over factors that very much influence the outcomes of care. Including clients in the development and use of tools to measure progress toward an objective is one way to assist with more client control. Accountability to the client is also demonstrated through the evaluation process. Although barriers to the demonstration of accountability exist in almost all practice environments, nurses can develop approaches that deal with the barriers while working to make long-term changes in organizations and systems.

Topics for Nursing Research
• What relationship does knowledge of a condition or health state have to behavior change of an individual?
• What types of teaching interventions by nurses are effective with what types of clients?

Study Questions

Choose the one or more best answer(s):

1. Evaluation is defined as:
   a. The appraisal of changes that are intended as the result of an intervention
   b. The determination of what is right or wrong
   c. A process that uses both objective and subjective information in making appraisals
   d. The measurement of success in reaching objectives
2. Why does a community health nurse need to know about evaluation at aggregate levels?
   a. This is a job expectation.
   b. The nurse is a more accurate data collector if knowledgeable about how data are to be used for evaluation.
   c. The nurse is likely to be involved in evaluation at aggregate levels.
   d. The community health nurse may be involved in committee work related to evaluation.
3. When is evaluation done as part of the nursing process?
   a. Only after implementing nursing actions
   b. Whenever it is needed throughout the nursing process
   c. As part of implementation

d. After the nursing process is completed
4. What are the essential criteria of an objective?
   a. Objectives do not need to meet specific criteria.
   b. Objectives must be broad, specify the nursing action, state an ultimate outcome, and be concise.
   c. Objectives must contain a verb in the active voice—that is, an action verb.
   d. Objectives must state a solitary aim, specify a single result, and include the expected time goal.
5. What is accountability?
   a. Responsibility
   b. The act of being answerable for the responsibilities that one assumes
   c. Meeting one's job description
   d. The act of meeting legal requirements
6. How are evaluation and accountability related?
   a. They are only indirectly related in that both are concerned with the practice of community health nursing.
   b. They are not related because evaluation is a scientific process and accountability is an individual professional concept.
   c. They are both based on the concept of professionalism.
   d. Evaluation is one mechanism through which the nurse demonstrates accountability.

References

American Nurses' Association: *A Plan for Implementation of the Standards of Nursing Practice.* Kansas City, Mo.: American Nurses' Association, 1975.

American Nurses' Association: *Standards of Community Health Nursing Practice.* Kansas City, Mo.: American Nurses' Association, 1973.

Bergman R: Accountability: Definition and dimensions. *Int Nurs Rev* 1981; 28(2): 53–59.

Braden CJ: *The Focus and Limits of Community Health Nursing.* Norwalk, Conn.: Appleton-Century-Crofts, 1984.

Donabedian A: *A Guide to Medical Care Administration, Volume 2: Medical Care Appraisal-Quality and Utilization.* New York: American Public Health Association, 1969.

Fromer MJ: *Community Health Care and the Nursing Process,* 2nd ed. St. Louis, Mo.: Mosby, 1983.

Mager RF: *Preparing Instructional Objectives.* Palo Alto, Calif.: Fearson, 1962.

Michigan Nurses' Association: *Position of Nursing Practice with Standards.* East Lansing, Mich.: Michigan Nurses' Association, 1980.

Paplau H: Responsibility, authority, evaluation and accountability of nursing in patient care. *The Michigan Nurse* 1971; 44(5): 5–7, 20–21, 23.

Passos JY: Accountability: Myth or mandate? *Nurs Adm* 1973; 3(3): 17–22.

Shortell SM, Richardson WO: *Health Program Evaluation.* St. Louis: Mosby, 1978.

Suchman EA: *Evaluation Research Principles and Practice in Public Service and Social Action Programs.* New York: Russell Sage Foundation, 1967.

Vengroski SM, Saarmann L: Peer review in quality assurance. *Am J Nurs* 1978; 78(12): 2094–2096.

Zimmer MJ: Quality assurance for outcomes of patient care. *Nurs Clin North America* 1974; 9(2): 305–315.

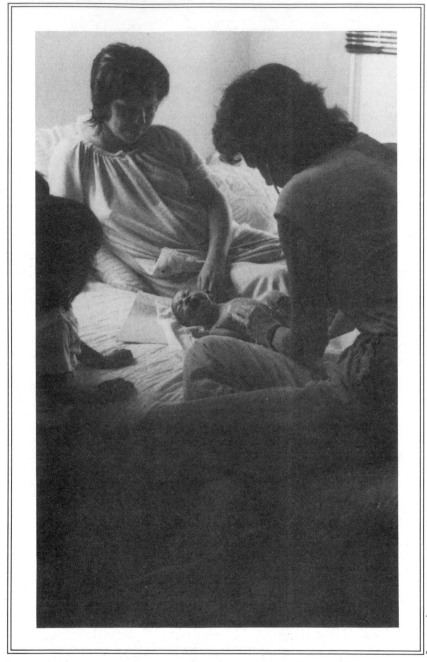

"Nurses of the future will have to be systems analysts as well as care-givers and counselors. They will have to see the family . . . as a group of individuals belonging to different generations with competing, constantly changing needs which should be negotiated in an atmosphere of love and good will." (McBride AB: Can Family Life Survive?" Am J Nursing *(Oct) 1975; 75 (10): 1653.)*

3

Family-Centered Community Health Nursing Practice

Chapter 16

Family-Centered Nursing Across the Life Span

Barbara Bryan Logan

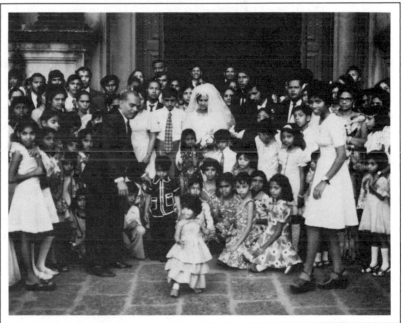

Steve McCurry, Gamma-Liaison

As the source of values and behaviors, and as the mediating influence between the individual and the world, families have a strong effect on health habits and wellbeing. A community health nurse must practice with the awareness of how families grow and develop over time and how they influence the individual.

Chapter Outline

Chapter Objectives

After completing this chapter, the reader will be able to:

- Explain how developmental theory, crisis theory, and the concept of wellness are related
- Contrast social systems and symbolic interactionist analysis of each stage of the life cycle
- Identify (1) the stages of family development as outlined by Duvall and (2) Erikson's eight stages of psychosocial development, and discuss how they are related
- List the situational crises a family is most likely to experience at each stage of family development
- Describe at least two strategies community health nurses can use to promote wellness at each stage of family development
- Explain the concept of anticipatory guidance, and give at least one example of its application to community health nurses

Community health nurses, more than many other groups of health care professionals, are likely to encounter families at varying stages of life-span development. For example, community health nurses enter the home when they visit a family for routine checkups following the birth of a child, or they encounter the family in health institutions or neighborhood clinics when different family members come for health care. Whatever the stage of the family's development, the ultimate goal for families is achievement of their highest state of wellness (see Chapter 13).

Health care's current focus on wellness has evolved as a more holistic perspective than the dominant medical model, which emphasizes disease prevention and treatment. The primary concern of this perspective is the maintenance of wellness and life-styles that promote optimum health—not just the prevention of disease or the treatment of symptoms. Nurses have long recognized the role of the family in maintaining health and healthy life-styles, from conception through old age, for its individual members. Adopting the social systems perspective that sees the family as a group of interdependent, interacting individuals (see Chapter 2), nurses recognize that poor health practices of one family member influence the health of the entire family system. At the same time, good health practices of one member are likely to have positive influences on the entire family system.

The family can serve as a buffer for its members against the dehumanization or impersonalization of bureaucracies and other social institutions (Leavitt, 1982; Pratt, 1976). This protection offered by the family helps to prepare family members for life in a very stressful environment (Friedman, 1981;

Leavitt, 1982). But families can also be a *source* of stress for individual members. For example, they may pressure individual members to succeed in the external competitive environment, or they may impose role expectations that lead to role conflicts among individual members. One of the nurse's most important goals in working with the family is to preserve it as a unit capable of strength and support for its members rather than as a unit of stress and anxiety.

To accomplish this goal requires that nurses have adequate knowledge of (1) how families grow and develop over time, (2) the critical tasks and normal crises they face as a result of development, and (3) the effects these experiences have on their health. This chapter is concerned with families' health across the life span. An overview of the life-cycle perspective is presented first as a framework to view the family as it develops over time. The concept of wellness is discussed as the primary goal of family-centered nursing. An overview of crisis theory also provides a framework whereby nurses can understand, assess, and plan interventions that can minimize the effects of critical life events that can cause family stress and disorganization and, thereby, bring about illness. The chapter looks at families at different developmental stages in the life cycle. Systems theory and symbolic interactionist theory (both introduced in Chapter 2) are also used to show how families may respond to the various crises they face in their developmental cycles. The chapter concludes with a discussion of health promotion strategies that community health nurses can use in helping families to achieve wellness throughout the life span.

Theories and Concepts

The family unit is not static; it changes over time in response to individual members' needs and to outside influences. At each stage of a family's life-cycle development, the community health nurse has an opportunity to promote changes in health behavior and to increase wellness.

The Life-Cycle Perspective

The life-cycle perspective has been defined as the explanation and optimization of developmental processes in the human life course from conception to death (Baltes, Reese, & Lipsitt, 1980). This perspective is rooted in the individual's changing life history, evolving in stages such as marriage, parenthood, and work life (Elder, 1978). The parallel between the life course of the individual and that of the family has led to the concept of family life cycle (Glick, 1957). Family life cycle is viewed in terms of the independent courses or life histories of its various members.

Duvall identifies sequential "stages" of family development throughout the life cycle as well as critical events and developmental tasks families are expected to accomplish at specific stages. The stage analysis basically delineates stages of parenthood and refers to changes in family composition that result from the addition and departure of children from the family (Duvall, 1977). It is important to emphasize that full understanding of a stage (for example, childhood) requires knowing its life-span implications; full understanding of the life span requires understanding of a stage as a unit. The idea of stages is at the heart of the family developmental approach (Hanson, 1983).

With its emphasis on stages, the life-cycle perspective enables community health nurses to (1) anticipate what to expect from families at each stage of development; (2) compare how families at the same stage of development differ from one another; (3) analyze family growth and health promotion needs at different points in the family life cycle; and (4) anticipate families' needs and provide them with support as they develop over time (Friedman, 1981). The family life-cycle perspective, particularly its emphasis on developmental tasks and stages, applies best to traditional families whose development over time is fairly consistent with normative expectations. Consequently, while this framework is useful to nurses, it may not be applicable to all the families nurses encounter. Alternative family structures, such as single-parent families and families without children, are discussed in Chapter 17.

The Concept of Wellness

The concept of wellness is often confused with the concept of health promotion. This is partly because the terms are abstract and people tend to define and interpret them differently. However, it is important to distinguish between them.

Distinguishing Wellness from Health Promotion   Whereas wellness is a state of well-being individuals and families strive (or should strive) to achieve, health promotion can be viewed as a strategy used to achieve wellness. Chapter 13 summarized Brubaker's (1983) review and analysis of the concept of health promotion. With respect to health promotion and wellness Brubaker emphasized that health promotion aims at high-level wellness by encouraging alterations in personal habits or the environment in which people live. Disease prevention and health maintenance are not primary goals, but rather prerequisites or by-products. That is, the health promotion client may not be in perfect health but has achieved a stable state of health without active disease. Brubaker conceives of health promotion as directed toward increasing levels of wellness to the ultimate achievement of high-level wellness. Her conceptualization of wellness is illustrated in Figure 16-1.

High-Level Wellness   According to Brubaker's model, high-level wellness is the ultimate goal of health promotion. This state, defined by Halbert Dunn, a pioneer of the wellness movement, represents a state in which the individual's potential capacity for integrated functioning in his or her environment is maximized (Dunn, 1961).

The state of maximum wellness is achieved through an integrated and dynamic life-style, whereby individuals pursue the highest level of health within their capability by incorporating some aspect of each wellness dimension such as self-

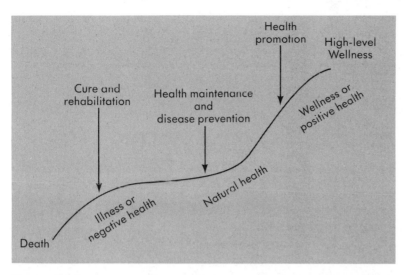

Figure 16-1 Types of health care in relation to areas they address on the health continuum. (Brubaker B: Health promotion: A linguistic analysis. *Adv Nurs Sci* 1983; 5(3): 13. Reprinted with permission of Aspen Systems Corporation, © 1983.)

responsibility, nutritional awareness, stress management, physical fitness, and environmental sensitivity (Ardell, 1977). High-level wellness, therefore, necessitates a life-style whereby individuals are consciously aware of mind and body functioning as a harmonious, integrated whole to achieve a maximum state of health. Family life-style is a key factor that can either promote or impede the maximum state of health individual members achieve.

Family life-styles consist of the family's:

- *Values,* the system of ideas, attitudes and beliefs that bind them together in a common culture
- *Roles,* which define how family members function vis-à-vis each other
- *Communication network,* the way they transmit feelings, ideas, and information among each other within the system and between the system and the rest of society (Hill, 1965)

Achievement of wellness often necessitates lifestyle changes among individuals within families. Such changes—diet modification, weight control, physical fitness, and institution of stress reduction techniques—may be difficult for families to initiate and sustain. Strategies community health nurses can use to help families make these difficult and challenging changes are included in the last section of this chapter.

Crisis Theory

Crisis theory grew out of the need to build a conceptual framework useful to community (preventive) psychiatry (Caplan, 1964), and was influenced by the works of theorists and researchers such as Lindemann (1965) and Erikson (1950), and by studies conducted at the Harvard School of Public and Community Mental Health. The theory was developed with a public health focus that emphasized the concept of prevention of illness in the community. Community health nurses have long used this theory to guide their practice with individuals and families.

Crisis has been defined as an "upset in a steady state"; a situation that occurs when an individual faces a problem he or she cannot solve and, as a result, experiences a rise in inner tension and manifests signs of anxiety; inability to function; and extended periods of emotional upset (Caplan, 1964; Rapoport, 1974). According to Caplan (1964), the person "faces an obstacle to important life goals, that is, for a time, insurmountable through the utilization of customary methods of problem-solving. A period of disorganization ensues, a period of upset during which time abortive attempts at solutions are made" (p. 15). Customary coping strategies and problem-solving methods do not work and the person becomes "upset." (See Box 16-1.)

Crisis Resolution The outcome of crisis depends on the state of the individual at the time of the critical event, the chance aspects of the development of extreme stress, the availability of resources, and the personality of the individual, including whether or not the crisis event is linked symbolically to past events in the person's life and whether or not the individual perceives the situation as stressful (Aguilera & Messick, 1982).

The individual perception is of utmost importance, since the same event may have different meaning to different individuals depending upon cultural, environmental, and personal circumstances. If the crisis event is symbolically linked with a situation the individual or family coped with successfully in the past, the family or individual is likely to cope successfully with the new situation. The opposite is also true. If coping was unsuccessful in the past, it is likely to be unsuccessful in the new situation.

Rapoport (1974) states that three things are likely to happen in response to crisis: the problem may be solved, the problem may be redefined in order to achieve need satisfaction, or the problem may be avoided by ignoring needs and relinquishing goals. If the problem cannot be solved in any of these ways, a major disorganization may ensue. She reports (Rapoport, 1974) that healthy crisis resolution involves:

1. Correct cognitive perception of the situation
2. Management of affect through awareness of feelings and appropriate verbalization leading toward tension discharge and mastery
3. Development of patterns of seeking and using help with actual tasks and feelings by using interpersonal and institutional resources

Community health nurses can assist individuals and families achieve healthy crisis resolution through these three steps.

Types of Crises The family unit experiences different types of crisis in much the same way as individuals. Most families face numerous troubles or stressful life events, and they work out procedures and division of responsibilities for dealing with these crisis events as they arise. However, the outcome of the situation for the family unit will depend on the meaning of the event that precipitated the crisis, the family's definition of the event as stressful, and the adequacy of family function or role performance in relation to the event (Hill, 1965). Crises have been delineated into two primary types: situational and maturational.

Situational crisis refers to unavoidable stressful events or life changes that occur in every individual's life course. These life change events threaten the individual's biological and social integrity, and cause some degree of disequilibrium (Aguilera & Messick, 1982). Examples of such events or crisis situations are death of a loved person, loss or change of a job, and traumatic accidental injuries or surgical procedures (Caplan, 1964).

One of the most widely used scales for studying life's changes as they relate to stressful life events is the Social Readjustment Rating Scale (SRRS) (Elder & Rockwell, 1979). The SRRS, developed by Holmes and Rahe (1967), was discussed in Chapter 8 (see Table 8-1) in the context of family assessment. The scale includes judgments of forty-three life-event changes, ranging from family relationship and economics to social activities. These life events require changes in individual adjustment. They can evoke faulty adaptive efforts by

Box 16-1   What Is a "Crisis"?

A crisis has several characteristic features. First, a crisis does not go on indefinitely—that is, a relatively short period of psychological disequilibrium accompanies the process. Usually it lasts from one to six weeks. Second, the period is divided into certain typical phases such as beginning, middle, and end (Rapoport, 1965). This phase characteristic is illustrated by Bowlby (1960) and Lindemann (1965). Bowlby studied hospitalized young children and found that their responses to the crisis of hospitalization could be identified by three distinct phases: protest, despair, and detachment. Lindemann (1965) studied bereavement and described the crisis of grief reaction in three stages: Stage 1, or beginning phase, when the bereaved starts to emancipate himself or herself from the bondage to the deceased; Stage 2, or the middle phase, when the bereaved makes a readjustment to the environment in which the deceased is missing; and Stage 3, or the end phase, when the bereaved forms new relationships or patterns of interaction that brings reward and satisfaction. Finally, crisis is both a *danger,* because it threatens to overwhelm the individual or family, and an *opportunity,* because it increases the individual or family's receptivity to therapeutic influence (Aguilera & Messick, 1982).

The characteristic of crisis as an opportunity was well demonstrated in the pioneer work of Erick Lindemann (1965), who was concerned with promoting good mental health and preventing emotional disturbances. As a result of his studies on bereavement reactions, Lindemann concluded that whereas bereavement or grief could be followed by emotional disturbances in a considerable proportion of the population, such disturbances could be prevented through crisis intervention supplied at the appropriate time by trained members of the clergy and appropriate community representatives. Thus the crisis situation presents an opportunity to intervene in order to prevent mental disturbance and may even allow people in crisis to develop more effective coping strategies, and function at a higher level of equilibrium than before the crisis (Aguilera & Messick, 1982).

The characteristic of crisis as an opportunity for growth has great relevance for community health nurses, who can supply the skillful intervention that will restore family equilibrium and prevent ill health. Depending upon the situation and nature of the crisis, community health nurses can themselves provide such intervention or refer individuals or families to appropriate sources who can.

---

the individuals and lower their bodily resistance, thereby enhancing the probability of disease. There is a strong positive correlation between the magnitude of life change (life crisis) and seriousness of the illness experienced. Illness or health changes observed (following a life-event change) covered a wide range of psychiatric, medical, and surgical disorders (Holmes & Masuda, 1974).

Elder and Rockwell (1979) contend that the effects of life changes on individuals depend on the timing of such change within the life course. For example, death of a spouse is given a maximum score on the SRRS scale, but if it occurs in young adulthood immediately after marriage and with young children present, it is likely to be more upsetting to the surviving spouse than if it occurred in old age after a prolonged, difficult illness.

The SRRS has achieved a high level of consistent agreement across different cultures and across varied groups of old and young, and males and females (Askenazy, Dohrenwend, & Dohrenwend, 1977). It is of use to community health nurses in that it provides a background of the types of crisis-producing events that can occur throughout a family's life course and the expected impact of such events. When assessing the impact of such events, nurses should consider the following: (1) the nature of the change (whether it brought about drastic alterations in customary habits, whether it resulted in loss or gain, and whether the change was expected); (2) the expectations and adaptive skills that one brings to the change and its position in the life course in relation to other events (Elder, 1974; Elder & Rockwell, 1979). It should be emphasized that there will be differential responses to life-change events depending on variability in individuals' and families' personal and situational circumstances.

Maturational crises are conflicts encountered by all human beings as they develop and are faced with transitions, or normal biological periods of growth throughout the life cycle. These periods of growth are characterized by marked physical, psychological, and social change, and are associated with a certain set of tasks that must be faced and mastered with a reasonable degree of effectiveness if the next transition or maturational stage is to yield its full potential for further growth and development.

Erikson (1950) devised an eight-stage model of growth and development, which is based on the notion that psychosocial development proceeds in an orderly sequence of stages from infancy to senescence. These stages are characterized by a series of crises or critical periods. Certain developmental tasks must be solved at each stage as a result of the individual's personal development and encounters with the social environment. A person's degree of

success in passing through one stage will influence his or her ability to move to, and pass successfully through, the next stage. The stages delineated are:

1. Trust versus mistrust
2. Autonomy versus shame and doubt
3. Initiative versus guilt
4. Industry versus inferiority
5. Identity versus identity diffusion
6. Intimacy versus isolation
7. Generativity versus stagnation
8. Integrity versus despair

Erikson's theory emphasized the normal rather than the pathological and integrated the biological, cultural, and self-deterministic points of view. The conflicts or tasks delineated are targeted to the individual as she or he encounters and interacts with the sociocultural environment. Maturational crises as highlighted by Erikson's eight stages of development, Duvall's conceptualization of stages and developmental tasks, and the concept of situational crisis together provide a good framework for understanding and analyzing the process of individual and family development over time. This process is illustrated by Table 16-1. The table, which has been adapted from Duvall, Erikson, and the SRRS scale, provides examples of the types of family developmental tasks and possible situational crises individuals face as they progress through the various stages of psychosocial development. Each stage is discussed in the following section.

Families Across the Life Cycle

This section provides an overview of families at different stages in the life cycle. The stages, which have been adapted from Duvall (1977) (see Chapter 2), include:

1. Beginning families
2. Families with very young children
3. Families with school-age children

4. Families with adolescents
5. Families launching young adults
6. Families with middle-aged members
7. Aging families

These families are discussed in terms of the life-cycle perspective and the family developmental tasks they face, and in terms of the possible maturational

Table 16-1 Family Developmental Tasks, Maturational and Situational Crises in the Family Life Cycle

Stage of Family Development[a]	Approximate Age/Year in Developmental Period	Major Family Developmental Tasks[a]	Stage of Psychosocial Development[b]	Likely or Typical Types of Situational Crisis[c]
Beginning families	(2 years)	Establishing a mutually satisfying marriage (finding a mate, getting married)	Intimacy vs. isolation	Marriage
Families with very young children		Establishing a mutually satisfying home for parents and infants		Pregnancy Gaining a new family member
		Adapting to parenthood	Trust vs. mistrust (infants)	Birth defects
Families with preschool children	Oldest child 30 months to 6 years	Adapting to needs and interests of preschool child; coping with energy depletion; lack of privacy	Autonomy vs. shame and doubt (toddler)	Personal injury or illness (accidents in children) work-related changes
Families with school-age children	Oldest child 6 to 18 years (7 years)	Encouraging children's education achievement; fitting into the community of school-age families	Industry vs. inferiority	Changing to a new school Divorce Marital separation Residential change
Families with adolescents	Oldest child 13–20 years (7 years)	Balancing teenage responsibility and freedom, establishing postparental interests	Identity vs. role confusion	Major business readjustment Major change in financial state Son/daughter leaving home
Families launching young adults	First child gone to last child leaving home (8 years)	Rebuilding marital relationship; maintaining ties with other generations	Intimacy vs. isolation	Onset of chronic illness Intergenerational conflicts
Families with middle-aged members	(15 years)	Maintaining ties with other generations	Generativity vs. self-absorption	Physical problems—onset of cancer, heart disease, diabetes, etc.
Aging families	10–15 years	Adjust to retirement, loneliness, and old age	Integrity vs. despair	Death of a spouse

SOURCES:
[a]Adapted from Duvall; depicts stages of family development throughout the life cycle.

[b]These conflicts (as defined by Erikson) or tasks are maturational crisis experienced by individuals within the family unit. Their successful accomplishment or resolution depends on effective functioning of the family system.

[c]These are examples of life changes or crisis from the SRRS that are likely to occur at particular stages of family development. Their timing in the developmental cycle is likely to influence the severity of their impact on the family system (e.g., death of spouse typically occurs in aging families, but can be more traumatic if it occurs in beginning families).

Duvall E: *Marriage and Family Development,* 5th ed. Philadelphia: Lippincott, 1977.

Erikson E: *Childhood and Society.* New York: Norton, 1950.

crises (as outlined by Erikson) and situational crises that can occur at each stage.

In addition, each phase of family development is discussed from the symbolic interactionist and social systems perspectives (see Chapter 2). Community health nurses can draw upon the traditions of the symbolic interactionists by looking upon each stage of family development from the perspectives of the families themselves and by understanding the meanings families attach to particular stages and the crises and other events surrounding them. In order to help individuals and families adequately meet their needs, nurses have to understand how those individuals and families view their world. On the other hand, social systems theory contributes to nurses' understanding that individuals and families function and interact within a network of people and institutions, and that such interactions can affect health.

Beginning Families

According to Duvall's stages of family development, married couples initiate the beginning of a family. The marriage ceremony can be considered as the ceremonial rite of passage that signals the beginning of a family. The relationship that the couple establishes as they form a couple system is of utmost importance. This fact has been emphasized by noted family therapist Virginia Satir who describes married couples as the "architects" of the family system. They are the people-makers who promote feelings of self-worth in the family system. It is their relationship that influences the homeostasis of the entire family system and creates "the axis around which all other family relationships are formed" (Satir, 1967, p. 1).

Life-Cycle Perspective and Developmental Task　This particular developmental stage in the life cycle is when couples must accomplish the task of establishing a mutually satisfying marriage. Consistent with the life-cycle perspective is the notion that the ease or difficulty with which couples face and successfully accomplish this task depends on its timing in the life cycle and the context in which it takes place. This includes the couple's preparation for the event. Apparently some couples prepare to accomplish the task of establishing a mutually satisfying marriage for varying periods before their marriage ceremonies. Based on sixty interviews of twenty engaged couples, Bernstein, Dixon, and Knafl (1978) report that in the process of committing themselves to a life together, couples go through three broad stages of couple relationship:

1. *Initiation stage*—individuals first encounter one another and begin casual social interactions and actual dates
2. *Sustaining stage*—couples move from a fun-oriented dating relationship to a commitment to permanence during which they systematically evaluate each other as possible marriage partners
3. *Commitment stage*—couples decide to marry and communicate this decision to family and friends.

These stages are illustrated in Figure 16-2. In addition to the couple's readiness for marriage, other factors that may affect their adjustment to this period are age, career development, financial and personal circumstances, and their personal development.

Maturational Crises　To establish a mutually satisfying relationship as a couple, young adults must have successfully resolved the maturational crisis described by Erikson (1950) (see Table 16-1) as "intimacy vs. isolation." Successful mastery of this stage increases the ability of each partner to experience the true intimacy that makes it possible for the couple to have a sense of identity of their own and at the same time establish a mutually satisfying marriage.

Situational Crises　During this time the couple could experience any number of stressful crisis-producing events (examples and their magnitudes are listed in the Social Readjustment Rating Scale in Table 8-1). Nurses should be aware that situational crises will affect couples differently, depending upon their unique set of circumstances and their interpretation of the crisis event. For example, some deeply religious black families may interpret a crisis (such as a serious illness) to be an act of God. Accordingly, they will turn to God through prayers and other religious activities to help them cope with the crisis. This is particularly true if they have limited resources and have experienced racial discrimination and other negative experiences in the health care system. Health care professionals may misinterpret these families' behaviors as helplessness, disinterest, and apathy when, in reality, the

Developmental stages in the process of becoming engaged.

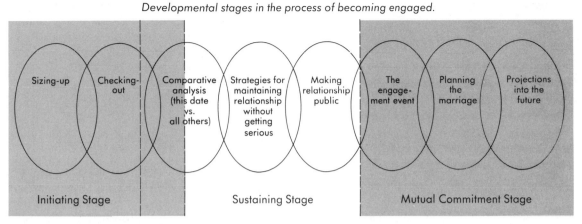

Figure 16-2 Developmental stages in the process of becoming engaged. (Knafl K, Grace H: *Families Across the Life Cycle.* Little, Brown, 1978, p. 30.)

families' energies are turned inward—devoted to reliance on their religious faith.

Symbolic Interactionist Perspective   A nurse's knowledge of the beginning stage of family development is only speculative until the knowledge is applied to, and verified by, specific families. When using the symbolic interactionist perspective, nurses can obtain individual partner's and families' views and analysis of this period, and the symbolic meanings they attach to the events surrounding it. Nurses cannot assume that a spouse holds the same meanings and definitions of events as his or her marital partner. Obtaining individual partner's and families' own perspective on marriage and beginning family development necessitates questions that are consistent with the symbolic interactionist perspective. These questions would yield a wide range of responses, and are likely to vary from family to family as well as from one spouse to another. For example, each of the following questions could yield a variety of responses:

- *What is the meaning of marriage?* (status symbol; fulfillment of societal expectations; a close, meaningful relationship; culturally accepted tradition; an institution necessary for sexual fulfillment and reproduction)

- *What do you expect from marriage?* (children; close relationship; emotional and financial security; a wife or husband to take care of or who will care for me)
- *What is the meaning of a child (children) to you?* (someone to love and care for; someone to be dependent on me; someone I can depend on or dominate; someone to perpetuate the family name and traditions; source for fulfillment of needs and fantasies)
- *How do you define wellness?* (absence of symptoms; feeling good; a program of good diet and regular exercise; psychological well-being; not having to go to the doctor)
- *How do you define illness?* (presence of symptoms; inability to function or execute daily responsibilities; not being able to get out of bed)
- *How do you define a healthy life-style?* (regular balanced diet, rest, and exercise; maintenance of a sense of well-being; absence of illness)

Responses to these questions will allow the nurse to:

1. Clearly see variations among spouses and among different couples in terms of the meanings they attach to a significant event such as marriage

2. Understand each partner's hopes, expectations, and fears concerning marriage, and how, if at all, the individual communicates these to the other spouse
3. Clarify each partner's definitions of health, illness, and wellness, and identify areas for therapeutic intervention
4. Identify misfitting expectations that may cause conflict in the marital relationship
5. Identify potential areas for ill health (psychosocial or physical), and promote wellness through anticipatory planning and guidance

Couples can become disillusioned when they discover that their spouse is different from what they expected during courtship. Community health nurses can encourage young couples to openly discuss differentness and role expectations in order to promote harmony in the spouse relationship and head off long-term family problems and ill health.

Social Systems Perspective The social systems framework allows nurses to examine both intrafamilial and extrafamilial relationships that are characteristic of the beginning stages of family development, and that facilitate or hinder successful resolution of maturational crises and family developmental tasks. Intrafamilial relationships include a network of interactions between the marital couple such as their communication system, or their method of dealing with separateness and differentness as well as their unity as a couple system. Resolution of these issues may depend on values and expectations learned within their own families of origin that might have been carried on for generations.

Interfamily relationships involve the couples' interactions and relations with other systems and networks outside the immediate family unit. Beginning families are particularly involved with systems such as extended family networks (in-laws), friendship networks, coworkers, and health systems. The new couple faces the task of establishing themselves as a unit, separate from their families of origin, while at the same time redefining their relationship with families of origin and friends.

Community health nurses are in excellent positions to examine family linkages with extrafamilial systems, and to serve as a conduit effecting good open communication between families and these systems (see Case Example 16-1).

Families with Very Young Children

One of the biggest decisions beginning families face concerns children—whether to have them, how many to have, and when. Some couples make these decisions during their courtship, while others come to the decision through negotiations during the early stages of marriage and beyond.

Life-Cycle Perspective and Developmental Task According to Duvall (1977), families with young children face the developmental task of establishing a satisfying home for both parents and infants. Parents learn to adapt to parenthood and to the needs and interests of their young children. While this task is primarily that of the spouse system, there are simultaneous situational crises children face as they are added to the family and grow and develop. Parents are responsible for creating a home environment conducive to the successful accomplishment of their task as well as to the successful resolution of developmental milestones their children face. This means that parents are alert to the safety of their physical environment, and that they teach children self-care skills as they grow and mature.

Maturational Crises A critical event during this period is arrival of the first child. Erikson defines the developmental task for the new infant (birth to eighteen or twenty-four months) as the establishment of "trust vs. mistrust." Achievement of this task requires maternal bonding—a close interactional relationship between the infant and constant mother figure. This relationship allows the infant to fulfill dependency needs and develop a sense of security, which fosters development of trust in the mother and, consequently, in the environ-

Case Example 16-1: Nursing Assessment and Intervention With Beginning Family.

Mrs. Jones, a community health nurse with the Visiting Nurses' Association, made her regularly scheduled visit to Ms. Carter, a fifty-year-old black woman who has been a chronic diabetic. Ms. Carter told Mrs. Jones that she was doing well, but added, "Frankly, nurse, I'm worried about my daughter. She is supposed to be married in one month and she is a nervous wreck. She is jumpy, jittery, and on top of it all she broke out in this terrible rash. Could you talk with her? She won't talk to me. Being a nurse, maybe you can help." Mrs. Jones agreed to talk with Brenda, Ms. Carter's twenty-four-year-old daughter.

Community health nurse's entry in the family system is with one member, but she recognizes the opportunity to help another family member.

In the initial phase of the meeting between Brenda and Mrs. Jones, Brenda was quiet. She said, "Nothing is wrong. I'm just running around a lot to get everything done for the wedding. My mother worries too much. This rash is nothing but overexposure to the sun." Mrs. Jones sat quietly, smiled at Brenda, and said, "Tell me about your wedding." Brenda said nothing. Gradually her hands began to shake and tears rolled down her cheeks. She said, "It's just that things are moving so fast. My fiancé, Tom, all of a sudden he starts talking about when you quit your job, and when you are at home taking care of our home and our baby, you're going to be so happy. I never told him I want to quit working, and I certainly don't want a baby, not anytime soon!"

The nurse adopts nonjudgmental attitude to encourage client to express feelings.

Client is facing a critical event—marriage.

Client and fiancé have different perceptions and expectations of marriage including different ideas about roles.

Based on information Brenda shared, Mrs. Jones concluded that Tom comes from a traditional family where his mother never worked outside their home. His father was the breadwinner, and his mother always remained at home taking care of the family. Brenda's situation was opposite—her mother always worked. She expected that she, like her mother, would continue to work and would have children but "some time in the future." She and Tom never discussed these issues. They concentrated mostly on their love for each other, which Brenda admits is very strong, but now she is worried.

Families of origin influence couple's expectations in forming their own family system, demonstrating interfamily relationships.

Mrs. Jones recommended that Brenda and Tom attend a premarriage enrichment seminar for couples in their community. Brenda talked with Tom, and the couple made the arrangements and decided to attend the sessions. The seminars provided information as well as allowed the couple the opportunity to discuss feelings and issues with other couples in a group setting.

Nurse capitalizes on the knowledge of crisis as an opportunity for growth.

Couple's decision is a move toward establishing groundwork for a mutually satisfying relationship.

---

ment. Maternal bonding is a reciprocal relationship. As the infant develops trust, the mother becomes secured in her mothering skills, thus raising her feelings of self-esteem.

As the infant grows older and moves into toddlerhood, Erikson believes that the child faces the maturational crisis of "autonomy vs. shame and doubt" (from about eighteen months or two years to about three and a half to four years). During this time toilet training begins as the young child learns to develop bowel and bladder control. The young child can move toward successful resolution of this conflict if he or she developed an overall sense of trust, including trust in self and the environment during the period of infancy. The toddler is, therefore, able to learn self-control. If the task is accomplished successfully, the toddler can emerge from this period self-assured, proud rather than ashamed, and can move to the preschool stage. At this stage the child faces the developmental crisis of "initiative vs. guilt." Erikson believes this is the play stage (from about age three and a half to entry into formal school). The child broadens skills through play and fantasy. If the child resolves this crisis successfully, he or she faces the world with confidence, high self-esteem, and initiative to begin and experience new things. The parents can feel proud that they have created and fostered an environment in which their young child feels safe, and can develop a sense of trust, autonomy, and initiative. They can become more secured in their parenting skills and continue to develop their relationship as an interdependent couple system.

Situational Crises   The period of early childhood can be fraught with accidents. As the infant develops through preschool years and begins to explore the environment, he or she may encounter such accidents as falling, ingestion of toxic substances, and burns from fire or other substances. Such accidents may cause serious injuries and/or illness to the child, thus creating a crisis for the family. Other childhood illnesses may become evident at this time, such as those derived from birth defects, injuries, or developmental maladjustments. In addition, parents may encounter crisis situations such as death of loved ones, job or career changes, or even marital difficulties. A nurse's understanding of wellness, growth and development, and crisis theory can be utilized to assist families develop and practice measures to prevent some of these crisis situations from occurring. Or the nurse can apply anticipatory guidance to minimize the effects of such crises should they occur. The nurse can also work with community groups to achieve this goal (see Case Example 16-2).

Symbolic Interactionist Perspective   Whereas theories concerning childbearing families can greatly facilitate the nurse's knowledge of this period, it is important to validate theoretical formulations with specific families. The symbolic interactionist perspective requires that nurses explore with each family the meaning of the childbearing experience. The

Case Example 16-2: Health Promotion with Young Families

A group of housewives who are also mothers of preschool children organized a network of young mothers for the improvement for community services to mothers and their preschool children. They organized play groups for the children, diet and exercise groups for the mothers, child care services on an exchange basis, and group sessions on child development and child care. They invited Ms. Penn, a community health nurse, to speak to one of their sessions on child development and on recognizing and dealing with young children who are sick. Ms. Penn capitalized on the opportunity for health teaching and health promotion with this special population and negotiated and planned with the mothers to present ongoing seminars particularly emphasizing safety and accident prevention among young children.

Community health nurse networks with community group for improved services to families with young children.

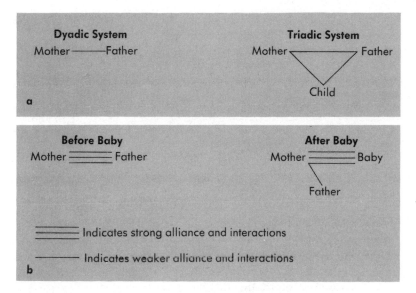

Figure 16-3 (a) Dyadic and triadic family system. (b) Strong and weak family alliances and interactions.

family's own definitions and meanings should be a significant part of nursing assessment and subsequent interventions.

Social Systems Perspective This perspective allows the nurse to examine intrafamilial and interfamilial relationships. The arrival of the first child creates a triadic (three-person) instead of a dyadic (two-person) system. See Figure 16-3a. The triadic system creates demands for new interactive patterns and, consequently, new role relationships. One person may feel left out as interactions are intensified and alliances are formed between two people in the family system. In young families the father may feel left out as the mother spends most of her time with the baby and develops a stronger alliance with the child. See Figure 16-3b.

This points to the need for couples to recognize their need for personal time and space as children are added to the family and their demands increase. Couples should share time with each other as well as with the child.

With respect to interfamily systems, the couple with their new baby must work out relationships with extended kinship networks (particularly grandparents), friends, child care systems, and health systems. The health care system exemplified by a nurse practitioner, community health nurse, private physician, or clinic personnel can encourage regular physical examinations to monitor the infant's health, to detect health problems and correct them before irreparable damage is done, to establish immunity against certain infectious diseases, and to continue to monitor the health of parents, particularly the mother who must have postpartum checkups to restore her optimum health. Daycare centers or other child care systems may become important for single-parent, dual-career, and other types of families who use them daily or occasionally. Many families at this time become involved with the families of other children with whom their children play. Community health nurses can help new families recognize the importance of establishing boundaries around their family unit yet have these boundaries flexible enough to facilitate communication between extrafamilial systems. This is important for the continued growth and development of the family unit.

Families with School-Age Children

According to Duvall (1977), this period begins when the oldest child reaches age six and (in American culture) enters elementary school. It is the busiest period for many families. During these years the child's world expands beyond the family. Formal school, organized sports, and peer group activities become a significant part of the child's life. He or she now learns the values, rules, and regulations of others outside the family. As children question their family values vis-à-vis those of others, parents may feel pressured to adjust their own values to conform to accepted community values common to school-age children. They may also feel reluctant to let their children go as they press for increased freedom to develop other interests outside the home. During this time parents, like their children, are apt to be very busy with their own career and/or other civic activities. They are responsible, however, for helping their child to complete developmental tasks and maintain the integrity of the family unit.

Life-Cycle Perspective and Developmental Task   Duvall (1977) outlines the developmental task for families of school-age children as encouraging children's education and achievement and fitting into the community of school-age families. The successful accomplishment of this task depends on other events that are occurring in the family. Negative events that could affect the family at this time are illness of any family member, marital conflicts and marital separation, unemployment, and job or career conflicts of one or both spouse. Some mothers who remain home to raise their children during the early years return to work at this time. Whereas this change may increase the financial stability of the family, it may call for changes in role relationships and division of labor, which could disrupt the family system. However, if there are flexible role relationships and allocation of tasks, the family can accomplish developmental tasks with little difficulty.

Maturational Crises   Erikson (1950) defines the developmental conflict of school-age children as "industry vs. inferiority." Although many school-age children in American society would have had some experience outside the home in daycare centers or other child care facilities, the development of true industry begins when the child enters formal school at the elementary level. The child must now learn to listen to the teacher, conform to rules and regulations, learn good work habits, and further develop cognitive capabilities. The child faces numerous challenges as he or she participates in organized sports and learns to excel in competition. The child also learns to relate to others— peers, teachers, and other adults—in socially acceptable ways. Parents should provide opportunities for the child to be challenged in learning and doing; this can be done by allowing for participation in activities that are carefully selected and monitored for the child's safety and protection. The family should provide an environment whereby the child learns discipline, not as punishment but as a mechanism that protects her or him from physical and emotional harm.

The child who successfully masters this stage has a positive self-concept, a sense of responsibility and belonging, a sense of confidence rather than inferiority, and the ability to accept successes as well as failures or disappointments.

Situational Crises   Like the preschool child, the school-aged child is subjected to injuries caused by accidents and can manifest physical handicaps. For example, injuries may result from motor vehicle accidents, drowning, fires, and other chemical substances. Physical handicaps may result from diseases such as cancer, diabetes, and various respiratory conditions. The school-aged child may also be prone to nutritional deficiencies, obesity and lack of physical fitness; smoking and drug and alcohol abuse may begin at this time. Such situations coupled with any number of crisis events that may beset other members of the immediate and extended family may create strain on the family system and may inhibit successful accomplishment of family and individual developmental tasks. Marital dissatisfaction has been reported to be high during this stage (see Rollins & Feldman, 1970). Consequently, school-age families are likely to experience the situational crises of marital separation and even divorce. Some researchers (Menaghan, 1983) call for additional studies to substantiate the marital dissatisfaction theory. However, it is still important that within the family unit there are opportunities for each parent to continue his or her own growth and development. It is essential that their personal needs are met and that they work on strengthening the spouse relationship.

Symbolic Interactionist Perspective The meanings and responses to children approaching school age will differ among families. Some children could view this stage as freedom from overprotective families and approach it with eagerness to participate in the world outside the family. Others may fear leaving the protection of the family unit, because they anticipate fear and frustration in learning and handling new relationships outside the family system. To some children, this period may signify increased growth and therefore increased responsibilities. Parents could view this period as symbolic of their losing some control over their children or as increased financial security if the wife is returning to the work force. It is clear that in order for community health nurses to adequately address their client's health needs, they need to understand their clients' interpretation and definition of these significant life events.

Social Systems Perspective The social system's perspective facilitates examination of the interrelationships between the various units or other systems with which the family is involved. The school is the primary child-focused system with which the family interfaces. The child is also likely to be involved in religious activities such as church school. Children may also be involved in other organized systems in the community such as Boy Scouts, Girl Scouts, or 4-H clubs. These systems are avenues whereby the school-age child can learn new things and gain recognition for his or her accomplishments. These systems, some of which

are organized along sex lines, also allow children to learn accepted gender-role behavior, and continued development of a sense of self as male or female as they prepare for adolescence.

Parents are also likely to be involved in occupational and other community systems. Input they gain from interacting with these various systems may cause them to adjust or change their own child-rearing practices or modify their family rules and norms. Examples of primary systems that the family is likely to be involved with are illustrated in Figure 16-4. Parents may be involved in related religious and community activities with their children. For example, one or both parents may participate in teaching church school or in coaching Little League baseball or as leaders in child-focused community activities. Community health nurses are in excellent positions to interface with the family and related systems. The pivotal role of the school nurse in promoting health of families with school-age children is discussed in Chapter 19.

Families with Adolescents

Adolescence is said to be the most difficult period for parents and children, perhaps because of conflicts and power struggles between them. According to Duvall's (1977) theory, this period begins when the oldest child reaches age thirteen and ends about six to seven years later when he or she leaves home. Many theorists describe this period as a transition from childhood to adulthood.

Life-Cycle Perspective and Developmental Task Duvall's family developmental task for this period is balancing teenage responsibility and freedom, and establishing postparental interests. There are numerous processes occurring simultaneously within the family unit. First, the adolescent is growing and developing rapidly. The body is changing physically, and with the onset of puberty, there is increased sexual awareness and interest in, as well as attraction to, the opposite sex. These inner changes are compounded by the demands of the educational system for satisfactory academic

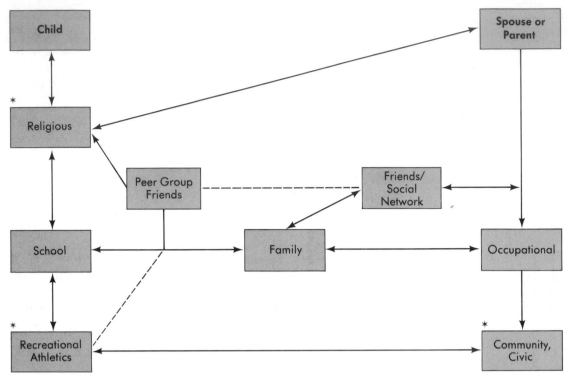

* Parents and children may be simultaneously involved in these subsystems, although assuming different roles.

Figure 16-4 Intrarelationships of primary systems in families with school-age children.

performance and peer pressure to conform to social values and norms of the peer group. The adolescent is pulled outside of the family to seek independence and to meet expectations of the peer group. His or her attempts at independence and self-expression may be acted out in rebellious activities, which then cause conflicts with parents.

Second, parents at this time may be dealing with personal issues such as health problems as their own bodies begin to change, career concerns, or community involvements, in addition to dealing with teenagers and perhaps younger children in the family. The timing of other events in their lives will affect how families accomplish their task and manage this period. Such events may include absence or presence of illnesses; satisfaction or dissatisfaction with career; adequate or inadequate finances; successful or difficult parent-child rela-

tionships at previous stages of family development; established plans for the future and chances of activating these plans; and location of the family in a community with desirable available or unavailable resources.

Maturational Crises While parents begin or continue to establish postparental interests, they are also involved in helping their teens to resolve the adolescence crisis Erikson defines as "developing identity vs. role confusion." In their quest for a sense of identity, teenagers typically break away from their families, which have been the center of their existence, and turn to their peer group for support and security. They tend to have greater feelings of belonging with their peers than with their families. The peer group allows them freedom from parental supervision and the opportunity to decrease their emotional attachment to parents and at the same time gain a sense of independence. To develop a sense of identity, it is important that the accelerated physical and psychosocial changes adolescents experience are integrated into a whole. They need to devise ways to cope with physical changes, increased sexual awareness, and peer pressure and learn to balance freedom and independence with responsibility. Erikson believes that a child who emerges successfully from this period has a clear sexual identity of manhood or womanhood. He or she develops a sense of "who am I" both in terms of sexual identity and in selection of a career or occupational role.

Situational Crises Automobile accidents and athletic injuries are very common in adolescence. Substance abuse resulting in injuries and ill-health and other health concerns such as suicide may also occur. Chapter 25 is devoted to adolescent pregnancy, which is another major problem at this time. In addition, parents of adolescents may be at risk to certain health conditions such as coronary heart disease, cancer, and hypertension. Death of loved ones and changes in job, career, or place of residence may also occur at this time. These stressful life events are likely to cause illness in the family.

Symbolic Interactionist Perspective This perspective facilitates understanding this period in terms of the meaning parents and adolescents attach to it. Having a teenager may signify to some parents that they are growing old, to some that they will soon encounter financial demands of a college education, and to some that their children will soon be launched in the adult world with their own responsibilities, thus leaving the couple time to devote to their marital relationship, career, and/or other interests. Other parents may want to keep teenagers at home so they can continue to invest in them rather than in their marital relationship. For some adolescents the teenage years may present opportunities to explore and "try on" new identities or cultural life-styles contrary to their families. To some they may mean confusion over one's interpersonal relationships, sexual identity, and/or career

paths. The predominant meanings adolescents and their parents attach to this period will influence their overt actions.

Social Systems Perspective Systems theory is particularly useful in examining intrafamilial relationships, particularly communication patterns of parents and adolescents, and interfamilial relationships, specifically adolescent peer group and parent interaction. Communication between parents and adolescents may be inhibited because of misunderstandings between parents and adolescents over a number of issues. Adolescents may challenge parental norms and values by their increased self-expression of sexuality and by acting out other peer group values. There may be misconceptions and misperceptions because of what is termed the "generation gap" between American teenagers and their parents. It is said that because of this gap parents and their adolescents seldom discuss issues and feelings openly and meaningfully. Failure to communicate openly could cause increased tension, stress, and ultimately ill health in the family system. Through anticipatory planning nurses can assist parents and their teenagers to communicate effectively and devise more open ways of working through sensitive feelings and issues. Parents should understand that despite their apparent distance and rebelliousness, teenagers still need parental guidance, support, and limit setting in a warm, accepting family atmosphere.

Because teenagers tend to go outside the family and look to their peer group for support and guidance, the peer group can be considered one of the most important systems in the lives of adolescents. Often there is conflict between the values of the peer group and those of the family. Nurses can help parents understand that teenagers turn to peer groups partly because of their quest to become independent and to be launched from the family to assume adult roles. The peer group can function as a constructive socializing agent in this process. As adolescents become more involved in peer group relationships, parents can continue to develop other nonchildbearing interests. Case Example 16-3 shows how parents are included in a teen clinic.

Case Example 16-3: Nursing Intervention During Adolescence

Ms. Bennet is a young community health nurse who works in a middle income community with a large population of teenagers. Working in collaboration with a teacher at a local high school, Ms. Bennet started an early evening "teen clinic" for teenagers at the health center in the community. The clinic was open from 4 to 6 P.M. Tuesdays and Thursdays. Every Thursday from 4 to 5 P.M., coeducational rap session groups were held for teens to discuss any issue of concern to them including: coping with physical changes, parents, the opposite sex, relationships, school, teachers, and the drug culture. Sessions on college preparation, job preparation, and self-management skills were also included. On Tuesdays teens could make individual appointments for physical checkups, family planning counseling, and any other matters of importance to them. Parent sessions were held monthly for parents to discuss (in a group atmosphere) personal concerns and concerns related to their relationship with their own teens or teens in general. In addition once per month at scheduled times, teens could invite their parents or parent representative for teen-parent rap sessions.

Community health nurse works in collaboration with high school teacher to develop innovative "teen clinic."

Group approach capitalizes on the power and importance of the peer group in adolescence.

Clinic is organized to address issues of concern to teens.

Clinic recognizes need for parent participation and need to establish good communication between parents and teenagers.

Families Launching Young Adults

The adolescent task of developing a sense of identity—a sense of who one is and where one is going—is in preparation for the next stage when that adolescent leaves the protection of the family to assume independent living. Duvall (1977) describes this period of family development as the launching stage. It begins when the first child leaves home, and ends when the last child leaves home, creating the "empty nest." The period lasts approximately eight years, depending upon how many children are in the family and when they leave home. Because of the current economic situation in the United States and other parts of the world, increasing numbers of young adults may remain at home or continue to require economic and other types of supports from their families. This factor will lengthen the number of years families remain in the launching stage.

Life-Cycle Perspective and Developmental Task Duvall (1977) outlines the family developmental task for this period as rebuilding marital relationships and maintaining ties with other generations. The simultaneous processes occurring in the family at this time are: (1) the children leave home to establish family units of their own with unique life-styles and values, and (2) the family shifts from a child-centered household to a primarily couple (husband-wife) unit. During this time both the young adults and the parents are faced with their own unique maturational crises. Consequently, how the family manages the launching depends on how they resolve individual crises and the nature of events surrounding their lives at that time.

Maturational Crises Erikson (1950) outlines the task of the young adult as learning "intimacy vs. isolation." This was discussed previously in terms of beginning families. It is discussed here in terms of the dynamics of the launching stage. To experience true intimacy, which is necessary to establish a good marriage or true friendship, the young adult must have achieved a good sense of self-identity as well as a certain level of independence and disengagement from the family unit. Issues raised in adolescence such as solidifying a career choice, selecting a mate, and establishing a new life and a new family are now reality and must be confronted. The capacity for intimacy allows the young adult to enter a partnership with someone with whom he or she can make a commitment to share life's experiences, meet life's demands, and thereby establish a framework for marriage. This results in compromise and joint decision making.

Meanwhile the parents of young adults are likely to be experiencing midlife crises, a situation described by Sheehy (1974) in her popular book, *Passages,* as a period of time when men (ages forty to forty-five) and women (ages thirty-five to forty) experience acute discomfort as they reach the midpoint of their lives and come to a crossroad where they face the discrepancies between earlier youthful ambitions and actual achievement, and the realities of their current situations. People at this stage are often dissatisfied with the way life has developed and they are ambivalent and uncertain about the future. These feelings are compounded by the realization of physical deterioration or signs of aging evidenced by graying hair, wrinkled skin, diminishing eyesight, and approaching menopause and climacteric. Sheehy also views this period as having the potential for personal development and growth if men and women critically reexamine and reassess their lives. They can move "away from institutional claims and other people's agenda . . . away from external valuations and accreditations, in search of an inner validation. [They] are moving out of roles and into the self" (p. 251). She contends that the midlife crisis offers individuals the "opportunity to emerge reborn, authentically unique, with an enlarged capacity to love ourselves and embrace others" (p. 251). This achievement would greatly enhance the potential of marital couples to readjust to, and strengthen, the spouse system following the absence of their children. Suc-

cessful launching of the children, and the continued integrity of the spouse-system is highly dependent on whether or not the marital relationship remains fulfilling for each spouse.

Situational Crises   During this period the family is most likely to experience critical events such as death of a loved one (as parents begin to lose their own parents), the birth of a grandchild, changes in jobs or careers, and business or financial readjustment. The young adult's leaving home is also a stressful event that can produce crises in the family. Parents may now be diagnosed as having life-threatening diseases such as heart conditions or cancer, and other chronic disabling conditions such as hypertension or diabetes. All of this could create great stress for the family.

Symbolic Interactionist Perspective   As with the other stages of family development, family members' perception of the stage will greatly influence how they make the transition. For example, some parents may interpret their young adult's bid for freedom not as a part of their continued development, growth, and maturity but as a rejection of them. Consequently, they hinder rather than encourage and facilitate this progress. The launching of the young adult may cause parents to reexperience some of their own unresolved conflicts related to this stage. Consequently, the meaning they attach to the event may be related to these old conflicts rather than to the current situation. Young adults may also attach various meanings to the situation. Whereas for some it could mean fear due to increased responsibilities, to others it could mean a desired time of challenge to establish new ideas and relationships with potential spouses and friends. It can even mean a time to begin new relationships with parents since some young adults can now provide their parents with support and understanding, thus reversing their previous role relationships.

Social Systems Perspective   This perspective can be used to examine structure and function, communication networks, and power hierarchy in

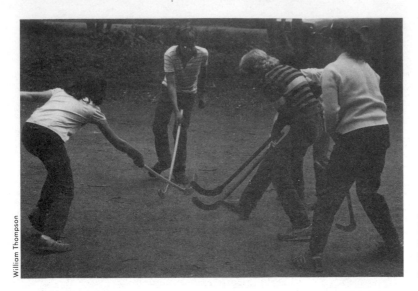

William Thompson

As school-age children become increasingly active and independent, the potential for their experiencing serious injuries also increases.

the intrafamilial system and relationships between the generations once the children are launched. The overall structure and function of the family system are changing in the launching stage of family development. Whereas the family previously had been structured around the inclusion and nurturing of children, the current system is now structured around the needs of the spouse-system and how it functions to facilitate the launching of children who are becoming adults. This means that parents no longer have complete decision-making power, but young adults share hierarchical power with their parents, who should now support them in their new decision-making capacity. Parents must be open enough to accept their young adults—their values and life-styles, including their choice of occupation, marital partner, residence, and other factors. This level of acceptance requires regular, open effective communication between parents and children.

When young adults leave home and form their own family systems, they decide on the type of intergenerational relationship they will maintain with their family of origin. Minuchin (1974) contends that young adults may, on the one hand, remain either too enmeshed or too disengaged from their families. On the other hand, they may establish clear boundaries flexible enough to promote

the young family's own growth and development, and at the same time facilitate effective communications and good relationships with other generations. Undoubtedly the outcome will be influenced by years of explicit and implicit negotiations that occurred previously in their daily routines while growing up in their families (Minuchin, 1974).

Families with Middle-Aged Members

This stage of family development consists essentially of the couple. Duvall (1977) describes it as beginning with the empty nest (when the last child leaves home) and ending with retirement or death of one of the spouses. With the couple's child-bearing and child-rearing responsibilities essentially over, the couple now has time to reexamine their lives and make suitable changes. They can turn from being other-oriented to being self-oriented (Diekelmann & Galloway, 1975).

Life-Cycle Perspective and Developmental Task According to Duvall (1977), the family developmental task at this stage is to maintain ties with other generations. This may entail redefining or establishing a satisfying and meaningful relationship with one's children and grandchildren, parents, and siblings. The middle-aged couple, who are now at the end of the reproductive cycle (menopause in women, climacteric in men), may suddenly come to the realization that they as well as their parents and siblings are aging. This necessitates adjustment to changes in body image and acceptance of these changes not only in oneself but also in one's peers, siblings, and parents. However, successful accomplishment of the developmental task depends on other events or situations in the couple's lives at this time (i.e., satisfaction or dissatisfaction with career; presence or absence of illness; meaningful or unsatisfactory intergenerational relationships; financial status).

Maturational Crises From Erikson's (1950) perspective the middle-aged adult faces the conflict of "generativity vs. self-absorption or stagnation." Successful accomplishment of this task requires middle-aged adults to remain creative and productive, and show concern for future generations by contributing to their development and guidance. Accomplishment of this task will depend on the adult's level of self-esteem, and degree of comfort with oneself. This self-awareness may require a self-orientation that involves assessment in four areas outlined by Diekelmann and Galloway (1975, p. 997) as:

1. Increasing one's self-esteem by developing more self-awareness
2. Separating from one's parents and children by slowly becoming a more independent and secure adult
3. Reviewing one's own values by confronting one's own existing value system
4. Initiating plans for the future by recognizing the aging process, and planning for aging as part of the future (this involves preparation for retirement)

Whereas all middle-aged adults face these tasks, their methods of accomplishing them may differ.

Situational Crises Middle-aged adults are predisposed to numerous situational crises. With aging parents, spouses, and siblings, they are particularly prone to experience the death of a loved one. Physical disabilities and/or chronic illnesses may be prevalent and very stressful at this time. Loss of employment and other undesirable job or career and residential changes can also be very traumatic and produce crises. This is also a time when a family could gain a new member (an aging parent). Such a situation can be stressful but can also be rewarding if carefully planned.

Symbolic Interactionist Perspective For some couples the empty nest may mean loneliness and isolation, while others may view it as a period of rediscovery when they are free from child-rearing activities and can pursue new hobbies, travel, join different clubs, or engage in other types of leisure-time activities. Some couples may define this stage as a time to pay attention to a healthier life-style of diet and exercise, while others view it as a time when they and others around them are susceptible and vulnerable to illnesses over which they have no control. It is important that the meanings families attach to middle age are explored so that they can be assisted with meaningful planning and development of effective coping strategies to meet the challenges of this and the subsequent stage.

Social Systems Perspective The systems framework can be used to understand the network of intergenerational relationships with which the middle-aged couple is involved. (See Figure 16-5. Relationships with the couple's children, parents, and siblings are illustrated.)

It is important that an effective open communication system is maintained with all family networks. This may necessitate working through conflicts derived from different beliefs, values, and life-styles that each unit has adopted over the years. The relationship and communication patterns of the couple system are of themselves most important. This is perhaps the first time that the couple have had so much time to spend together. A mutually satisfying marital relationship can help couples adjust to aging parents, deal with children whose life-styles may be in conflict with their fam-

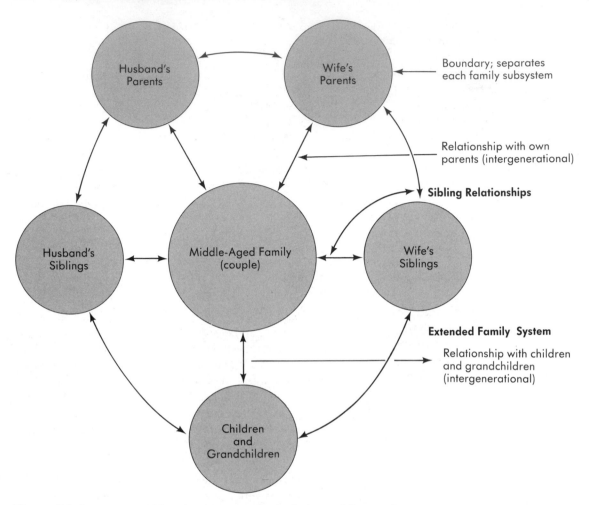

Figure 16-5 Network of family systems with which the middle-aged family is involved. Each unit is a subsystem of the extended family system and is separated by its own boundaries.

ily values, maintain kinship ties, and, in general, meet the developmental tasks of the middle years (see Case Example 16-4).

Aging Families

This stage of family development begins with the retirement of one or both spouses, ends with the death of the other spouse, and lasts for approxi-

mately ten to fifteen years. According to Duvall (1977) this is the last stage of family development. Erikson (1950) defines the maturational crises for this period as "integrity vs. despair." This requires having the wisdom to accept what has gone on without resentment and disappointment so that the present and future can be lived with integrity. (See Chapter 23 for a full discussion of families at this developmental stage.)

Case Example 16-4: Assessment and Referral of a Middle-Aged Couple

Fifty-three-year-old Mrs. Johnson came to the neighborhood health center complaining of heart palpitation and frequent crying spells. After taking Mrs. Johnson's vital signs and obtaining a brief history of her personal and family life situation, Mrs. Cole, the community health nurse discovered that Mrs. Johnson has been a housewife all her life. She has three children: a son who is married and out of the home; a daughter who has completed college, is currently working, and is also out of the home; and the youngest child, Maryann, who is about to leave home for college. Mr. and Mrs. Johnson maintained close relationships with all their children, but Mrs. Johnson, has been closer to the children, particularly to her youngest, Maryann. At the same time she has become increasingly distant from her fireman husband who had been very busy with his job the last few years. However, recently, Mr. Johnson who is sixty years old has been thinking about retiring and moving to another state as their youngest child prepares to leave home for college. Mrs. Cole recognized that Mrs. Johnson was facing a critical stage of family development: launching her youngest child, the empty nest, and her husband's retirement as well as possible residential relocation. In addition, Mrs. Johnson's relationship with her husband had deteriorated as she became more involved with the children and he with his job. Mrs. Cole discussed these issues with Mrs. Johnson and her feelings related to them. They arrived at a mutual decision that Mr. and Mrs. Johnson could benefit from family counseling to work through these issues and better adjust to the normal crisis they face. Mrs. Johnson discussed the recommendation with her husband who after much encouragement from Mrs. Cole agreed to the family sessions. Mrs. Cole made the referral and the family followed through. Mrs. Cole also arranged for Mrs. Johnson to have a thorough physical examination and heart disease was ruled out. Mrs. Johnson was in excellent physical condition.

Community health nurse assesses client situation.

Family is in the launching stage. Youngest child is about to leave home, creating "empty nest."

Family must prepare for retirement of husband and father and possible relocation.

Community health nurse's knowledge of human growth and development and crisis theory enables her to make accurate assessment and referral.

Nurse's action is an example of anticipatory guidance. Family counseling instituted now can promote a better couple relationship and therefore avoid more serious problems later.

Implications and Strategies for Community Health Nurses

Based on this overview of families at different stages of the life cycle, community health nurses can develop strategies to promote family health. While the main thrust of this chapter has been the family whose development most closely fits the pattern and sequence of the life-cycle perspective and developmental task model, the implications and strategies are also applicable to families with alternative structures and development such as those discussed in Chapter 17.

The strategies discussed are directed primarily toward health promotion and achievement of high-level wellness as opposed to disease prevention. They include promotion of self-responsibility and self-care for individuals and families and consumer advocacy for community groups. (See also Chapter

13 for general health promotion strategies that can be applied to families.)

Promotion of Self-Responsibility and Self-Care

A wellness perspective requires that families take responsibility for their own health. Some families may be reluctant to assume self-responsibility and self-care, and in order to motivate them nurses may need to point out risk factors—the probability that a family member may develop an illness and the consequences of that illness for the individual as well as for the family. Assuming self-responsibility may require life-style changes such as cessation of smoking, reduction of alcohol intake, weight control, regular physical exercise, regular self-examination of the body (particularly those areas susceptible to disease), and healthier relationships and communication patterns in the family system. To maintain life-style changes, families may need to establish self-contracts, whereby they plan to learn and practice behaviors that promote wellness on an ongoing basis. Community health nurses can be very instrumental in helping families to achieve this goal. Strategies that can be effectively used in this endeavor are: (1) *anticipatory guidance*, (2) *assessment* that is complete and culturally relevant, and (3) *health teaching*.

Anticipatory Guidance Community health nurses' knowledge of predictable stressful life events and their characteristic behavioral patterns, including their potential to cause crisis and ultimately illness, allows the nurse to anticipate when a family is likely to experience crisis, the nature of the crisis, and the problems likely to be associated with it. Nurses can use their knowledge of crisis theory to help families problem-solve, thereby strengthening their coping skills, reducing the impact of the crisis, and preventing illness. If the stressful event leads to crisis, the nurse can use crisis intervention techniques to solve the crisis. According to Aguilera and Messick (1982), these

techniques include "helping the individual to gain an intellectual understanding of the crisis, assisting the individual bring his feelings into the open, exploring past and present coping mechanisms, finding and using situational supports, and anticipatory planning to reduce the possibility of future crisis" (p. 26). Basic steps of crisis management include: (1) assessment of the family in crisis; (2) development of a plan with the family in crisis; (3) implementation of the plan drawing on personal, social, and material resources; (4) follow-up and evaluation of the crisis management process and resolution of the crisis (Hoff, 1984, p. 27). These steps are illustrated in Case Example 16-5. Through anticipatory guidance, community health nurses can, therefore, provide families with skills that can maximize their potential for healthy living and move them up on the health continuum toward high-level wellness.

Assessment Assessment is an important strategy in health promotion. As discussed in Chapter 8, baseline data are obtained from the family to determine the quality of family functioning, strengths and weaknesses of both the family unit and each individual member, and the specific health status of each family member. A holistic assessment would address the five components described in Chapter 8: physical, psychosocial, sociocultural, nutritional, and environmental. It is important to remember that the family is an active participant in the nurse's assessment, with both nurse and family reaching consensus about the assessment outcome. The nurse shares the assessment with the family and listens to their concerns and explanations. Together they arrive at common agreements about their current health status, life-styles, level of function, overall strengths and deficits, and information concerning what they need for optimum growth and development of their members. Once the assessment has been completed, family problems or health needs are identified, and plans and implementation strategies are instituted by the family to meet these needs or alleviate the problems. The community health nurse works with the family in these processes.

Table 16-2   Health Education Programs for Families Across the Life Span

Stage of Family Development	Areas for Health Education Programs
Beginning families	Marriage enrichment, marriage counseling Family planning Pregnancy; preparing for parenting
Families with very young children	Growth and development of infants and young children Care of infants and young children Detecting early signs and symptoms of illness in infants and young children Maternal/infant bonding Safety in the home
Families with school-age children	Immunization Safety and school-age children Teaching children self-care Sex education Human reproduction; menstruation Managing work and family
Family with adolescents	Sexuality and Responsibility Reproduction, contraception, pregnancy, and childbirth Managing independence Peer-group relationships Male-female relationships Driving safely to prevent accidents and death Parent-adolescent communication
Families launching young adults	Dealing with the empty nest Marital relationships after children leave home
Families with middle-aged members	Stress management Weight reduction and control Self-examination Dealing with aging parents Being a grandparent
Aging families	The aging process: physical and psychosocial changes Health and physical fitness Retirement

Health Teaching   Health teaching, which has been discussed in Chapter 13, is one of the most important strategies community health nurses can employ to educate families about health promotion and wellness. Through health education families can gain the knowledge necessary to establish patterns or behaviors that can have lifelong positive impact on their health. To educate families concerning their health, community health nurses may employ a variety of methods such as dissemination of health information, group discussions, and lectures. Nurses can reach families through schools,

Case Example 16-5: Nurses' Knowledge of Anticipatory Guidance Helps Family Avoid Full-Blown Crisis

Mrs. Benson, a community health nurse, made a home visit for follow-up assessment of one of her clients, forty-two-year-old Mrs. J. and her eight-week-old baby son Jason. Mrs. J. has three other children: Dana, age twenty-two, who is away at college; John, age sixteen, who is in high school; and Gloria, age thirteen, who is nearing completion of elementary school. When Mrs. Benson arrived at the J. family home, she observed that Jason was apparently developing well, but the house was in some disarray and Mrs. J. appeared sad. She asked Mrs. J. how she was feeling. Mrs. J. began to cry while telling Mrs. Benson that her sixty-eight-year-old mother had died shortly after the birth of her child. She explained, "It's just so hard for me. I just can't seem to cope; we were so close." Mrs. Benson allowed Mrs. J. time to discuss her feelings and the events related to them. She learned that Mrs. J.'s mother was sick for a long time with cancer of the breast, but her death was unexpected. Mrs. J. has three sisters with whom she is very close; two of them live in the same neighborhood. Mrs. J.'s husband is a long-distance truck driver who "earns a good living" but spends much time away from home. Mrs. J. has been a housewife and worked part-time in a dry cleaning facility until Jason's birth. She is now at home. She always took good care of her family and coped well with a variety of situations in the past. "But now I'm having so much trouble, all I want to do is cry. I can't even take care of Jason the way I should." (Her son and daughter at home are fairly self-sufficient.)

In the assessment of the J. family done conjointly with Mrs. J., Mrs. Benson also learned that the J. family is very

Client (mother) has experienced child-birth—a developmental crisis.

Family is still in child-bearing stage while launching young adult.

Community health nurse assesses family. Family has experienced a situational crisis or stressful event in the death of a loved one—Mrs. J.'s mother.

Family is in a state of disequilibrium.

Nurse facilitates open discussion of feelings and events.

Potential support systems and areas of strengths and weaknesses are identified.

Mother's previous level of functioning and coping skills are identified.

Mother's previous coping skills are not working successfully.

occupational settings, community groups and organizations, local health departments and health centers, and families' homes. Information families need will depend on their unique circumstances and particular stage of development including the psychosocial development of individual members. A comprehensive health education program for families should cover the following areas: (1) human growth and development to establish a base of normalcy; (2) nutritional awareness, including the relationship of food to health; (3) personal hygiene and physical fitness; (4) dental health, including the relationship of diet to good dental health and the role of fluoridation in reducing tooth decay in young children; (5) stress reduction and stress management; (6) detection and management of common health problems; and (7) the role of self-care and self-responsibility in achieving wellness. Community health nurses may devise and conduct health education programs specific to particular stages of family development as illustrated in Table 16-2.

Various private and government organizations compile consumer-oriented health education materials that community health nurses can use in religious. Their pastor and church members are always supportive of one another, but the J.'s have a strong family belief—to rely only on themselves to solve their problems. Mrs. Benson realized that Mrs. J. was experiencing several stressful events simultaneously: the death of her mother, the birth of a baby (while Mrs. J. is approaching the middle years), launching a young adult, and Mr. J.'s absences from home. Mrs. Benson also noted that Mrs. J. was very overweight and was paying little attention to her diet. Recognizing the potential for Mrs. J. to experience a full-blown crisis that could seriously affect her physical and emotional health as well as that of her family, Mrs. Benson took action to help Mrs. J. resolve her problems. She enlisted consultation from the community mental health nurse specialist and together with Mrs. J. they devised a plan: (1) realistically appraise her situation; (2) identify her resources (her children, her sisters, church members, her husband, and his good income); and devise ways to use these resources (e.g., provide her with companionship so she is not alone for long periods, assist with the baby, allow her to discuss her feelings of loss related to losing her mother, and assist with household chores). With encouragement from Mrs. Benson, Mrs. J. was able to accept assistance from church members most of which was in the form of emotional support—prayer meetings consistent with their religious beliefs. These were most helpful to Mrs. J. in working through the death of her mother.

Within a few weeks Mrs. J. was feeling in control of herself, and family equilibrium was restored. Mrs. Benson then initiated the issue of Mrs. J.'s overweight condition. They reached consensus that it was a problem affecting Mrs. J.'s overall health. A self-contract was initiated whereby Mrs. J. agreed to initiate and closely follow a weight control program with periodic follow-ups.

Religious background and church members are resources and potential sources of support that family may ignore because of family values.

Anticipatory guidance is employed to resolve problem before full-blown crisis is experienced.

Collaboration is set up with psychiatric nurse.

Plan of action is developed.

Plan is implemented with help from personal resources.

Nurse employs strategy of anticipatory guidance—to help client institute self responsibility to improve her health status with follow-up and evaluation.

health teaching. Examples of such organizations are the March of Dimes, the American Cancer Society, the American Health, Lung, and Diabetic Associations and the Department of Health and Human Services. These organizations may be contacted for their most current information.

Consumer Advocacy

Community health nurses can advocate for individuals and families at the community level. This can be accomplished in several ways. They can act as liaisons between families and numerous community agencies to families. Nurses can bring to families' awareness the existence of health information through the media and through consumer and government reports. They can also assist families to locate as well as obtain access to health facilities and other resources necessary to maintain health. They can let families know what to expect from these agencies and how to ensure that their rights are not violated. In other words, community health nurses support families' efforts in acting in their own behalf in order to maintain healthy lifestyles. This is particularly important for families at high risk to health problems such as those ethnic minority groups whose members may be in socioeconomic disadvantaged positions with limited access to quality health care.

Community health nurses can also participate in a wide range of social actions that can lead to improved health of families. For instance, nurses can lobby their local and state legislators to obtain community resources such as accessible quality health services for all citizens and adequate housing and recreational facilities. Nurses can add vital support to community drives such as campaigns for car seat belts to curtail fatal accidents; movements for safety caps on medicine and other toxic substances to protect children from accidental poison-

ing; and support for food stamps, school lunch, breakfast, and WIC (Women, Infant and Children) food supplementary programs for women, infants, children, and other groups in need of health and health-related services. Nurses can also participate in community drives to protect families from unsafe drinking water, nuclear wastes, and other environmental health hazards. Nurses can also organize and participate in communitywide health fairs, conduct health screening for prevention and early detection of diseases that are common at various stages of the life cycle, and distribute health promotion information. Nurses can also work closely with their governmental representatives to provide input to be included in bills and other legislative processes that shape social policies affecting families' health.

Summary

This chapter described the family life-cycle perspective, the concept of wellness, and crisis theory as a background for understanding the various types of families community health nurses encounter in their practice. Knowledge of family development (stages and tasks), Erikson's eight stages of psychosocial development, maturational crises, and situational crises allow the nurse to plan anticipatory guidance and other wellness strategies that can be implemented in terms of each family's specific level of development. Nurses' increased knowledge of families will enhance their efforts to implement family-centered nursing.

Topics for Nursing Research

• How do families define, interpret, and respond to stressful life events?

• Compare health promotion measures of families with young children with those of families with school-age children.

• What are health education needs of first-time parents?

• Compare the adjustment young couples make to accommodate their new baby in two different ethnic groups.

• How do families teach their children self-care measures?

• How do middle-aged families deal with loss (i.e., the death of a spouse compared to the death of a parent)?

• What adjustments do middle-aged couples make in preparation for retirement?

• Design a pre- and posttest to evaluate the effectiveness of a two-hour health education program for teenagers.

Study Questions

1. Which of the following statements accurately describes the life-cycle perspective?
   a. It enables nurses to anticipate what to expect from families at each stage of development.
   b. It is concerned primarily with families as a group, not with individuals.
   c. It is applicable to all families.
   d. It does not permit analysis of roles in domains such as marriage and occupation.

2. Twenty-two-year-old Terry, who is about to get married, came to a neighborhood health center for her blood test. She encountered the community health nurse, who saw that Terry was very upset. The nurse took time to explore with Terry the reason why she was upset. Terry's response was, "It's this wedding. I don't know if I want to go through with it." The nurse then explored with Terry the meaning of the wedding to the young woman, her feelings and perceptions of the upcoming event, and other circumstances surrounding the wedding as perceived by Terry.
   Which of the following theoretical perspectives is *most* likely to be the one guiding the nurse's interaction with Terry?
   a. Social systems
   b. Symbolic interaction
   c. Crisis theory
   d. None of the above

3. Achieving a state of wellness depends on which of the following?
   a. Exercising self-responsibility
   b. Maintaining a healthy life-style
   c. Ability to manage stress
   d. All of the above

4. Mrs. Jones is a forty-eight-year-old mother of three whose own mother recently died. Mrs. Jones is very upset. Which of the following is *least* likely to affect the outcome of this stressful event for Mrs. Jones?
   a. Type and nature of available resources
   b. Mrs. Jones's own personality and previous method of handling stress
   c. Mrs. Jones's perception and interpretation of her mother's death
   d. The socioeconomic status of Mrs. Jones's family

5. A community health nurse visited Mrs. Jones in her home for postpartum checkup and realized that she was depressed and having difficulty mourning the loss of her mother. Recognizing the need to help Mrs. Jones avoid a full-blown crisis that could seriously affect her health, the community health nurse referred her for psychological counseling. The nurse's action is an example of which of the following?
   a. Tertiary prevention
   b. Anticipatory guidance
   c. Life-style change
   d. Secondary prevention

References

Aguilera D, Messick J: *Crisis Intervention: Theory and Methodology*, 4th ed. St. Louis: Mosby, 1982.

Ardell DB: *High Level Wellness*. Emmaus, Pa.: Rodale Press, 1977.

Askenazy AR, Dohrenwend BP, Dohrenwend BS: Some effects of social class and ethnic group membership on judgements of the magnitude of stressful life events: A research note. *J Health Soc Behav* 1977; 18: 432–439.

Baltes PB, Reese HW, Lipsitt LP: Life span developmental psychology. *Ann Rev Psychol* 1980; 31: 65–110.

Bernstein BJ, Dixon DM, Knafl KA: Relationships in process: forming a couple identity. In: Knafl K, Grace H (editors), *Families Across the Life Cycle*. Boston: Little, Brown, 1978.

Bowlby J: Separation anxiety. *Int J Psychoanal* 1960; 41: 89–113.

Brubaker BH: Health promotion: A linguistic analysis. *Adv Nurs Sci* 1983; 5 (3): 1–14.

Caplan G: *Principles of Preventive Psychiatry*. New York: Basic Books, 1964.

Duvall E: *Marriage and Family Development*, 5th ed. Philadelphia: Lippincott, 1977.

Diekelmann N, Galloway K: The middle years: Emotional tasks of the middle adult. *Am J Nurs* 1975; 75 (6): 997–1001.

Dunn HL: *High Level Wellness*. Arlington, Va.: R.W. Beatty Co., 1961.

Elder G: Family history and the life course. In: Hareven TK (editor), *Transitions: The Family and Life Course in Historical Perspective*. New York: Academic Press, 1978.

Elder GH, Rockwell RC: The life-course and human development: An ecological perspective. *Int J Behav Develop* 1979; 2: 1–21.

Erikson E: *Childhood and Society.* New York: Norton, 1950.

Friedman MM: *Family Nursing: Theory and Assessment.* New York: Appleton-Century-Crofts, 1981.

Gilliss CL: The family as a unit of analysis: Strategies for the nurse researcher. *Adv Nurs Sci* 1983; 5 (3): 50–59.

Glick PC: *American Families.* New York: Wiley, 1957.

Hanson SL: A family life-cycle approach to the socio-economic attainment of working women. *Journal of Marriage and the Family* 1983; 45 (5): 323–338.

Healthy People: The Surgeon General's Report on Health Promotion and Disease Prevention. US Department of Health, Education, and Welfare, 1979.

Hill R: Generic features of families under stress. In: Parad HJ (editor), *Crisis Intervention: Selected Readings.* New York: Family Service Association of America, 1965.

Hoff L: *People in Crisis: Understanding and Helping.* Menlo Park, Calif.: Addison-Wesley, 1984.

Holmes TH, Masuda M: Life change and illness susceptibility. In: Dohrenwend BS, Dohrenwend BP (editors), *Stressful Life Events: Their Nature and Effects.* New York: Wiley, 1974.

Holmes T, Rahe R: The social readjustment rating scale. *J Psychosom Res* 1967; 11: 213–218.

Knafl KA, Grace HK: Family beginnings: Premarital relationships. In: Knafl KA, Grace HK (editors), *Families Across the Life Cycle.* Boston: Little, Brown, 1978.

Leavitt MB: *Families at Risk: Primary Prevention in Nursing Practice.* Boston: Little, Brown, 1982.

Levinson DJ: *The Seasons of a Man's Life.* New York: Ballentine Books, 1978.

Lindemann E: Symptomatology and management of acute grief. In: Parad H (editor), *Crisis Intervention: Selected Readings.* New York: Family Association of America, 1965.

Logan BB: The nurse and the family: Dominant themes and perspectives in the literature. In: Knafl KA, Grace HK (editors), *Families Across the Life Cycle.* Boston: Little, Brown, 1978.

Menaghan E: Marital stress and family transitions: A panel analysis. *Journal of Marriage and the Family* 1983; 45 (5): 371.

Miller JR, Janosik E: *Family-Focussed Care.* New York: McGraw-Hill, 1980.

Minuchin S: *Families and Family Therapy.* Cambridge, Mass.: Harvard University Press, 1974.

Norton AJ: The family life cycle: 1980. *Journal of Marriage and the Family* 1983; 45 (5): 267.

Pratt L: *Family Structure and Effective Health Behavior.* Boston: Houghton Mifflin, 1976.

Rapoport L: The state of crisis: Some theoretical consideration. In: Parad HJ (editor), *Crisis Intervention: Selected Readings.* New York: Family Service Association of America, 1965.

Reinhardt AM, Quinn MD: *Family-Centered Community Nursing: A Sociocultural Framework.* St. Louis: Mosby, 1973.

Rollins BC, Feldman H: Marital satisfaction over the family life cycle. *Journal of Marriage and the Family* 1970; 32(1): 20.

Satir V: *Conjoint Family Therapy.* Palo Alto, Calif.: Science and Behavior Books, 1967.

Sheehy G: *Passages: Predictable Crisis of Adult Life.* New York: Dutton, 1974.

Tinkham C, Voorhies E: *Community Health Nursing: Evolution and Process,* 2nd ed. New York: Appleton, 1977.

Chapter 17

The Changing Family

Barbara Bryan Logan and Cecilia E. Dawkins

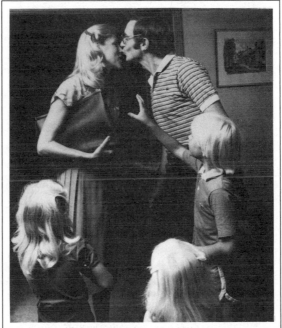

Erika Stone

Contemporary society affords a family with many more opportunities than ever before. The structure of the family and the roles of its members are shifting away from traditional forms in response.

Chapter Outline

The Nature of Contemporary American Families
   Influences of Traditional Beliefs
   Contemporary Concerns
Social Forces that Affect American Families
   Industrialization and Urbanization
   The Women's Movement
   Divorce
   The Economy
   Poverty
Emergent Family Structures: Implications for Community Health Nurses
   Single-parent Families
   Dual-Career Families
   Stepfamilies
   Cohabitating Couples
   Gay and Lesbian Families
   Communal Families

Recommendations and Strategies for Community Health Nurses
   Anticipatory Guidance
   Health Education
   Crisis Intervention
   Counseling
   Networking and Advocacy
Summary
Topics for Nursing Research
Study Questions
References

Chapter Objectives

After completing this chapter, the reader will be able to:

- Outline traditional values that have influenced families
- Discuss four societywide changes that have affected the contemporary American family
- Describe at least four types of family structures that can be identified among contemporary American families
- Cite examples of the types of stresses contemporary American families face
- Identify strategies community health nurses can use in working with contemporary American families

Many American families follow traditional patterns: they become engaged, marry, have and raise children; they adjust to the empty nest of living alone without children; and they prepare for and adjust to old age and finally death. Research indicates, however, that growing numbers of families deviate from this pattern (Lamb, 1982; Scanzoni, 1983).

This chapter focuses on such changing family patterns and examines selected alternative family structures and life-styles. The chapter explores the nature of contemporary American families; predominant societal forces such as industrialization and urbanization, the women's movement, divorce, and the economy that have contributed to changes in the family; family structures that have emerged as a result of societal forces such as single-parent families, dual-career families, stepfamilies, gay and lesbian families, cohabiting couples, and communal family arrangements. Implications for community health nurses and recommendations and strategies useful to community health nurses in planning and providing care for such families will be presented.

The Nature of Contemporary American Families

Contemporary American families are not homogenous but rather regionally, ethnically, and organizationally diverse (White House Conference on Families, 1980). They vary in *structure* (how they are organized in terms of members present), in *function* (the activities they perform for, and among, one another), and in terms of their *interaction patterns* (how they communicate and relate).

Some critics argue that the family has changed to the extent that it no longer performs vital functions for its individual members. For example, some of the traditional services once provided by the family such as education and custodial care of children are being assumed by other social institutions. Critics also assert that social institutions external to the family are assuming economic functions (providing financial resources) for many families. Because of these changes and also because of changing roles and responsibilities occurring within modern families, these social critics question the role of the family as a vital social institution. As indications of disintegration of the contemporary family, some observers point to increased rates of juvenile delinquency, family violence, suicide among young people, divorce, out-of-wedlock births, and young children who spend a great proportion of their day in child care centers or come home after school to empty homes. Some contend that the family has outlived its usefulness, and as a viable institution, is in a state of crisis (Cooper, 1971; Moore, 1958).

Influences of Traditional Beliefs

Undoubtedly concern for modern American families stems from traditional beliefs about the family. For a long time Americans held an ideal conceptualization of the family as the nuclear type. This consisted of a husband-father, who is a breadwinner working outside of the home; a wife-mother, who is a full-time housewife concerned with domestic matters and emotional stability inside the home; and two or more children, who all live within the same household. Scanzoni (1983) summarized the elements or essence of this traditional family as follows:

1. The male head of the household, the father, is the sole economic provider.
2. The female head of the household, the mother, is the homemaker, and is responsible for domestic care and the socialization of the children. She is a helpmate to the husband, pro-

viding support for him in his struggle for the family's survival.

3. The children are helpless and dependent, vulnerable and malleable. They must be nurtured full-time by the mother (or mother-surrogate) only, because emotional stability is essential.

4. The family is a private institution and within it individuals can fulfill their most important needs. This fulfillment is based on the foundation of the economic income provided by the husband (where necessary, supplemented by the state). Only when economic and material needs have been met do expressions of psychological and social needs for love, esteem, self-expression, and fulfillment emerge within the family.

5. Healthy families produce healthy individuals, who adjust to social roles (p. 34).

Traditional views of the family (which are often more ideal than real) also have been shaped by religious doctrines. In the nineteenth and early twentieth centuries, for instance, Evangelical doctrine successfully repudiated women's sexuality, dictated reduction of their economic and occupational activities, and enforced patriarchy, obedience, and the sexual repression of women (Scanzoni, 1983). Thus, the family model of this period was strongly influenced by religious doctrines that dictated male-female relationships and role behaviors.

These beliefs and values have contributed to the traditional conceptualization of the family and also to the way Americans think about families even in modern times. They have contributed to concerns about the future viability of the contemporary American family and to labeling as deviant those families with alternative structures or life-styles that differ from the conventional model. This is seen among such groups as the so-called "Moral Majority," which has definite beliefs concerning the family and strongly negative views of issues affecting families such as abortion, homosexuality, divorce, and sex education. Such negative views contribute to their interpretation of the contemporary family as being in crisis.

Contemporary Concerns

Public concern about American families in crisis and about the future viability of such families has led to many conferences and forums about the family. One such notable event was the White House Conference on Families, called in 1980 by President Carter, to discuss the welfare of American families. Scholars, public officials, religious leaders, and ordinary American families came together to share insights concerning the nature and needs of American families (White House Conference on Families, 1980). Some conclusions reached as a result of this conference are:

Americans care passionately about their families. Families are our most important institution, the glue that holds this society together . . . families are under unprecedented economic, social and even political pressures. Many families are overcoming them and prevailing. Many others struggle and some have been overwhelmed and broken. . . . Families are enormously diverse. . . . Discrimination and poverty intensify the pressures facing families, but all families are finding it more difficult to cope with contemporary challenges (p. 9).

In general, the conference report indicates that the American family will survive and be a strong force in the future despite the many challenges it faces. It is clear, however, that the family of the future will differ from traditional definitions of the family.

We take the position that the family, defined as a group of two or more people living together who have a commitment to each other (see Chapter 2), is a viable institution whose structure is changing to accommodate the realities of modern society. Family households may or may not include a marital pair, children, or even both men and women. It might be a group bound by intention rather than by contract or it might also be a single-person household (Boulding, 1983). With longer life expectancy and growing emancipation of children from their families of origin, a great proportion of contemporary families may well consist of older adults without children. Changes within the family can be attributed to major societal forces or some of the changes occurring in society itself.

Social Forces that Affect American Families

Scientists have debated as to whether or not the family generates social changes or is merely affected by them. Regardless of whether or not the family is a producer or product of change, American families *have* changed and much of this change relates to movements or forces that have occurred in society at large. The movements that will be discussed are (1) industrialization and urbanization, (2) the women's movement, (3) divorce, (4) the economy, and (5) poverty. Although these forces are discussed separately, they are obviously interrelated. For example, divorce may be an outcome of some aspects of the women's movement, and divorce may also lead to unemployment or economic disaster for some families.

Industrialization and Urbanization

The shift in American society from primarily rural and agrarian to urban and industrial affected the family in many ways. Three effects that are particularly relevant to the community health nurse are the increase in mobility for the family and its members, the disruption of extended family structures, and the realignment of the family's ethnic identity with regard to the surrounding community and the society at large.

Geographical mobility increased as industrialization created factory jobs that drew family members, especially men, from the country to the city. As it was difficult to relocate entire families, only the nuclear, conjugal family would tend to migrate, leaving the extended family members such as grandparents behind. Extended family members thus became increasingly removed from the children and less available for assisting in their development and socialization.

Industrial jobs were highly specialized, creating a sharper division of labor between men and women, and thereby reducing the opportunities for family members to work together in occupational settings. Women, who had had significant roles on the family farm, were not readily incorporated into the factory labor force alongside men. This, in turn, sharpened the division of labor in the home, where women focused even more exclusively on housekeeping and child-rearing responsibilities. These roles, considered less important than the economic provider roles assumed by the husband and father, contributed to perceptions of women as childbearers and domestic servants and of men as protector-masters and economic providers (Nass, 1978).

The relocation from rural to urban areas also affected the family's relationship to the surrounding community and society with regard to culture and values. Public education, rather than extended family members, played an increasingly important role in the socialization and education of children. Television and other media exposed children to life-styles far beyond what they experienced within the family. Mass transportation and the concentration of diverse cultural elements within the confines of the city gave children access to activities and experiences outside the parents' control. The potential for children to become socialized in ways contrary to their families' values and expectations has been a source of intergenerational conflict in modern American families.

The city promoted exposure not only to new ideas and experiences, but to different groups of people as well. Within the great ethnic diversity found in most American cities, families often found themselves segregated in pockets characterized by poverty or ethnic affiliation. Whereas ethnic affiliation may be functional on some level, families sometimes experienced conflicts as they moved into the occupational or educational arenas of the larger society. How the family functioned as a unit affected its ability to buffer or minimize the damaging effects of these conflicts, and influenced its ability to make the necessary changes within itself to adapt to societal forces. These conflicts and adaptations applied not only to families moving from rural to urban areas, but also to the many waves of immigrant families that have entered the country from other parts of the world.

The Women's Movement

The women's movement resulted in increased awareness of tremendous opportunities and choices available to women in careers, marriage, childbearing, and other family roles. The movement did much to legitimize work and career options for women and successfully promoted the belief that women have the right to challenging and satisfying jobs and deserve educational opportunities equivalent to men (Maymi, 1982), and that women should have equal opportunity of employment in positions for which they were qualified (Lamb, 1982).

The increased participation rate of women in the labor force has been dramatic and one of the most significant outcomes of the women's movement. Women with preschool children have shown the greatest increase in labor-force participation over time, and there is every reason to believe that this trend will increase. Projections show that by 1990 two-thirds of all mothers with children under six years of age will be working outside the home. Both young and older women are expected to increase their labor-force participation in the future (Maymi, 1982).

Women are choosing to combine marriage, motherhood, and employment in various ways. For example, some begin their careers after graduation whether or not marriage is in their future. Some opt to delay marriage and build their careers. Others, taking advantage of available family planning methods, choose to marry and delay childbearing or continue in their careers as working mothers and wives. Whether college educated or not, women are working outside the home for several reasons. One is economic. According to Maymi (1982), two-thirds of the women in the work place are usually in the single, widowed, divorced, or separated categories or have husbands with salaries in low income brackets. Therefore, there exists an economic incentive for these women to participate in the labor force to supplement the family income or to support themselves and their families (Maymi, 1982). Women also work outside the home because they want to pursue careers or work roles. They value career pursuits over housework and childbearing. Increasingly women, particularly the well-educated, elect to wait and have children until their careers are well launched. In addition, having small families allows women more time to engage in occupational or career pursuits.

The women's movement has provided much of the impetus, in the form of practical and psychological supports, needed to move women out of the home in the work force and to keep them there. However, many of these women have families to which they are equally committed, and have therefore recognized the need for certain changes in the occupational arena. For example, the women's movement has been instrumental in dramatizing and publicizing the need for alternative work patterns—alternatives to the standard eight-hour day/five-day week schedules, flexible time schedules, funding of daycare centers, equal pay for equal time (equity in pay)—all of which are supportive to women who work outside the home.

As women workers who constitute a large percentage of the female labor force, nurses can be particularly sensitive to the needs of women who work and also manage families and can advocate for this group of which they are a part. (See Chapter 22 for additional information on the health needs of working women.)

Divorce

Divorce is becoming a common occurrence among Americans. Cherlin (1981) reports that "the divorce rates of the 1960s and the 1970s are much steeper and more sustained than any increase in the past century" (p. 23). While there was one divorce for every six marriages in 1940, there was one for every two marriages in 1980 (Waldman, 1984). The rise in divorce rates has long caused concern among Americans, and divorce itself has been viewed as "a symptom of general family illness due to vast social changes confusing to individuals" (Houdlette, 1939, p. 25). It has been regarded as a major factor in the deterioration of the family.

On the other hand, some people argue that divorce is not an indictment against marriage and the family but a welcome alternative to unhappy marriages. It is a way of escape for people who are oppressed in their marriages. In fact, most people who divorce eventually remarry within several years after the divorce, and one-third of all adults find themselves in remarriage situations following divorce (Cherlin, 1981). Consequently, whereas the divorce rate has increased, so has the marriage rate (Waldman, 1984).

Several reasons have been cited for the increase in divorce rates, the most predominant ones being changing attitudes toward divorce and liberalization of divorce laws. Since the mid-1960s the stigma against divorce has considerably declined, and for the most part, society no longer views divorce as the failure or disgrace it was in earlier decades, making it easier for people in unhappy marriages to leave their spouses. Many states have no-fault divorce laws that make it easier for couples to go through the legal process of obtaining the divorce.

Demographic variables such as race, income, education, and religious affiliation are important factors in divorce. Research indicates that divorce is lower among high income, educated groups; it is higher among lower-income nonwhite groups, particularly blacks, who also tend to cluster at the bottom of the socioeconomic ladder. A prevailing fact has been that economic stability also contributes to family stability.

Highly religious couples show less incidence of divorce than those who are less religious or with no religious affiliation (Booth, Johnson, & Edwards, 1983).

In general, even if the divorce is beneficial in the long run, the process entails adjustments that can be traumatic for some families. Couples may experience ambivalent feelings and increased anxiety as they face reorganization of their lives without the other spouse (see Box 17-1). For families with strong religious beliefs that include sanctions against divorce, the experience of divorce may result in religious conflict, guilt, and other spiritual dis-

Box 17-1   The Aspects of Divorce

Becoming divorced or terminating a marriage can be a complicated and difficult process. As described by Bohannan (1970), it consists of at least six aspects:

1. *Emotional divorce*—This aspect signifies the deterioration of the marriage relationship. The couple may continue to live together, but each is disappointed since the trust and the attention for one another have disappeared.
2. *Legal divorce*—Couples obtain the actual divorce decree.
3. *Economic divorce*—Settlement of money matters and division of property take place.
4. *Coparental divorce*—Continued involvement with children is determined. This includes custody issues, visitation rights, and parents' responsibilities.

5. *Community divorce*—Friends and community relationships change as a result of divorce.
6. *Psychic divorce*—Each partner develops a sense of identity without the other spouse—being uncoupled.

Divorcing couples may experience difficulties in any or all of these aspects; some areas may prove to be more problematic than others depending upon the couple's unique circumstances. For example, obtaining the legal decree may be easy for some couples. But it may be more troublesome for others or for one spouse who views the marriage as an emotional upheaval and a blow to self-esteem.

tress. Children of divorced couples are particularly vulnerable. They may become upset as they adjust to separation from a parent and changes in their daily routines and life-styles, or changes in their schools, neighborhood, and other familiar networks. Making the necessary changes such as learning to live apart from certain family members and establishing new relationships are all areas for nurses to plan anticipatory guidance and work with these families for better and easier adjustments. Specific strategies community health nurses can employ will be discussed later in this chapter.

The Economy

The nation's economy has a significant effect on American families. Factors such as unemployment, underemployment, and inflation can lead to increased costs for food, housing, transportation, energy, and health care. This, in turn, exerts severe economic pressures on families. Sustained economic pressures can lead ultimately to reorganization of family roles and functions. For example, it may become necessary for a housewife who has been out of the paid labor force for several years to seek reemployment so that the family can maintain a minimum standard of living when her husband becomes suddenly unemployed. Teenage children in such a family may also seek part-time work to help the family's economic status. On the other hand, the father in such a family may assume housework and child care functions formerly assumed by his wife and children. Families that can adapt to such economic pressures and subsequent family reorganization can grow emotionally and even become closer together as a result of those new experiences, while families that have difficulty adjusting to such changes can become disorganized to the point of disintegration.

In one study Easterlin (1980) illustrated the relationship between economic conditions and the family. Easterlin (cf. Cherlin, 1981) showed that male income has a direct impact on family function. Easterlin contends that men who are products of the "baby boom" (an era of dramatic increase in the birthrate following World War II) grew up during a time of relative affluence, but came of age in the late 1960s and 1970s to find a tightened labor market and increased competition for jobs. With high expectations for career and material well-being, these men had to settle for employment that offered less than they had hoped for. When they later married, their wives sought employment outside of the home to supplement their income; and as young married couples they postponed having children (Cherlin, 1981).

Thus, the lower income of young men was a strong reason for delay in having children and for wives to seek employment outside the home. Easterlin also contends, however, that increased wife employment can also lead to marital conflict and even marital dissolution.

While family economic pressure is certainly not the only motivation to work, it is undoubtedly a major incentive for women to enter the labor force even if other types of incentives keep them working. It should also be pointed out that whereas wife employment raises or helps to maintain the standard of living for some families, many families (particularly many uneducated, ethnic or racial minorities and younger families) are plagued with such high levels of joblessness and underemployment that they exist at poverty level or below, and their quality of life reflects this.

Poverty

In the United States poverty is officially determined by income level, but the concept of poverty is much more complex than whether or not a family's household income is at, above, or below the amount designated as the poverty level. For example, some families may have incomes above the poverty level and still *feel* poor and unable to maintain a satisfactory standard of living. Other families may have income significantly below the poverty level, if for example the breadwinner is temporarily unemployed, and may not *feel* poor even if they are unable to maintain their customary standard of living. For them, the loss of income and the accompanying adjustments they must make are temporary.

Some families experience generations of poverty, and for them poverty is a way of life. Their chronic poverty produces a life-style of hopelessness and despair because of consistent lack of access to needed American institutions and services such as good health care.

Sometimes hopelessness and despair among the chronically poor are misconceived as laziness or lack of ambition and initiative. However, families in the United States with the highest poverty levels—single-parent families maintained by women, older families, and disabled families—have legitimate reasons to be poor because they are disadvantaged in the labor market. Older and disabled families lose income because of retirement and/or reduced working capacity. Single women who maintain families generally completed fewer years of school than wives and are concentrated in lower-skilled and lower-paying jobs where there is a high turnover. At the same time, much of their energy is devoted to the responsibilities of caring for their children. Their chronic, higher unemployment rate keeps their economic status well below that of other American families (Johnson & Waldman, 1984). With each additional child, single-parent families maintained by women come closer to poverty (Johnson & Waldman, 1984).

Blacks are more likely than Whites or Hispanics to live in single-parent families maintained by women (Hayghe, 1984). A *New York Times* article (Norton, 1985) dramatized the condition of black families maintained by women in reporting that 70 percent of black children under eighteen who live in female-headed households are brought up in poverty. This condition was attributed to permanent joblessness among many young black men and racial discrimination and its accompanying effects. In other words, unemployed black men are unable to perform their historical role of support to their families. These families as well as other poor families and their young children develop life-styles where obtaining adequate food, housing, and health care is a daily struggle.

There are no simple solutions to the conditions families in poverty face. Community health nurses encounter these families often—in neighborhood health centers, clinics, and their homes. Yet it is a challenge to plan and implement health care for such families in our society, where there is a growing trend toward providing health services on a fee-for-service or for-profit basis. Collaborative efforts with other disciplines are needed to develop innovative health programs for poor families.

Emergent Family Structures: Implications for Community Health Nurses

Through anticipatory guidance and crisis intervention, community health nurses can help families meet daily challenges and cope with difficult life events. Concerned with all aspects of family life that affect health, community health nurses should understand the broad social changes that affect families and the changes that occur in families themselves in response to societal forces.

Single-Parent Families

Single-parent families are generating considerable public interest and concern (Gelman et al, 1985). Such families have existed throughout history, but increased divorce rates, increased choices available to women, and greater acceptance of single men raising their children have contributed to their increase in numbers—from 11 percent of families in 1970 to 22 percent in 1983 (US Department of Commerce, 1984). Recent trends indicate that single-parent families, particularly those headed by women, are growing rapidly and far outnumber those headed by men (US Department of Commerce, 1984). Such families, though not a new phenomenon, are the fastest growing family type in the United States. Their numbers have grown almost ten times as fast as two-parent families and are significantly outdistancing husband-wife and male-headed households (Ross & Sawhill, 1975). Single parents are often stressed, because most of them have sole responsibility for supporting themselves and their children, and often do not have the resources to manage effectively. Weiss (1978) identified three common sources of stress among single-parent families:

1. Responsibility overload—when parents become overwhelmed because of the decisions they have to make and needs they must provide for
2. Task overload—when parents have too much to do such that they have no time to meet unexpected demands because of the routine demanding activities of work outside the home, housekeeping, and parenting
3. Emotional overload—when they must provide emotional support to children whether or not they are depleted.

These stresses can make it difficult for single parents to manage their lives and those of their children.

Single-Parent Families Headed by Women

Approximately 10 percent of the 62 million family households in the United States in 1984 were headed by women, compared to only 2 percent headed by men (US Department of Commerce, 1984). In addition, by the mid-1970s, one out of every seven children in the United States lived in fatherless homes (Ross & Sawhill, 1975). This increase in female-headed families has paralleled such social changes as changing norms, changing economic conditions, shifts in government policies, and the individual decisions men and women are making

concerning their lives. Whereas female-headed families are found at all income levels and among all groups, the greatest increase in female-headed families has occurred among the youngest women and among nonwhite women (Johnson & Waldman, 1984).

Evidence suggests that most female-headed families are interim transitional units of short duration. This is because most women who head single-parent families are divorced or separated rather than widowed, and they eventually remarry and reestablish traditional husband-wife, nuclear type of family arrangements within a short time (Ross & Sawhill, 1975). Despite this trend toward remarriage, however, some families make it back to husband-wife family patterns very slowly, while some do not make it at all; others have no desire to reestablish husband-wife, nuclear type of family arrangements.

Single-parent families headed by women are reported to suffer greater hardships than any other family type, and are more susceptible to stressful life events (Guttentag, Salasin, & Belle, 1980). Most of their hardships are grounded in their lower economic status, since many single-parent families exist at the poverty or below poverty level, as was discussed earlier in this chapter. In a comparative study of 200 families living in different family structures (including traditional two-parent groups, unwed social contract family groups, single-mother family groups, and communal living groups) Eiduson (1983), reported that compared to children in the other family groups, the child who grows up in a single-mother family grows up in an environment that is financially downwardly mobile and frequently dependent on welfare. The single mother is very likely to be in the full-time work force by the time the child is two years old, and she is dependent on daycare or nursery school for child care.

Single mothers can also lack the social support and approval to sustain them in their struggle. Compared to single men who are applauded in this society for raising their children alone, single women involved in the same situation are often scorned or considered immoral, despite the tremendous effort

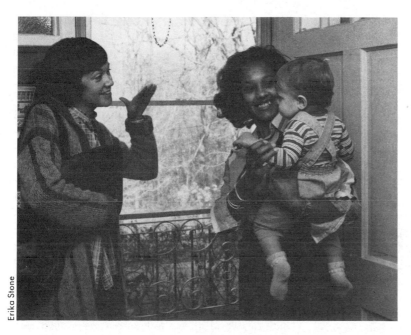

Erika Stone

Single-parent families face extraordinary pressures. Women working by choice or out of economic necessity may shift a considerable portion of their childrearing role to child care professionals.

they expend in raising their children. They often do this with fewer resources than most single-parent fathers, and they receive fewer awards.

Single-Parent Families Headed by Men   Traditionally, males in the United States have been socialized to identify with occupational rather than with child-rearing roles. Consequently, the role of father has been of secondary importance to the role of worker in a man's life. Accordingly, most child custody cases until recently have been settled in favor of mothers rather than fathers, who have been considered less competent in their performance of domestic roles and functions. This assumption is reflected in television commercials and other media productions that suggest that fathers are ineffective when performing domestic activities. This picture is rapidly changing as more fathers are gaining sole custody of their children and are electing to raise and keep them as single parents.

Fathers who are heads of single-family households are reported to be better off financially than single-parent mothers, but they experience some of the same difficulties, such as loneliness, social isolation, and guilt for not providing children with

a mother, particularly if the children are very young girls. The life-styles of single fathers raising young daughters are often scrutinized by community residents concerned that fathers be good role models and provide the moral guidance children need.

It is important to note that parent substitutes, relatives, or friends are available and interact regularly with many single parents and their children. On the other hand, a parent in a traditional two-parent family may be absent or unavailable to the family because of other involvements such as long working hours, time-consuming hobbies, and the like. One cannot, therefore, assume that traditional two-parent families are better off than single-parent families, except in one sense—financial stability. Studies consistently show that two-parent families are generally better off economically than one-parent families, particularly one-parent families headed by women. As Cherlin (1981) explains, "the lack of male income is the most detrimental circumstance that single-parent homes headed by women face" (p. 81). However, a growing number of professional women are *choosing* to have and raise children as single parents after they have launched their careers. These women may have less economic difficulties but are likely to experi-ence the same need for emotional support as all single parents.

Dual-Career Families

Dual-career families are families in which both the husband and the wife pursue active careers in addi-tion to their family lives (Moore, 1980). Rapaport & Rapaport (1969) are among the first researchers to use the term *dual-career family* to define these types of family structures. In such families the careers of both the husband and the wife are taken seri-ously, and career commitment and motivation are attributed equally to both partners (Moore, 1980).

Dual-career families are distinct from two-person career families. In the latter type, both husband and wife are devoted to the career success of the husband (Moore, 1980). Wives often work in the home and are totally devoted to the career success of the husband and rearing of their chil-dren. This family type is consistent with the cliché "Behind every successful man is a good woman." Dual-career families are also distinguished from another family type, two-job families (Moore, 1980). In two-job families both partners work, but the wife is seen as having a job that is dispensable and/or secondary to the husband's. Examples of dual-career, two-person career, and two-job families are compared in Table 17-1.

Whereas two-person and two-job families are more traditional forms, dual-career families are more consistent with a contemporary outlook on fami-lies, because they are based (at least in theory) on a belief in the career advancement of *both* members of the couple. There is also support for an egali-tarian couple relationship—equalization of power and decision making and shared domestic respon-sibilities and child-rearing. Both partners are, therefore, forced to make adjustments and adap-tations that may not occur in nontraditional fam-ilies. If the careers of the couple are pursued in different locations, as can be the case when one or both have academic positions at a university, long-distance commuting or a second residence may be necessary adjustments.

Despite the career satisfaction that can be gained by couples in dual-career family arrangements, these couples are likely to encounter such difficulties as role strain, (particularly on the part of the wife and mother), family vs. career conflicts, and competi-tiveness in terms of whose position is most impor-tant. Because of early socialization patterns, women are likely to be more concerned with domestic mat-ters and assume more responsibility for childcare and household tasks than their husbands, irrespec-tive of their careers. Consequently they can become "burned-out," suffer from role strains, and be forced to make sacrifices at the expense of their careers. This is especially true if the women have husbands who are not supportive.

On the other hand, some women who are totally dedicated to child-bearing, other domestic respon-sibilities, and their husband's careers may feel unfulfilled, bored, and resentful. Because of all the choices and alternatives available, families can work out arrangements that are mutually satisfactory not only to couples but to children as well. Some fam-ilies may need guidance and counseling to arrive at such arrangements.

Stepfamilies

Stepfamilies are complex family systems that result from disintegration of a marriage following death or divorce and subsequent remarriage (Visher & Visher, 1979). Stepparents and children in those family arrangements have to establish new kin rela-tionships that extend far beyond the boundaries of the family of the first marriage. Extended family relationships are created involving stepparents, stepchildren, stepgrandparents, and stepsiblings. In some instances, these relationships can be unclear, conflict ridden, and anxiety provoking.

It may be necessary to alter the way we define family and kinship in order to understand stepfam-ily relationships. For example, some children in stepfamily relationships may have contact with more

Table 17-1   Example of Career Influence on Family Structure and Function: Dual-Career Families Compared to Two-Person and Two-Job Families

	Dual-Career Family	*Two-Person Career Family*	*Two-Job Family*
Occupation or Activity	Dorothy Chen is an attorney, and her husband, Robert is a university instructor in sociology.	Mr. Wallings is the police commissioner of a small city. His wife Molly is a housewife.	Derrik Steele is a cardiologist teaching at a large medical school, and his wife Cathy teaches English at the high school level.
Domestic Management	The couple have delayed having children until their careers are further developed. They share equally in household and domestic chores.	Molly is totally dedicated to running the household and caring for the children. She also helps organize her husband's personal calendar and hosts social events for his business and political associates.	Two daughters attend the same high school where Cathy teaches. Mrs. Steele has primary responsibility for domestic and household chores. Her husband helps out when his schedule permits.
Career Decision	Robert was the first to receive an attractive job offer after both finished graduate study. When Dorothy could not find an acceptable offer in the same city, they both continued searching until they found reasonably attractive positions in the same city. Robert's position was with a less prestigious university than his first offer, but he accepted it to accommodate Dorothy's position.	Although she has a college education, Molly has not worked outside the home.	When Dr. Steele was offered a more attractive position in another state, the entire family prepared to leave. Cathy resigned her position without hesitation, and her husband sent her resume to his colleagues in the new city. Cathy was content to spend time taking care of the household and settling the children in school before taking on a new teaching position.

relatives than they did before their parents' divorce. Therefore they are exposed, and have ties to, households that they did not have before, thus making it difficult for them to determine who is "family" and what the nature of family relationships ought to be. Furthermore, society offers no institutionalized solutions to day-to-day problems stepfamilies face (Visher & Visher, 1979). How, for example, can a young girl explain why she has two mothers and three or four sets of grandparents?

The problems stepfamilies face are complex and, like those of other contemporary family structures, are often rooted in the clash between traditional values and expectations and contemporary realities. Stepfamilies substitute new individuals in old family roles, and the preceding spouse and parent-child relationships can make it difficult for new stepfamilies to interact openly with one another and establish close, meaningful relationships. Remarriage may join families with different social or cultural values and life-styles, thereby giving rise to conflict. Stepfamilies may also encounter difficulty integrating into community life and gaining community recognition.

Many of the problems that stepfamilies face can be addressed by promoting the well-being of the family unit itself. A strong, psychologically healthy relationship between the parent couple can provide stability for all the family members. Clear, open communication and expression of feelings can reduce divisiveness, minimize conflicts, and promote healthy family relationships. Toleration of differences can help the family make the cultural adjustments required to integrate persons from divergent backgrounds. Allowing children to continue family relationships established prior to the creation of the stepfamily—particularly relationships with grandparents, other siblings, aunts, and uncles—can help children maintain a stabilizing sense of continuity with their past. Using many of the strategies presented later in the chapter, the community health nurse can assist healthy family functioning for stepfamilies, thereby promoting the health of each individual member.

Cohabitating Families

Cohabitating families involve couples who live together in the same household without marrying (Cherlin, 1981). The number of these family arrangements has increased considerably and has more than doubled between 1970 and 1979 (Cherlin, 1981). The largest increase has been in the age group of twenty-five and under, and this trend is continuing into the 1980s (Spanier, 1983).

The Census Bureau counts cohabitating couples in terms of all persons living in households containing two unrelated adults of the opposite sex (Cherlin, 1981). Whereas many of these couples are involved in intimate relationships, it is possible that some are simply sharing apartments.

Data suggest that "living together," or cohabitating, is common among two distinct groups of urban adults—the better educated who live together before marriage and the less well-educated whose relationship includes at least one previously married partner. Living together has become common among a distinct subset of the better educated: college students. An estimated 25 percent of college students live with a dating partner at some point in their college career (Macklin, 1978).

Living together does not appear to indicate a lack of commitment to long-term relationships; a large percentage of cohabitating couples marry their partners, or plan to marry someone eventually (Macklin, 1978). Risman, Zick, and Peplau (1981) support these findings based on a two-year study of college dating couples. They concluded that cohabitating in college does not pose a threat to the institution of marriage, but seems to be more a part of the courtship process itself. The subjects in their study indicated that they planned to marry in the future.

By preceding marriage, cohabitation can facilitate an easier transition into marital roles and may even lead to a better marriage by serving as a form of "trial marriage."

In countries such as Sweden (and to a lesser extent France), the practice of cohabitation is very widespread, and has gained acceptance (Cherlin, 1981). Wider acceptance of cohabitation is also evidenced in the United States by the legal rulings governing these arrangements. Some couples elect to remain unmarried and continue to live together because they perceive the costs of traditional marriages to be greater than their rewards. Many such couples establish a social contract based on positive interpersonal relationships, strong emotional involvement, and egalitarian relationships. There is some danger, however, that without the formal ties or legal commitment, a partner in this type of arrangement can terminate the relationship at any moment, causing the family to break up (Eiduson, 1983).

Gay and Lesbian Families

As the gay community becomes more vocal, calling for recognition and acceptance of the gay lifestyle and institution of gay rights, gay and lesbian marriages are also becoming more visible. Many homosexual couples choose this union as an alternative to traditional marriage.

The terms *homosexual* and *gay* have been used interchangeably, but it is possible to identify differences in their meanings. The term *homosexual* refers to the emotional and sexual relationship between two individuals of the same gender. The term *gay* has been used to describe male homosexuals, but increasingly the term is being applied to all homosexuals and implies the life-style, the commitment, and the group identification of those who pursue their homosexuality openly, assertively, and with a sense of dignity and self-esteem. It may also imply a political commitment to seek equal rights (Scanzoni, 1976).

Gay marriages resemble traditional marriages in that gay couples establish ongoing relationships based on instrumental (material) and expressive (domestic and nurturing) exchanges and are both economically and sexually interdependent. Society has been slow to endorse and support homosexual marriages. For example, most states do not recognize same-sex marriages as valid and legal. This lack of approval may make it difficult for them to be strong, long-lasting unions. Furthermore, raising children in gay families may be problematic, both because it is difficult for homosexual couples to gain custody of their children and because society generally disapproves of raising children in gay families. In addition, gay individuals may conceal their sexual preference from their children for fear that their children may reject them, or that their "coming out" may have negative effects on their children such as causing them to experience turmoil or

uncertainties about their own sexual identity. Coming out has been defined as a process by which a gay individual identifies himself or herself as gay and accepts being gay as a positive state of being (Kus, 1985). Gay individuals are increasingly vocal and assertive, but gay families will continue to struggle with relationship and parenting issues until society becomes more accepting.

Communal Families

Communal families are like extended family systems that also serve as an alternative to the traditional nuclear family. People choose to belong to communes because of some common attraction, which may vary from a desired geographic location to a strong commitment to a particular ideology or religious doctrine. Like an extended family system, the commune is an intimate network where biologically unrelated persons come together to build a large family and fulfill functions traditionally assumed by biological extended kin. Scanzoni (1976) contends that communes serve as functional equivalents of the extended family in several ways:

- *Affection*—Commune acts as a source of primary relationships for its members such that they can experience a sense of belonging and feelings of sisterhood and brotherhood.
- *Interdependence*—There is a shared commitment to care for one another and a sense of needing one another and the group as a whole.
- *Rituals*—Members come together and participate in activities, ceremonies, and other events that symbolize commitment to the group and group solidarity.
- *Migration*—Movement of new members to new locations is facilitated when commune members break off, form new groups elsewhere, and serve as a natural support system for other members who follow them.
- *Influence or control*—The commune exerts influence and control over the lives of individual members.

Control over members inside the commune may be so strong that friendships and other connections outside the group may be very difficult or even impossible.

Communal families may vary in organization and function. For example, in some structures nuclear families may have separate dwelling units and function as a subsystem in close proximity to the larger family system of the commune, while in other systems no such division is allowed. Also, in some commune family structures, subunits may be economically independent, while in others all personal possessions and resources must be relinquished and pooled for the common consumption of all. Communal family life may, therefore, require that commune members make personal investments and sacrifices for the overall good of the group. Because of the numbers of individuals present, decision making may be complicated. Rivalries and resistances may emerge, personality clashes and conflicts of interest may result in quarrels (Eiduson, 1983), and open conflicts can ultimately lead to difficult interpersonal relationships within the commune.

Children in communal family structures have more adults and other children to deal with than they would in other family structures. These individuals may provide needed assistance and serve as allies, teachers, and socializing agents. In addition there may be multiple caretaking and sharing of tasks and assignments. Nevertheless, children may feel that they have no special person to care for them, to stand up for them, and for them to turn to when they are really in need. Furthermore, multiple caretaking and sharing of tasks may require constant negotiation and clarification of roles.

Because of general lack of privacy, persons living in commune family structures may feel that they are under constant scrutiny. This may make it very difficult to resolve problems and difficult relationships, particularly among couples and smaller family units or subsystems. Privacy to work out personal difficulties may be nonexistent, and people may feel that they are being watched and judged constantly. Consequently, although communal family living is an alternative to traditional nuclear family life, such structures may have negative consequences for their members.

Recommendations and Strategies for Community Health Nurses

Community health nurses will deliver care to families and individuals with customs, values and lifestyles that differ from conventional norms, or from the nurses' own conception of family. They may also find themselves working in communities with a preponderance of one or another type of nontraditional family—for example, a community in which a large commune family is located, a community with a large percentage of single-parent or gay families, or a community with a high incidence of divorce. Knowledge of the diversity of contemporary families and of the social forces that affect how such families are organized and function will help nurses to work more effectively with them.

As with other families, the primary role of the community health nurse with changing, nontra-

ditional families is health promotion. This means that the nurse functions in ways that help families improve their health and adopt life-styles that will increase their potential to achieve the highest level of wellness. When doing this, the nurse does not impose personal values on families but recognizes and respects all families as unique and valuable in their own right. He or she recognizes their strengths and assists them to identify ways to capitalize on their strengths and resources to achieve maximum health. This means that the nurse functions on all three levels of prevention—primary, secondary, and tertiary.

Primary prevention, however, remains the major goal of the community health nurse, who works to identify groups at risk of health problems and to plan nursing services that will reduce such risks. For example, based on knowledge of contemporary families, the nurse knows that children of recently divorced parents, single-parent families—particularly those who are poor and headed by women—and gay and lesbian couples, who are attempting to raise their children in communities hostile to their life-style, are all at risk of emotional difficulties, and as a result may be prone to other health problems.

There are many strategies that community health nurses can use in addressing the needs of contemporary families. These include:

1. Anticipatory guidance
2. Health education
3. Crisis intervention
4. Counseling
5. Networking and advocacy

These strategies are effective with *all* families, but in this section, their application to nontraditional families is emphasized.

Anticipatory Guidance

In Chapter 16, anticipatory guidance was discussed as a strategy that allows the community health nurse to identify and anticipate stressful life events that have the potential to cause crises, as well as plan and implement problem-solving mechanisms that can alleviate the harmful effects of such events. In similar fashion, the nurse can apply the strategy of anticipatory guidance to changing families. For example, entering first grade is a potentially stressful life event, not only for the new first grader but for the entire family. However, this stress may be intensified if the parents of this new first grader are in the process of divorce. Based on knowledge of crisis theory, of stressful life events and of community resources, a community health nurse can anticipate these events and mobilize community resources such as the teacher, school nurse, and family or school counselor to help the child with a smoother transition to first grade and to work

with the family to alleviate or minimize the effects of the crisis of entering school and divorce.

The nurse can also intervene personally to help such families harness the family's strengths and resources, to solve problems effectively, and ultimately to cope during these critical periods without undue stress and physical or emotional illness. For single mothers who are heads of households and also poor, the nurse can anticipate needs for emotional support, child care, and financial assistance.

Anticipatory guidance, therefore, enhances problem solving since prior knowledge of events and their circumstances allows the nurse to anticipate problems families could have at different points in time and take action beforehand to prevent or minimize such problems.

Health Education

Educating individuals, families, and communities about health is an ongoing function of community health nurses. This education may take place informally, such as when nurses are giving routine care or when they encounter people or potential clients in natural settings such as the home, church, community centers, or neighborhood gatherings. Health education may also take place formally through organized, structured classes or workshops. Case Example 17-1 illustrates the community health nurse's health education role in a formal and informal setting.

Community health nurses can provide health education not only at the individual and community levels, as illustrated in Case Example 17-1, but also at the family level. For instance, the nurse may teach a dual-career family time-management and stress-reduction techniques designed to help them cope with busy schedules in ways that minimize conflicts and emotional upsets.

Health education at the community level is obviously more effective in reaching large groups of people. Community structures such as YMCA, YWCA, churches, schools, and occupational settings are useful sites for such education. Community health nurses can educate community resi-

Case Example 17-1: Health Education

Informal Setting

Mrs. May works for a home health agency. In one of her routine follow-up visits to Mrs. Johnson after her discharge from the hospital, she found Mrs. Johnson and Lois, her twenty-seven-year-old daughter, engaged in an angry argument. Mrs. Johnson began to cry. Mrs. May soon learned that she was upset because her daughter had just revealed to her that she was a lesbian and was considering entering into a marriage situation with her roommate and partner. Mrs. Johnson was confused, upset, and angry. She blamed herself for Lois's life-style and said, "I must have done something wrong." After listening quietly to Mrs. Johnson, accepting her outburst and waiting for her to become calm, Mrs. May talked with her about society's openness to different types of life-styles. She talked specifically about gay and lesbian life-styles. She provided Mrs. Johnson with information about groups and organizations in the community that help people to cope with such life-styles. She also provided Mrs. Johnson with telephone numbers of such groups. Mrs. Johnson asked Mrs. May several questions about homosexuality and homosexual life-styles. Reassured by Mrs. May's frank, factual responses and calm, accepting attitude, Mrs. Johnson agreed to follow through with the telphone calls and to report the outcome to Mrs. May on her next visit. Mrs. Johnson also felt confident that she and her daughter, Lois, would eventually "work things out."

Mother finds daughter's life-style unacceptable.

Community health nurse provides mother with information about different family life-styles.

Nurse's attitude and factual information reassure mother, helping her to be more accepting of daughter's life-style.

Formal Setting

Mrs. Temple, a community health nurse, holds eight-week parenting seminars for single parents in the community center of a local church. Each week a different topic is discussed. Mrs. Temple presents information didactically followed by questions and answers for the group. Topics are suggested by Mrs. Temple and by group members. They include: parent-child relationships; coping without a partner; nutrition; exercise for the whole family; stress reduction and management; time management; child-care centers; discipline; and drug and alcohol abuse.

Nurse conducts education seminars in the community with the goal of health promotion for single-parent families.

dents about changing societal patterns, such as the women's movement and the economy, and their effects on the family. For example, communities can expect that increasing numbers of women with children will work outside the home, creating a need in the community for good daycare and other child care services outside the home. Being informed, community leaders and lay residents can take action to meet these challenges at the community and family levels. Community health nurses can play a vital role in helping families and communities to become informed in order to meet these needs. (See Case Example 17-2.)

Crisis Intervention

The nurse identifies when a family is in potential crisis and then helps the family to define the problem that has caused the potential crisis; identifies

Case Example 17-2: Meeting a Community's Educational Need

Ms. Blake is an energetic, innovative community health nurse who works in a family health center in a community with predominantly working parents. There are several daycare centers and nursery schools in the community. At a community forum Ms. Blake learned that child care and nursery school workers were "good with the children" but were limited in their knowledge of child development theory and issues. In collaboration with a pediatric nurse practitioner and the director of one of the child care centers, Ms. Blake planned and implemented a series of child development workshops offered to child care and nursery school teachers in one of the child development centers.

Community health nurse recognizes health education need.

Interprofessional collaboration leads to institution of workshop for better health of young children.

resources that are helpful in dealing with the problem; and devises and implements plans to alleviate the problem before a major crisis ensues. Before the nurse can devise an action plan, the family may need to list their priorities, list solutions that have been tried but have not been successful, and identify alternative solutions that are acceptable. In the problem-solving process the nurse's goal is to help the family to maximize their strengths and resources so that they can bring about the changes necessary to help them cope with and adapt to the situation.

Potential crisis periods for contemporary families are points of change, such as when parents of a two-parent family become divorced or when a dual-career couple begins childbearing. Community health nurses may encounter such families in clinics or health centers when they seek care usually because of physical symptoms, in the work setting, in homes when nurses make home visits for routine care, or in their neighborhoods because they are recognized as helping professionals. (See Case Example 17-3.)

Counseling

When counseling families with nontraditional patterns and life-styles, counselor-practitioners such as community health nurses must maintain a caring, accepting attitude. Such families may evoke the nurse's own personal feelings and family values, and differences between the nurse's own family life-style and that of the family may become blatant. In such circumstances it it important that the nurse be able to create a supportive environment and understand that meeting the needs of the family is the most important goal. It is also important that the relationship between the nurse and the family allows for the values of both to be respected and retained.

Community health nurses can counsel families directly or they can counsel groups of individuals from potentially high risk families. (See Chapter 12 for a discussion of group process as a strategy for reaching community residents.) For example, Bonkowski, Bequette, & Boomhower (1984) described their work in establishing a counseling support group designed to help children adjust to parental divorce. The group served as a peer support network for members by providing an open, therapeutic atmosphere and an opportunity for children to be with other children with similar experiences of family disruption. Community health nurses can collaborate with psychiatric mental health nurse specialists, social workers, psychologists, and other practitioners to conduct counseling groups with children with the goal of helping them adjust to their parents' divorce. Such groups can be established in such community facilities as schools, churches, and daycare centers.

Case Example 17-3: Early Crisis Intervention with Single Parent and Stepfamily

Clara Payton, a community health nurse, made a home visit to Cheryl Jones for routine follow-up and health assessment of Cheryl's three-year-old daughter and nine-month-old son. Ms. Payton noticed that Cheryl appeared depressed and seemed to have been drinking. Ms. Payton conducted a health assessment of the children and concluded that they were in good health. She explored with Cheryl what had happened and assessed her family situation.

Nurse observes potential family problem.

Ms. Payton discovered that Cheryl, a single parent, was very close to her divorced father who also constituted her major support system until he married a woman close to Cheryl's age three weeks ago. Cheryl was unable to accept her father's new, young wife as her stepmother, and she feared that she would lose his love and support. She responded by becoming very angry with her father and his new wife and quarreled with them to the extent that they no longer made her welcome in their home. Their last quarrel was a week ago, and since that time, she had not seen or spoken to her father. She had also been upset ever since. She began drinking two days ago. She had had a drinking problem for a brief period during her adolescence when her mother and father initially divorced.

Nurse conducts assessment of single-parent family with limited resources and supports.

Father's remarriage poses problem.

Client evidences inadequate coping.

Ms. Payton recognized that Cheryl was in a potential crisis situation that could develop into a full-blown crisis given her past history and current life situation and stresses—her father's remarried situation, perceived loss of her father, and the everyday stress and strain of single parenthood.

Nurse's knowledge is basis for planning anticipatory guidance.

Ms. Payton assisted Cheryl in clearly identifying her problems, planning ways to deal with them, and identifying all the actual and potential resources that could help her activate the plan. A vital step in the plan was to reestablish a relationship with her father and at the same time broaden her support network in order to be less dependent on her father. Cheryl, her father, and stepmother were able to work out their difficulties and build good relationships after a few visits to a family counselor who was referred to them by Ms. Payton. With Ms. Payton's assistance, Cheryl located and joined a self-help group for single mothers in her community. Ms. Payton evaluated Cheryl's progress periodically through follow-up visits.

Nurse helps to identify problems.

A plan is formulated.

The plan is implemented with additional professional resource.

Nurse conducts evaluation and follow-up.

Case Example 17-4 is an illustration of a counseling group in a community facility.

Community health nurses can also counsel families when some family members encounter role overload and misfitting expectations. They can help the family to clarify deep-seated values, formulate goals, and learn new, mutually acceptable role relationships.

Networking and Advocacy

Networking and advocacy, discussed in detail in Chapter 14, involves collaborating with formal and informal agencies and with families and their extended family networks to bring about positive changes in families and optimum health of family members. Employing these strategies with contem-

Case Example 17-4: Group Sessions for Single Parents

Mrs. Jones, a community health nurse, conducted weekly group sessions in the local YWCA for single parents. The group consisted of fifteen single-parent mothers and six single-parent fathers. Each week group members discussed issues of concern to them. These may have included social needs such as the need to overcome loneliness and lack of intimacy and also the need to deal with feelings of anger and abandonment (for those who have lost partners through divorce). Or they may have included financial needs such as the need to budget adequately in order to meet financial responsibilities, or the need to cope effectively in times of crisis. Mrs. Jones encourages sharing and discussing of feelings, provides factual information when needed, and assists the group to identify various resources to deal with practical everyday situations. The group itself was a supportive environment that met some of the participants' needs for social interaction as well as a testing ground for validation of feelings and problem solving.

Community health nurse uses group process to help single parents meet their needs.

porary families means that the community health nurse is knowledgeable about resources available to serve different types of families. If needed community resources are unavailable, then community health nurses have a vital role in networking with community residents, leaders, and other professionals to seek such services. It may be necessary for them to collectively lobby political representatives to sponsor and support legislation as well as appropriate funds to implement such programs.

Community health nurses can also participate on the community level in supporting broad issues that help contemporary families such as issues concerning the need for greater flexibility of work hours and for changes in the structure of work time such as extended maternity leave for mothers and fathers who are working parents.

On the family level, community health nurses can participate in establishing support groups or self-help network groups that provide the opportunity for families with similar patterns to share their experiences and problem-solve more effectively. Such groups could be established in community facilities and serve special family types such as stepfamilies, single-parent groups, gay and lesbian couples, or adolescents with divorced parents.

These groups differ from therapy groups because they provide a supportive atmosphere for sharing common or similar experiences and because they focus on problem solving rather than on working through emotional difficulties. Often contemporary families, stepfamilies in particular, have no institutionalized patterns to serve as guides for family members. Community support and self-help groups can serve such functions, and community health nurses are important resources for establishing such groups.

Working at the family level, community health nurses can also serve in advocacy roles for contemporary families by linking families to community agencies that provide needed functions and by coordinating the network of services families use when appropriate. While serving linking and coordination functions, community health nurses can also teach families how to use services effectively, how to deal with unresponsive agencies, and how to identify community supports. Community health nurses' knowledge of the array of formal and informal community services allows them to establish the networks that are necessary for them to function as family advocates, and to facilitate families' access to needed community service.

Summary

Several broad social forces such as urbanization, industrialization, the women's movement, rising divorce rates, the economy, and poverty have influenced the organization and function of modern American families. The outcome is that modern American families are changing, moving away from the traditional ideal of the nuclear two-parent family with the father as breadwinner and the mother as housewife and instrumental supporter. Diverse family structures have emerged including single-parent families, dual-career families, stepfamilies, cohabitating couples, commune families, and gay and lesbian families. It is important for community health nurses to be knowledgeable about various types of families that exist in society and to maintain an open, accepting, and nonjudgmental attitude toward families even when the nurses' own values and customs differ from those of the family. In spite of such differences, the nurse is able to plan and implement nursing care to meet the needs of such families. The strategies of anticipatory guidance, health education crisis intervention, counseling, and networking and advocacy can be useful to community health nurses in meeting the needs of contemporary American families.

Topics for Nursing Research

- Compare the life stresses and coping strategies of single-parent mothers and single-parent fathers.
- What are the adjustment patterns of preschool children compared to school-age children following divorce?
- Describe division of labor and role relationships in dual-career families.
- Explain parenting styles in gay and traditional families.
- What is the attitude of community health nurses toward the following nontraditional families: (1) male-headed single-parent families; (2) female-headed single-parent families; (3) dual-career families; and (4) gay families?

Study Questions

1. Which of the following trends is cited as a reason for the declining importance of traditional American families?
   a. The increasing importance of the women's movement
   b. Growing numbers of children cared for in daycare centers
   c. The leveling off of the birth rate
   d. Growing numbers of extended family units
2. Which of the following types of institutions has had the strongest influence on traditional values of the American family?
   a. Religious
   b. Educational
   c. Political
   d. None of the above
3. One of the conclusions of President Carter's White House Conference on Families is that American families:
   a. Have outlived their usefulness
   b. Represent a tangle of pathology
   c. Are becoming a drain on the nation's economy because of the numbers of families on welfare
   d. Are viable, but members are finding it difficult to cope with contemporary challenges
4. Which of the following statements about poverty would *not* be helpful to community health nurses in planning care for poor families?
   a. Poverty is related to chronic unemployment.
   b. Single-parent families maintained by women are the fastest growing poverty group.
   c. Poverty is a direct result of laziness and lack of initiative.
   d. Chronic poverty often produces hopelessness and despair.

5. A community health nurse is planning a seminar on the stresses of dual-career families in her community. It is important for her to know that which of the following could cause stress among dual-career families?
   a. Role strain
   b. Family vs. career conflicts
   c. Competitiveness
   d. All of the above
6. When working with changing, nontraditional families to promote their health, it is important that community health nurses do which of the following?
   a. Recognize and respect all families as unique and valuable
   b. Work only with families who have values similar to the nurses to avoid conflict
   c. Avoid secondary and tertiary prevention measures since their efforts should be concentrated on primary prevention
   d. None of the above

References

Bohannan P: *Divorce and After*. Garden City, N.Y.: Doubleday, 1970.

Bonkowski S, Bequette S, Boomhower S: A group design to help children adjust to parental divorce. *Social Casework* 1984; 65 (3); 131–140.

Booth A, Johnson D, Edwards J: Measuring marital instability. *Journal of Marriage and the Family* 1983; 45 (2): 387–393.

Boulding E: Familia Farber: The family as maker of the future. *Journal of Marriage and The Family* 1983; 45 (2): 257–266.

Cherlin A: *Marriage and Divorce*. Cambridge, Mass.: Harvard University Press, 1981.

Cooper D: *The Death of the Family*. New York: Vintage, 1971.

Easterlin R: *Birth and Fortune: The Impact of Numbers on Personal Welfare*. New York: Basic Books, 1980.

Eiduson B: Conflict and stress in non-traditional families: Impact on children. *Am J Orthopsychiatry* 1983; 53 (3): 426–435.

Gelman D et al: The single parent: Family Albums. *Newsweek* (July 15) 1985: 41–50.

Guttentag M, Salasin S, Belle D: *The Mental Health of Women*. New York: Academic Press, 1980.

Hayghe H: Married couples' work and income patterns. *Families at Work: The Jobs and the Pay*. Washington, D.C.: Government Printing Office, 1984.

Houdlette H: *The American Family in a Changing World*. Washington DC: American Association of University Women, 1939.

Johnson B, Waldman E: Most women who maintain families receive poor labor market returns. *Families at Work: The Jobs and the Pay*. Washington DC: Government Printing Office, 1984.

Kus, RJ: From grounded theory to clinical practice: Cases from gay studies research. In: Chenitz WC, Swanson JM (editors), *From Practice to Grounded Theory: Qualitative Research in Nursing*. Menlo Park, Calif.: Addison-Wesley (in press).

Lamb M: *Non-traditional Families: Parenting and Child Development*. London: Lawrence Erlbaum, 1982.

Macklin E: Non-marital heterosexual cohabitation. *Marriage and Family Review* 1978; 1 (2): 1–12.

Martin E, Martin J: *The Black Extended Family*. Chicago: University of Chicago Press, 1978.

Maymi C: Women in the labor force. In: Berman P, Ramey E (editors), *Women: A Developmental Perspective*. Hyattsville, Md. US Department of Health and Human Services, 1982.

McLanahan S, Wedemeyer N, Adelberg T: Network structure, social support, and psychological well-being in the single-parent family. *Journal of Marriage and the Family* 1981; 43 (3): 601–611.

Messinger L, Walker K, Freman S: Preparation for remarriage following divorce: The use of group techniques. *Am J Orthopsychiatry* 1978; 48 (2): 236–272.

Moore B: Thoughts on the future of the family. In: Moore B Jr (editor), *Political Power and Social Theory*. Cambridge, Mass.: Harvard University Press, 1958, pp. 160–178.

Moore D: Equal opportunity laws and dual-career couples. In: Pepitone-Rockwell F (editor), *Dual Career Couples*. Beverly Hills, Calif.: Sage Publications, 1980.

Murdock G: *Social Structure*. New York: Macmillan, 1949.

Nass, G: *Marriage and the Family*. Menlo Park, Calif.: Addison-Wesley, 1978.

Norton E: Restoring the traditional black family. *The New York Times Magazine* (June 2) 1985: 42.

Rapaport R, Rapaport R: The dual career family. *Human Relations* 1969; 22:3–30.

Risman B, Zick R, Peplau L: Living together in college: Implications for courtship. *Journal of Marriage and the Family* 1981; 43 (1): 77–83.

Ross J, Sawhill I: *Time of Transition: The Growth of Families Headed by Women*. Washington, DC: The Urban Institute, 1975.

Scanzoni J: *Shaping Tomorrow's Family: Theory and Policy for the Twenty-First Century*. Beverly Hills, Calif.: Sage Publications, 1983.

Scanzoni L: *Men, Women and Change: A Sociology of Marriage and Family*. New York: McGraw-Hill, 1976.

Seward R, Lantz H: *The American Family: A Demographic History*. Beverly Hills, Calif.: Sage Publications, 1978.

Spanier G: Married and unmarried cohabitation in the United States: 1980. *Journal of Marriage and the Family* 1983; 45 (2): 277–288.

Stack C: *All Our Kin*. New York: Harper and Row, 1974.

US Department of Commerce, Bureau of the Census: Households, families, marital status, and living arrangements. In: *Population Characteristics: Current Population Reports*. Washington, DC: Government Printing Office, August 1984.

Visher E, Visher J: *Step-families: A Guide to Working with Step-parents and Step-children*. New York: Brunner/Mazel, 1979.

Waldman E: Labor force statistics from a family perspective. *Families at Work: The Jobs and the Pay*. Washington, DC: Government Printing Office, 1984.

Weiss R: *Going It Alone: The Family Life and Social Situation of the Single Parent*. New York: Basic Books, 1978.

White House Conference on Families: *Listening to America's Families: Action for the 80's*. Washington, DC: Government Printing Office, 1980.

Chapter 18

Family-Centered Nursing in the Home

Judith M. Cattron, Jean Gala, and
Robah Kellogg

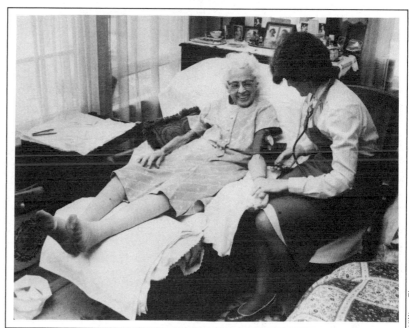

William Thompson

*Receiving care in the home setting has proved to be beneficial for
many clients. The psychological security and continued family functioning are positive factors in health improvement and maintenance.*

Chapter Outline

Chapter Objectives

After completing this chapter, the reader will be able to:

- Describe the community health nurse's role in the home
- Identify steps in preparing for and conducting a home visit
- Describe how the nursing process is applied to the home visit
- Outline assumptions that guide family-centered nursing in the home
- List factors that ensure personal safety
- Outline trends in home health care
- Describe agencies that provide home health services
- Evaluate a nursing home visit

Community health nurses provide health care in home and clinic settings throughout the United States. This chapter focuses on family-centered nursing in the home and illustrates health promotion, health maintenance, and home health care services provided to families by community health nurses. The text also incorporates the essence of the community health definitions found in Chapter 1.

Nursing students are probably most familiar with the hospital setting and the concept of delivering individualized care to the person termed "patient"; some incidental or planned teaching may be provided to family members about the patient's care or condition. A different perspective is advocated and practiced by community health nurses. Why should the community health emphasis be on *family*-centered nursing and within the home setting?

The home is the historical setting for the care of the ill. When nurses began caring for the ill family member in his or her own environment, using home resources in daily nursing care activities, and observing effects of illness upon others within the home, they acquired superior skills for family health and environmental assessment. As health promotion and health maintenance nursing services were funded by health agencies, the family-centered concept became the model for community health nursing practice.

Community health nurses have constantly observed that the health and welfare of individuals within the family depend upon the functioning of the basic family unit. Environmental resources within the home and surrounding community directly influence health states. Family selection of sources for health care is further influenced by general community resources, the family's means of transportation, and the public transportation available within the community. Mode of payment may limit access to health care.

Compared to other modes for health delivery, the home environment alters the setting for nursing care. The nurse must recognize the home's territory is owned by the family; by contrast, in the clinic setting, the nurse influences use of the building, equipment and the timing and flow of patients. The knowledge and skill base of the nurse are not diminished in the home setting; however, the power base of family members is enhanced by being in a familiar setting. It follows that greater family participation in decision making most likely occurs when the nurse provides health care in the home.

To create a change in health behaviors the individual and family members need to "own" their health problems and be goal-directed toward resolution of health problems and attainment of optimum health states. The nurse and family work together to identify the problem, allocate resources to alleviate the problem(s), delineate nurse and family actions to resolve the problem(s), and measure the outcomes in health states following the agreed-upon interventions. These actions best typify the partnership between the family and the community health nurse.

The following assumptions are the guiding framework for nursing students and community health nurses as they provide family-centered nursing in the home setting:

1. The family is the basic unit of nursing services.
2. The family home is a natural setting for the delivery of health care.
3. The family's well-being and self-determination are the principles guiding decision making.
4. Health care decision making is an active and shared process between family and health care provider.
5. The community health nurse is a provider of primary health care services for the family's health maintenance and promotion needs.
6. Secondary and tertiary health care services are provided when home health care is required by the family.
7. The nursing process facilitates health care decision making.

8. Contracting is a methodology illustrating the active shared process of decision making between family and nurse.
9. Counseling and health education principles guide interaction of the family and nurse.
10. The basic preparation for community health nurses is provided within a baccalaureate nursing program.

This chapter begins by defining the community health nurse's role in the home. Next we follow the steps of the nursing process in the home setting. We also describe the organization of home health services, and the chapter concludes with a national update on the home health care services movement.

The Community Health Nurse's Role in the Home

For most of us in community health nursing, the first home visit is one of those events that can be recalled vividly. The extremely high level of anxiety commonly associated with the first home visit seems to be related to some of the unanswered questions generated in anticipation of the experience, such as: Who am I? What is my role? What if they don't let me in? What will I do after I get in the home? Who can help me if I don't know what to do or say? Is this neighborhood safe? All of these questions are valid, and a concerted effort to get some answers to the questions is time well spent, even if it means postponing the actual experience of going out into the community. The "sink or swim" approach may be an effective way to teach a person to swim, but it is not a very efficient way to teach a nursing student to implement the role of the community health nurse.

If nursing students visit their families for the first time with a staff member who has been responsible for the caseload, their fear may be reduced and they may develop a collegial relationship with the community health staff nurse. Sometimes faculty choose to assign students to make home visits in pairs, such that one student is a primary deliverer of nursing care and the other acts as a peer reviewer. Other faculty may recommend that the students make solitary visits to a family from introduction to closure of the case.

The particular characteristics of the nurse's role in the community, as opposed to other settings such as acute care, have been described in Chapter 1 and elsewhere in this text. Two characteristics that need to be stressed when discussing the community health nurse's role in the home are (1) the emphasis on the family as the locus of decision making, and (2) the independent and collaborative aspects of the nurse's role in providing home care.

The Family as the Locus of Decision Making

In the hospital setting where the "medical model" prevails, the individual autonomy of the patient is restricted; that is, all the information about the individual is given to the physician, who in turn makes the decisions regarding the services that should be rendered. With the medical model, the physician and the nurse have more information about the patient than the patient has about himself or herself, thus ensuring the patient's dependency and lack of qualifications to be involved in making the decisions affecting him or her (Tinkham & Voorhies, 1977). It is noteworthy that the consumer movement and the patient's Bill of Rights are gradually causing some erosion of the sanctity of the medical model.

The family and its needs are the focus of the nursing home visit, regardless of the purpose of the visit. The family makes its own decisions about the nursing and other services it needs, wants, and will use. The operating model for the community health nurse is the family model. All of the information about the family is directed to the family so that *the family* may make sound decisions about the services it receives. The following are basic assumptions underlying the practice of community health nursing (Tinkham & Voorhies, 1977):

1. The family has the right and the responsibility to make its own decisions.
2. The community health nurse works *with* the family to assist the family in determining its health needs and problems, in developing the plan of action, and in evaluating the outcomes (sometimes referred to as either "implicit or explicit contracting").
3. The family is involved early in the decision-making process.
4. In order to be effective in their nursing practice with families, community health nurses must trust in the ability of families to solve their own health problems with the support and guidance of the nurse.

Ultimately, the goal of community health nursing practice with families is to assist families to grow in independence to the point where the services of the nurse are no longer needed. Paradoxically, community health nurses gratify their own needs through the growth process that they foster in the people served.

Independent and Collaborative Aspects of the Nurse's Role in the Home

The community health nurse functions under broad and quite general agency policies, procedures, and guidelines. For example, the agency may establish criterion for financial eligibility for the use of a child health conference. The nurse would refer only those families who meet the financial eligibility requirements. However, for the actual counseling and guidance of mothers with young children, the nurse *independently* utilizes professional knowledge and skill. If the nurse identifies a handicapped child in the home, he or she may refer the child to a crippled children's agency for diagnosis and treatment. To work effectively with the family on an ongoing basis, the community health nurse collaborates with the professional staff of the crippled children's clinic so that care for the child is coordinated, thus avoiding the pitfall of the nurse, the family, and the crippled children's clinic working at cross purposes. In this example, the community health nurse is functioning *collaboratively* in relationship to the professional staff of the crippled children's clinic. A similar relationship is established with physicians in the nursing care of the chronically ill and disabled in the home. (See Chapter 14 for further discussion of multidisciplinary collaboration.)

The Nursing Process and the Home Visit

In the home visit the nurse follows certain basic steps, beginning with the preparation for the visit and ending with an evaluation of the visit. Following these steps can make the visit proceed smoothly.

Preparation

In general there are two methods of preparing for the home visit (Leahy, Cobb, & Jones, 1977). The first method consists of thoroughly reviewing the record of previous nursing contacts with the family, studying the assessment data including medical reports, and acquiring an initial understanding of the overall family dynamics. Further information about the family is gathered through discussions with nurses and other personnel who have worked with the family in the past. The second method consists of only a very brief perusal of the family's record to become acquainted with the family constellation and to make note of the reason for the visit; the latter is done by reading the preceding nurse's plan for the next visit.

There are pros and cons for each of the two methods. Less experienced nurses are well advised to choose the first method, because they will go into the home with a sense of security that they already know the family—at least from the perspective of others who have come before them. The sense of security is further enhanced by reviewing theoretical material relevant to the family's particular health problems. A drawback to this method is that it helps to form preconceptions about the family that may be difficult to change. The second method avoids the danger of developing a predetermined, biased opinion about the family. Nurses free themselves to use their own skills to make their own assessment and to get the family's perceptions of events that have occurred in the past. Later, nurses can check their own observations against the observations recorded in the family folder by previous personnel. Which method is chosen is a matter of personal choice and style and depends upon the individual nurse's perception of how he or she functions more effectively.

In some situations, as in Case Example 18-1, there is no school nurse and there has been no previous public health nursing contact with the family. Consequently, there is no family folder to review. All that is known prior to the visit is the teacher's observations of Mary Phillips and the nurse's observations, which are essentially the same as the teacher's. (We'll return to the Phillips family in Case Example 18-4.)

First Contact with the Family

In the past, and even today in rural America, it may still be acceptable to just "drop in when you are in the neighborhood." Standards of courtesy prevalent in the area should be observed along with "what's possible." Ideally, if the family has a telephone, it is best to call in advance of your visit, explain the purpose of your visit, and arrange a mutually agreeable time. This action demonstrates respect for the family by giving them an opportunity to prepare for your visit in a way that makes them most comfortable when outsiders call upon them; gives the family an opportunity to think about the purpose of your visit; gives them an opportunity to accept or reject service; and avoids the wasteful and expensive problem of finding the family "not at home." If the family has no telephone, nurses must find another way to initiate the first contact, preserving as many as possible of the advantages just described to arranging for a mutually agreeable visiting time. For example, nurses might write the family a letter explaining why they would like to visit, noting the day and time they plan to come. The nurse might also send a note home with a

---

Case Example 18-1

The second grade teacher in the local public school district called the community health agency and requested that a home visit be made to the family of Mary Phillips, one of her pupils. She explained that Mary has seemed unusually irritable recently, has trouble sitting still. In addition, for about two weeks, the teacher has observed quick, twitching, involuntary, uncoordinated movements of Mary's face, trunk, and extremities. The teacher requests that a nurse observe the child in the classroom before making the home visit. The nurse's observations of Mary coincide with the teacher's observations.

Community health nurse requested to conduct health assessment in the home.

child. However, even the most reliable and responsible child has been known to lose notes on the way home from school.

Assuming that arrangements have been made with the family for the first visit, another important consideration is nurses' personal safety while visiting.

Personal Safety

Nurses and families alike fear for their personal safety in some neighborhoods. Although incidents involving crime against community health nurses are the exception rather than the rule, naiveté and lack of attention to potential dangers would be foolhardy. Perhaps crime against community health nurses is relatively low because community health nurses have become "street-wise" and take precautions to ensure their own safety. In addition, the uniform is recognizable and respected in most communities.

On the other hand, the community health nurse may need to deal with fears that have no basis in reality. An international and a national example of this type of fear may give student nurses courage to verbalize to faculty and classmates their concerns about visits to persons of different races or ethnic groups, religious practices, and life-styles in rural and urban areas (see Case Examples 18-2 and 18-3).

In general the community health nurse is seen as a friend to the community, not a threat, except in situations where people mistakenly connect the nurse with an agency they fear or distrust, or in situations where the family is afraid the nurse may report them to one of those agencies, such as the Department of Immigration or the Department of Public Assistance. Especially in high-crime areas, the personal safety of community members can become a nursing concern. In some neighborhoods, the incidence of break-ins is so high that people routinely hire sitters to guard their belongings while they go shopping or go to the doctor's office (Gala & Reisch, 1979). The elderly and infirm are especially vulnerable to attacks, because they frequently carry substantial amounts of money on their person for the feelings of security the money gives them. An elderly person living alone may leave the door unlocked during the day because they fear that "something may happen" to them and, if the door were locked, no one would be able to get in to find them.

In instances such as these, the nurse can help the person think through various plans that protect the person and his or her belongings. For example, some hospital emergency departments now provide telephone hookups to the home of elderly people living alone. With this system, each subscriber has a communicator unit attached to the phone and a portable button that can be worn on clothing or carried about in a pocket. The user can be as far

Case Example 18-2: International Experience

A community health nursing student who grew up in a southern province of Ethiopia had been told since early childhood that the people living in a northern province of Ethiopia were cannibals. The public health college and training center was located in this northern province, and needless to say, the student was terrified about making her first home visit. Fortunately, she was able to verbalize the source of her fear in student-faculty conference and was reassured that she had received false information.

Student's fears are related to perceived cultural differences.

Case Example 18-3: Local Experience

A nursing student of middle-class background and values was aware that her background was quite different from that of a family she was visiting. She was extremely anxious and afraid that this difference would present an insurmountable barrier to developing a therapeutic relationship with the family. When this was explored further, it was learned that the family's home was infested with bold cockroaches. The student stated that she jumped in fear when several of the cockroaches walked across some material she had in front of her on the table. She "just knew" the family would not be able to be comfortable having her in their home again and that she must be able, somehow, to control her own reactions to assaults from cockroaches in the future. Another student asked, "Do you think the family likes living with cockroaches?" This question precipitated an open discussion of differences in life-styles, and coping with poverty, which was clearly helpful to the student. In the next home visit there was a frank discussion between the family and the student about cockroaches and how the family had fought a losing battle with them over the years. After that, the cockroaches did not interfere with the relationship that was developing between the family and the student.

Student's fears are related to perceived socioeconomic class differences.

away as 200 feet from the telephone. At the first sign of trouble, the subscriber pushes the button, which sends an electronic message (via telephone) to the hospital's emergency department, where trained personnel immediately call back to find out the problem. If the subscriber does not answer the telephone, measures to investigate the apparent problem are set in motion by the hospital. The system allows an extra sense of "security" for those who have cardiac problems or who are prone to stroke, falls, or fainting, and extends the time that disabled, elderly, or medically fragile persons can live independently in their homes.

Another system, the "Carrier Alert Program," endorsed in 1983 by the U.S. Postal Service, the National Association of Letter Carriers, the United Way, the American Red Cross, and the Agency on Aging, is an alternative alert program for persons throughout the United States. Registered persons in the program have a "Carrier Alert" decal posted on the inside of their mailbox. The letter carrier will automatically notify his or her supervisor if mail of registered persons remains undisturbed for a day. The postal supervisor institutes contact with the coordinating agency (either the American Red Cross or the Agency on Aging), who then attempts to contact the residence. If this is unsuccessful, designated contact persons are telephoned. If none of the three designated contact persons can be reached by telephone, either a staff person from the coordinating agency or the police visits the home to determine the status of the individual.

Agencies have employed various ways to protect the safety of their nursing staff. Some provide escort services to nurses going into neighborhoods considered to be dangerous (the escorts may be students or local residents paid by the agency). Others have nurses visiting in pairs, which is a rather expensive way to utilize scarce nursing personnel. Whether visiting in pairs or utilizing an escort service, following a personal safety checklist such as the one provided in Box 18-1 may be useful.

Assessment and Establishing Rapport

In the first visit to the Phillips family (in Case Example 18-4), the nurse's plan for the visit will

Box 18-1 Personal Safety Checklist

I. Avoid corners where groups (gangs) congregate.

II. If someone wants your nursing bag, let them have it. It will probably be found later and returned to the agency.

III. Trust your intuition. Cues that have not yet been identified at the conscious level such as vague feelings of discomfort or a sense that "something" is different in the building than on previous visits should be trusted. No medals are given for bravery!

IV. Know the greetings common to the neighborhood, and accept the greeting for what it is—don't be frightened or offended. For example, "What's happening?" may be a way of saying "hello" in some neighborhoods. Maintain eye contact just long enough to return the greeting, and then look away, which indicates no desire for a conversation, and continue on your way.

V. Always have an escape route.

VI. Whenever possible, avoid the use of elevators in tenement buildings.

VII. If you have never learned to scream, practice it! Don't be afraid to call attention to yourself and a danger you may find yourself in.

VIII. Dogs may be dangerous—some are trained to kill. If the dog is a stranger to you and you are unsure of its character, it is better to err on the side of mistrust than trust. You can always telephone the family and go back after the dog has been leashed.

IX. Maintain watchful vigilance at all times when on streets or in dark hallways of buildings. Always have an escape route!

X. Always have enough money on your person (in a shoe or a pocket) to make at least one telephone call. Don't carry your purse in the neighborhood.

XI. Follow the uniform code of the agency so that people in the community know you are a community health nurse.

XII. If you are a victim of a crime, know what to do ahead of time. Ask your clinical instructor, or supervisor, what the guidelines are. Do you first call the police and then your instructor? Or do you first call your instructor and let him or her notify the police?

XIII. Involve the family in plans for your individual safety. They will not be offended. They share in the same reality.

XIV. Give your clinical instructor or supervisor a list of the homes you plan to visit in the order you plan to visit, along with the addresses and telephone numbers of the homes. Indicate the time you plan to call into the office and the expected time of return to the office.

XV. Don't be alarmed if a patrol car stops beside you and an officer asks what you are "doing in *this* neighborhood." Explain briefly and thank the police officer for his or her concern.

XVI. When rival gangs are "at war," take special precautions to avoid being caught in the crossfire. The families you visit will be alert to what is going on and the location of the warring gangs. Follow their advice about the best route to reach their home and to return to the office.

XVII. Additionally, alert police when you are working in certain districts of the city. They prefer to be alerted and will provide surveillance support.

emphasize establishing rapport and beginning to assess the family's health problems and related needs. The assessment process is a continuous, ongoing process; one should not expect, therefore, that all possible assessment data will be collected on the first visit. Data will be gathered over time in the following assessment categories as needed (American Nurses' Association, 1973):

1. Growth and development (individual and family)
2. Biophysical status

3. Emotional status
4. Cultural, religious, socioeconomic, and occupational background
5. Performance of activities of daily living
6. Patterns of coping
7. Interaction patterns; family dynamics
8. Family's perception of and satisfaction with health status
9. Relevant codes, statutes, regulations, contracts, and agreements
10. Environment (physical, social, emotional, and ecological)
11. Available and accessible human and material resources

Through continuous assessment and ongoing analysis of assessment data, the nurse identifies the family's health problems. This, in turn, helps to delineate the nursing needs of the family. As defined by Tinkham and Voorhies (1977), a nursing need is the contribution nursing can make to the solution of a health problem. This may also be called the nursing diagnosis (Yura & Walsh, 1973). This area is expanded further within the Phillips case study in Case Example 18-4.

Families usually have multiple needs, some of which may be nursing needs. One of the first things community health nurses determine on their home visit is the relationship of nursing needs to other family needs. Are nursing and health high on the family's priority list or are they somewhere at the bottom? Are the health problems as seen by the family different from those seen by the nurse? If health needs are given a low priority because of other needs, such as marital difficulties or economic problems, what do you as a nurse do about it?

Community health nurses are concerned with all aspects of family life. They are able to help families with needs, other than nursing needs, by making appropriate referrals to other agencies so that the problems preventing a health need from having a place of high priority may be alleviated.

Although the community health nurse's ultimate goal in the work with families in their homes is to help them to become independent of the need for nursing service, the family may need to first experience the nurse as a person who can be trusted and relied upon for support and understanding, a person on whom one can be dependent for a period of time, and a person who can be looked to for timely advice. This therapeutic or helping relationship with the nurse enables individual family members to meet the needs of others in the family. The capacity to give genuine caring and concern to others in interpersonal relationships seems to be in direct proportion to the amount received. Therefore, it is important that nurses receive an adequate amount of caring and concern in their own lives so that they, in turn, can share it with the families they serve. Adult family members can then share themselves more fully with each other, their children, their elderly parents, and other relatives. Through genuine caring relationships people can grow and be more fully that which they are capable of becoming (Buber, 1970).

The role of community health nurses in relationship to families is dynamic—it changes as the family changes. It is important that nurses start where the family is, not where they would like the family to be. The role is probably best interpreted through what is done with the family rather than what is said to the family.

If the health problems as seen by the family are different from those seen by the nurse, the nurse's responsibility is to try to modify attitudes, beliefs, values, and knowledge about the body and its functions through education and counseling so that the family is able to recognize a health problem that exists—and then to do something about it.

Obviously it is not possible for the family and the nurse to solve all health problems at the same time; therefore, priorities of goals must be established. Nurses rely on their knowledge, skill, and judgment in coming to a decision with the family about priorities of nursing goals. The family's active involvement in the process contributes to the growth potential of the family and, at the same time, communicates something very specific about the nurse's role to the family. That is, the nurse's role is not to control the family's life and health, but rather to help the family gain more control over its own

Table 18-1   Sample Plan

Health Problem	Nursing Need	Nursing Goals (Long and Short Term)	Nursing Action
Post cerebral vascular accident	Provide teaching and guidance in management and rehabilitation	Family will be able to provide nursing care and assist patient to do passive and active exercises between home visits.	Demonstrate passive and active (range of motion) exercises to family and patient Observe family and patient doing passive and active range of motion exercises

life, health behaviors, and health problems. Ultimate decision making is the family's responsibility.

The nursing goals may be equated with the destination of a planned trip. The long-term goal is a statement of where you want to end up. The short-term goals are the little steps along the way that help you to reach your long-term goal.

The short-term goals give immediate direction to the ensuing nursing action and make it possible to periodically evaluate the nursing contribution and to reevaluate the long-term goal and restate it if necessary (Tinkham & Voorhies, 1977).

Consistent with the concepts discussed earlier, the nursing goals are established jointly by the nurse and the family. Although they may originate with the nurse, they must not remain only the nurse's goals. If the family is not involved in establishing the goal, or does not even know the goal exists, how can the family be expected to work with the nurse to attain the goal? The main focus of the stated goals is on the family and what it can do, not the nurse and what the nurse does.

The nursing action is planned by the nurse with the family before initiation of the plan of action. The plan for the nursing action may be stated in a variety of ways, and the goal may require more than one type of nursing action. A sample plan of care is shown in Table 18-1. This decision-making process carried out by the family and the nurse may be either a verbal agreement, referred to as an "implicit

contract" or the agreement may be more formalized as in a written agreement or "explicit contract."

Planning: Written and Implicit Contracts

Community health nurses have traditionally maintained written family or individual records in folders at the agency office. Contents of the written records vary among agencies, but the usual contents are (1) data collected in the initial assessment phase and at periodic intervals thereafter, (2) list of needs or problems of the family, and (3) documentation of the interventions.

Few families visited in the home by community health nurses have received a written agreement, hereafter called a contract, which serves as the framework for health care. Contracts have been described in Chapter 7. As conceptualized in this chapter, a contract consists of:

1. Family needs or problems list
2. Outcome criteria stated in measurable terms for each need or problem on the list
3. Identified interventions associated with the names of family members and provider responsible for implementation of the intervention
4. Evaluation schedule for determining the degree of goal attainment achieved at a specified date for each need or problem of the family

Case Example 18-4

The bus stop is two blocks from the Phillips home, so you have an opportunity to observe their surroundings. You note that the houses are mostly one- and two-story frame houses dating back to the 1930s. The houses have not been painted recently; they are covered with soot, and porches and wooden steps are in need of repair. In general, though, the lawns are well kept and there is no noticeable accumulation of litter in the streets. It is a warm day and many children are out playing in the yards. It is apparent that the people living in this neighborhood are of mixed ethnic and racial background. You see some black children, some Latinos, and some white children.

Note: The nurse begins the assessment process before entering the Phillips home.

Two of the children run up to you and say, "Hi! You're a nurse, aren't you?"

What else might you observe about the children or the environment?
What do you respond to this?

As you approach the Phillips home, a German shepherd tied to the porch railing greets you with a loud bark.

What do you do about the dog?

Mrs. Phillips comes to the door when she hears the dog bark. She is carrying a small boy about two years of age on her left hip. Mrs. Phillips is neatly groomed, wearing a clean apron but she appears tired and pale. She smiles warmly, holds the dog so that you may pass him, and asks you to please come in. The entrance way is dark, but when you enter the living room, you are impressed with the fact that the blinds are not drawn, and that the sun coming through the window adds some cheer to what would otherwise be a dreary room. The furniture is shabby, the carpet is worn, but the room is clean and tidy.

If Mrs. Phillips does not ask you to sit down, how do you handle it?

Mrs. Phillips invites you to have a chair and then she sits down in a chair opposite you, holding little Johnny on her lap. Johnny, curious about you and the bag you placed beside you, is not satisfied to sit on his mother's lap, wiggles off, and comes over to you. He is content to stand by you for a short time, but is obviously very interested in your bag. When he reaches for it, Mrs. Phillips says, "No, no Johnny, come back here."

If Mrs. Phillips pays no attention to what Johnny is doing, how do you handle it?
What do you think about the way Mrs. Phillips handles this situation? How do you respond?

She gets up to get a small box of ABC blocks from the bookshelf and empties them on the floor in front of her chair. Johnny sits down with them and begins to play.

You then ask Mrs. Phillips if she has noticed anything unusual about Mary's behavior and muscular activity at home.

How do you begin your interview aimed at accomplishing the purpose of your visit to the Phillips family?

Mrs. Phillips says she has also observed Mary's symptoms but has been hoping it is just a transient problem that will soon pass. She thinks perhaps it is just a nervous habit that she has developed for some reason.

Why do you inquire about this?
How do you interpret this?

She goes on to say that a lot of things have been happening in the family recently and that she herself is upset and nervous.

Mrs. Phillips says it seems like everything goes wrong at the same time. Her husband's union went on strike about a month ago and the strike still isn't settled. The longer he's off work, the more depressed he gets, and the more depressed he gets, the more he drinks. She goes on to say, "He is so hard to get along with when he is drinking—he acts like it is my fault that he is off work and we don't have enough money to buy food, pay our bills, and make the house payment. If he didn't drink so much, we wouldn't be as short as we are." Her parents made the house payment for this month. "He is even angry about that."

You say, "It sounds as though it is very important to your husband to be able to support his family."

This is apparently a new insight to Mrs. Phillips, and her facial expression loses some of the tightness and anger she was showing as she was talking about the effect of her husband's drinking on the family relationships and budget.

You then say, "Mrs. Phillips, you said everything goes wrong at the same time. Was there anything else?"

Mrs. Phillips answers, "Yes, Mary and Johnny both got sick just after my husband went out on strike. Mary had a sore throat and a high fever, and Johnny had diarrhea and a high fever. While they were both sick, Robert, our fourteen-year-old, was caught smoking marijuana in the bathroom at the high school. The principal called us and said if it happened one more time, Robert would be expelled from school. We went 'round and round' with Robert about that. He's always so devilish—always getting into some kind of trouble. We've tried everything and nothing seems to help."

You say, "Perhaps together we can take some of these problems one by one and begin to find some solutions to them."

Mrs. Phillips says, "When everything piles up like this, I just don't know where to begin or what to do."

You direct the interview to further assess Mary's problem. Mrs. Phillips replies, "Mary never gave us a bit of trouble up to now—now she's so strange." Mrs. Phillips says Mary had been a very healthy and happy baby, was never ill except for an occasional upper respiratory infection (URI) and measles when she was about four years old. You then explore Mary's most recent episode of illness (sore throat and high fever) with Mrs. Phillips. Mrs. Phillips did not call the doctor because money was so tight and she always paid

How do you facilitate further discussion about this?

What are the feelings expressed by Mrs. Phillips? How do you respond?
Is this an appropriate response? Explain why or why not.

Do you try to deal with all of these needs now? If so, how? If not, why not?

How do you respond to this?

Note: The Phillips family has multiple problems and will need the nurse's help in establishing priorities for meeting their nursing needs.

(continued)

Case Example 18-4 (continued)

her doctor bills before leaving the office. Mrs. Phillips's mother advised her on home remedies for both of the children, and they got better. She gave Johnny "milk" made from the water in which rice had been boiled and boiled carrots. She did not give him regular milk or any other foods except scraped apple until the diarrhea stopped. For Mary, she tried to keep the fever down with aspirin, gave her a lot of juice to drink, and had her gargle with salt water. Thinking back about it, Mrs. Phillips says it was around this time that she first noticed how Mary was so irritable and twitching in such a strange way. She wonders if you think this had anything to do with Mary's sore throat and fever.

What is your response?

You go on to say that you feel it would be a good idea for Mary to be examined by a physician to determine the cause of her symptoms. Aware that there are economic problems, you mention that the family could take Mary to the Pediatric Clinic at the County Hospital for an evaluation. At this point Mr. Phillips comes in from outside where he has been repairing the car. Mrs. Phillips asks him if he can sit down with us for a minute "because this is the nurse who called to say she wanted to come and talk with us about Mary." Mr. Phillips says, "Oh, yes, what do you think is wrong with Mary?"

How do you answer Mr. Phillips's questions?

Mr. Phillips says he has been thinking that Mary should see a doctor, but "money is tight now. I've been wondering if maybe my union could help. We have something called an 'emergency medical fund,' but I don't know if they would call this an emergency." After some more discussion about this Mr. Phillips says, "Well, I can call and ask about it. They can't do any worse than say no, and they might say yes." The alternative plan of taking Mary to the Pediatric Clinic

Note: Every effort to include the father in your work with families should be made. When the father is employed, this may entail planning an evening visit when he is at home.

A written contract, which becomes joint property of the family and agency, is useful in many instances.

As just described, the contract is analogous to the nursing process. The contract phases include assessment, planning, implementation, and evaluation. The contract negotiation between family and nurse occurs initially within the assessment and planning phases. In the assessment phase the nurse and family members jointly review the individual member's health status, the home environment, and general aspects of the work environment. From the assessment data base the nurse and family members identify the health needs or problems of the family. During the joint planning phase, additional community resources and potential fam-at the County Hospital is also discussed with Mr. Phillips. The parents agree that their first step will be to call the union to see if they can get help there. If not, they will make an appointment at the Pediatric Clinic. You write down the number of the clinic, give it to them, and begin to terminate your visit.

Which aspect(s) of the nursing process is in operation here?

Terminating your visit, you tell Mr. and Mrs. Phillips that you will plan to come back to see them next Tuesday morning if that time is suitable for them. If, in the meantime, they want to get in touch with you, they may call you. You give them a piece of paper on which you have written your name, the name of the agency you represent, the phone number, and the days when you can be reached. You indicate that on your next visit you will be interested in finding out the results of Mary's checkup. You also say, "We might talk some more about the problems that Robert has been having."

Note: Agencies are encouraged to provide business cards.

Mr. Phillips seems surprised and says, "Oh, Jennifer told you about the trouble Robert got into at school? We've tried everything with that boy and nothing seems to help. Sure hope this little guy [meaning Johnny, whom he has bouncing in his arms] doesn't give us so much grief!"

You say, "I see you both feel very discouraged about Robert."

Mr. and Mrs. Phillips look at each other and say simultaneously, "We sure do." Both thank you for coming and you say again that you will see them again next Tuesday. Mr. Phillips laughs and says, "I hope you won't see me—I hope our strike will be settled by that time!"

You say, "I can understand how you must be anxious for things to get back to normal again."

Evaluate the termination of this visit.

Reproduced from *The Home Visit: A Learning Module* by JA Gala with permission from the Board of Trustees, University of Illinois, copyright ©1975.

Note: For readers whose curiosity about Mary's condition has been aroused: Mary's "strange behavior" was chorea, resulting from an episode of acute rheumatic fever.

ily networkings may be explored, the needs and problems are prioritized, alternative interventions for needs or problems are examined, an intervention plan that is mutually acceptable to the family and the nurse is developed, and the outcomes with an evaluation schedule are projected. The assessment and planning phases may take two or three home visits and additional telephone calls prior to a plan of health care being instituted and written as a contract between the community health nurse and the family. Implementation and evaluation phases occur as projected, unless a family need or problem emerges, necessitating modification of the contract. The methodology of the community health nurse may be similar in the original illustration where the agency has sole possession of all components of the record; however, the value of the shared written contract between the community health nurse and the family is the shared expectation being formalized and serving as a guide to the family as well as to the nurse.

Contracting can promote goal-oriented practices by both family members and community health nurses. Adherence to improved health practices by families can improve health for the individual, family, and community. The hows, whys, and values of contracts are depicted by many providers in a variety of health settings (Hays & Davis, 1980; Herje, 1980; Leavitt, 1982; Maluccio & Marlow, 1974; Steckel, 1980, 1982; Zangari & Duffy, 1980). In selected studies with chronic illnesses those who have contracted with health providers have shown greater adherence to the therapeutic regimen and improved health states (Aragona, Cassady, & Drabman, 1975; Etzeiler, 1974; Hackney, 1974).

Steckel's *Patient Contracting* (1982) provides the nurse with the methodology for contracting. Leavitt (1982) lends support to the value of and process of contracting with families in the community. Her models of contracting depict the family and nurse roles in the process of negotiation, implementation, and termination of family contracts.

Implementing the Nursing Plan

The case of the Phillips family (Case Example 18-4) simulates a home visit so that readers can evaluate their responses to their potential role as community health nurses. The case example emphasizes the implementation phase of the community health nursing process.

To facilitate your analysis of the implementation phase of the nursing process in the first home visit to the Phillips family, respond to the questions in the right-hand margin before proceeding to the next segment and questions. In addition, evaluate the extent to which:

1. Nursing actions are purposefully directed toward promotion, maintenance, and restoration of the family's health potential.

2. Nursing actions provide for the family's active participation in health promotion, maintenance, and restoration.
3. The family care plan is implemented within the framework of the nurse-family relationship, ensuring mutual responsibility for the plan and the family's maximum independence.

Evaluating the Home Visit

Evaluation follows the implementation of actions designated in the family care plan. While elements of evaluation, like those of assessment and planning, are concurrent and recurrent with other components, evaluating the effect of actions during and after the implementation phase determines the family's response to nursing actions and the extent to which short- and long-term goals are achieved (Yura & Walsh, 1973).

The family care plan, which includes all aspects of the nursing process, is dynamic and flexible. It changes as nursing needs, priorities, and goals change. The evaluation process is extremely important in keeping the nurse in step with, and responding effectively to, the family's nursing needs.

The checklist for evaluating community health nursing services to families presented in Table 18-2 was developed by converting the ANA statements of *Standards for Community Health Nursing Practice* (1973) into evaluation questions. Useful for self-evaluation, this tool lists the complexities of providing services to families in their homes so that the omission of important assessment data or nursing actions can be readily identified. It is important to remember that the various categories of assessment data are collected over a period of time. Novice nurses can feel pressured to get answers to all of the questions in the first visit, thus damaging the beginning relationship with the family. At the end of the community health nursing experience, the tool can be used to measure accomplishments in work with an entire caseload of families.

Home Health Services

The historical review of nursing and its development given in Chapter 1 illustrates that all of public health nursing has its origins and roots in care of the sick in their homes. This care was initially provided by voluntary agencies, and gradually official health agencies (health departments) joined in this effort.

One of the most profound changes to affect public health nursing and care of the sick in their homes was the 1966 enactment of Title XVIII of the Social Security Act, "Health Insurance for the Aged and Disabled," Public Law 89-97 called "Medicare." This law established "Home Health Agencies" as providers in the health care system with reimbursement for "home health services" given to Medicare-eligible beneficiaries. These home health services include nursing, physical therapy, speech therapy, occupational therapy, nutrition guidance, home health aide and social work services. In order to be reimbursed by Medicare for care given to eligible patients, agencies providing care-of-sick to people in their homes (see Table 18-3) are certified as home health agencies by meeting the "Minimum Standards of Conditions of Participation for Home Health Agencies." Thus, this new "home health" nomenclature became firmly established.

Types of Agencies Providing Care

The earlier established visiting nurse associations were most common in New England, the Middle-Atlantic, and East North-Central states, with others scattered primarily in large cities of the remainder of the country. These "voluntary" agencies are autonomous; a board of directors selects an administrator to be directly responsible for the agency's operation. They may provide other community services—for example, maternal and child health care. In the 1960s, some voluntary agencies joined with local health departments and were called "combination agencies" (see Table 18-4). Thus, a single nursing service might provide health promotion,

disease prevention, and care-of-the-sick services for both agencies. This was done to decrease costs, promote efficiency and continuity of services, and prevent duplication (two sets of staff and cars travelling long distances). Complexities in administration within the past decade have led to the decline of "combination agencies."

Local health departments, or "official agencies," constituted over 59 percent of certified home health care agencies by 1969. They are established by state law and provide disease prevention and detection and health promotion services as determined by state mandate and local need. After Medicare was established, many health departments expanded their programming to include home health services.

With the advent of Medicare and its assurance of reimbursement, new forms of home health agencies appeared—the private agencies. These agencies are either "not-for-profit" or "proprietary" depending on their administrative eligibility for Internal Revenue Service tax exemption. Some are a part of franchise chains or other types of nationwide corporations such as Homemakers-Upjohn. These private agencies are fee-for-service units with some serving only Medicare patients. Many health care providers viewed this development with grave concern, having observed some unfortunate results with private business ownership in the nursing home movement.

Private home health agencies have demonstrated many helpful practices; for example, business acumen, efficiency of administrative practices, marketing skills, and the ability to meet the needs of their patients and families with nursing services offered twenty-four hours a day. On the other hand, it has primarily been private companies that have instigated congressional hearings on fraud and abuse in the Medicare home health program (Mundinger, 1983). These practices have included:

- Increased administrative overhead costs
- Bribes, rebates, and referral fees

Table 18-2 Checklist for Evaluation of Community Health Nursing Services to Families

Directions to Student: Check (✓) "Yes" if you think the behavior has been met; check "No" if you think the behavior has not been achieved; check "DNA" if the behavior does not apply.

NOTE: DATA FOR EVALUATION IS ACQUIRED OVER AN EXTENDED PERIOD OF TIME, REQUIRING *MANY* VISITS TO THE FAMILY!!!

	Yes	No	DNA
PREPLANNING			
Did I review all available information:			
a. From the family record			
b. By discussion with agency personnel having knowledge of the family			
c. By discussion with *other* agency personnel if appropriate			
Did I have a plan for this visit?			
Did I review scientific literature relevant to anticipated, or previously documented, needs of the family?			
THE HOME VISIT			
Did I interpret my role to the family so that they know:			
a. I am a student?			
b. My name?			
c. How long I will be available to work with them?			
d. The name of the agency I represent?			
e. The function of the agency I represent?			
f. The purpose of my visit?			
Did I get feedback from the family to determine that they actually do understand my role?			
Has rapport been established with the family?			
ASSESSMENT			
Was I able to facilitate a discussion of the family health status?			
Were any health problems identified that were not previously noted in the family record?			
Do I need to know any more information in any of the Assessment Categories:			
a. Growth and development			
b. Biophysical status			
c. Emotional status			
d. Cultural, religious, socioeconomic, and occupational background			
e. Performance of activities of daily living			
f. Patterns of coping			
g. Interaction patterns and family dynamics			
h. Family's perception of and satisfaction with health status			
i. Family's health status			
j. Relevant codes, statutes, regulations, contracts, and agreements			
k. Environment (physical, social, emotional, and ecological)			
l. Available and accessible human and material resources			

Table 18-2 *(continued)*

	Yes	No	DNA
ASSESSMENT (continued)			
Groups and Communities:			
a. Community dynamics			
b. Power structures (legislative, political, and decision-making)			
c. Economic and cultural considerations or values			
d. Demographic data			
e. Information derived from current local national and international studies of disease surveillance.			
Health status evaluation was based on the identification of health needs.			
Health status evaluation included the availability of resources and the patterns of delivery of health care.			
Potentials and limitations of resources within the family and community were identified.			
The health status data were analyzed and selectively applied in arriving at a diagnosis.			
Was I able to identify nursing needs (i.e., make a nursing diagnosis)?			
PLANNING			
In the planning stage of this visit:			
Were priorities assigned to the nursing needs?			
a. Did the family understand what I can do about their nursing needs?			
b. Did the family understand what I cannot do about nonnursing needs?			
Did I identify any differences in the priorities as I see them and as the family sees them?			
In the planning stage of this visit:			
If the priorities were different, was I able to help the family remove the barriers preventing a health need from having a place of high priority?			
Were goals mutually set with family and relevant others?			
Were goals congruent with other planned approaches?			
Were goals stated in realistic and measurable terms?			
Were goals assigned a time period for achievement?			
Were goals consistent with human and material resources?			
Was a contract clearly established with the family?			

(continued)

Table 18-2 *(continued)*

	Yes	No	DNA

PLANNING (continued)

In determining nursing actions:

a. Are primary, secondary, and tertiary preventive measures planned to meet specific family needs, and are they related to nursing diagnosis (the nursing needs and nursing goals)?

b. Are teaching-learning principles incorporated into the plan of care? (Objectives for learning are stated in behavioral terms; reinforcement is planned; readiness is considered, and the content at the learner's level?)

c. Does the plan include the utilization of available and appropriate human and material resources?

d. Is the plan flexible, and does it include an ordered sequence of nursing actions?

e. Are nursing approaches planned on the basis of current scientific knowledge?

IMPLEMENTATION

In determining progress toward goal achievement with the family:

a. Were baseline and current data about the family used in measuring progress toward goal achievement?

b. Were nursing and family actions mutually analyzed and evaluated for their effectiveness toward goal achievement?

Nursing actions involve ongoing reassessment, reordering of priorities, new goal settings, and revision of the nursing plan. In this visit:

a. Was reassessment an ongoing process in evaluating goal achievement or lack of goal achievement?

b. Were alternative actions identified and mutually initiated?

In the termination of this *visit:*

a. Did I summarize the visit with the family?

b. Did I reach an agreement with the family on a plan for the next visit?

c. Did I arrange for a mutually agreeable day and time for the next visit?

d. Is the family aware of how much time remains before I will make my *final* visit?

If service was terminated:

a. Was termination of service based on reassessment and evaluation?

b. Was provision made for follow-up of the family to determine the long-term effects of nursing service?

Based on your responses in the checklist, how do you evaluate your work with the family at this point?

SOURCES:
JA Gala
Adapted from American Nurses' Association: *Standards for Community Health Nursing Practice.* Kansas City, Mo.: Author, 1973.

Table 18-3   Types of Home Health Agencies—Number and Percent, Years Before Medicare

Type of Agency	Prior to 1945	1945– 1954	1955– 1959	1960	1961	1962	1963	1964	1965– 1966
					Number				
Official health	167	228	271	286	318	455	527	569	612
Visiting Nurse Association	464	568	589	592	594	599	602	604	611
Combined government and voluntary	27	41	50	55	56	69	76	82	32
Other nonofficial	27	37	38	40	40	46	49	50	51
Total	685	874	948	973	1,008	1,169	1,254	1,305	1,356
					Percent				
Official health	24.4	26.1	28.6	29.4	31.5	38.9	42.0	43.6	45.1
Visiting Nurse Association	67.8	65.0	62.1	60.8	58.9	51.3	48.0	46.3	45.1
Combined government and voluntary	3.9	4.7	5.3	5.7	5.6	5.9	6.1	6.3	6.0
Other nonofficial	3.9	4.2	4.0	4.1	4.0	3.9	3.9	3.8	3.8
Total	100.0	100.0	100.0	100.0	100.0	100.0	100.0	100.0	100.0

SOURCE:
Ryder C, Stiff P, Elkin W: Home health services: Past, present, future. *Am J Public Health* 1969; 59(9): 1721.

- Overutilization of services (with concurrent loss of patient independence)
- False recording (for example, billing for services not provided or when service was not medically necessary)
- Wasteful practices (for example, home health aide four-hour minimum assignment when many patients need only one to two hours of care)
- Exorbitant rental fees for medical equipment
- Inordinate overall per patient costs for services (with higher per visit charge and many more visits per patient than other types of agencies find necessary)

The multiplicity of Medicare regulations and documentation required of agencies in the federal effort to forestall these abuses have added to the frustration and overhead costs experienced by all home health agencies (*Medicare and Medicaid Frauds*, 1977; *Study of Home Health Services Under Medicare*, 1976).

The philosophy of hospitals in recent decades has increasingly expanded to cover community-wide responsibility for health services. This includes the development of hospital-based home health agencies. Advantages of this sponsorship include continuity of patient care, immediate availability of special resources, increased utilization of home care by physicians for their patients, facilitation of discharge planning, and/or readmission planning (Stewart, 1979). Disadvantages that may be experienced in hospital-based home health agencies include high overhead costs, cost sharing of hospital cafeteria and other institutional administra-

Table 18-4   Medicare-Certified Home Health Agencies by Number and Type, Selected Years 1966–1983

Year	Official Health Agency[a] No.	%	Visiting Nurse Associations No.	%	Combined Government and Voluntary Agency No.	%	Hospital-Based No.	%
1966	579	45	506	40	83	7	81	6
1968	1,035	54	562	30	97	5	148	8
1970	1,334	58	552	24	102	4	202	9
1975	1,228	55	525	23	46	2	273	12
1976	1,218	51	515	22	42	2	280	12
1977	1,213	51	493	21	44	2	272	12
1978	1,272	47	502	18	45	2	316	12
1979	1,269	46	504	18	49	2	327	12
1980	1,260	43	515	18	63	2	359	12
1981	1,189	37	512	16	57	2	456	14
1982	1,215	33	516	14	59	2	511	14
9-1-83	1,216	30	519	13	58	1	541	13

SOURCES:
US DHEW, Health Resources Administration: *Health Resources Statistics: Health Manpower and Health Facilities, 1976–77*, p. 394.

Moran, M US DHHS, HCFA. Personal communication, September 22, 1983.

[a]An agency administered by a state, county, or other local unit of government.

tive expenses, limited out-of-hospital and competing hospital referrals, governance by hospital administration that may have institutional bias, financial limitations on clients served, service limited to those who have used the hospital's facilities, and overlap of services and expenses when community-based home health agency exists in same geographic area.

Whatever its sponsorship, the nurse considering employment in a home health agency should, in addition to general employment concerns, determine:

- Agency philosophy—Is it primarily patient-focused with a family health care concern?

- Utilization of services per patient—Do these fall within accepted norms?
- Team relationships among staff and the variety of professionals and auxiliaries providing home care
- Adequacy of the range of home health services provided by the agency
- Reputation of the agency as reflected within the community
- Costs of services to clients—Do they reflect the going rate in the area?
- Licensure, Medicare-certification, and accreditation status of agency
- Limitations of services—Does the agency practice patient "dumping" when funds (patient's and/or third-party) are exhausted?

Table 18-4 *(continued)*

Skilled Nursing Facility Based[b]		Proprietary[b]		Private Nonprofit[c]		Other		
No.	%	No.	%	No.	%	No.	%	Total
—	—	—	—	—	—	26	2	1,275
—	—	—	—	—	—	48	3	1,890
—	—	—	—	—	—	121	5	2,311
5	<1	47	2	—	—	118	5	2,242
5	<1	68	3	—	—	233	10	2,361
7	<1	75	3	—	—	261	11	2,365
8	<1	145	5	—	—	435	16	2,723
8	<1	147	5	408	15	50	2	2,762
9	<1	186	6	484	17	47	2	2,923
12	<1	432	13	537	17	46	1	3,241
36	1	651	18	632	17	51	1	3,671
112	3	871	22	671	17	59	1	4,047

[b]Included in "Other" through 1970.
[c]Included in "Other" through 1978.

- Utilization of other community resources for patients

Home health agency ownership has changed markedly in the recent decade as illustrated by a comparison of Table 18-3 with the home health agencies in Table 18-4.

Official agencies (health departments) quickly expanded their services to include home health care in the first three years of Medicare. The more recent decline in this type of home health agency sponsorship reflects both mergers of small county health units into single multicounty health departments and discontinuity of home health programs when agencies of other sponsorship became available and/or shrinking of tax fund support resulted in cancellation of home health services (Kuhns & Kellogg, 1982).

The number of visiting nurse associations (VNA) has remained relatively stable. Although numerous small VNAs, especially in the Northeast, have merged into larger, stronger single organizations (Kuhns & Kellogg, 1982), new VNAs have also been established. The graphic expansion of home health agencies based in hospitals can be expected to grow even larger with the advent of Medicare reimbursement legislation based on Diagnosis-Related Groups (DRGs). The most conspicuous development is the marked increase in private, not-for-profit and proprietary agencies.

Proprietary and private not-for-profit home health agencies including both individual agencies and nationwide organizations with many agencies have so expanded as to now be the major suppliers of home care personnel throughout the nation (Spiegel, 1983).

The Multidisciplinary Health Team

The home health agency of high standard provides a broad array of coordinated health services through agency-employed staff, contractural arrangements, or a combination of administrative patterns. According to the "Proposed Model for the Delivery of Home Health Services" (National League for Nursing, 1974b) developed by a national group of nurse administrators, essential home health services, even to remote, sparsely populated areas, should reflect a multidisciplinary health team including:

• Nursing or home health aid (homemaker)
• Nutrition services
• Occupational therapy
• Physical therapy
• Social work
• Speech pathology services

Other essential services that may be provided directly or by arrangement include:

• Audiological
• Dental
• Ophthalmological
• Physician
• Podiatry
• X-ray
• Respiratory therapy
• Home-delivered meals
• Housekeeping services
• Patient transportation and escort service
• Laboratory services
• Medical supplies and equipment
• Prescription drugs
• Prosthetic or orthotic services

Additional desirable environmental support services, some of which may be provided on a voluntary basis, include:

• Barber or cosmetology
• Handyman or heavy cleaning
• Legal and protective
• Pastoral
• Personal contact or friendly visitor
• Recreational
• Translation

The developing network of home health agencies in this country is moving us toward the goal of a full-service home health system. Together with the primary health services provided by ambulatory care providers, home health care services become the basic source of health care. The alternative is institutional care for those acutely ill patients needing intensive, high technology health services.

Coordination of services among the professional home health team members, with close-knit service coordination with their colleagues in ambulatory and institutional care settings, is mandatory in a quality health care system.

Financing Home Health Services

For many home health agencies, Medicare and Medicaid (federal support for health services needed by public aid clients) are the sole source of reimbursement, and these resources provide the largest source of income for most agencies—a tremendous boon to the elderly population. The frequent changing of eligibility requirements and diversity of interpretations given by fiscal intermediaries (organizations designated by the federal government to manage Medicare reimbursement) within and among states serve to limit needed services to some clients and is costly in time and documentation to provider agencies.

Private insurance companies increasingly provide home health coverage. Corporate groups appreciate the cost-effectiveness and value of this service to employees and their family members. The National League for Nursing and the Health Insurance Association of America cooperated to develop and distribute a uniform "Home Health Care Benefit Request Form" (National League for Nursing, 1978a), which not only enhances reimbursement to agencies but has served to legitimize home health in the health insurance industry. Both the national Blue Cross Association (1976) and the Health Insurance Association of America (1976) have published model home health benefit programs and guidelines helpful to agencies in marketing their services to corporations and unions. Those Health Maintenance Organizations that are federally-certified are mandated to provide home health benefits to their members. Agencies are wise to establish contracts with local health maintenance organizations to provide these services.

Many clients pay directly for all or a portion of their home health services. Supplementary funding is provided to many agencies through United Way funds, private foundation support, bequests, and memorials.

Community health nurses have long had the advantage of excellent guidelines for determining precise service time and cost data (Levenson, 1964; National League for Nursing, 1964; U.S. Department, 1964).

The Division of Nursing of the U.S. Public Health Service and the National League for Nursing cooperated in the early 1970s to launch and support the development of management information systems in public or community health agencies, greatly enhancing their fiscal management practices. The publications series documenting these cosponsored conferences and workshops outline the whys and wherefores of management information systems—how to plan and implement them, errors to avoid, and guidelines to follow (National League for Nursing, 1974a; 1975; 1976; 1978b).

Networking for Continuity of Care

The crucial link in the chain of health care services is the philosophy and practice of continuity of care. Whenever and wherever a patient needs nursing or other health care services, inherent in providing this care should be planning for how this care will be provided in the future. This means teaching the client or his or her family or neighbors how to give this care or how to initiate a referral with needed medical orders and care information to an appropriate community- or institution-based support service. It is no platitude that "discharge planning begins at the time of admission." It would serve patients and their families well if the home health agency were given referral for future care *before* the patient leaves the hospital so that the community health nurse can plan for home care with mutual assurance of the patient, family, and nurse. A predischarge assessment home visit can be made to prepare for the patient—for example, determining width of doors or height of beds and securing such appropriate durable medical equipment as wheelchairs, raised toilet seats, overbed lifts, commodes, or bed siderails. With a predischarge assessment hospital visit, the community health nurse can learn new techniques to support the family in providing complicated therapy. Within the continuity of care concept, discharge planning is the vehicle moving the patient to the proper level of care and/or facility (Bristow, Stickney, & Thompson, 1976). Whoever is responsible for discharge planning in the hospital—community health nurse, social worker, or preferably a team of both disciplines—it is the individual professional's responsibility to contribute to that effort by providing his or her continuity of care plan when that plan involves use of continuing health care support from another provider service in the health care system.

Communication and collaboration are the interdependent factors enhancing discharge planning—uniting the patient, the family, the primary planners who make discharge plans, and the community health nurse (McKeehan, 1981). Any nurse experienced in home health care has encountered the unforgettable nightmare of individuals suffering lifelong handicaps after health professionals failed to ensure continuity of patient care. Neglect has often resulted in more injury to the patient than the original disease. All nurses must incorporate continuity of care concerns into their practice. The cost of discontinuity is too great physically, emotionally, and financially.

With their intimate knowledge of the community and its resources community health nurses must continually redemonstrate and teach by example continuity of care skills to their nursing peers in institutional settings where continuity of care may be limited by institutional constraints.

Trends in Home Health Care

What is ahead for home health services and community health nurses? The last few years have seen the emergence of some alternative forms of health services, such as the hospice and daycare services for adults. In addition, the nursing community itself is actively involved in working with other associations and agencies to create new standards for the home health industry.

Hospice In 1974, hospice care, patterned after the English movement, was initiated in the United States in New Haven, Connecticut. It refers to a coordinated, interdisciplinary program of palliative and supportive services for terminally ill persons and their families (National Hospice Organization, 1982). Early hospices tended to be institution-based with home health care provided via contract with the local home health agency. The full range of home health services may be utilized in hospice care, and clergy, volunteers, and others may join the hospice team.

A new era of hospice, as well as home health care, began in 1982 when Congress enacted legislation to approve Medicare funding for hospice care. Although final regulations have yet to be promulgated, in draft form they include the stipulation that in the aggregate no more than 20 percent of hospice care may be "inpatient" days with at least 80 percent of care given in the patient's home. The probable requirement that all core services must be provided by hospice staff (not by contract) has resulted in a wave of new hospices being established under the auspice of home health agencies.

The hospice care plan is designed so that the patient may live until he or she dies, free from pain and other physical symptoms. Both patient and family are provided the psychological, social, and spiritual support they need before and after the death of the patient. Frequently nurses have spearheaded the organization of a local hospice, and a nurse often is the coordinator of the hospice care team (National Hospice Organization, 1982). The team provides nursing care, pastoral care, emotional support, and other specialized services as required. Many communities await the leadership required to start a hospice program.

Extended Hours of Home Health Services Traditional home health agencies commonly provided their services only during daytime hours. As private not-for-profit and proprietary agencies assessed community need, they determined that the demand for twenty-four hour services, especially in larger metropolitan areas, warranted provision of round-the-clock care. Contributing to this change were the increasing numbers of elderly; the need for surrogates for people living alone; the increased prevalence of chronic, long-term illness; the hospice movement; the earlier hospital discharge of patients with need for the intensive care level of home care; and the expansion of elderly citizens' political clout. Smiraglia (Snellman & Smiraglia, 1978) describes guidelines for assessing community need and steps in planning the extended service system as experienced in five East Coast agencies. Snellman (Snellman & Smiraglia, 1978) describes similar expansion of home health aide services.

Daycare Services Throughout many communities in our country there is a great need for organized daycare services for the elderly. Nursing care in the daycare center includes providing needed nourishment and stimulating opportunities for socializing and learning. Working men and women are assured that their elderly parent is cared for during the day. Home health agencies are among the organizations that have established Adult Day-care Centers especially in larger cities. The nurse, social worker, therapist, nutritionist, and health aide team provide the daycare services as well as home health care.

Mergers By the mid 1970s, over 50 percent of the Medicare-certified home health agencies employed fewer than four full-time staff nurses. Many factors served to accelerate the demand for more efficient and effective home health agencies:

- Limited availability of well-prepared nurse supervisors and administrators
- Demand for comprehensive home health services by the public, physicians, Health Maintenance Organizations, and insurance companies
- Sophisticated documentation and service demands required by Medicare, private insurance, and other third-party payment sources

In response to these and other stimuli, many smaller agencies, especially those sponsored by voluntary boards, have sought to provide program strength through agency mergers. Kuhns and Kellogg (1982) have documented this process and cited recent successful mergers among smaller agencies. The people served, agency staff, and boards sense many gratifications through unification of effort in a stronger merged agency.

The competition among home health providers, especially in metropolitan areas, has served to further stimulate the movement for merger-for-strength among smaller agencies.

Accreditation of Home Health Agencies and Community Nursing Services In 1966, the National League for Nursing (NLN), in cosponsorship with American Public Health Association (APHA), established the national program for Accreditation of Home Health Agencies and Community Nursing Services. This program and the standards it established have since served as beacons for quality services in the home health industry. The list of accredited agencies is published annually in *Nursing and Health Care.* Nurse consultants with this program assisted the Joint Commission on Accreditation of Hospitals in developing standards for home health programs and criteria for accreditation study in those hospitals with home health programs.

In 1982 the National Association for Home Care was established by the merger of NLN's Council of Home Health Agencies and Community Health Services and the National Association of Home Health Agencies. The National Association for Home Care passed a resolution, without dissent, in support of the previously described NLN/APHA Accreditation program. Whereas, the American Nurses' Association is still endeavoring to secure direct participation in the JCAH accreditation programs for institutional health organizations, community health nurses are gratified that the described NLN/APHA accreditation program, designed by nurses with ongoing support and involvement of national organizations representing the core disciplines involved in home health care, demonstrates nursing's contribution to assurance of quality services in the American health care system.

Summary

The functioning of the basic family unit greatly contributes to the health and welfare of family members. In the home setting, the nurse and family work *together* to resolve health problems. Community health nurses are concerned with all aspects of family life, not just nursing.

In the practice of community health nursing, nurses will be challenged to apply all of their theoretical and clinical nursing skills to provide family-centered nursing in home settings. Community health nurses can experience many professional and personal rewards as families respond positively to a jointly-established therapeutic plan, enjoy improved health states, and reach the eventual goal of becoming independent in health care decision making.

Topics for Nursing Research

• Evaluate the use of "implicit contracting" and "explicit contracting" with families in the home setting.
• Audit a family folder (record) from a community health agency with the ANA standards "Checklist for Evaluation of Community Health Nursing Services to Families" (Table 18-2). What quality of care did this family receive from the community health nurse?
• How does the accreditation process influence the delivery of community health nursing services in the home?

Study Questions

1. As Sally Jones, a student nurse, prepares for her first home visit, she is apprehensive about getting the family to cooperate with her treatment plan. Which of the following statements best explains how Ms. Jones should regard the family's input?
   a. The family's input is solicited at the end of the home visit after Ms. Jones decides and prioritizes the family's needs and presents her plan to them.
   b. Ms. Jones works with the family in identifying their own needs and determining a plan of action.
   c. It is not necessary to involve the family in determining the plan of care since the family depends on Ms. Jones's skills and knowledge to plan and implement nursing care.

d. Ms. Jones determines a plan of action before making the home visit and explains the plan thoroughly to the family as she goes through its implementation.

2. Which of the following is an appropriate method for preparing for the home visit?
   a. Thoroughly review the family's case record of previous nursing contacts with the family and gather additional information from all who have worked with the family in the past.
   b. Briefly review the family's case record and make note of the reason for the visit.
   c. Neither A nor B are appropriate.
   d. Both A and B are appropriate.

3. Ms. Jones is not familiar with the family's neighborhood and is concerned about her personal safety as she prepares for the home visit. Which of the following actions can ensure her personal safety?
   a. Avoid corners where groups (gangs) congregate.
   b. Avoid using elevators in tenement buildings.
   c. Let the family know the time she expects to arrive.
   d. All of the above.

4. It is important that community health nurses emphasize which of the following aspects of the nursing care plan at the initial home visit?
   a. The implementation phase of the nursing process as outlined in the plan
   b. The assessment phase of the nursing process including growth and development, and cultural and psychosocial assessment of family members
   c. Establishing rapport with the family
   d. Formulating nursing diagnosis of the family's health problems in order to establish the basis for a family-nurse contract.

5. Which of the following factors was most responsible for the development of home health agencies.
   a. The need for primary prevention in communities
   b. Political activities of consumer and community action groups
   c. The advent of Medicare and its assurance of reimbursement
   d. Push for better health services among professionals

References

American Nurses' Association, Division on Community Health Nursing: *A Conceptual Model of Community Health Nursing*. Kansas City, Mo.: Author, 1980.

American Nurses' Association: *Standards for Community Health Nursing Practice*. Kansas City, Mo.: Author, 1973.

Aragona J, Cassady J, Drabman RS: Treating overweight children through parental training and contingency contracting. *J Appl Behav Anal* 1975; 8: 269–278.

Archer SE, Fleshman RP: *Community Health Nursing Patterns and Practice*, 2nd ed. North Scituate, Mass.: Duxbury Press, 1979.

Bristow O, Stickney C, Thompson S: *Discharge Planning for Continuity of Care*. New York: National League for Nursing, 1976.

Blue Cross Association: *Home Health Care: Model Benefit Program and Related Guidelines*. Chicago: Blue Cross Association, 1976.

Buber M: *I and Thou* (Trans. Walter Kaufman). New York: Charles Scribner's Sons, 1970.

Dever GEA: *Community Health Analysis*. Germantown, Md.: Aspen Systems Corporation, 1980.

Etzeiler D: Why not put your patients under contract. *Prism* 1974; 1: 26–29.

Freemen RB, Heinrich J: *Community Health Nursing Practice*, 2nd ed. Philadelphia: Saunders, 1981.

Fitzpatrick ML: *The National Organization for Public Health Nursing, 1912–1952: Development of a Practice Field*. New York: National League for Nursing, 1975.

Gala JA: *The Home Visit: A Learning Module*. Copyright 1975, Board of Trustees, University of Illinois.

Gala JA, Reisch HR: Urban family health care. In: Hymovich DP, Barnard MV (editors), *Family Health Care*. Vol. 1. New York: McGraw-Hill, 1979.

Hackney H: Applying behavior contracts to chronic problems. *The School Counselor* 1974; 9:23–30.

Hanlon JJ: *Public Health Administration and Practice*. St. Louis: Mosby, 1974.

Hays WS, Davis LL: What is a health contract? *Health Values: Achieving High Level Wellness* 1980; 4:82–89.

Health Insurance Association of America: *Insurance Benefits for Home Health Services*. New York: Health Insurance Association of America, 1976.

Helvie CO: *Community Health Nursing: Theory and Process*. Philadelphia: Harper and Row, 1981.

Helvie CO, Hill E, Bambino CR: The setting and nursing practice, Parts I and II. *Nurs Outlook* 1968; 8:27–28 and 9:35–38.

Herje PA: Hows and whys of patient contracting. *Nurse Educator* 1980; 1:30–221.

Illinois Department of Public Health: *Standards of Health Departments in Illinois*. 1977.

Kuhns P, Kellogg R: *Agency Mergers: A Cost Effective Approach to Improving Quality Care*. New York: National League for Nursing, 1982.

Leahy M, Cobb M, Jones C: *Community Health Nursing*, 3rd ed. New York: McGraw-Hill, 1977.

Leavitt MB: *Families at Risk: Primary Prevention in Nursing Practice*. Boston: Little, Brown, 1982.

Levenson G: *A Guide for Time Studies*. New York: National League for Nursing, 1982.

Maluccio AB, Marlow WD: The case for contract. *Social Work* 1974; 1:28–36.

McKeehan KE: *Continuing Care: Multidisciplinary Approach to Discharge Planning*. St. Louis: Mosby, 1981.

Medicare and Medicaid Frauds. Hearing Before the Special Committee on Aging, U S Senate, in cooperation with the Subcommittee on Health and the Subcommittee on Oversight of the Ways and Means Committee, House of Representatives, 95th Congress, 1st Session, March 8, 1977. Washington, DC: Government Printing Office, 1977.

Mundinger M: *Home Care Controversy: Too Little, Too Late, Too Costly*. Rockville, Md.: Aspen Corporation, 1983.

National Hospice Organization: *The Basics of Hospice*. McLean, Va.: National Hospice Organization, 1982.

National League for Nursing: *Cost Analysis for Public Health Nursing Service*. New York: National League for Nursing, 1964.

National League for Nursing: *Home Health Care Benefit Request Form*, rev. ed. New York: National League for Nursing, 1978a.

National League for Nursing: *Management Information Systems for Public Health/Community Health Agencies*. New York: National League for Nursing, 1974a.

National League for Nursing: *Proposed Model for the Delivery of Home Health Services*. New York: National League for Nursing, 1974b.

National League for Nursing: *Selected Management Information Systems for Public Health/Community Health Agencies*. New York: National League for Nursing, 1978b.

National League for Nursing: *State of the Art in Management Information Systems for Public Health/Community Health Agencies*. New York: National League for Nursing, 1976.

Pan American Health Organization: *Teaching of Community Health Nursing*, Scientific Publication No. 332. Washington, DC: Pan American Health Org., 1976.

Public Health Nursing Section, American Public Health Association: *The Definition and Role of Public Health Nursing in the Delivery of Health Care*. Washington, DC: Author, 1980.

Ryder C, Stiff P, Elkin W: Home health services: Past, present, future. *Am J Public Health* 1969; 59(9): 1720–1729.

Snellman L, Smiraglia C: *Extended Hours for Home Health Services.* New York: National League for Nursing, 1978.

Spiegel A: *Home Healthcare.* Owings Mills, Md.: National Health Publishing, 1983.

Steckel SB: Contracting with patient: Selected reinforcers. *Am J Nurs* 1980; 9:1596–1599.

Steckel SB: *Patient Contracting.* Norfolk, Conn.: Appleton-Century-Crofts, 1982.

Stewart J: *Home Health Care.* St. Louis: Mosby, 1979.

Study of Home Health Services Under Medicare. Hearing before the Subcommittee on Health and the Subcommittee on Oversight of the Committee on Ways and Means, House of Representatives, 94th Congress, 2nd Session, September 13, 1976. Washington, DC: Government Printing Office, 1976.

Tinkham W, Voorhies R: *Community Health Nursing: Evolution and Process,* 2nd ed. New York: Appleton-Century-Crofts, 1977.

US Department of Health, Education and Welfare: *How to Determine Nursing Expenditures in Small Health Agencies,* Rev. ed. Washington, DC: HEW-Public Health Service, 1966.

Wensley E: *The Community and Public Health Nursing.* New York: Macmillan, 1950.

Wilner DM, Walkley RP, O'Neill EJ: *Introduction to Public Health,* 7th ed. New York: Macmillan, 1978.

Winslow OEA: *Man and Epidemics.* Princeton, N.J.: Princeton University Press, 1952.

Yura H, Walsh B: *The Nursing Process: Assessing, Planning, Implementing, Evaluating.* New York: Appleton-Century-Crofts, Educational Division, Meridith Corporation, 1973.

Zangari ME, Duffy P: Contracting with patients in day-to-day practice. *Am J Nurs* 1980; 3:451–455.

Chapter 19

School Health

Linda H. Edwards
and Julia Muennich Cowell

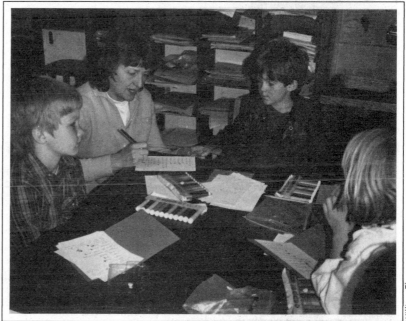

The school nurse is in a unique position to support the health of families. By promoting wellness and monitoring the child's health, the nurse can provide ongoing care and guidance.

Chapter Objectives

After completing this chapter, the reader will be able to:

- Describe the evolution of school nursing practice and relate the influence of early events and mandates on school nursing practice today
- Demonstrate the utilization and integration of the nursing process and
  the school health program component
- Identify the levels of prevention as they relate to the school health
  program and provide examples of the school nursing role in each level
  of prevention
- Discuss the role of school nurses and identify appropriate preparation
  for school nursing practice
- Describe and discuss current practices and trends in school nursing
  practice

Since its early days, school nursing has built its practice around children and their families. School nurses have historically identified families as the critical care-givers and have recognized that the success of school health programs is contingent on the cooperation of families. Thus, the school nurse is in a pivotal position in the school health program, acting as liaison between the child, family, and school and the available community resources.

The relationships formed between the school nurse and families of schoolchildren are crucial in effecting meaningful care. Indeed, a family-centered approach acknowledges and enhances the family as a focal point for nursing intervention. Wold (1981, p. 16) cites two important reasons for the school nurse to adopt a family-centered approach in school health services:

1. It fosters better understanding and assessment of children's needs and capabilities.

2. The family unit is a system, with each part interacting and affecting other parts.

This chapter describes school nursing as it has developed historically and as it is shaped by legal constraints and mandates. We look at the three major components of a school health program and see how they are integrated with the nursing process. Next is a general discussion of the educational preparation needed for school nursing and the roles and functions of the nurse in the school. The fourth section examines several trends and their potential for the future. The last two sections cover strategies for school health nursing practice, such as tactics for establishing client and team relationships, and strategies for health promotion in schools.

Defining School Nursing

School nursing developed in the United States as a specialization within public health nursing (Buser, 1980). Like public health nursing, school nursing in its ideal form has always focused its attention across the health care continuum—from care of the sick to health promotion. What *is* unique about school nursing is the client and setting focus. School nursing is focused on the child in an educational setting and meets the child's needs by recognizing that the family, as well as the school community, is critical to any plan of care.

Historical Perspectives

To gain a clear understanding of school nursing as it is today, one must trace its origins and identify the important historical influences. Florence Nightingale's establishment of an independent school of nursing had a profound impact on all of

nursing. From this early point the expanded educational opportunity prepared nurses for many roles. Though Miss Nightingale did not accept the "germ" theory, her strong focus on asepsis and hygiene had a great impact on health promotion (Goodnow, 1943).

In England, early school nursing programs focused attention on students' nutritional problems, while French programs were directed to improvement of sanitary conditions (Wold, 1981). These early programs shared a common dilemma with school health programs of today in that they were constantly struggling for financial security.

The first American school health program was in the Boston schools in 1894. This program provided medical inspections to identify and exclude from schools children with communicable diseases. These early "inspections," however, did not provide for follow-up; consequently, many children were excluded from school for long periods. The

463

nurses at the Henry Street Settlement House in New York found examples of exclusion for extremely long periods of time. In one case a twelve-year-old boy had never been in school (Wold, 1981). Given the compulsory attendance laws, Lillian Wald, founder of community health nursing in America, had little trouble negotiating a school nurse position for one of her nurses, Lina Rogers. The goal of the nursing intervention was to follow up individual cases, work with their families, and provide health education. As a result of this intervention, school absence decreased tenfold. The outcome of this first effort was so dramatic that twenty-five nurses were placed in the schools of New York City (Wold, 1981).

This example in the New York City schools illuminates a general change in the focus of school health programs: from health inspections for exclusionary sake to examination for case finding with subsequent health education and medical supervision. Though many school nurses today subscribe to purposeful health examinations that allow for education and medical supervision, it is interesting to observe the impact of the school financial constraints on the philosophy of school health programs. As money grows tight, many schools are shifting the responsibility for school-identified health care problems to the family. The contemporary family, on the other hand, is putting new demands on traditional institutions such as schools. As the single-parent family and the family with two working parents become more commonplace, families turn to outside resources, like the school, for help and support in providing for their children's needs. Furthermore, the American family has become a better consumer of health care and weighs a variety of considerations when making health care choices. This phenomenon provides a unique challenge to school nurses today.

Legal Mandates

Since education falls under the jurisdiction of state government, individual states rather than the fed-

eral government determine legal mandates (Buser, 1980). Hence, there is much variation from state to state.

In some states, the required educational preparation of school nurses is spelled out. The school nurse may be mandated to hold certification for school nursing. In addition, school nursing certification may require courses in education and special training in screening services. Mandates may also define programs in the health services. The most commonly mandated screening programs are vision and hearing and, increasingly, scoliosis (Gruber, 1981). Assessment through review of health records rests upon legal mandates for physical examinations and immunizations. Although the laws are not new, the federal immunization initiatives of the 1970s have resulted in increased emphasis in this area.

Screening activities are also affected by legislation related to confidentiality of school records. The Family Education Rights and Privacy Act of 1974 gives parents the right to examine their children's school records upon request (Oda & Quick, 1977). As part of the school record, health records are included in the provisions of this act. Results of screening tests, identification and follow-up activities, and nurse-student interactions, while rarely controversial, need to be recorded accurately and systematically.

Implementation of P.L. 94-142 (Education for All Handicapped Children Act) may also shape the practice of school health services (see Box 19-1). This law requires that all children (ages three to twenty-one) have appropriate educational opportunities. Further, it requires that all children's needs be assessed thoroughly so that impediments to successful education are identified and appropriate individualized interventions are planned. Health care needs affecting educational opportunity must be identified and treated.

Legal mandates may also define health education curriculum and require its utilization in the schools. The school nurse's role in health education is discussed later in the chapter.

Box 19-1 Public Law 94-142

Public Law 94-142, The Education for All Handicapped Children Act, was passed in 1975 to guarantee appropriate services and free public education for all handicapped children, regardless of the particular handicap. Handicapped—or exceptional—children are those who require special education and related services in order to reach their maximum potential. Every possible effort must be made to identify these children, who are to be educated with no more restriction or segregation than is absolutely necessary (a concept known as *least restrictive environment*).

The law requires that an Individualized Educational Plan (IEP) be written for each special education student between the ages of three and twenty-one (individual state laws, court orders, or actual educational practice might narrow these years to ages six to seventeen) once a year. The IEP is developed by a team consisting of, at a minimum, the student's parents or guardians, current teacher, school administrator, child (if appropriate), and any other individual designated by the parent or county/district educational office (such as a nurse).

The IEP consists of a formal statement outlining the child's present level of educational performance and a statement listing both the annual goals and the short-term objectives to be obtained through educational services. The IEP lists those services and the date they will go into effect, as well as their duration. Special evaluation procedures for determining whether or not the student is reaching the short-term objectives are also stated in the IEP.

What services are to be made available to handicapped children? PL 94-142 includes services such as language and speech assessment and remediation, audiological services, mobility instruction, counseling and guidance, physical and occupational therapy, social work services, parent counseling and guidance, transportation, adaptive physical education, vocational education and *nursing services*.

The law protects both parents (or guardians) and students in the following ways. Parents have the legal right for an independent educational assessment to be performed with the child; the right to review and inspect all educational records; the right to give written consent to the assessment plan, to refuse consent to an assessment, and to have a full explanation of the procedural safeguards for the child. In addition, parents have the right to inspect and obtain copies of all information regarding their child. Of course, all results of assessment data and placement are kept confidential.

The student's rights ensure that all evaluations and tests are conducted in the student's own language (or mode of communication); that a variety of achievement tests and teacher recommendations, as well as any other background information, are used for placement procedures; and that an evaluation shall be conducted every three years, or upon request of the teacher or parent.

SOURCE: Lewis K, Thomson H: *Manual of School Health.* Menlo Park, Calif.: Addison-Wesley (in press).

Program Components

Identifying client needs provides the nurse a sound basis for program development. Nonetheless, the basic program components, which remain constant in any community, are (1) health services, (2) health education, and (3) environmental health and safety (Wold, 1981). The purpose of the school health program is to promote optimal health, thereby maximizing each child's potential for learning

(Mayshark, Shaw, & Best, 1977; Rustia, 1982). The goals of the individual program focuses support this general purpose.

School Health Services

The goal of the health services component is to assess and provide adequate medical and/or health care. School health services are directed to the health care needs of healthy children as well as those with problems. In this traditional role the nurse provides care for the child or interprets a medical regime to school personnel. Where medical care needs are identified, the school nurse serves as an advocate for the child and family in ascertaining appropriate care. The chronically ill child may be managed in the school setting with medication or even more sophisticated treatment. Other services to students are screening and special education activities including staffing by a pupil personnel service team. In addition, the school health services should be designed to include school personnel. While not often recognized by school administrators as part of school nursing services, nevertheless, school nurses frequently find themselves unofficially serving the entire school community, including teachers and administrators.

Health Education

The goal of the health education focus is to offer an understanding of optimal health behavior. This goal is achieved both formally and incidentally.

Formal implementation of health education is carried out in the health education curriculum. The nurse's participation here varies: He or she may take part directly in the classroom settings and/or act as consultant to a health educator. In addition, the school nurse can indirectly support the teacher's efforts in health education. The nurse can most effectively affect the formal health education program as a content expert rather than as a curriculum expert. The nurse might help to define

priorities for health teaching, identify resources on specific topics, and review materials for accuracy and completeness. Health education, in and of itself, is an education specialty. School nurses often refer to their educational roles as health counseling or health teaching. Health education is a function of primary prevention and is discussed thoroughly in that context.

Incidental implementation is carried out as a thread of the health service focus. That is, the school nurse incorporates an educational goal in every interaction so that a broader health understanding can be fostered. For example, a well child may be referred to the school nurse for a hygiene problem. The school nurse works with the child to discover and clarify the problems underlying poor hygiene habits and subsequently sets some goals with the child to improve hygiene.

Environmental Health and Safety

The environmental health and safety goal is to attain and maintain a healthy and safe environment. This goal is also achieved formally and incidentally. The formal implementation could be carried out through the activities of an environmental health and safety committee. This committee may inspect the general physical plant for problems and recommend solutions.

The incidental implementation is carried out as a thread of the service focus as it relates to specific student needs. For instance, one school nurse observed that during a two-week period in January, four sixth-grade girls had come to her office with burns on their arms or legs. Careful questioning revealed that the burns were the result of contact with a radiator while waiting in line to see the teacher. The nurse took the problem to the safety committee of the school who then recommended a barrier around the radiator to prevent further contact between students and hot surfaces. More permanent alternatives such as other heating arrangements or relocation of the class to another building, were also explored.

The entire school community may become the focus of school nursing activity when matters of policy and environment arise. To the extent that the nurse has developed ongoing relationships with all levels of school personnel, from the school board to the crossing guards, concerns about health may be considered and acted upon.

The Program Components and the Nursing Process

The nursing process provides a logical approach to nursing activities in any programmatic area (see Table 19-1). In a mature program the programmatic focuses are closely integrated by the nurse.

Table 19-1 illustrates the relationship of the nursing process to the school health program components. In this model the phases of the nursing process form the vertical strands. Horizontal strands within each step of the nursing process encompass the various program components. It is an interactive model with feedback loops to the beginning of a new cycle in the nursing process.

The school nurse's primary client is the child. As a nurse progresses through the nursing process, the child as client merges with significant others until "client" evolves to mean child and the significant others, such as family, school, and community, who are important to the child's health and educational needs.

Various roles of the nurse emerge in progressing vertically through the nursing process as shown in Table 19-1. Consider the nursing role as it relates to vision screening. As casefinder, the nurse surveys the student community to identify children with vision problems. Once identified, the nurse works with the family to remedy problems and may well become a "resource person" to families in need by referring the child to appropriate resources. Once the diagnosis and treatment are provided, the nurse may well assume the role of "coordinator" between medical resource and school. At the evaluation point of the process nurses draw on their clinical base to make judgments about the effectiveness of a program and may well assume the role of "problem solver" to analyze problems.

Horizontal movement between program elements in Table 19-1 illuminates the managerial functions of the school nurse. In addition to being a generalist in the clinical sense, the school nurse must have skills in management to address programmatic needs horizontally. In the vision screening example, the school nurse, as consultant to the health education curriculum, would coordinate the health instruction content on topics related to vision. Further, the nurse may well encourage the environmental health and safety committee to assess and reevaluate the environmental considerations related to vision conservation. The ability to stand back from the direct student-nurse relationship and gain the programmatic perspective is critical to the well-managed school health program.

Teachers often refer children who are at-risk to the school nurse. Children whose parents are divorcing may have nonspecific problems such as

Table 19-1   School Health Program

Nursing Process	Health Service	Health Education	Environmental Health and Safety
Assessment			
Diagnosis			
Planning			
Implementation			
Evaluation			

decreased attention, increased absence, or other symptoms that indicate a potential health problem. The school nurse is in a position to recognize the effects of family stress on the child's health behavior. Part of the assessment process includes contact with the family. When this occurs, the client as family is then incorporated in the plan of care. As a resource person, the school nurse may suggest counseling resources available and acceptable to the family. The nurse may well assume a counseling role by helping the family see the effects of stress on the child's health behavior and by facilitating family coping skills.

The implementation of plans that include support require that the nurse maintain a relationship with the family in the role of coordinator so that the referring teacher is kept abreast of progress and appropriate classroom support. The evaluation of nursing activities is ongoing through the process, allowing for analysis of success and failures. Ulti-

mately, evaluation of the nursing process is based on resolution of the identified problems.

This example illustrates vertical movement through the nursing process as the nurse works with an individual family. The school nurse analyzes such individual cases as an index to school-community problems as well. If an increasing number of students with comparable problems are identified, the school nurse assumes the role of planner and may well move horizontally to incorporate schoolwide education programs for families in stress. By drawing on expertise within the school, the nurse can develop programs to serve a larger segment of the school population rather than one or two individuals.

Further horizontal movement would require an analysis of stress factors in the school environment. Minimizing stress in the environment serves to reduce stress in general and provides a modeling focus for students.

Preparation, Roles, and Functions of the School Nurse

School nursing preparation is not standardized. In some states a school nurse needs only to be registered (an RN) to practice as a school nurse. The educational preparation is not prescribed. In other states, in addition to being an RN, the nurse must have a degree. But the type of degree is not specified, so again an associate degree or diploma training may well be the only nursing preparation. Many states require "certification" by a state board of education, which may include post-bachelor's degree, education courses, as well as an internship in school nursing.

Preparation

Proponents for school nursing typically agree on several points. Associate degree and diploma programs do not provide nurses with the community health nursing skills to develop school health programs that have a strong emphasis on health promotion and wellness (Marriner, 1971). Nurses with

a minimum of a baccalaureate in nursing (BSN) education have a theoretical basis and clinical experiences not only in community health but also in rehabilitation and leadership. These curricular areas are the basic building blocks of school health programs. Considering the independent practice setting and the management and administrative responsibilities of school nursing, many professionals advocate a master of science in nursing (Marriner, 1971).

This lack of standardized entry level is even more complicated in school nursing than in other areas of nursing. Like other areas, employers are often concerned about costs and feel the cost savings of a lesser prepared nurse outweigh the gains. School nurses often fail to recognize the practice of accountability skills gained in upper-division baccalaureate nursing programs and choose to "specialize" in other nonnursing fields. Further, school nurses may tend to align themselves with teachers and teacher organizations in an effort to develop peer relationships and financial equality in the school. Though these considerations are important for many reasons, this alignment may occur at the expense of professional nursing development.

The school nurse is often assigned to the pupil personnel services. These services are highly specialized and are designated as the support services in the school. These support services include diagnosis and placement of special education students. The nurse's responsibility may well be that of a diagnostic screener for special services, and therefore, the population served is the entire school community. The psychologist, social worker, and nurse approach placement decisions through a team effort. The psychologist and social workers are professionals with masters degrees or doctorates, while the nurse may or may not have comparable educational preparation. This often results in role disparity and/or devaluation of the nurse's contribution.

Roles and Functions

School nursing may be a service provided by an agency whose primary purpose is education rather than health service, or it may be obtained or purchased by a school from a health care agency. Regardless of the source of service, the functions of the nurse generally are comparable. The influence of school administration on delivery of service is an important consideration in the interpretation of school nurses' functions. For example, if administration identifies the nursing role as purely first aid, the nurse might be limited in terms of time to develop a health promotion program.

Several agencies supporting the role of the school nurse provide frameworks for nurse functioning. The American Nurses' Association (ANA) has utilized the nursing process to develop standards for school nursing functions (ANA, 1983, Standard III). These standards were developed by a special Task Force on Standards of School Nursing Practice consisting of representatives from the following organizations: National Association for State School Nurse Consultants, American School Health Association, American Nurses' Association, National Association of Pediatric Nurse Associates and Practitioners, National Association of School

Nurses, and American Public Health Association. Specific functions are identified for each step of the nursing process: data collection, nursing diagnosis, planning, intervention, and evaluation. Structure, process, and outcome criteria provide a framework for practice. Figure 19-1 illustrates the systematic functions of the school nurse.

Internalization of the systematic functions in Figure 19-1 enables the school nurse to develop confidence and competence as a health professional and allows the nurse equal standing among other school faculty.

In many communities school nurses have felt that they must have faculty standing to ensure financial equality and job security. Furthermore, they have felt that faculty standing has put them in a position to promote health services in a more comprehensive manner. Because of this attitude, many school nurses are members of traditionally educational organizations, such as the National Education Association (NEA).

The American School Health Association (ASHA) membership is made up of persons concerned with school health programs. The membership includes a variety of personnel, from health education teachers to health service personnel. Thus, the base of support for school health programs within this organization is broad and reflects a multidisciplinary approach to school health.

All these organizations describe the nurse as the person responsible for identifying the health needs of the school population. The American Nurses' Association and American School Health Association specifically mention students and school personnel as the recipients of nursing care. The organizations all identify health education as a nursing responsibility. The manner in which the nurse participates in formal health education certainly is controlled, to some extent, by the institutional policy, but more importantly by the nurse's own interpretation of the health education role. The extent to which the school nurse interacts with family and community is also related to the nurse's identification of the appropriate role.

To the community, the school nurse is a highly visible member of the nursing profession (Hawkins, 1971). Thus, the school nurse often reflects

A. Collection of Data—Process Criteria
    The nurse—

    1. collects health status data including:
        a. growth and developmental history
        b. health history
        c. screening results
        d. physical assessment
        e. emotional status
        f. performance level of activities of daily living
        g. interactional patterns
        h. nutritional status
        i. immunization status
        j. student's perception of his or her health status
        k. student's health goals
        l. cultural variance
    2. collects data from: student, family, significant others, school personnel, and health care professionals
    3. obtains data by: interview, screening procedures, observation, physical assessment, and review of records and reports
    4. systematically records data on the student's cumulative school health record
    5. interprets data by comparing it to norms and standards

B. Nursing Diagnosis—Process Criteria
    The nurse—

    1. formulates a nursing diagnosis based on a comprehensive assessment
    2. coordinates efforts with those of other providers and school personnel for the student to decrease duplication of care
    3. identifies the relationship between health status and the student's ability to learn

    4. formulates a nursing diagnosis in emergency situations based on selected components of assessment

C. Planning—Process criteria

    1. When establishing nursing care plans, the nurse collaborates with the students, family, health care-providers, and school personnel
    2. The nursing care plan—
        a. is based on identifiable school nursing principles, utilizing theories and research findings in search of alternative solutions
        b. is individualized to meet the physical, mental, emotional, social, cultural, and educational needs of students
        c. is based on measures of prevention and health promotion
        d. incorporates the students' and parents' goals and priorities
    3. When developing a care plan, the nurse—
        a. identifies skills necessary for self-care
        b. identifies interdisciplinary approach to care
        c. identifies priorities of care
        d. identifies the impact of health needs on educational programming
        e. identifies the impact of cultural variance on educational programming
        f. states goals and measurable behavioral objectives based on identified health needs and specific services and resources to meet the needs
        g. proposes an ordered sequence of nursing action
        h. gives options to meet stated needs

Figure 19-1 Functions of the school nurse. (American Nurses' Association: Standards of School Nursing Practice. Kansas City, Mo.: Author, 1983, pp. 5-11.)

      i. plans physical measures to prevent or control specific student problems that clearly relate to the nursing diagnosis

      j. provides that teaching-learning principles are incorporated. Objectives for learning are stated in behavioral terms, reinforcement is planned, readiness is considered, and the content is at the learner's level

      k. indicates which student needs will be the primary responsibility of the school nurse and which will be deferred

D. Intervention—Process Criteria
The nurse—

1. intervenes appropriately for individuals and populations at risk for preventable, potential health problems

2. intervenes for a normal well child who evidences an acute illness, injury, or temporary handicapping condition

3. provides for teaching the student skills for self-care or assists in modifying the environment to allow the student to use self-care skills

4. ensures that the student and family are informed about current health status, roles of health care and school personnel, and health care and educational resources

5. structures each student encounter to provide a learning opportunity for self-care

6. employs principles of learning theory and teaching to ensure the student develops decision-making skills to attain optimal wellness

7. encourages students to collaborate in the development of a self-care plan of positive health practices

8. informs school personnel about adaptations of the comprehensive school program, interventions, or environment required by students to meet their individual health needs

9. provides necessary health counseling and refers to an appropriate professional when indicated

10. engages in appropriate and necessary nursing care to ensure optimal education opportunity for:

      a. handicapped: set goals to habilitate or rehabilitate to highest potential for specific disability

      b. chronically ill: educate client, family, and school personnel regarding the specific condition; monitor treatment regime and ensure continuity of care

      c. terminally ill: arrange for physical care, medication, and treatments; offer anticipatory guidance to student, family, school personnel, and peers in preparation for death

E. Evaluation—Process Criteria
The school nurse—

1. pursues validation, suggestions, and new information

2. analyzes observations, insights, and data with colleagues

3. documents the results of nursing care

4. provides for follow-up of selected cases in order to assess long-term effects of nursing care

5. determines new priorities and goals in collaboration with the student, family, and school personnel if appropriate

positively or negatively upon the profession as a whole. Also, since they cultivate relationships that may have a lasting impact upon the school health program and upon nursing, school nurses extend their influence far beyond the immediate arena of the school.

Future Perspectives

Projections into the future are always risky; however, several approaches currently in use have not yet reached their full potential and are likely to be of value in school health programs for some time to come. Those described in this section are increased emphasis on school nurse practitioners, use of auxiliary personnel, managerial roles, and commitment to excellence in practice.

School Nurse Practitioner

The first of these trends received renewed vigor with the advent of the school nurse practitioner model. Originally designed to improve availability and accessibility to primary care, the school nurse practitioner stimulated new interest in health assessment of schoolchildren (Robinson, 1981). Continued education offerings and short-term coursework on the expanded role of nursing grew increasingly popular for all school nurses.

Assessment of a student's health begins with collecting known health information that is readily available. This includes information on the health records, results of screening tests, fitness tests, teacher observations, and other pertinent information. A comprehensive health history from students and their families completes the background data. Next in order is a general inspection of the child by the school nurse, utilizing skill in observation of body characteristics, nutrition, development, and emotional health. The final step is a physical examination and developmental assessment (Wold, 1981). Obviously the depth of these latter appraisals is limited by the training and experience of the nurse, since educational preparation in assessment may vary from a single course in assessment techniques to a master's level practitioner. However, health assessment is a vital function of all school nurses. While new skills may affect the depth and detail of the assessment, the basic modes of observation, interviewing, and record analysis have always contributed to the nurse's plan of care.

In addition to health assessments, the school nurse practitioner has specific training in managing minor illnesses of school-aged children, in health promotion, and in identifying factors associated with learning difficulties (Igoe, 1980a). This relatively new type of nurse practitioner can contribute much to the effectiveness of the school health program (Wold, 1981). Due to defined legal constraints upon nursing practice, the school nurse practitioner may not prescribe medications; however, nursing rather than medical treatments has always been within the realm of school nursing practice. For instance, children with poor nutritional practices can be appropriately managed by counseling from the nurse, group activities, or other health promotion and treatment modalities.

Use of Auxiliary Personnel

Studies of the amount of time spent on various activities by the school nurse have indicated large amounts given to clinical and/or technical duties (Dale et al, 1981). The use of a health aide to accomplish some of the nonprofessional functions has found growing acceptance in school districts across the country. Some of these nonprofessional tasks include maintenance of health records, routine first aid, notification of parents when a child is ill, and scheduling screening programs. While there are potential benefits in employing a health aide to assume these tasks, there are acknowledged problems in role confusion, supervision, and delegation of tasks. Many school districts view the health aide as a replacement for the school nurse. On the other hand, when role expectations are clearly delineated and appropriate tasks delegated to the nonprofessional, school nurses are able to function more efficiently and effectively for optimum care to children (Dale, et al, 1981).

Wold (1981, p. 443) challenges the school nurse to the following responsibilities when working with auxiliary personnel:

1. Participate in development of clear and appropriate job descriptions
2. Encourage recruitment of qualified and motivated school health aides
3. Participate in the development of guidelines for delegation of specific responsibilities to the school health aide
4. Provide appropriate orientation and supervision of school health aides
5. Document through research the efficiency and impact of employing school health aides

Managerial Role

The evolving role of the school nurse as manager of the school health program is often overlooked and underrated. While ultimate responsibility for all programs within the school rests with the administrator, the school nurse "takes on the role of manager as she participates in planning, implementation, and evaluation of the school health program" (Wold, 1981, p. 23). In previous discussions of the importance of team relationships, the school nurse was depicted as coordinator and facilitator of team processes. In addition to team responsibilities, the school nurse must participate in decisions on the purpose and goals of the health program, as well as providing input for the allocation of resources to implement goals (Wold, 1981).

The 1983 ANA *Standards of School Nursing Practice* speaks to Program Management in Standard II: "The school nurse establishes and maintains a comprehensive school health program" (p. 4). Criteria related to active participation in all aspects of the school health program are defined in this section. Wold (1981) states that the management process is one of the "most important keys to the future of school nursing" (p. 434).

One of the distinguishing characteristics of the nurse in a managerial role is the ability to initiate the nursing process in relation to the school health program. Rather than a crisis-driven program, responding to "immunization initiatives" and cries for "first-aid," the school health program becomes a coordinated plan of services individualized for a particular school and established in response to identified needs (Wold, 1981). Thus, the school nurse provides leadership in assessing needs, planning programs and services to meet those needs, implementing a comprehensive program based on identified needs, and evaluating the outcomes of programs and services in conjunction with the school administration.

During the process of planning for health services, the school nurse utilizes managerial skill to the greatest degree. A difficult but crucial planning task is setting program goals and objectives. This process allows the school nurse to assume control of program direction. Without clear-cut goals, the school health program becomes subject to each new externally imposed demand.

Commitment to Excellence

School nurses can enhance their value in the school system through documentation that nursing practice makes a difference in the health of the school child. The connection between school nursing activities and learning outcomes, the primary focus of the school, is even more critical to document. Chinn (1973) studied the relationship between health problems and school achievement and reported the link between learning and health, with both infectious and noninfectious health problems. This study needs to be repeated and applied to other school populations. Chinn found a serious lack of research documenting outcomes of school health services and school nursing. Although school nurses are aware that their contributions are often overlooked, most do not realize that data on the impact of health services to school children are sorely needed if that impact is to be believed and valued (Wold, 1981).

Research is needed in many areas of school nursing. In addition to the cost benefits of nursing services, there are issues relating to the quality of care given in the school, clarifications of the school nurse's role, use of health aides, and relationships with the many health team members (Wold, 1981). While many school nurses have not engaged in systematic study, they do see the need for proving the value of school nurses. Therefore, it is up to school nurses to begin to define and document their practice, providing their own evidence that school nursing is essential to health and learning.

Proponents of school nursing services adhere to the belief that the school nurse is vital to an effective, coordinated program of services to schoolchildren and, ultimately, to the health of the community. Because of the interdependent relationship between the members of the school community and the community-at-large, knowledge of community, family, and child dynamics enables nurses to enlarge the scope of their practice for the benefit of all. Emphasis on health promotion and health protection have given the school nurse a wellness perspective, focusing on health rather than disease. The systematic processes discussed in the following sections provide the nurse with tools to document this expanded scope of practice. Within this family- and community-centered context, excellence in practice grows and thrives.

Strategies for School Nursing Practice

To increase the likelihood of successful outcomes in school health, the school nurse will approach problems with a well-planned action or sequence of actions. Because of diverse populations found in most schools, effective strategies must consider ethnic and cultural aspects of the school community, the families of schoolchildren, and the community at large. These will be discussed in the following pages as well as some general strategies utilizing interpersonal and group relationships, which will prove helpful in maximizing outcomes of nursing practice.

Ethnic and Cultural Factors

School nurses are in a position to recognize the influence of ethnic factors on health care needs and adjust their care plan accordingly. The demographic composition of many cities means that large numbers of children who come from various ethnic

minority groups, such as blacks and Hispanics, are present in school classrooms. Consequently, it is important for the school nurse to be aware of how culture influences the health behavior of children and their families. Because school nursing services often necessitate visits to the home, sensitivity to these influences often assists the nurse in communicating with families and interpreting data from assessments. By first recognizing the nurse's own value system and that of the school as an institution, the school nurse is then able to recognize and affirm strengths of diverse cultural value systems (Friedman, 1981). The nurse may then incorporate these understandings in planning and delivering future health services. For instance, pamphlets depicting the predominant minority group may be selected for classroom use during a health education session.

The fact that one or more parents do not speak English may go unrecognized without the nurse's intervention. The parent may be labeled uncooperative or indifferent if the language barrier is unknown. Once aware of the language barrier, the school nurse may seek to obtain health education materials in the family's native tongue (see Case Example 19-1).

General Strategies

The following general strategies for school nursing practice are based on the nurse's assessment of the local school's own needs. It is a planned set of services individualized for each school population, taking into account community demographic variables, school characteristics, and common health problems.

Establishment of Client Relationships   One strategy for successful practice as a school nurse is the establishment of relationships with the individual, the family, the community-at-large, and the school community. The recipient of nursing care—that is, the "client"—may be any or all of these. Each influences the school health program and, in turn, is influenced by it. Therefore, the type of relationship developed by the school nurse with each has a direct bearing on the program scope and impact.

Although the school nurse generally is well prepared in interpersonal skills, special attention may need to be given to family relationships. The changing nature of family constellations makes the establishment of relationships with parents more difficult and challenging for the school nurse. Unlike several decades past, there is often no adult at home when the child becomes ill during the day, when the child requires noontime medication, or when the child arrives home from school. Conferences and health histories must be scheduled around the parent's work hours. A young child ill at home may pose a serious dilemma for parents who cannot take off work without jeopardizing their employment status. Often that dilemma is transferred to the school nurse when the child comes to school ill.

The school nurse frequently has occasion to contact parents who are in the process of divorce, those who have recently been divorced, or those

engaged in transitory relationships. Stress caused by these family disruptions are often manifested in a student by behavioral disturbances, anxiety, or depression. Joint custody arrangements may further intensify the conflict within the schoolchild (Liebow, 1984).

The rising proportion of single-parent families intensifies normal stresses upon the family and often places children at increased risk of physical and emotional problems. In addition, single-parent families headed by women are more likely to have incomes below the poverty level. Children from these families have higher than average absences from school due to chronic illness (Gephart, Egan, & Hutchins, 1984).

Because these families are often isolated from school personnel and events, relationships fostered by the school nurse may be the only link between parents and the educational program. Support, counseling, and/or referral from the school nurse may be needed in each of these situations.

These same societal forces affect the school community and the community-at-large. When planning strategies for groups of teachers and parents, for example, the nurse must consider aspects of single parenting, family disruption, and population mobility.

Establishment of Team Relationships   A second strategy for implementing school nursing services draws upon resources of other school and community personnel. Whether the primary focus is education or health, the nurse participates on multidisciplinary teams to further goals of positive well-being.

The group most immediately concerned with health needs of pupils is the *school health team*. It includes all persons within the school community and significant others who directly influence the student's health—from school administrator to building maintenance engineer to classroom teacher. The school nurse coordinates the activities of this loosely knit group and plans for effective use of each member.

Although often ill-prepared in health matters, the teacher, nevertheless, is the key member of the

Case Example 19-1: Noncompliant or Non-English-speaking Family

Waldi Zalankovitch, a fourth grader at Rosenberg School, was excluded by the health aide, Mrs. Ramiro, for the fourth time in six weeks for head lice because nits were found in her hair. The aide brought this to the school nurse's attention. The nurse, Ms. Newman, asked the aide what steps had been taken at the time of each exclusion. Mrs. Ramiro reported that a letter was sent home each time explaining the school exclusion policy regarding head lice as well as the directions for treatment.

Ms. Newman telephoned the Zalankovitch family. A young child, who identified herself as Waldi, answered the call. Waldi reported that her mother could not come to the phone. Ms. Newman decided to stop by the Zalankovitch home on her way to her afternoon school. When Ms. Newman drove onto Greenwood Street, she noticed the well-kept row of town houses. She approached the Zalankovitch house and noticed a young girl playing on the steps. Ms. Newman introduced herself and the child responded, with somewhat of an accent, that she was Waldi. As they went into the house and entered a small living room, Ms. Newman asked Waldi to get her mother. After a few minutes the child returned from another room with a young woman dressed in black.

Making a thorough assessment

Waldi told Ms. Newman that her mother did not speak English. Ms. Newman asked Waldi if any of the neighbors could act as interpreter with her. Waldi ran outside and returned in a few minutes with an old woman. Within a short time Ms. Newman uncovered a tragic history. The Zalankovitch family arrived in the United States six months ago from Yugoslavia. Mr. Zalankovitch was able to find work through his cousin. Two months after his arrival, however, he and his cousin were killed in an automobile accident. Mrs. Zalankovitch and Waldi were left alone, unable to speak English and without income. The family house was in a Yugoslavian neighborhood and most of the neighbors were helping out, but Mrs. Zalankovitch did not know to whom to turn when Waldi was excluded from school. She was embarrassed and frightened by the little information Waldi gave her.

Use of home visit and neighborhood resources

Developing a trusting relationship

Ms. Newman explained what head lice are and showed Mrs. Zalankovitch how to shampoo, rinse, and comb Waldi's hair. In the months following Ms. Newman was able to identify many important resources for Waldi and her mother.

Demonstrating a practical solution

school health team. He or she observes children day by day and can detect any changes in appearance, alertness, or behavior that often precede overt health problems. The school nurse can support this role and encourage the teacher's contribution of observation to the health assessment process.

Parents are also considered members of the extended health team because of their responsibility and interest in the child's health. In addition, the school health team may utilize parent volunteers to assist with screening programs, health fairs, career days, and some aspects of record-keeping, and to be members of school health advisory committees.

Physicians and other providers in the community may also be part of the school health team, either as representatives on a medical advisory committee or as the primary care-giver for a specific child's health problem. The medical advisory committee usually consists of school administrators, local physicians, and school nurses. They serve as a liaison group between the school and other medical providers, and they advise the school administration on medical aspects of the school health program.

Since the passage of PL 94-142 (The Education of All Handicapped Children Act) in 1975, the concept of *pupil service teams* has expanded rapidly (Rose, 1980). The school nurse, once a tangential member of this group, has now been accepted as a fully contributing member. Pupil service teams are formed to assess and plan for educational needs of students who demonstrate learning difficulties in one or more areas. Since this description includes students with physical impairments that interfere with learning potential, the nurse obviously needs to be involved in planning for modified school programming whether that includes administration of medicines, classroom seating, or more intensive nursing care such as tracheostomy care, catheter care, and dressing changes. Other special education students may have no overt physical defect, but a thorough health history by the nurse often reveals illness patterns, minor health problems, or inadequate health behaviors.

The pupil service team is composed of school nurses, psychologists, social workers, guidance counselors, and special education teachers. Children with learning difficulties are referred to the team for a diagnostic work-up. The nurse is usually responsible for ascertaining the student's health status through a health history, screening tests, and other measures from the health record. After the completion of assessments by all the team members, a joint meeting or "staffing" is held by all relevant parties including the parents. An individual educational plan (IEP) is developed for each child, detailing specific educational objectives and interventions (Rose, 1980). The ANA *Standards* (1983) call for the nurse to assume "leadership in the individualized educational plan when primary service for the student is health related" (p. 12). In each plan, annual goals are established with the child; these are then evaluated and new goals are set based on the evaluation. The school nurse should be an integral part of this process (see Case Example 19-2).

A third team relationship that the school nurse should cultivate is based in the community and includes parent organizations, clinics, other health agencies, local health departments, and social service organizations. In some cases it may include mental health centers and/or police departments. The *community health team* may be formally structured or informal, but serves as a network of resources available for promoting and protecting health.

The community health team is a major ally of the school nurse because of its linkages to services needed for the health care of individual schoolchildren with identified health problems. The team also serves as a forum for school nurses to demonstrate the effectiveness of school health programs and, especially, health promotion activities. The support and backup of health professionals from the community is an important asset in creating a climate in which school health services can flourish (Jerrick, 1978; Lowe, 1977; Paustian, 1983).

Establishment of Support Groups A third strategy identifies children with health conditions in common and attempts interventions through utilization of group process. One such group may include overweight teenagers who work together to reinforce positive attempts to lose weight. Because peer relationships are so important to the growing child, these support groups can make a positive impact on health behaviors.

The initial step in forming support groups begins with an epidemiological assessment of the school population to determine the prevalence of certain types of disease patterns and to identify groups at risk of common health problems. This initial step, therefore, presupposes a familiarity with epidemiological principles and other public health concepts. Once identified, students in these groups

Case Example 19-2: Nurse as Member of Pupil Service Team

Linda Homan, the school nurse at Hickory Hill School, read through the schedule of special education staffings for the next month. She had completed the health histories of all but one child, Benjamin Garver. When Ms. Homan read the school psychologist's report, she noted the six-year-old child was very bright, but was being evaluated for a special education placement because of his tracheostomy.

The special education evaluation consists of work-ups from each specialty area.

Before going to the Garver home, Ms. Homan touched base with the preschool teacher and social worker to see if they had any particular questions. The social worker was concerned about the medical support the child would need in a regular classroom, and the teacher reported that she thought the child should be referred to a school for children who were profoundly impaired both physically or mentally.

Ms. Homan found the Garver house sparsely furnished but well kept. Mrs. Garver reported that Benjamin had the tracheostomy since he was six months old for sleep apnea. He was under care at the University Medical Center and might have the trach for another year or two. Ms. Homan had Mrs. Garver sign the release of information forms necessary to request Ben's history from the Medical Center. She observed Ben actively playing with his one-year-old sister in the living room. He was able to verbalize well and was obviously a bright child.

The hospital staff reported that they had attempted to wean Ben from the trach six months before, but that he had an episode of sleep apnea. The decision had been made to wait another year before attempting to wean him again. The mother had been given instructions for suctioning, providing adequate moisture, and caring for the trach.

Ms. Homan identified two sets of nursing problems. One set related to the child's needs to have an appropriate school experience that was safe, and one set of problems related to the school staff's fear of the child's care. At a team meeting prior to the special education staffing, Ms. Homan described the two sets of problems and suggested that the team could resolve their problems by gaining knowledge and skill about Ben's health care. Ms. Homan arranged for home visits for those concerned so that they could personally observe his independence. Ms. Homan had not cared for a pediatric trach in some time, so she accompanied Ben and his mother to the hospital for a "refresher." At the staffing, the entire pupil personnel team and Garver family agreed that Ben could be placed in a normal classroom. The Individual Educational Plan (IEP) was developed to focus on his health care needs since he was not handicapped educationally.

The team includes parents as well as team of experts.

Nurse assumes leadership role when the educational need is health oriented.

can be brought together for health teaching, counseling, and peer support.

Successful groups have been established with pupils who have chronic diseases, such as juvenile diabetes, hypertension, ulcers, asthma, and others.

Children at-risk of health conditions may benefit from groups centered on overnutrition, smoking cessation, loss of a parent or sibling, divorce, and/or family alcoholism. Resources, strategies, and mutual concern can be shared during group sessions.

Strategies for Health Promotion

Most strategies for effective school nursing practice use the concept of levels of prevention. In its *Standards of School Nursing Practice* (1983), the American Nurses' Association emphasizes the importance of participating with the community for health services. Standard VII reads: "The school nurse participates with other key members of the community responsible for assessing, planning, implementing, and evaluating school health services and community services that include the broad continuum of promotion of primary, secondary, and tertiary prevention" (p. 14).

The school nurse needs to direct the philosophical development of a school health program that includes primary, secondary, and tertiary prevention. The objectives of a prevention program relate to all levels of prevention and to health promotion.

Health promotion and disease prevention have remained the cornerstones of school nursing practice despite the fads in health care. A comprehensive school nursing program addresses all the levels of prevention and recognizes the importance of the family in effective prevention programs (Wold, 1981).

A main reason for the school nurse to be firmly grounded in child development is evident as the nurse seeks to establish rapport with children of different ages and backgrounds. It is important for the school nurse to recognize overall patterns of growth and development and each child's unique growth and maturation phases. An understanding of the range of individual differences in maturation can often prevent the mislabeling of a child progressing at his or her own rate.

Because of the level of physical and cognitive development, the school nurse may relate quite differently to children in primary grades than to adolescents. For instance, the school nurse interacts with family members to a much greater extent with young children than with adolescents. Conversely, the direct counseling role of the nurse receives greater emphasis in dealing with high school students than with younger ones. This counseling emphasis at high school grade levels does not preclude other aspects of school nursing or involvement with family members.

Primary Prevention

Since the basic assumption that healthy children learn better has been established, the school nurse faces the important task of facilitating each student's optimal level of wellness. This approach to school nursing requires a careful analysis of the school health program philosophy and resources. The skill with which a nurse approaches this analysis is often critical to its success, because a limited focus upon one level of prevention does not allow a full spectrum of health programming.

Primary prevention of health problems includes prevention of psychosocial and physical health problems. The objectives of this preventive level are to promote health and welfare in the school and provide specific protection from health and safety hazards. The family and school community play important roles in this level of prevention because success is contingent on their cooperation.

The specific protection provided by compulsory immunization laws is an important example of primary prevention, in which the nurse plays a pivotal role by providing for the coordination of parent reporting of immunizations. The interaction of the school nurse with family members is vital if the goals of the school health program are to be met.

Health Education Mandated comprehensive health education programs provide an illustration where school support of primary prevention is essential. These programs typically identify relevant curricular health education areas and mandate the inclusion of such areas. Parental support often can provide an impetus for such programs. The school nurse may develop a role in primary prevention by providing faculty with support in regard to classroom health habits. Identifying the relevant aspects of a healthful environment (e.g., hand washing, facilities, classroom temperature, etc.) would be an example of nursing support of primary prevention.

Teachers and other school staff assume the status of client when they express their own health needs, whether it takes the form of information-seeking or whether direct services, such as first aid, are sought. Such occasions for contact afford the school nurse with opportunities to assess, and perhaps modify, the information gaps and attitudes toward health and well-being. Since much of the incidental, as well as planned, health teaching in the classroom reflects the teacher's own attitudes about health, the nurse can exert an indirect influence on the health of children. Relieving personal anxieties about specific health concerns also enables school staff to function in a more relaxed and open manner.

The anticipated outcomes in primary prevention are increased knowledge about health content; therefore, the nurse could anticipate the health behaviors related to that area and provide for measurement.

Self-Care The child is supported by a variety of systems, such as family and teachers, and as those systems raise their members' level of health, one could anticipate the same for the child. An important concept related to high-level wellness is the idea of responsibility of the individual. In a school health program designed for high-level wellness, the child is taught responsibility for health rather than focusing on a passive "patient" role. Many times this requires an entirely new approach to health services and education. The long-range goal of this type of strategy aims to develop a sense of responsibility for self-care and create positive attitudes toward health.

One such system of care was initiated in an elementary school in Los Angeles (Lewis, 1974; Lewis, et al, 1977). The intervention was designed to actively involve children in decision-making processes related to their own health care. Students were able to initiate visits to a school nurse practitioner and participate in selection of treatment and/or referral alternatives. An evaluation of this program found significant changes in health orientation—namely, a reduction in perceived vulnerability as well as an increased value placed on self-care (Lewis et al, 1977).

A Colorado project was developed to prepare school-age children to assume new roles and responsibilities as health consumers (Igoe, 1980b). Known as Health PACT (Participatory and Assertive Consumer Training), this program is focused on visits to a physician, clinic, or hospital as well as to the school nurse. Students are encouraged to practice the following five steps:

1. Ask questions
2. Personally communicate information about themselves to the health professional
3. Encourage the health professional to provide them with health instruction
4. Participate with the health professional in making decisions about their own health; express their opinions about the acceptability of the health professional's advice so that the health plan developed meets their special needs
5. Clarify what responsibilities they are to assume for their own health on a day-to-day basis before leaving the health facility (p. 2016).

Case Example 19-3: Incorporating the Community in High-Level Wellness Programs

Lindbloom High School was a new magnet high school for physical education in the center of the city. The students came from a wide metropolitan area to attend. At a faculty meeting the entire faculty group voiced their concerns about involving parents and developing parental support in the high-level wellness focus of the health curriculum. The school nurse suggested a community fitness program as a vehicle to involve parents as well as reinforce the High-Level Wellness concept included in the school's health education curriculum.

The school nurse serves as problem solver for health promotion focus.

A survey of interest was forwarded to the PTA for circulation. A variety of wellness topics were offered as possible program components: weight control, exercise and the working woman, fitness and diet. Parents were asked to make recommendations as well. A meeting time was selected so that the faculty and working parents could attend.

The faculty initially thought that there would be little parental interest in fitness. The nurse suggested that focusing a fitness program toward parents would engage their personal interest, subsequently enlarging the fitness resources for the students. A professional ballplayer, active in the community, was recruited to join the organizational efforts.

The school nurse identifies a wide grass roots interest in fitness.

When the meeting night arrived, the Community Fitness Program Task Force was delighted to find a large number of parents interested. A "before-school exercise program" was organized, since many parents drove students to school. Within a short time, a weight control and exercise class was organized to meet one night a week. The initial fear that a wellness approach might not work was dispelled.

The program is implemented.

Through encouragement of participatory decision making, these and similar programs can promote positive health behaviors and facilitate development of healthier life-styles. Any program encouraging a student's self-care should include the nurse-family relationship. This relationship would provide for parental support by keeping the family informed about self-care goals and outcomes. It can have an indirect outcome of developing the entire family's self-care potential. Families can be included in other ways. For example, a fitness program for teachers, which may provide a quit smoking program, exercise, and/or diet counseling, often can be enlarged to include parents. Another approach would be to incorporate the PTA (Parent Teacher Association) as volunteers in school health programs. (See Case Exampe 19-3.)

Secondary Prevention

Secondary prevention is directed toward preventing health problems by means of early identification and prompt intervention. The school nurse uses secondary prevention measures when he or she identifies children at risk of educational failure because of health problems. Epidemiologic skills are used to determine appropriate screening procedures to identify the risk factors of a particular school community (see Chapter 6). Examples of these procedures include review of health history and examinations. Children typically have physical examinations at varying periods throughout their school experience, and the examinations are usually accompanied by health histories. These data provide for early identification and intervention.

Since families are sometimes not aware of the important relationship between health and learning, the school nurse first must develop this understanding to maximize parental cooperation. The nurse may also explain that one of the goals of early intervention programs is to alleviate the burden of special education expenses, which are often quite high (Gruber, 1981).

A study by Pelizza in 1973 looked at parent perceptions of school health services. He found that parents consider health services to be a vital function of the school and recommended that school nurses extend their efforts to the family "so that parents as well as children may be better informed about the health functions of the school" (p. 179). The Pelizza study was updated by Winkleman and McKaig (1983). They concluded that parents were knowledgeable about school health programs and do "expect and accept school health services as part of their child's total health care management" (p. 402). They suggest that these positive perceptions can aid health personnel when programs are threatened by fiscal constraints.

Often contacts with parents are made in the school, either as formal or informal conferences. It may be necessary, on the other hand, to visit family members in the home. Assessments of family interaction patterns, environmental conditions, health knowledge and attitudes, and communication are best observed in the family's own life setting. Parents are frequently more relaxed in the home and able to participate more fully with the school nurse than at the school or other locations. The nurse's willingness to step into the family's territory demonstrates a recognition of and interest in the total family (Wold, 1981).

Personnel within the school may assist the school nurse in meeting the health needs of school-aged children or may be the recipients of services to meet their own health needs. Jenne (1970) found a significant correlation between the amount of nurse-school contact and the number of observations by teachers of health problems in the classroom. These findings suggest that school nurses can influence the number of children identified with health problems through increased contact with teachers.

Screening Programs　Among the most visible of the school nurse's activities are screening programs encompassing specific grade levels and, at times, the entire school. Most screening programs seek to identify health problems at an early, correctable stage and therefore fall into secondary prevention. At times the nurse does not participate directly in the screening, but is responsible for the program's planning and administration. Usually follow-up of suspected problems is the nurse's direct responsibility. Vision and hearing screening (as mandated in most school codes) underscores the public support of early identification.

Nearly all screening programs are a part of the overall assessment of each student's health status. The most common types of programs are vision and hearing, hypertension, developmental, and scoliosis screening. Less common are dental, streptococcal, lead, and diabetes programs. For the most part, these are annual events that are discrete and apparently unrelated to each other; however, the objective of these screening programs is to contribute to the total health assessment of the child. Nurses should be attuned to this concept and plan screening programs that accomplish a comprehensive health assessment in a cost-effective manner.

Not often considered a type of screening, but contributing to the assessment of a child's health, are the data gleaned from review of health records. Although often incomplete, information may be gathered from the physical and dental examinations, family health history, and immunization levels. Unfortunately, research studies have revealed a poor correlation between a student's health status and the school physical examination (Lan et al, 1976; Sweeney, 1982). Sweeney (1982) studied 756 schoolchildren from low income, minority neighborhoods who went through the required physical examinations. She concluded that the low rate of detection of adverse medical conditions was of questionable benefit, given the costs incurred. Instead Sweeney recommended replacement of the physical by a school health assessment. The proposed assessment would consist of data from a dental check, vision screen, hearing screen, psychometric screen, immunization record, observable deviation from ideal body weight, and copy of a physical exam obtained within a three-year period.

This more comprehensive approach has appeared in many schools in recent years, combining many of the separate screening activities mentioned, as well as the health history and general overall inspection of the child. Nurse practitioners or other specifically trained school nurses often perform these health assessments (Hill, 1971). To the extent that specific training or experiential skill permits, each school nurse is able to conduct an assessment of the child.

Referral and Follow-up Screening tests, such as those found in most school health programs, serve to differentiate normal children from those suspected of having a health problem. It is important to note that a screening test is neither definitive nor diagnostic; it merely indicates the need for further testing and diagnosis, usually through the traditional medical care system. Often parents and teachers misinterpret the results of screening programs and jump to the conclusions that either (1) the child is impaired or (2) the test is at fault. The nurse, then, must carefully interpret the purpose and results of screening tests to those concerned.

The follow-up school nursing role is much less visible and not as defined as that of the role in assessment. For example, the child who fails a vision test in school is referred to the family's care-provider for diagnosis and treatment. Given that there are no financial problems, the treatment is only as good as the child's compliance with the treatment regime. With this in mind, the nurse then becomes coordinator of care between physician and school. In cases where family economic problems are limiting, the school nurse may well provide the resources to ameliorate these problems.

In addition to the influences generated within the family grouping, the schoolchild is related to a community. The nurse needs special skills to see the health problems of an individual child within a larger context and to be able to communicate across many levels of care-givers and services (Snyman, 1981). The resources of the community play a significant role in meeting the goals of the school health program. Effecting a successful referral may be facilitated by relationships based on mutual respect and shared goals between the school health professional and community health care services.

Follow-up of identified health problems has been characterized as "the greatest lack in school health programs" (Lan et al, 1976). Careful and successful follow-up necessitates an accurate system of record-keeping so that the outcomes of referrals are known. Often a "promise" or an appointment date is accepted as evidence of successful completion of a health care referral. Unless the children identified through screening programs receive adequate follow-up and treatment, the time and effort spent on screening activities are wasted.

Tertiary Prevention

The tertiary prevention role involves limiting the alteration of health, taking corrective and restorative measures and promoting maximal adaptation. PL 94-142 (The Education of All Handicapped Children Act, 1975) places this level of prevention at high priority by requiring a free and appropriate education for all children despite any handicapping problem. The school nurse is many times the only person on the school team with a thorough understanding of the child's health needs and acts as advocate for the child as well as coordinator of service between school, family, and care-provider.

Mainstreaming Since the enactment of PL 94-142, education for handicapped children is mandated to take place in "the least restrictive environment possible." This means that the school activities of each identified child should be as close to that of a normal child as possible (Buser, 1980).

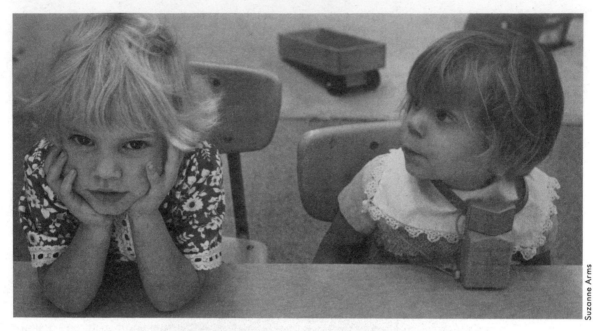

Children with an identified disability can benefit from remaining in the usual school setting. The practice of mainstreaming is particularly effective when follow-up and coordinated care can be provided by the school nurse.

The concept of "mainstreaming" is an attempt to carry out the intent of the law by placing handicapped children in regular classrooms whenever feasible. The school nurse can assist the assimilation process by providing input on the necessity to modify school structures to allow handicapped students access to necessary components of the educational program. Often the nurse acts as a mediator between needed changes and costs to the school (Rose, 1980).

The nurse can also intervene in plans for adaptive physical education for handicapped students. As a source of health information, the nurse is able to plan with the physical education department for recommended changes and evaluation of progress (Rose, 1980). Frequently classroom teachers need health information and counseling about particular children with chronic disease or other disabling conditions. The nurse is the primary source of such information.

Summary

The development of school nursing from its historical roots in public health nursing is characterized by increasing emphasis on health promotion and prevention in a multicultural setting with increasingly diverse family constellations (see Chapters 5 and 17). In the future school nurses will need to be highly skilled in interpersonal and family relationships, environmental concerns, educational programming, and management of health services. They must also be familiar with legal mandates affecting health and educational programs.

Effective strategies to accomplish goals of the school health program include establishment of effective relationships with the student, family, school personnel, and community persons. A knowledge of the ethnic and cultural factors affecting health behaviors is critical in this respect. Nurses should also understand how to apply the levels of prevention to assist with health programs.

As the key health professional in the school, the school nurse must be able to articulate the needs of schoolchildren and their families to the educational specialists within the system and also to the larger community. It is this ability to influence both internal and external systems for the attainment of better health that makes the role of the school nurse so pivotal.

Topics for Nursing Research

• How often are school nurses called upon to provide health services to teachers and other school staff?
• How is school nursing practice affected by the professional identification of the nurse?
• What is the role of school health aides? What is the association between the level of a child's health and learning?
• How does the school health program contribute to a child's health?
• What strategies does the school nurse utilize in working with minority or culturally diverse families?
• How does the school nurse contribute to the cost-effectiveness of early intervention programs?

Study Questions

1. In addition to school health services, the other major components of a school health program are:
   a. Health assessment and health education
   b. Health education and environmental health
   c. Environmental health and safety
   d. Pupil services and levels of prevention
2. Which of the following sentences best describes the relationship of the nursing process with the school health program components?
   a. The program components are dependent upon the nursing process.
   b. The nursing process is dependent upon the program components.
   c. The nursing process is tangential and independent of the program components.
   d. The nursing process is interactive and interdependent with the program components.
3. A panel discussion by students on the topic of student safety patrols is an example of:
   a. Primary prevention
   b. Secondary prevention
   c. Tertiary prevention
   d. Self-care
4. The role and functions of the school nurse as defined by the American Nurses' Association (ANA) reflect which of the following:
   a. Advanced preparation in school nursing
   b. Current practice norms of school nurses
   c. Nursing process
   d. Innovative evaluation plans
5. The school nurse can contribute to the health of a mainstreamed child most effectively by:
   a. Instituting adaptive physical education
   b. Close communication with the classroom teacher
   c. Planning of special classes for such students
   d. Forming a school health program to monitor a students' academic progress
6. The primary reason for utilizing support groups as an effective nursing strategy is because groups:
   a. Are economical of nurse's time
   b. Utilize peer relationships
   c. Are noninvasive
   d. Utilize all members of the school health team

7. The Gonzalez family has three school-aged children. First grader, Rosaria, has been a frequent visitor to the nurse's office with numerous vague complaints. The first step the school nurse should take in formulating a plan of care is:
   a. Consult the pupil service team
   b. Make a home visit
   c. Contact the parents by phone
   d. Contact the classroom teacher

References

American Nurses' Association: *Standards of School Nursing Practice.* Kansas City, Mo: Author, 1983.

Buser BN: The evaluation of school health services: New York and nationwide. *J Sch Health* 1980; 50: 475–477.

Chinn P: A relationship between school and health problems: A nursing assessment. *J Sch Health* 1973; 43: 85–92.

Clemen SA, Eigsti DG, McGuire SL: *Comprehensive Family and Community Health Nursing.* New York: McGraw-Hill, 1981.

Dale S, et al: The effects of health aides on school nurse activities. *J Sch Health* 1981; 51: 547–551.

Friedman MM: *Family Nursing: Theory and Assessment.* New York: Appleton-Century-Crofts, 1981.

Gephart J, Egan MC, Hutchins VL: Perspectives on health of schoolage children expectations for the future. *J Sch Health* 1984; 54: 11–17.

Goodnow M: *Nursing History in Brief,* 2nd ed. Philadelphia: Saunders, 1943.

Greenhill ED: Perceptions of the school nurse's role. *J Sch Health* 1979; 49: 368–371.

Gruber MA: Why screen for scoliosis? *Edu-Facts* 1981; 3 (2): 1.

Hawkins NG: Is there a school nurse role? *Am J Nurs* 1971; 71: 744–751.

Hill AE: School health services today: Some reflections and comments. *Clinical Pediatr* 1971; 10: 620–623.

Igoe JB: Changing patterns in school health and school nursing. *Nurs Outlook* 1980a; 28: 486–492.

Igoe JB: Project health PACT in action. *Am J Nurs* 1980b; 80: 2016–2021.

Jenne FH: Variations in nursing service characteristics and teachers health observation practices. *J Sch Health* 1970; 40: 248–250.

Jerrick SJ: The facts of life. *J Sch Health* 1978; 48: 312–313.

Lan SM et al: Screening and referral outcomes of school-based health services in a low-income neighborhood. *Public Health Rep* 1976; 91: 514–520.

Lewis CE et al: Child initiated care: The use of school nursing services by children in an 'adult-free' system. *Pediatrics* 1977; 60: 499–507.

Lewis MA: Child initiated care. *Am J Nurs* 1974; 74: 652–655.

Liebow PR: The new-look school nurse. *J Psychosoc Nurs Ment Health Serv* 1984; 22 (3): 37–41.

Lowe CU: Health opportunities in schools. *J Sch Health* 1977; 47: 431–434.

Marriner A: Opinions of school nurses about the preparation and practice of school nurses. *J Sch Health* 1971; 41: 417–420.

Mayshark C, Shaw DD, Best WH: *Administration of School Health Programs.* St. Louis: Mosby, 1977.

Oda DS, Quick MJ: School health records and the new accessibility law. *J Sch Health* 1977; 47: 212–216.

Paustian BJ: Stand up! Speak out! Show off! *J Sch Health* 1983; 53: 326–327.

Pelizza JJ: A comparative study of how parents from different social classes perceive health services. *J Sch Health* 1973; 43: 176–180.

Robinson T: School nurse practitioners on the job. *Am J Nurs* 1981; 81: 1674–1676.

Rose TL: The education of all handicapped children act [PL 94-142]: New responsibilities and opportunities for the school nurse. *J Sch Health* 1980; 50: 30–31.

Rustia J: Rustia school health promotion model. *J Sch Health* 1982; 52: 108–114.

Snyman N: The community health nurse in school health services. *Curationis* 1981; 4 (3): 39–40.

Stanhope M, Lancaster J: *Community Health Nursing.* St. Louis: Mosby, 1984.

Sweeney KA: School health screening: Costs, benefits and alternatives. *Urban Health* 1982; 11 (10): 46–48.

Thompson F: *Health Policy and Bureaucracy: Politics and Implementation.* Cambridge, Mass.: MIT Press.

Winkleman TA, McKaig C: Parental expectations of school health services. *J Sch Health* 1983; 53: 400–403.

Wold SJ: *School Nursing: A Framework for Practice.* St. Louis: Mosby, 1981.

Chapter 20

Occupational Health

Carol A. Frazier

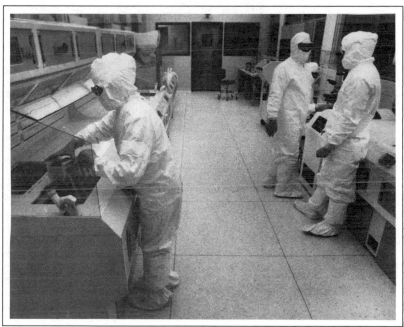

Sam Forencich/Times Tribune

While work can provide economic security and fulfill higher-level needs, it can also jeopardize health by exposing workers to noxious substances or high levels of stress.

**Chapter
Outline**

**Chapter
Objectives**

After completing this chapter, the reader will be able to:

- Identify the role of the occupational health nurse
- Recognize the impact of work on the health of the client, family, and community
- Discuss the application of nursing theory to the practice of occupational health nursing
- Identify federal legislation that impacts occupational health
- Identify members of the occupational health team
- Discuss some specific work exposures affecting the health of the individual client through the life cycle

Work in modern society provides not only economic security to an individual and/or family but also status and prestige within the community. Work offers an individual respect, social interaction, and a sense of usefulness, moreover, it allows the person an outlet for creative ideas, a means of gaining self-actualization, involvement in decision making, or a means of fulfilling goals and dreams. Through their work individuals gratify some of the needs identified by Maslow in his hierarchy of needs (Maslow, 1954).

While work can potentially help people fill their higher-level needs, it is also capable of jeopardizing human requirements for physiologic well-being, safety, and security. This chapter examines the subject of occupational health by looking at the governmental impact on occupational health, the role of the occupational health nurse and the occupational health team, occupational health hazards through the life span, and strategies for health promotion.

Occupational Health: An Overview

During the past century health care professionals have made major scientific discoveries that have eliminated many of the communicable diseases and other health threats that lead to early morbidity and/or mortality. The communicable diseases of the past have been replaced with a host of chronic diseases; cancer, heart disease, respiratory disease, and liver and kidney disease are new major targets of medical science. The chronic diseases of today appear to be caused by, or augmented by, our environment and life-style. The work environment contributes significantly to the incidence and prevalence of these diseases.

In addition to illness, job injuries cause major alterations in health status. Statistics show that one out of ten workers suffers a job injury during the course of the year. Job accidents kill about 13,000 workers a year and disable 2.3 million workers per year; of these latter workers, about 80,000 will be permanently disabled (Greenwald, 1980).

The incidence of occupation-related disease has not been as well recognized as occupational accidents. Statistics now being accumulated suggest that occupational disease and deaths cost about $23 billion a year in lost wages alone. This does not include the cost of medical care and hospitalization or the pain to the individual and family (Greenwald, 1980). The U.S. Public Health Service estimates

that 390,000 new cases of occupational disease appear annually. Epidemiologic analysis suggests that as many as 100,000 deaths occur each year as a result of occupational diseases (Levy, 1983). Occupational factors may have a significant impact on the causation of the major diseases and health problems, such as cancer and pulmonary disease, that confront the health care professions (see Table 20-1). Many of the exposures of the workplace have prolonged latent periods. For instance, a worker may be exposed at the worksite to agents such as asbestos or benzene, but symptoms may not appear for five, ten, or twenty years. Thus, when workers reach retirement, instead of enjoying the latter years, they can be confronted with a major chronic and often debilitating disease.

In the early part of the twentieth century, several states began to examine the problem of disability among workers and by 1920 forty states had enacted workers compensation laws. The increased technology that developed in the postwar era created a need for knowledge about health and safety hazards to workers. Today all fifty states have workers compensation laws, each with its own specific requirements and level of compensation. Despite the diversity of individual state laws, all have the following basic characteristics in common: (1) limited liability without proof of fault, (2) compulsory

Table 20-1   Occupational and Nonoccupational Factors Contributing to Major Health Problems

Health Problem	Nonoccupational Factors	Occupational Factors

Arthritis	Age
	Genetic makeup
	Nutrition
	History of trauma
	Stress
	Infection
		Repeated articular movement
		Trauma
		Cold humid environment
		Poor body mechanics
		Improper work design—
		    Inappropriate work
		    Awkward tool design

Cancer	Age Genetic makeup Smoking Nutrition DES	Exposure to carcinogens Radiation Asbestos Benzidine and its salts 2 acetylamino fluorine 4 aminodiphenyl 3,3 dichloro benzidine and its salts 4 dimethylaminoaxo benzene alpha-naphthylamine beta-naphthylamine 4 nitro biphenyl n-nitrosodimethylamine beta-propriolactone bis-chloromethylethyl ether methyl chloromethyl ether 4,4 methylene (bis) 2-chloroaniline

insurance, (3) automatic benefits, (4) health care, (5) income protection, (6) death benefits, and (7) a process for resolving disputes (LaDou, 1981).

The workers compensation system is based on the theory that

(a) employers and employees in industry are engaged in a common venture for the furnishing of goods or services to society, anticipating profits or wages, as the case may be, as a reward; (b) their relationship is not solely one created by simple contract with each other, but amounts to a kind of industrial status; (c) the risk of injury and financial burden resulting therefrom should be borne by the industry as a whole rather than fall solely upon the employee involved; and (d) the burden of the wearing out and destruction of human, as well as inanimate machinery should be borne by industry just as other costs of production are assumed by the employer and ultimately passed on to the public. It is in effect a special tax and a part of the operating expense, just as truly as any other cost of repair or operation (Stertz, 1918, p. 256).

Safety in the work environment has continued to be an important concern for legislators and the public. The single most influential factor affecting health care delivery at the worksite was the passage of the Occupational Safety and Health Act in 1970. This act was the first comprehensive attempt to ensure safe and healthful working conditions for the working population. The act encourages "employers and employees in their efforts to reduce the number of occupational safety and health hazards at their places of employment, and to stimu-

Table 20-1   *(continued)*

Health Problem	Nonoccupational Factors	Occupational Factors
Dermatitis	Age	Pressure on skin
	Genetic makeup	Friction
	Pigmentation	Sweating and wet work
	Systemic drugs	Exposure to a primary irritant
	Sex	Alterations in pH
	Nutritional status	Solvents
	Personal cleanliness	Plasticizers
	Hobbies	Petroleum products
		Epoxy resins
		Synthetic rubber
		Insecticides
		Agricultural chemical
		Use of protective equipment
Heart Disease	Age	Solvents
	Genetic makeup	Gases
	Sex	Pulmonary irritants
	Nutritional status	Temperature extremes
	Stress	Stress
Pulmonary Disease	Age	Dusts
	Genetic makeup	Gases, mists
	Smoking	Use of respirators
	Sex	Temperature
	Hobbies	Humidity

late employers and employees to institute new and perfect existing programs for providing safe and healthful working conditions" (OSH Act, Section 2 (b) (1)). The OSH Act established the Occupational Safety and Health Administration (OSHA), which is the agency responsible for administering the act. The primary functions of OSHA are to promulgate and enforce standards governing the work environment, to monitor the adherence to these regulations, and to obtain accurate and uniform information about workplace injuries and illnesses for statistical analysis.

A second agency established by the OSH Act is the National Institute for Occupational Safety and Health (NIOSH). Housed in the Department of Health and Human Services, this agency carries out the research and educational functions designated in the original OSH Act. NIOSH provides consultation, advisement, and evaluation of health hazards within industry upon request by management or labor. NIOSH also offers information concerning specific hazards in a consultant capacity.

The institute is also responsible for the development of educational opportunities for health professionals in the area of occupational health. In keeping with this charge, NIOSH has developed a variety of short-term courses in industrial hygiene, safety, and nursing. NIOSH also provides funding to a number of Educational Resource Centers for Occupational Health and Safety (ERC). ERCs provide graduate level education for nurses, physicians, industrial hygienists, safety personnel, epidemiologists, toxicologists, and other professionals who work in the area of occupational safety and health.

Research, hazard evaluation, and the development of criteria documents are a major focus of NIOSH activities. Specific occupational hazards are identified and studied as to their potential impact on human health. After intensive research, including animal and human studies, a criteria document is developed. The document includes a careful review of the literature concerning the substances, results, and evaluation of research studies and recommendations for safe exposure levels. The institute presents a plan for health care of workers exposed to the substance. This plan delineates screening, monitoring, diagnostic tests, educational programs, and protective equipment. The criteria document is sent to the Assistant Secretary of Labor, and during a review process, all interested parties (management, labor, and the scientific community) are invited to participate in a critical analysis of the document. After extensive review, the document can then be promulgated as a standard, adherence to which is enforced by OSHA. Several hundred criteria documents including those on lead, noise, benzene, hot environment, asbestos, carbon monoxide, and anesthetic gases have been developed. Most of the documents have not reached the point of becoming standards.

Recently, OSHA has issued a standard on hazard communication that requires manufacturers and employers to disclose to employees, emergency personnel, and appropriate community groups information about the hazards of toxic substances. This is the first piece of federal legislation that acknowledges the employees' right to know the potential health effects of agents with which they are working. Many states and communities have enacted their own right-to-know legislation that includes specifics the federal legislation does not address.

The federal law requires that a material safety data sheet (MSDS) be in the workplace for each hazardous chemical in the plant. These sheets must be accessible to all employees (McElveen, 1985). An employer may withhold the specific chemical name of a substance if it is a trade secret. In an emergency a physician can gain access to the information. The federal standard does not, however, allow occupational health nurses access to the Material Safety and Data Sheets, a point that has been energetically protested by the American Association of Occupational Health Nurses. Occupational health nurses have been vocal in explaining the professional role of the nurse in emergency situations and have been successful in having the nurse identified as a health professional who has access to the information in many of the states' right-to-know laws.

Employees need to know the specifics of legislation at the local, state, and federal level and be educated as to the degree of hazard of chemicals with which they are in contact (McElveen, 1985). Workers need to be able to identify specific hazards and the acute and chronic effect to their health status. The results of animal studies in the area of toxic effects, mutagenesis, teratogenesis, and carcinogenesis should be available for the individual worker, the union, management, and health professionals. Programs can then be developed to inform the workers of current technology available to protect the employee from hazardous effects. All workers are responsible for participating in their own care. The occupational health nurse can effectively plan, implement, and evaluate employee health education programs that allow workers to be responsible for their own health state.

In 1980 the U.S. Department of Health and Human Services set forth a list of objectives to be achieved by 1990. Those pertaining to occupational health nurses can serve as one set of guidelines for nurses practicing in work settings (see Box 20-1).

Occupational Health Nursing

While there is an ANA certification program for generalists in community health nursing, the American Board for Occupational Health Nurses (ABOHN) directs the certification process specifically for occupational health nursing. The ABOHN certification program is designed for the registered nurse practicing in occupational settings, irrespective of the nurse's previous education, whether at the diploma, baccalaureate, or master's level. After completing the required number of continuing education courses and obtaining verification of expertise in occupational health nursing, the nurse may sit for the board examination. Successful completion of the exam results in certification as an occupational health nurse.

The field of occupational health nursing is just beginning to emerge as a specialty for nursing practice. Educators responsible for nursing programs are beginning to integrate concepts of occupational health into basic nursing programs. Twenty years ago, when McCain published a nursing assessment tool, only one question concerned the client's occupation (McCain, 1965). Today health care professionals are aware of the need for a detailed occupational health history. Knowledge of the client's occupation is vital in developing a nursing diagnosis, and planning nursing care and subsequent return to home and job.

Educational Preparation

The nurse who chooses to enter the specialty of occupational health nursing is equipped with basic skills such as communication, fundamental physical assessment and counseling skills, and basic knowledge of such subjects as pathophysiology, health education, and rehabilitation. If the nurse assumes the role of a clinical specialist in occupational health nursing, increased skills and knowledge must be developed in such areas as advanced physical assessment, epidemiology, occupational health, safety, toxicology, research methodology,

and computer technology. Additional preparation in management, personnel relations, and labor relations is desirable. Such a program requires a master's level education. The "Standard Interpretation and Audit Criteria for Performance of Occupational Health Programs" recommends a master's degree in occupational health nursing or in public health nursing for nurses in supervisory positions or nurses in one-nurse units in industry.

Scope of Practice

In order to practice the specialty of occupational health nursing, one must work within the framework of a theory applicable to that practice. As a profession, nursing focuses on the whole individual, not just a particular illness or injury. A holistic approach to health is an appropriate philosophy for occupational health nursing practice. The nurse takes a primary health care approach, viewing workers as healthy individuals and facilitating that health process by helping them avoid illness and injury. Occupational health nurses must be prepared to deliver nursing care to workers who may have problems with oxygen transport, nutritional status, chemical abuse, mobility, coping, and other physiologic and psychologic manifestations of altered homeostasis. Occupational health nurses can counsel workers about approaching retirement, initiate emergency care for a worker who has been burned, or deliver a baby.

Along with a holistic nursing approach, the philosophy, goals, and objectives of the particular industry are important concerns for health care delivery within the occupational setting. Health care, after all, is not the primary product of the organization. Completion of the technological process within a preordained budget and profit system is the primary goal.

Within this framework, the occupational health nurse must be able to provide managers with essential data that document the need for the provision

---

Box 20-1 1990 Objectives for the Nation in Occupational Safety and Health

1. By 1990, work place accident deaths for firms or employers with eleven or more employees should be reduced to less than 3,750 per year.
2. By 1990, the rate of work-related injuries should be reduced to 8.3 cases per 100 full-time workers.
3. By 1990, lost workdays due to injuries should be reduced to 55 per 100 workers annually.
4. By 1990, the incidence of compensable occupational dermatitis should be reduced to about 60,000 cases.
5. By 1990, among workers newly exposed after 1985, there should be virtually no new cases of four preventable occupational diseases—asbestosis, byssinosis, silicosis, and coal worker's pneumoconiosis.
6. By 1990, the prevalence of occupational noise-induced hearing loss should be reduced to 415,000 cases.
7. By 1990, occupational heavy metal poisoning (lead, arsenic, zinc) should be virtually eliminated.
8. By 1985, 50 percent of all firms with more than 500 employees should have an approved plan of hazard control for all new processes, new equipment, and new installations.
9. By 1990, all firms with more than 500 employees should have an approved plan of hazard control for all new processes, new equipment, and new installations.
10. By 1990, at least 25 percent of workers should be able, prior to employment, to state the nature of their occupational health and safety risks and their potential consequences, as well as be informed of changes in these risks while employed.
11. By 1985, workers should be routinely informed of life-style behaviors and health factors that interact with factors in the work environment to increase risks of emotional illness and injury.
12. By 1985, all workers should receive routine notification, in a timely manner, of all health examinations or personal exposure measurements taken on work environments directly related to them.
13. By 1990, all managers of industrial firms should be fully informed about the impor-

---

of health care services to employees, identifying not only occupational but also nonoccupational risks affecting the employees' health and productivity. Employers are aware of the rapid increase in health care costs that they must pay when employees succumb to other nonoccupationally related acute or chronic illness or injury. Primary prevention in health care is one way to provide cost-effective health care. The work place provides an ideal setting for developing a primary health care program, since the occupational health nurse can develop and implement health care programs that provide screening, education, and counseling to workers, thus detecting risks to health and intervening before illness results (LaLonde, 1977; Saward & Sorenson, 1978). The occupational health nurse must have the nursing and management skills necessary to carry out such a program effectively. Knowledge of current literature relating to the cost effectiveness of a primary health care program is mandatory in negotiating the scope of the occupational health program.

Expanded Roles

As the specialty of occupational health nursing has grown, health professionals and health educators have recognized the need for expert training and education in the area of occupational health nursing. Traditionally the occupational health nurse tance of, and methods for controlling, human exposure to the important toxic agents in their work environments.

14. By 1990, at least 70 percent of the primary health care providers should routinely elicit occupational health exposure as part of patient history, and should know how to interpret the information to patients in an understandable manner.

15. By 1990, at least 70 percent of all graduate engineers should be skilled in the design of plants and processes that incorporate occupational safety and health control technologies.

16. By 1990, generic standard and other forms of technology transfer should be established, where possible, for standardized employer attention to such major common problems as: chronic lung hazards, neurologic hazards, carcinogenic hazards, mutagenic hazards, teratogenic hazards, and medical monitoring requirements.

17. By 1990, the number of health hazard evaluations being performed annually should increase tenfold; the number of industry-wide studies being performed annually should increase threefold.

18. By 1985, an ongoing occupational health hazard/illness/injury coding system, survey and surveillance capability should be developed, including identification of work place hazards and related health effects, including cancer, coronary heart disease, and reproductive effects. This system should include adequate measurements of the severity of work-related disabling injuries.

19. By 1985, at least one question about lifetime work history and known exposures to hazardous substances should be added to all appropriate existing health data reporting systems (e.g., cancer registries, hospital discharge abstracts, and death certificates).

20. By 1985, a program should be developed to: (a) follow up individual findings from health hazard and health evaluations, reports from unions and management, and other existing surveillance sources of clinical and epidemiological data; and (b) use the findings to determine the etiology, natural history, and mechanisms of suspected occupational disease and injury.

SOURCE:
Department of Health and Human Services: *Promoting health/preventing disease: Objectives for the nation.* Washington, DC: US Government Printing Office, 1980, pp. 39–43. Taken from Millar JD, Myers ML: Occupational safety and health: Progress toward the 1990 objectives for the nation. *Public Health Reports* 1983; 98 (4): 324–336.

has been viewed as a "bandage and aspirin" person. In the 1980s this role has evolved into practice at more of a clinical specialist level. The occupational health nurse still provides direct care to the workers for minor lacerations, burns, headaches, and other complaints, and is still the coordinator of health care in cases of major trauma to the worker. In addition, however, the occupational health nurse of the 1980s has assumed such roles as occupational health nurse practitioner, consultant, educator, researcher, and administrator.

The nurse consultant has developed special skills in the consultation process as well as knowledge of occupational health and can provide the industry with specific information about the type of program need in the area. The consultant works with the occupational health team to facilitate the problem-solving process of the program. The consultant should be a nurse from outside the industry who would contract with the industry for a specific task. The task may be to develop a program, evaluate a current program, or overhaul an existing program.

The role of the nurse researcher in occupational health is to help identify areas of nursing research and to assist in the planning of the research project, the development of hypotheses, the selection of the population, the determination and collection of necessary data, and the tabulation and reporting of those data (Silberstein, In Press).

The educative role of the nurse is common to all areas of nursing. Some nurses specialize in the preparation of students in the area of occupational health, but all nurses in occupational health function as educators for the workers (Patterson, 1983).

Occupational health nurses also may assume the role of administrators of the occupational health unit. As such, the nurse is responsible for the administrative functioning of the unit including budgetary decision making, policymaking, advancement of nursing practice, and the innovative and comprehensive care of the working population (Whitney, 1983).

Future Perspectives

Nursing as an emerging profession is deeply involved in the identification of a unique base of knowledge, and in the development of concepts and theories delineating the scope of nursing practice. The specialty of occupational health nursing is actively involved in the process of professional identification and as such has much to offer to the development of concepts and theories of nursing. The development of the occupational health nurse clinical specialist has helped increase awareness of the need to identify nursing concepts and nursing theories that address the impact of the occupational environment on the health of the individual worker.

Nursing theory helps direct the occupational health nurse toward a holistic approach to nursing care of the worker. The occupational health nurse clinical specialist is familiar with the recent literature on the development and utilization of nursing theories, and uses a systematic approach to decision making. The occupational health nurse clinical specialist develops and utilizes a conceptual model of nursing practice that reflects the standards of the profession, the nurse's personal philosophy, and the identification of the work place as a unique site of nursing practice. Finally, the occupational health nurse clinical specialist should test the success of the conceptual model in terms of nursing care delivery, client satisfaction, successful implementation, and cost effectiveness. The results of these findings are communicated to the specialty group of occupational health nurses and to professional organizations as a whole at meetings, conferences, and workshops, and through the publication process.

Research is an essential activity for the growth of any profession. The occupational health nurse clinical specialist must be able to evaluate existing research in occupational health and implement nursing activities based on sound research data. Information derived from research studies can be used to initiate changes in health care delivery within the occupational health setting, to identify nursing diagnoses unique to the work place, and to provide consultation to improve health care to individual workers (Lister, 1983).

As the profession of nursing grows, so grows the speciality of occupational health nursing. The occupational health nurse can effectively and efficiently manage the total occupational health unit. As health care costs continue to rise, maintaining the health of the individual will be far more cost effective than restoring it. Nurse researchers are providing new knowledge into the behaviors of workers exposed to agents within the work environment and are implementing this knowledge in the practice setting. These data will provide information to expand the practice of occupational health nursing and benefit industrial workers and their families. The work place then may become the ideal environment to practice primary health care under the supervision of a clinical nurse specialist in occupational health.

Third-party payers, insurance companies, pension plans, and government programs are becoming aware of the excellent quality of health care provided by nurses and are negotiating the feasibility of paying nurses for their expertise. It is not unrealistic that within the next decade there will be a rapid increase in the number of nurses establishing private practice clinics. Ideally this practice model would include a group of nurses certified in specific practice areas: maternal-child nursing, medical-surgical nursing, psychiatric nursing, and occupational health nursing. With this model, clients would benefit from an effective interdisciplinary nursing team who could assess, plan, implement, and evaluate an effective nursing care program for clients and their families.

The Occupational Health Team

Occupational health is an unique discipline requiring an interdisciplinary effort to bring about program development. Nursing, medicine, labor, management, industrial hygiene and safety must develop a peer relationship that fosters the discriminating development of programs to best serve the needs of the industry, the worker, and the consumer.

Each member of the occupational health team brings unique skills and experience to the planning, implementation, and evaluation of the occupational health program. The industrial hygienist is prepared to assess the work environment for the recognition, evaluation, and control of potential health hazards. Monitoring and evaluation of the presence of dusts, fumes, vapors, noise, and other factors are of prime concern. The safety officer will focus on the safe and efficient use of machinery, as well as on educating the worker to use protective equipment such as masks, respirators, and protective clothing to their maximum efficiency to protect the worker and avoid injury. The physician specializing in occupational medicine focuses on the diagnosis and treatment of diseases whose origins are in the work place.

The composition of the occupational health team will vary according to the size of the industry and the type of hazards involved. In large corporations the team may be expanded to include (1) a toxicologist, who focuses on determining the toxicity of new chemicals introduced into the work place and their interactions with existing chemicals; (2) a psychologist or psychiatric nurse, who may develop stress reduction programs or employee assistance programs; and/or (3) an epidemiologist, who may examine established data bases to determine the prevalence and incidence of occupationally related illness.

A small company may have none of these health professionals and may rely on consultation activities from a local health department or other community agency. In larger companies, while the nurse may be the principal health professional, he or she may work with a safety officer and consulting occupational physician. In this situation a team approach is still essential to decision making. The nurse, physician, managers, and workers must all be involved in the problem-solving process. Consultation from other occupational health experts is sought when appropriate.

Communication facilitates the effective functioning of this team. The dissemination of information about new tests, techniques, or research findings within one area to other members of the occupational health team provides individual team members with the ability to recognize when to seek consultation from other team members. Similarly, when new procedures, screening measures, or processes are initiated, input from other members of the occupational health team can help determine short- and long-range impact. Occupational health nurses bring a special expertise to this team approach since they are skilled in assessment, planning, implementation, and evaluation within the work environment. Case Example 20-1 demonstrates the function of the interdisciplinary health team.

Effects of Work on the Family

As mentioned previously, work at its best can provide the individual with status, prestige, and role satisfaction and at its worst can facilitate disease, disability, and death. From conception to death, work affects the health of the individual with specific consequences for the family as a whole.

Case Example 20-1: The Occupational Health Team

Mrs. J came to the occupational health nurse complaining of back pain during the workday. The occupational health nurse took a health history and assessed the appropriate systems. The nurse referred Mrs. J to the occupational health physician for further evaluation. Finding no pathologic condition, the nurse and physician went to the worksite to observe Mrs. J's work routine. Here they saw that Mrs. J had to reach across a moving conveyor belt to obtain parts. The conveyor belt was designed for the average man, and is too high for Mrs. J. It was concluded that the back strain was due to poor body mechanics on the job.

Nursing assessment

Medical assessment

The occupational health nurse then contacted the industrial hygienist and a specialist in ergonomics (the science of designing the work place to fit the worker) to determine if the worksite could be adapted. These individuals were able to redesign the packing process to adapt to Mrs. J's height. Management was notified of the adaptation and the cost. The union was informed of the needed adaptations. Following the implementation of the new process, the occupational health nurse visited the worksite to be sure that the adaptions were indeed meeting Mrs. J's health needs.

All members of the health team involved

Communication is essential

Evaluation and follow-up

The Beginning Years

Human propagation, and hence family development, depends on the ability of the male and female to effectively produce healthy children. Drugs such as thalidomide, diethylstilbestrol, and aminoglycoside antibodies have tragically led to fetal death or permanent disability (Doull, 1980). Women exposed to lead, mercury, and other metals have increased fetal loss. Dioxins, which are now being found as contaminants in the soil of many communities, also pose a threat to a successful reproductive history. Exposure to radiation, either on the job or as part of a diagnostic or therapeutic regime, has long been known as a threat to fetal life. Other agents such as lead cross the placental barrier and affect fetal growth (Khera, Wibberley, & Dathan, 1980; Lee, 1961; Levy, 1983).

Concern for the impact of work on the reproductive functions of men and women is becoming a very real issue. As more women have identified employment as a priority in their life-style, an increasing number of women are maintaining that employment during the pregnancy. A Public Health Survey found that 59 percent of all women bearing their first child were employed and that 50 percent of that group maintained their employment until at least the seventh month of pregnancy (Stellman, 1977).

Although much attention is focused on women of childbearing age, equal attention is needed on male reproductive hazards related to spermatogenesis. Occupational exposures that affect the reproductive process in man have been identified. Dibromochloropropane (DBCP) has been cited as a cause of sterility in men who work with this chemical. Exposure of men to anesthetic gases, vinyl chloride, chloroprene, and other hydrocarbons has been associated with an increased spontaneous abortion rate among nonexposed wives. Cadmium exposure in men can lead to testicular degeneration and damage to the seminiferous epithelium resulting in sterility (Doull, 1980).

Reproductive health in the work place is a controversial area of public and corporate concern. The current practice of some industries of excluding fertile females from jobs involving exposure to particular toxic substances such as lead is highly debatable. The Equal Employment Opportunities Commission has not yet provided guidelines as to whether or not this practice is discriminatory.

Studies on reproductive hazards have clearly identified that both males and females are at risk from chemical and physical agents in the work place. Until regulations and employment practice consider the reproductive risks involved in the work setting and act to minimize or eliminate the hazard, there will remain continued conflict within this area of occupational health (Levy, 1983).

The occupation and the occupational environment of the parents also have significant effect on the early development of the young child. The type of work will determine the salary level of the family and hence the economic status. This, in turn, will help to decide the family's type of housing and the child's external and internal environment. If that housing is in a largely industrial area where the family is exposed to the effluent of local industries, the location could pose a hazard to the child. With the economic philosophy of the 1980s much of the long sought environmental legislation has been allowed to run out or enforcement is at a minimum, thus exposing families to a variety of agents that may have significant health effects. De la Burde's (1972) study of children living near lead smelters found that school-age children had increased blood levels and manifested decreased verbal and motor skills. David (1974) has reported numerous studies of children with blood lead levels in the 24–35 μg/dl range who manifest learning problems and/or behavioral problems such as hyperactivity. Lead is frequently a problem in older homes where lead pipes and lead paint were used in the original construction and continue to pose health problems.

The work practices of the parents may also impact the child. Many industries provide uniforms for their employees as well as shower facilities. Many others do not. There are frequent reports in the literature of family members, wives, and children developing occupational diseases because of such contaminants as beryllium, lead, asbestos, and polyvinyl chloride being brought home on the work clothes of the parent (CDC, 1977). Workers need to know the potential health effects of the agents they work with and how to protect themselves and their family.

The School Years

It may seem strange to address the school years in a discussion of work. Nonetheless children do spend twelve years in a kind of work environment that may pose health hazards. The playground has long been seen as an area where accidents and injuries are commonplace. It can also be an ideal opportunity for teaching children the concept of safety.

As children advance in school they frequently choose courses in vocational training or the science laboratory. Both of these areas may expose the student to health hazards well recognized in the occupational setting but frequently ignored in the school setting. Vocational shop machinery must be properly guarded and ventilated. Machines made for adult males are not always adaptable to teenagers, male or female. Likewise, protective equipment such as masks, gloves, or safety glasses are made for adults and frequently do not fit the young adults properly and therefore do not provide the necessary protection.

The science laboratory also poses a variety of biologic and chemical hazards to the student. Safety measures must be taken to ensure the student's health. Too few science teachers are aware of the National Institute for Occupational Safety and Health's (NIOSH) guidelines for science laboratories. Whenever possible, the least hazardous chemical should be used to illustrate the concept. If hazardous materials must be used, the teacher may perform the experiment as a demonstration rather than having all students complete the laboratory task. Ventilation in the science laboratory is also crucial, and such ventilating systems must be installed and maintained by qualified individuals.

Another area of concern for young people is the use of video display terminals (VDTs) in the school. Contradicting studies have been published concerning the health effects of VDTs. Eye strain, postural problems, and stress have been related to use of these devices. Further research in this area needs to be done, however, to determine if problems exist.

The Work Years

General Assessment   Upon entering the full-time work force as independent adults, workers become exposed to a variety of physical, chemical, and psychological stressors that can affect their health status for years to come. The majority of workers are oblivious to the health hazards present in their place of employment or, worse still, accept the adverse effects as part of the job. For example, young workers beginning employment in a foundry may succumb to a syndrome called metal fume fever. The syndrome results in the worker having flu-like symptoms, elevated temperature, myalgias, and leukocytosis after exposure at work. Older workers may explain that it is a harmless syndrome, which appears to be true, and that the symptoms will subside as the worker adjusts to the job. Similarly, workers exposed to chromium (electroplaters, lithographers, metal workers, and welders) may develop painless ulcers on the nasal septum resulting in a "chrome hole." Many workers accept this health deviation as part of the job. Effective engineering controls would eliminate both of these conditions from the work place.

When developing health programs for workers, occupational health nurses are concerned with the use of substances in the work place within a specific margin of safety. In this context, safety is defined in terms of the probability that exposure to a substance will not produce pathophysiologic damage to the worker under specified conditions. Many factors directly or indirectly affect the physiologic response to a chemical, physical, or biologic agent. These factors include the biologic system itself, the unique properties of the agent, any chemicals or formulation factors used in combination with the agent, factors related to exposure, factors related to the internal environment of the individual exposed, and external environmental factors.

When determining which factors are relevant to each particular worksite, occupational health nurses must be familiar with the current literature concerning the specific agents to which the workers in the plant are exposed. Analysis of the literature should be done in terms of the types of studies presented (case studies, case control, experimental); the study sample (animals or people); the study design; and the utilization of appropriate statistical analysis for interpretation of the data. After careful analysis of the literature the occupational health nurse can determine the scope of the problem and develop an appropriate health program to meet the health needs of the workers.

In order for a physiologic or pathophysiologic response to occur upon exposure to a potentially toxic agent, several factors must be present:

1.   The toxic agent, its metabolite, or its conversion product—any of which may cause physiologic alterations—must reach a susceptible target organ.
2.   There must be sufficient concentrations of the agent to cause a physiologic response.
3.   The time of exposure must be long enough for an effect to occur.

Many chemicals used in the work place are combined with other substances called *formulation factors*, which may alter the physiologic effects of the agents. Formulation factors usually have little or no chemical activity of their own but enhance the utilization of the chemical in the process for which it is essential. Examples of formulation factors are water, starch, gels, saline, polyethylene glycols, vegetable oils, and various organic solvents. Formulation factors may increase or decrease the toxicity of an agent either directly or indirectly by altering the chemical nature of the agent or by altering its rate of absorption by the host.

Many of the principles initially gained in the study of pharmacology are applicable to determining the effect of exposure to a potentially toxic agent on the worker. All processes within the work place should be carefully evaluated in terms of the potential hazards to the worker. The occupational health nurse is aware of all chemical, physical, or biological agents to which the workers are exposed. This information is available from the industrial hygienist or from the company that manufactures the product. Any changes in a process, which would alter the amount of exposure to the worker, must be communicated to all members of the occupational health team. The nurse should have copies of all of the safety data sheets provided by the manufacturers of the agents. The nurse also maintains accurate, current information as to the volume of each agent used, the concentration in which it is used, the current threshold limit value of that agent, the acceptable standard (if one exists), and the potential dose received by the average worker involved in that process.

In addition, the occupational health nurse is aware of the route of exposure, whether the worker will be exposed by absorption through the skin or by inhalation, and what protective measures can be taken to protect employees. Identification of the site of action and the target organ is also important. By being familiar with the manufacturing process the occupational health nurse will be able to determine the duration and frequency of exposure as well as factors such as particle size and the presence of smoke or fumes, which may affect the exposure level.

External environmental factors are also important in determining the amount of exposure a worker receives during a workday. The rate of work of the individual worker will determine his or her level of metabolic activity and may provide for an increased exposure. Environmental factors, such as heat, humidity, and barometric pressure, will further affect the individual worker and the exposure level. Other exposures in the work setting, such as

ultraviolet light, noise, pesticides, or ionizing radiation, may influence the worker's physiologic response to specific agents. The adherence to good personal hygiene practices and attention to general principles of housekeeping also help control the worker's level of exposure.

The type of exposure the worker receives, acute or chronic, is also of prime importance in evaluating the impact of an agent. An acute exposure may be of very short duration as in an emergency situation where a ceiling level exposure occurs, or it may be a single exposure over a period of hours.

A chronic exposure, on the other hand, results in continuous long-term exposure of the worker to a specific amount of the agent. The effects of the exposure will usually be determined by the ability of the individual worker to effectively metabolize, detoxify, store, or eliminate the substance from the body. If the rate of metabolism, storage, or elimination is decreased, then the pathophysiologic response may be increased.

Several factors must be considered relating to the internal environment of the subjects. These include age, sex, body build, genetic makeup, immunologic state (sensitive, hypersensitive, or idiosyncratic), nutritional status, hormonal status, maturity, emotional status, and the presence of any disease and/or organ pathology that may influence the metabolism or excretion of a potentially toxic agent.

Based on a thorough assessment of the workers and the work place, the occupational health nurse can develop, implement, and evaluate an occupational health program that will protect the worker, the family, and the community from harmful exposure to agents used or produced at the worksite. This includes identification of all individuals exposed, recognition of those workers who may be more sensitive, and development and implementation of educational programs for exposed workers. All of this information must be accurately recorded and maintained in a record system that provides for ready accessibility for data analysis and interpretation. Box 20-2 illustrates the type of data that should be maintained on all physical, chemical, and biological agents in the work place.

Box 20-2   Hazard Information File

1. Name of Substance
   Chemical Name:
   Brand Name:

2. Routes of Exposure:

3. Number of Workers Exposed:

4. Recommended Exposure Level:

5. Monitoring Process
   Who is Responsible for Monitoring:
   Frequency of Monitoring:
   Date and Results of Last Monitoring:

6. Target Organ of Exposure:

7. Signs and Symptoms of Exposure
   Acute:
   Chronic:

8. Nursing Diagnosis:

9. Nursing Care of Acute Exposure
   Emergency Measures to be Taken:
   Instructions to Transporters:
   Instructions to Hospital Emergency Room
   Personnel:

10. Nursing Care of Chronic Exposures
    Screening Programs:
    Biological Monitoring:
    Educational Programs:
    Protective Equipment:

Dermatologic Hazards   Occupational dermatitis represents about 65 percent of occupational disease and is considered a major health problem in the industrial setting. The cost of occupational skin disease is high in terms of lost work time for the employee, lost production time to industry, and increased costs in terms of workers compensation and health care (Rom, 1983).

Occupational hazards that may result in the occurrence of occupational dermatitis can be divided into four major categories: (1) mechanical injuries caused by friction, trauma, or pressures; (2) chemical insults that result in the absorption of toxic materials through the skin and result in local or system responses; (3) physical insults to the skin such as temperature extremes or radiation exposure; and (4) biologic hazards such as bacteria, fungi, parasites, or virus.

As with other organ systems the skin has only a limited number of responses to insult or injury. Pathologic or defensive responses include the pro-

liferation of skin cells, atrophy, the formation of ulcers, scaling, an inflammatory response, and the formation of blisters.

Prevention is the key to controlling occupational dermatitis. Good housekeeping and personal cleanliness help to sustain the integrity of the skin. Showers should be available to workers and the general maintenance of the plant must be excellent. Workers must be informed about the proper measures for protecting the skin from undue exposure to dermatologic hazards. An interdisciplinary team approach to education of the workers and enforcement of protective programs is essential. Workers should be provided with protective equipment such as aprons, gloves, sleeves, face shields, and coveralls, and a program of screening and monitoring should be developed by the occupational health professional. Table 20-2 illustrates a nursing diagnosis related to dermatologic hazards as well as some of the agents and jobs that expose workers.

Table 20-2   Nursing Diagnosis Related to Occupational Exposure to Dermatologic Hazards

Nursing Diagnosis	Defining Characteristics	Agents	Occupation
Potential for skin breakdown	Exposure to toxic agent	Ultraviolet light	Construction Aircraft worker Hairdressers Welders
		Microbes	Animal handlers Bakers Dairy workers
	Heat Altered sensation Itching Blisters	Wood	Cabinet workers Forest workers
	Rash	Solvents	Garage workers Laboratory workers Painters Chemists Electricians Health care workers

Respiratory Hazards   The respiratory system has a distinct position in the structure of the human body. The lung is the only organ in which there is direct contact between the environmental air and the functional elements that allow for the transport of oxygen and carbon dioxide across the alveolar membrane. Because the lung tissue does have direct contact with inspired air, it also has direct contact with those substances in the air of the work environment. Any substance the worker inhales may have the potential of causing a physiologic reaction in the lung. As with the skin, there are a limited number of responses that may occur. Excess exposure to toxic agents such as irritant gases or vapors may produce an inflammatory response in the lung tissue. This response will increase secretions in the lung and may progress to pleural effusion or pulmonary edema. Chronic exposure may result in a chronic inflammatory process that may cause destruction and/or fibrosis of the lung tissue. Tumor formation is also possible in the lung after exposure to carcinogens.

Occupational pulmonary disease is a major cause of disability among workers in certain industries such as mining, asbestos, and sandblasting. The exact magnitude of the problem is difficult to pinpoint since other factors such as home exposure and life-style habits (smoking) also impact the response of the lung to substances in common use in the work environment. As with other occupational exposures, several factors impinge on the pathogenicity of toxic agents. One set of factors includes the physical properties of the potentially toxic agent: the particle size, the mass diameter, and the concentration. Another set of considerations relates to the chemical properties of the agent: the solubility, the concentration, the molecular weight, and the pH. Environmental conditions such as heat, moisture, and ventilation must also be accounted for. The individual worker also needs to be considered in terms of the impact of the substances on his or her health status. Age, sex, general health, genetic factors, current and past exposure to respiratory insults, occupational history, and

Case Example 20-2: Respiratory Hazards in the Work Place

Mr. Y is a thirty-seven-year-old man who works in an automotive plant. He is in good health and has had no identified health problems. He is a smoker. His job involves testing motors and requires that the engines be run. The testing area is enclosed, located away from other workers, and has its own ventilating system to minimize exposure to carbon monoxide.

One day Mr. Y was working in his area alone and developed a severe headache. He decided to go to the occupational health clinic to obtain an analgesic and return to work. The occupational health nurse did an initial assessment including a brief health and job history. Familiar with Mr. Y's job, she was concerned that the headache and drowsiness were due to carbon monoxide exposure. The health assessment includes respiration rate, depth, quality, sound chest movement, pulse rate, regularity, quality, blood pressure, skin temperature, color, moisture, level of consciousness, sensory status, mood, and thought process.

Nursing assessment provides data for nursing diagnosis.

The nurse decided that the nursing diagnosis was impaired oxygen-exchange related to exposure to carbon monoxide.

The occupational health nurse establishes a nursing diagnosis.

The immediate nursing interventions included removal of Mr. Y from the contaminated environment, determination of carboxyhemoglobin level, and administration of oxygen. The occupational health nurse also asked the industrial hygienist to monitor the room to determine the carbon monoxide levels and check the ventilation system for effectiveness. No workers were allowed in the room until these safety measures had been taken.

The nurse initiates immediate nursing action.

The nurse has responsibility for individual workers and the total working population.

Once this information had been obtained, the occupational health nurse could decide if further tests needed to be made to determine the safety of the work environment. The nurse could also provide opportunities for educational programs regarding worker protection when in a potentially hazardous environment, smoking cessation programs, and information programs regarding early signs of carbon monoxide exposure and immediate first aid.

The nurse has responsibility for worker education.

In addition the nurse met with other members of the occupational health team, the physician, and representatives from management, labor, industrial hygiene, and safety to establish a plan to avoid this type of exposure in the work place.

The nurse is a change agent.

---

lung functions should be noted and assessed before a job assignment is made.

The lung is primarily responsible for the exchange of gases between the human and the environment. As a biologic barrier between the two, the lung is so effective in that it is normally sterile from the first bronchial division to the terminal lung units.

The lung is vulnerable to infectious agents, air pollutants, allergens, industrial materials, and cigarette smoke. The occupational health nurse has several strategies for addressing respiratory problems in the work place, as illustrated in Case Example 20-2.

Several pulmonary diseases are specifically

attributed to occupational exposure. Here we'll discuss silicosis, pneumoconiosis, byssinosis, and asbestosis.

Probably the oldest recognized occupational pulmonary disease is *silicosis*. Writers from Hippocrates to the present have identified the problem of workers exposed to silica dust. Silica is a common element in the earth's crust and, in combination with oxygen, forms silicon dioxide, commonly referred to as silica. Workers in such occupations as mining, quarrying, sandblasting, chipping, grinding, molding, stone cutting, and abrasive blasting are exposed to respirable free silica.

The onset and severity of clinical symptoms of silicosis vary with the intensity of the exposure. Individual workers who have had long-term low dose exposure may not develop the disease until late in life, while other younger workers who have had heavy exposure to silica dust may develop disabling and rapidly progressive symptoms. Workers with silicosis usually present with dyspnea on exertion, prolonged and slowed expiratory phase, and an enlarged thorax. Coughing is not uncommon and may be related to the dust itself, smoking, or the occurrence of a complicating infectious process such as tuberculosis, which is a common infection in workers with silicosis.

The treatment of these workers is to remove them from the exposure, screen and treat for complicating infections, and counseling the worker regarding life-style habits such as smoking, which would further compromise the respiratory status.

Another major occupational pulmonary disease is coal workers' *pneumoconiosis*, or what is commonly called Black Lung disease. It is estimated that 10 to 20 percent of active miners have some pulmonary impairment due to exposure to coal dust and 50 to 75 percent of retired workers have significant impairment as a direct result of exposure to coal dust. The incidence of coal workers pneumoconiosis varies with the type of coal (seen more frequently in miners working bituminous coal) and with the process of mining (strip mining or underground mining).

The mechanism by which the coal dust produces the physiologic response is unclear, but the coal dust accumulates throughout the respiratory tree—in the alveoli, the macrophages, and the lymph nodes (Parkes, 1982). As with other pulmonary exposures, the onset of symptomatology will vary with concentration and duration of exposure. Twenty-five percent of workers will usually present with a productive cough soon after initial exposure in the mines. As the disease progresses, the cough increases and the worker begins to complain of breathlessness and dyspnea on exertion. Pulmonary function studies will show significant decrease in lung volume. The workers will produce profuse black sputum and have decreased breath sounds and an enlarged barrel-shaped chest. Workers who are smokers should be instructed to stop smoking. Prevention is the real solution to controlling coal workers' pneumoconiosis. Once the disease has developed, the only treatment is supportive for the respiratory symptomatology.

Byssinosis is an occupational pulmonary disease common among textile workers. Inhalation of cotton textile dust, flax dust, and soft hemp dust produces symptoms of respiratory distress in exposed workers. The worker complains of shortness of breath, tightness in the chest, cough, and wheezing after exposure to the dust. Complaints are more common in workers in the picking, blending, and cording areas of the mill since these are the dirtiest areas of the plant. Prevention of exposure and surveillance of the workers become the prime responsibility of the occupational health nurse in this setting.

A discussion of occupational pulmonary disease would not be complete without addressing the problem of asbestos exposure. Asbestos is a fibrous mineral with unique physical properties including (1) insulation material against heat, cold and noise; (2) incombustibility; (3) good dielectric properties; (4) tensile strength; (5) flexibility; and (6) resistance to corrosion.

Asbestos causes a parenchymal fibrosis of the lung *(asbestosis)*. The cardinal symptom of asbestosis is dyspnea, which is usually progressive. Cough and sputum production are common, and the worker may complain of pleuritic chest pain and chest tightness. Characteristic changes are noted on

Table 20-3   Nursing Diagnosis Related to Occupational Exposure to Respiratory Hazard

Nursing Diagnosis	Defining Characteristics
Potential for Suffocation	Reduced olfactory sensation Lack of safety precaution Lack of compliance with safety precautions Presence of asphyxiant
Ineffective Breathing Patterns	Shortness of breath Cough Altered respiration Change in mental status Presence of dusts, fumes, vapors Lack of compliance with respirator protection program
Impaired gas exchange	Confusion Somnolence Restlessness Irritability

X-ray. Numerous studies cite exposure to asbestos as being significantly associated with lung cancer and mesothelioma of the lung. Workers who smoke and are exposed to asbestos have a higher incidence of tumors than nonsmokers (Rom, 1983).

For all respiratory hazards the role of the occupational health nurse is one of primary prevention. Worker education programs, counseling programs, screening programs, pulmonary function studies, monitoring programs, and smoking cessation programs are essential in maintaining a healthful work environment for workers exposed to pulmonary hazards. Table 20-3 illustrates some of the nursing diagnoses related to occupational exposure to respiratory hazards.

Neurologic Hazards   The human nervous system is exposed to an increased number of chemical substances capable of producing reversible and/or irreversible changes in neurologic function. The industrial revolution has resulted in the potential exposure of humans in the work place and in the general environment to a wide variety of neurotoxicants. While some of these chemicals were developed primarily for their toxic action on the nervous system (nerve gases), the majority were developed to increase the quality of our life-style.

Although the central nervous system is the target organ for many neurotoxic agents, some chemicals' toxicity is manifested by peripheral neuropathy. Inorganic lead, acrylamide, and some organophosphates appear to cause injury directly to the peripheral nerves.

Some neurotoxic agents cause both polyneuritis and central nervous system effects. Carbon disulfide is an industrial toxicant used in the rubber and rayon industry. Workers overexposed to this substance may manifest symptoms of psychosis, tremor, and polyneuritis. Chronic exposure results in lower extremity weakness and paresthesia. The metal mercury in its inorganic form may produce psychological changes, deposition of mercury in the anterior lens of the eye, tremor, and increased salivation (Rom, 1983).

When determining the nervous system's response to potentially toxic substances, occupational health nurses must take into consideration the duration of exposure and the concentration of the substance. The ability of the nervous system to compensate for nerve damage must also be considered. The individual worker may have had a large exposure with significant amounts of damage but have little functional loss. The circumstances of exposure or potential exposure must also be considered.

Carcinogens in the Work Place   As the incidence of cancer rises, there is an increasing effort to identify the causative agents and develop a cure. One of the major problems with pursuing this goal is that most cancers have multiple causes. The relationship between one exposure and the synergistic effects of exposure to other chemicals has not been clearly defined. Individual susceptibility to the development of cancer can be altered by genetic, congenital, or acquired biological host factors. Cancer manifests itself in a variety of clinical syndromes and in most organ systems. It is now estimated that 80 percent of all cancers occur as a result of environmental exposure to carcinogens. Environmental risk factors include life-style habits such as smoking or dietary intake, occupational exposures, and cultural differences. Scientific studies are under way to identify the host factors that interact with environmental carcinogens, with particular emphasis on identifying the intrinsic host factors that protect some individuals from cancer.

Two approaches are commonly used in the control of cancer related to occupational exposure. The first approach is primary prevention through the identification of the multiple etiologic factors of carcinogenesis through epidemiologic and laboratory studies. The second approach is the identification and screening of workers at risk of developing cancer because of occupational exposure.

A carcinogen may be defined as an agent that results in the development of a cancer after human exposure to it. Characteristics of a carcinogen include the fact that the action is irreversible, that an undetected single dose may have an additive effect, that most carcinogens have a long latent period, and that many carcinogens have synergistic effects with other chemicals. Chemical exposure to a carcinogen may initiate a change in the DNA structure of the cell, thus resulting in malignant

growth. Malignant change may also occur by indirect action—that is, the activation of a latent oncogenic virus, depression of genetic activity, or interference with normal immunologic defense. Physical hazards such as ionizing radiation or ultraviolet light may also directly affect the DNA structure and result in the formation of malignant cells.

It seems appropriate at this point to identify some of those chemicals identified as carcinogens. Polycyclic aromatic hydrocarbons are products of incomplete combustion of hydrocarbons and are components of gas-engine exhaust, tobacco smoke, and incinerator and combustion stack effluents. The most potent of these carcinogens are benz [a] anthracene and benzo [a] pyrene. Workers in the coal and coke industry, steel plants, and metal working industries are at risk because of this exposure. Vinyl chloride has been identified as a carcinogen, and workers exposed to the vinyl chloride monomer are at risk to developing angiosarcoma of the liver. Carbon tetrachloride and chloroform, commonly used organic solvents, have both been found to be carcinogenic in animals, producing liver or kidney tumors in rats. Bladder cancers in industrial workers have been associated with aromatic amines. Asbestos has been identified as a carcinogen whose exposure results in mesothelioma of the lung. Inorganic compounds such as arsenic, cadmium, chromium, and nickel are all suspected to be carcinogenic.

In light of these data it is vital that occupational health nurses be experienced in implementation of screening programs for workers exposed to known or suspected carcinogens.

Other Occupational Health Issues   Occupational stress has become a major health problem among workers today. Studies presented at the Reducing Occupational Stress Conference in May, 1977 suggest that occupational stress derives from three major sources: anxiety over joblessness, anxiety over work place accidents and/or work-related illness, and anxiety over work-role insults to one's adulthood. Stress reduction programs are a valuable, cost-effective mechanism by which the worker can be educated to cope with stressful situations

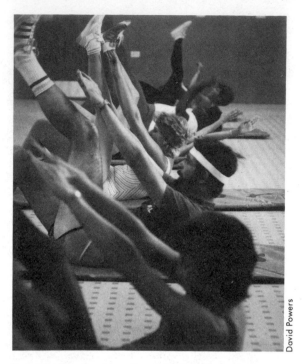

David Powers

Recognizing the benefits of health promotion in the workplace, many employers offer on-site exercise facilities and incentives for attendance.

related to the home or work situation. Employee assistance programs, stress reduction programs, and life-style programs are being introduced into health plans within the occupational setting. Occupational health nurses function as resource people and coordinators in the development, implementation, and evaluation of these worthwhile programs.

Another area essential to health promotion in the work place is the study of *ergonomics*. The discipline studies the interaction of people with tools, machines, and other physical and behavioral factors in the work environment. The proper use of body mechanics when lifting and moving bedridden clients is an example of the application of the principles of ergonomics. Workers need to be taught

how to effectively use their muscle structure in adapting to the work environment so that they avoid musculoskeletal injury that results in disability and lost work time (Chaffin, 1978).

The Senior Years

In many cases the full impact of exposure to occupational health hazards is not recognized until later in life, when the worker retires. With the increase in longevity comes questions about the quality of life in older adulthood. Retirement is viewed as a period in one's life when one is able to enjoy the harvest of one's labors. In reality retirement is a stressful event in one's life pattern and requires major adaptation. Exposures in the work place particularly to chronic respiratory hazards or carcinogens may leave the employee ill or disabled during the retirement years. The occupational health nurse can intervene by helping to provide a work place that minimizes health hazards.

Retirement programs may also be included in an occupational health care program. Older workers are usually well informed by the company of the benefits package that they have accumulated over the years of employment. Health issues related to aging are only recently being addressed. Education programs planned and implemented by the occupational health nurse can provide valuable information to this long-term employee. Information should be provided on the physiology of aging (Coyne & Hojlo, 1985), sexuality and the aging, leisure time alternatives (Evans, 1985), psychological impact of retirement, and exercise (Johnson, 1985) and the identification of support groups and resources are most appropriate (Evans, 1985). Family members, spouses, and children should be invited to attend these sessions so that anxiety-provoking issues can be discussed in a therapeutic, nonthreatening environment. See Chapter 23 for a more detailed discussion of the health of the older adult.

Strategies for Health Promotion

Health promotion is the main focus of any occupational health program. Industry must have a healthy work force to produce effectively and efficiently. Well-designed health promotion programs support industry's aims by reducing absenteeism, lost work time, and health care costs.

Primary Prevention

The occupational health nurse can develop programs in the area of health education in the work place, which will provide the worker with essential knowledge of potential health risks. Programs should be designed to give information about attaining and maintaining high-level wellness; avoiding physical, chemical, biological, and psychological stressors in the work setting, using protective equipment for decreasing exposures to toxic substances, and understanding life-style changes.

Companies should be encouraged to support health programs based on the worksite. Wellness programs focus on the employees' responsibility for maintaining their own individual high levels of wellness. Health education measures may include programs in smoking cessation, exercise, diet control, and stress reduction. Some companies provide incentives to workers who participate and successfully achieve their goals: monetary rewards for quitting smoking, vacation trips for weight reduction, and extra vacation time for other activities. In cooperation with other members of the team, occupational health nurses can be creative and imaginative in developing incentives for healthy behavior.

The occupational health nurse's contribution can begin even before the workers start their employment. Preemployment examinations as well as routine physical examinations would help identify actual and potential health problems that might affect performance. Such screening measures would include pulmonary function testing, audiometry, lipid profiles, and strength testing. Workers would

be assessed for their health level and would be placed in a job compatible with their health status.

Another area of primary prevention requiring action by occupational health nurses is the development of local, state, and national legislation regarding occupational health. As discussed earlier in this chapter, the process of setting standards is a rigorous one. Occupational health nurses must be prepared with the research skills needed to accumulate, analyze, and interpret data that contribute to the knowledge base in standard setting. The nurse also needs to have the political skills to present testimony that can support or reject the legislation.

Finally, the occupational health nurse needs to function within the political system in terms of networking and lobbying with those groups who have similar interests and needs regarding legislative decision making.

Secondary Prevention

In the occupational setting, secondary prevention is frequently the most important goal. As the new employee enters the work force, the assessment and screening process begins. Baseline data are accumulated to identify the employee's current health status, and a program is implemented that will continually monitor the individual's health status. For example, new employees are screened to determine their hearing levels upon employment. If exposed to a noisy environment, they will have yearly audiograms to determine any hearing loss as well as to teach them how to utilize hearing protection.

Based on the assessment, nursing diagnoses are derived and focus on potential health problems due to exposure on the job, poor health habits, or risk factors identified in the initial history. Such risk factors might include history of hypertension, smoking, obesity, or hereditary diseases. Plans of nursing care would include interventions not only for work exposures, but also for risk factors such as diet control and smoking cessation programs. In this way, signs and symptoms of early disease may be identified and referred to the primary care physician practicing within the community before a major illness occurs.

Once seen by the physician, the worker can then be followed in the occupational health setting to facilitate compliance with the prescribed regime. Communication between the occupational health nurse, the primary physician, and the occupational health physician facilitates the worker's health care. Other members of the health team would also be informed if appropriate. Early diagnosis helps to control not only the pain and suffering of the workers but also the cost of health care. The worksite is the ideal situation for the practice of primary health care, since the emphasis can be placed on wellness rather than illness.

Employee assistance programs can also be offered through the occupational health unit. An essential role of occupational health nurses is in counseling and guiding the workers with mental health problems. Nurses see workers routinely and can easily detect signs and symptoms of stress. For this reason they should be aware of appropriate community resources that can be utilized by the worker and the family. It may mean referral to a local mental health clinic, a finance officer for budget problems, or a community group for help with dependency behaviors such as chemical abuse (Brennan, 1983). Occupational health nurses may also develop a program that trains first line supervisors to recognize changes in an employee's behavior that may indicate increased stress. Late arrival, increased absenteeism, moodiness, change in work pattern, or inattention may indicate potential health problems. The supervisor then consults with the nurse regarding these observed behaviors and the nurse would determine if the worker should be seen for further assessment. Supervisor training programs have proven very effective in the success of employee assistance programs (Weisensee, 1985).

Assessment programs centering on women in the work place are needed. With close to half of the employed individuals in the United States today being women it is important to gather data on exposure levels in women. The current threshold limit is based on a consensus standard established by the American Conference of Governmental Industrial Hygienists, which set values for the "average" man working a forty-hour week. Insufficient data are available to determine if these exposure levels are safe for women. With the changing social system many industries are working ten- or twelve-hour shifts rather than the previously accepted eight hours. The effects of increasing the time of exposure on men or women has yet to be determined. The occupational health nurse can facilitate the collection of this vital information by careful assessment and documentation of worksite exposure and individual workers' reactions. (See Chapter 22 for a more detailed discussion of the health concerns of women.)

Assessment of the work place is also a vital component of secondary prevention. Monitoring of noise levels, temperature extremes, dust levels, and air levels of metals as solvents within the plant are all examples of information that must be obtained, usually by the industrial hygienist, and communicated to the occupational health nurse who will determine the frequency of monitoring programs. Monitoring programs will facilitate early case finding and the initiation of treatment for the detection of signs and symptoms of disease.

Secondary prevention should also include an assessment of the impact of the plant on the community. Such factors as employment rate, impact of plant closure, and the effect of pollutants from the plant in the air, water, or soil of the community must be discussed with community groups. Plans to control emissions that are potentially harmful to the population should be carefully designed. Emergency plans need to be instituted with appropriate health care facilities.

Tertiary Prevention

Finally, caring for the ill and/or injured worker is the shared responsibility of the occupational health professional and the health professionals within the community. Plans for rehabilitation of workers are important. All fifty states now have workers' compensation laws that have some provision for rehabilitation. Companies may have training and retraining programs within their own health units. Sheltered workshops within the company provide employees the opportunity to reevaluate their jobs and see if adaptation can be made so that they may return to the same job. If that is impossible, then retraining can take place.

Summary

Occupational health is a specialty area demanding expertise in problem solving, decision making, nursing process, and occupational health. A working career spans two-thirds of a typical life span, and therefore affects both physical and mental health. Workers have the right to know the potential effects of work upon their health status and the effect on their families. Occupational health nurses have the expertise to identify health problems in the work setting and to implement appropriate changes that protect the worker, the family, and the community.

Topics for Nursing Research

• In a particular worksite, what are the appropriate primary prevention measures an occupational health nurse can employ?

• Demonstrate the effectiveness of health screening programs at specific worksites. What are the frequently identified health problems? What referral sources are needed to handle these health problems?

• What is the family's response to the exposure of one of its members to occupational hazards?

• What are the responses and health care needs of men compared to women exposed to occupational hazards that affect the reproductive system?

Study Questions

1. Which of the following statements concerning chronic diseases and the work environment is true?
   a. The ultimate cause of chronic disease can be traced to the work environment.
   b. The work environment can contribute to the incidence and prevalence of chronic diseases.
   c. There is no relationship between chronic diseases and the work environment.
   d. Statistics show that very few workers suffer chronic conditions that can be traced to their jobs.

2. Which of the following is the primary concern of occupational health nurses?
   a. Legislation to regulate the working environment
   b. Health care of the working population
   c. Health education programs for primary prevention
   d. Workers who become injured in the work place

3. Which of the following legislative acts was designed to ensure safe and healthful working conditions for the working public?
   a. Occupational Safety and Health Act
   b. Standard Interpretation and Audit Criteria for Performance of Occupational Health Programs
   c. Employee Health Surveillance Evaluation Act
   d. The Health Maintenance Organization Act

4. Occupational health nurses may assume which of the following roles?

a. Counseling
b. Management
c. Provision of emergency care
d. All of the above

5. Occupational health usually requires interdisciplinary collaboration. Which of the following factors is a prime concern to the occupational health nurse when engaging in interdisciplinary collaboration?
   a. Power and control
   b. Discipline expertise
   c. Communication
   d. None of the above

References

Agricola GG: De Re Metallica 1556. Translated by Hoover HC, and Hoover LH in Min Mag London, 1912.

Ashford, WA: Crisis in the workplace: A Report to the Ford Foundation. MIT Press, Cambridge, Mass.: 1977.

Ashford N: Framework provides path through right to know law. Occup Health Saf (October) 1983; 52 (10): 11–19, 25–27.

Brennan AJ: How to set up a corporate wellness program. Management Review (May) 1983; 72 (5): 41–47.

Burke M: The older employee and preretirement. Occupational Health Nursing (March) 1985; 33 (3): 113–114.

Cahall J: The history of occupational nursing. Occupational Health Nursing (October) 1981; 29 (10): 11–13.

Center for Disease Control: Lead poisoning in children of battery plant employees. Morbidity and Mortality Weekly Report 1977; 26: 1.

Chaffin D: Localized muscle fatigue: Definition and Measurement. J Occ Med 1978; 15: 346.

Coyne M, Hojlo C: Physiologic aspects of aging. Occupational Health Nursing Journal (March) 1985; 33 (3): 117–122, 150.

David OJ: Association between lower level lead concentrations and hyperactivity in children. Environ Health Perspect (Max) 1974; 7: 17–25.

de la Burde B: Does a symptomatic lead exposure in children have latent sequelae? J Ped 1972; 81: 1088.

Dickinson L et al: Lead poisoning in a family due to cocktail glasses. American Journal of Medicine 1972; 52: 391–394.

Doull J, Klaassen C, Amdur M: Casarett and Doull's Toxicology: The Basic Science of Poisons, 2nd ed. New York: Macmillan, 1980.

Dyal L: Plant profile: A contemporary interpretation of the nursing process. Occupational Health Nursing (March) 1982; 30: 17–21.

Evans L: Over the back fence. Occupational Health Nursing (March) 1985; 33 (3): 127–131, 152.

Faber M, Reinhardt A: Promoting Health Through Risk Reduction. New York: Macmillan, 1982.

Greenwald HP: Work and Health: Inseparable in the Eighties. Western Institute for Occupational/Environmental Science Inc., 1980.

Johnson J: Exercise, aging, and health. Occupational Health Nursing (March) 1985; 33 (3): 137–139, 151.

Khera AK, Wibberley PC, Dathan JC: Placental and stillbirth tissue lead concentration in occupationally exposed women. Br J Ind Med 1980.

La Dou, J: Occupational Health Law: A Guide for Industry. New York: Marcel Dekker, 1981.

Lappe M: Ethical issues in testing for differential sensitivity to occupational hazards. Journal of Occupational Medicine (November) 1983; 25 (11): 797–808.

LaLonde M: New Perspectives on the Health of Canadians: A Working Document. Ottawa: Minister of Supply and Services of Canada, 1977.

Lee J: Occupational Health Services for Women Employees. 1961.

Levy B, Wegman D: Occupational Health. Boston: Little Brown, 1983.

Lister DW: The nursing diagnosis movement and the occupational health nurse. Occupational Health Nursing 1983; 31 (2): 11–14.

Maslow AH: Motivation and Personality. New York: Harper and Row, 1954.

McCain F: Nursing by assessment not institution. Am J Nurs 1965; 65: 82.

McElveen J: Despite pre-emption threat local right-to-know laws increase. Occup Health Saf (January) 1985; 54 (1): 20–26.

McKechnie MR: A descriptive study of the scope of practice of occupational health in one-nurse units. Occupational Health Nursing 1983; 31 (3).

Millar JD, Myers ML: Occupational safety and health: Progress toward the 1990 objectives for the nation. Public Health Reports (Jul-Aug) 1983; 48 (4): 324–336.

Murphy SA, Hoffer B: Role of the specialties in nursing science. Adv Nurs Sci 1983; 5 (4): 31.

Parkes WR: Occupational Lung Disorders. London: Butterworth, 1982.

Patterson D: The occupational health nurse as a health educator. Occupational Health Nursing 1983; 31 (2).

Rammazzini B: De Morbis Artificiin (1713). Translated by Wright WC. Chicago: University Press, 1940.

Rom W: Environmental and Occupational Medicine. Boston: Little, Brown, 1983.

Saward E, Sorenson A: The current emphasis on preventative medicine. Science (May 26) 1978; 200: 884–894.

Schorsch A: Images of Childhood. The Main Street Press, 1979.

Sicherman B: Alice Hamilton. Harvard Medical School Alumnae Magazine (Spring) 1985.

Silberstein C: The role of the occupational health nurse

researcher. *The Proceedings of the NIOSH Symposium. The State of the Art and Directions for the Future.* NIOSH, Department of Health and Human Services. In Press.

Solomon C: The effects of a master's degree in occupational health on the delivery of services to workers. *Occupational Health Nursing* 1982; 30 (8): 9–24.

Standards, Interpretation and Audit Criteria for Performance of Occupational Health Programs. Report to the National Institute for Occupational Safety and Health. Chicago: Occupational Health Institute, 1975.

Stellman JM: *Women's Work, Women's Health.* New York: Pantheon, 1977.

Stertz V: Industrial Insurance Commission, 91 Washington, 588, 158, p. 256 (1918).

The Nurse in Industry: A History of the American Association of Industrial Nurses, Inc. New York: American Association of Industrial Nurses, 1976.

Weisensee M: Evaluation of health promotive. *Occupational Health Nursing* (January) 1985; 33 (1): 9–14.

Weisensee M: *Work and Health: Inseparable in the '80s.* Bethesda, Maryland: US Department of Health and Human Services, National Institute of Health, 1980.

Weisensee M: *Reducing Occupational Stress.* US Department of Health, Education and Welfare, Public Health Service, 1977.

Whitney F: Winning: The art of successful negotiation. *Occupational Health Nursing* 1983; 31 (5): 31–34.

Chapter 21

Rural Health

Nancy Dolphin

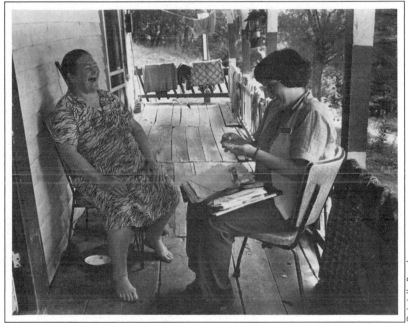

Community health nursing in the rural setting can provide a high level of satisfaction for nurses who enjoy holistic care and who approach opportunities for leadership and change with confidence.

Chapter Outline

Characteristics of Rural Families
- Family Structure
- Family Income and Employment
- Social Interaction
- Sex Roles

Characteristics of Rural Communities
- Political
- Economic
- Social
- Environmental
- Religious and Other Values
- Ethnic

Health Care in the Rural Community
- Types and Organization of Health Services
- Health Care Needs
- Resolution of Health Care Problems and Needs
- Use of Health Care Services and Health Care Providers
- Characteristics of the Delivery System

Nursing in Rural Communities
- Generalist Role
- Management Role
- Partnership Role
- Marketing Role
- Perceptions of Rural Nursing Practice
- Ethical and Legal Considerations

Strategies for Health Promotion
- Primary Prevention
- Secondary Prevention
- Tertiary Prevention

Summary
Topics for Nursing Research
Study Questions
References

Chapter Objectives

After completing this chapter, the reader will be able to:

- Identify four major characteristics of rural families that differentiate these families from urban families
- Describe the effects of political, economic, social, environmental, values and religious, and cultural characteristics of the rural area on the health care of the rural family
- Evaluate possible nursing solutions to the problems in the rural health care system using common descriptions of the scope of nursing care
- Apply each type of prevention to descriptions of generalist nursing activities in rural areas
- Analyze rural nursing situations to identify components of the nursing management roles

The health needs and the delivery of health services to individuals and families who live in rural communities are of concern to community health nurses, many of whom work in rural areas. Biegel (1983) defines *rural nursing* as: "the diagnosis and treatment of a diversified population of people of all ages and a variety of human responses to actual (or potential) occupational hazards or (actual or) potential health problems existent in maternity, pediatric, medical/surgical and emergency nursing in a given rural area" (p. 46).

For the purposes of this chapter, Biegel's definition has been modified to define rural *community* nursing as rural nursing that takes place outside hospitals or nursing homes. Conducting clinics and/ or making home visits are the main vehicles for the delivery of direct nursing services by the rural community health nurse. Such a nurse is most likely to be a government-funded employee. Occasional school nurses, occupational nurses, or nurses in physicians' offices in rural areas may meet the clinic or home visit criteria, but most of the nurses described will have positions with the health department. Although community health nurses in rural settings function more as generalists than community health nurses in urban settings, nurses in both settings function within the same nursing process and nursing care standards.

What is "rural"? The most common definition of *rural* is, places that are either incorporated or unincorporated, contain less than a population of 2,500, are low in population density, and are peripheral to cities (US Bureau of the Census, 1983). The problem with this definition is that some towns of that size are immediate suburbs of cities and are entirely urban in characteristics. Another definition of *rural* is based on the designation of an area as metropolitan versus nonmetropolitan. A Standard Metropolitan Statistical Area (SMSA) based on census data is a city of 50,000 or more plus adjoining counties that are an integrated social and economic unit (Roemer, 1976). When statistical data in this chapter are labeled "rural," the first definition of rural will be used unless the term "nonmetropolitan" is included, in which case the second definition is being used. Figure 21-1 indicates which states are more "urban" and which are more "rural" by ranking them by population density.

Community health nursing in rural areas can provide a high level of satisfaction for nurses who are confident of their skills and judgment, who enjoy holistic care, and who find pleasure in becoming a leader and change agent in a local setting. This chapter describes the uniqueness of community health nursing in the rural setting. Since the setting is so important to the work, the text outlines characteristics of rural families and rural communities. To prepare nurses for actual work experience, the chapter offers skills and strategies for community health nurses working with individuals and families in rural communities.

Characteristics of Rural Families

Before exploring the complexities of rural communities, we need to look at the components of rural families. As you might expect, every family is composed of unique qualities, but some common characteristics do exist.

Family Structure

Like families in other settings, rural families can be either nuclear or extended. The nuclear rural family is likely to be husband and wife (92.3 percent of rural households) with either one or two children (69.2 percent) or three to four children (26.8 percent). Rural populations contain more children under the age of seventeen than urban populations (US Bureau of the Census, 1983). The family lives in a single-family dwelling or mobile home (Murphree, 1976). Extended family members may also live together in the same household, or so close by that family holiday gatherings are

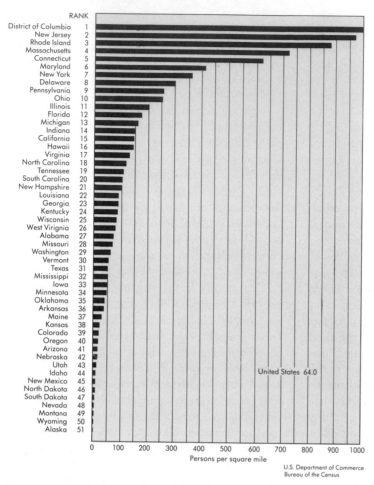

Figure 21-1 States ranked by population density.

bigger than most houses can hold. Some neighbors are regarded as "family" and are likely to be lifelong acquaintances.

Other types of families found in rural areas include female-headed, transient, and newcomer families. The latter two types of families are not usually well liked in rural communities primarily because they have no roots in the area. Some may be hiding from legal authorities, and others may be people who move frequently to find jobs. Newcomer families usually are accepted in rural communities and

asked to be a part of community institutions such as the church, only after it is clear that they can conform to community standards (Hanton, 1980).

Family Income and Employment

A high percentage of all rural families live in poverty (US Bureau of the Census, 1981). The percent varies by race. For example, higher percentages of rural Hispanic (45 percent), black (32 percent), American Indian (29.2 percent), and Asian/Pacific Islander (10.7 percent) families compared to white (9.1 percent) are below the poverty line in rural areas. The family may be made more aware of its low economic status when wealthy urban families purchase middle-class farmers' land for recreational purposes. The addition of these wealthy families creates a wealthy elite not previously prominent in rural areas (Travel, 1970). The wealthy elite and those in power may be willing to help low-status families in a crisis, even though those families with permanently low status lasting for generations are usually not well liked in rural communities.

The family income level will be perpetuated by the children's educational and occupational aspirations. Since there are few community role models of jobs that require a college education, the children probably will finish high school but not go beyond that. In rural areas 60.4 percent of the adult population have completed high school and 11 percent have four or more years of college. In urban areas, 68.8 percent completed high school and 18.1 percent have four or more years of college (US Bureau of the Census, 1980).

According to the 1980 census (US Bureau of the Census, 1983) 40 percent of the rural population over the age of sixteen are employed. Table 21-1 shows the percentage of employed workers in various occupations. There is no way to determine from the table whether the employment is in a rural or urban setting, only that the workers reside in a rural area. Of the rural people who live on farms, one out of six has nonagricultural employment (US Bureau of the Census, 1981) that contributes two-thirds of the family income (Associated Press, 1984a). This worker is probably the male head of household, and in Table 21-1 he would not be counted as an agricultural worker since agriculture (farming) is not his primary source of income.

Social Interaction

Rural families are usually heavily involved in the church, and churches and schools are major set-

Table 21-1 Types of Employment of Rural Population

Type of Employment	% of Total Employed Rural Population
Agriculture	9
Forestry or fisheries	.4
Mining	2
Construction	8
Manufacturing	25
Public utilities	7
Wholesale trade	4
Retail trade	14
Finance, insurance, and real estate	4
Services	23
Professional (health care, law, and education)	17
Public administration	4[a]

SOURCE:
US Bureau of the Census: *General Social and Economic Characteristics: 1980.* Washington, DC: Government Printing Office, 1983.
[a] Total is greater than 100 due to rounding.

tings for social activities and interaction. For example, family members are often identified in the community according to the church they attend. Junior high and high school sports activities are central entertainment activities in rural communities. Hunting and fishing, if available, can serve both as leisure time activities as well as sources for food. A favorite social activity in rural communities is visiting with other community members.

Sex Roles

In rural communities, traditional sex roles are emphasized; women are wives and mothers, and men are authority figures, fathers, and primary breadwinners (Wodarski, 1983). Daughters play with dolls and kittens; sons climb trees and play with trucks. Interestingly enough, sick roles also vary by sex. Women are expected to be ill often, but men must keep working and not "give in" to illness (Murphree, 1976b).

If the family is headed by a single woman who is not a widow, social isolation is likely due to the family orientation of rural society. Because a rural woman is primarily defined in relation to other family members, especially "her man," the single woman may have no social status. There is great pressure to marry (LaGodna, 1981). Having a female head of household increases the chances the family lives in poverty to 27 percent if they are white, and to 53 percent if they are black or Hispanic (US Bureau of the Census, 1981).

An interesting merger of economics and sex role is occurring among some farm families. Women are becoming more prominent as farm owners and managers. Ten percent of the nation's farms are now run by women (US Bureau of the Census, 1980). The pattern of acquiring these positions reinforces the male dominance pattern. In New England, most farms run by women were acquired from fathers or husbands. The average size is ninety acres—suitable for greenhouses, truck gardens, berry farms, or horse raising (Christian Science Monitor, 1984). Thirty-one percent of all women in the farm population are employed as nonmanager agricultural workers including unpaid family workers (US Bureau of the Census, 1980).

Characteristics of Rural Communities

Families are influenced by the communities in which they participate. To understand the family, one must understand the community. Because rural communities are characteristic of the culture and the ethnic origins of the residents, rural culture for all America must be described in general terms. Characteristics of rural communities will be described in six sections: political, economical, social, environmental, religious and other values, and ethnic. Health care implications and adaptation of nursing skills for the rural community will be described for each area.

Political

The rural family operates as a member of a political subunit of the state and nation. For the purposes of this chapter, that unit will be considered to be the county. (Counties are called by other names in some states—for example, "parish" in Louisiana.)

Political Organization   The county is likely to be governed by an elected commission that makes laws and ordinances and supervises budgetary matters. Some counties employ managers who run the day-to-day operations of government. The members of the rural family are likely to be personal acquaintances of one or more members of the commission.

Within the county there may be townships. There may also be one or more towns or villages of less than 2,500 people within the county. These towns and townships may have their own governmental structure. The towns serve the rural areas as centers for church, school, postal service, and some commerce and health care. Travel to cities and towns of larger size is required for complex services.

Political Power   *Political power* is the ability to influence events and policies in rural areas. The small population in rural areas makes it more likely that all members of the community know each other.

Through discussion at places such as the grocery, church, and school sports events, members of rural families share with other community members information and opinions on local issues (Stuart-Burchardt, 1982). Members of the county commission are influenced by the input of community opinion.

In some (but not all) rural areas there are community leaders (who are not commission members) whose formal or informal power is so great that these leaders are able to control the outcome of commission decisions in which they are interested (Travel, 1970). Rural nurses report that these leaders are most often male physicians or judges (Dolphin, 1984). The smallness of the population group makes commission members more accessible to less influential members of the community as well. Since members of the commission are likely to be acquaintances of the rural family, a personal discussion with the commissioner is likely to be the way to resolve an issue of interest to the family (Wodarski, 1983). Starting the process by writing a letter of request or appearing at a commission meeting is more formal of an approach than needed in rural areas (Dolphin, 1984). For example, if the family is concerned about getting paving for the road in front of the house, a family member (probably the head of the household) will likely approach a commissioner directly and informally to seek action.

The community nurse who understands the informal decision-making process can make input into the system to influence decisions for the improvement of health care. Speaking to appropriate community leaders and involving community members are likely to be the best actions to promote change in rural areas (Dolphin, 1984).

Economic

The economic elements of rural communities to be considered include employment, tax base, and exchange of goods and services.

Employment During the time in American history when "rural" meant "working the land" as a farmer, rancher, logger, or trapper, employment was not a problem in the rural culture. Rural work was not mechanized. All hands, including women and children, were needed at least on a seasonal basis. Rural families were large, in part to provide farm workers. There has been a change in the employment of rural populations. In 1910, one in three Americans lived on a farm or ranch, but in 1982 the ratio was one in forty-one (Associated Press, 1983a). Much of this decline represents migration to urban areas. The remainder of the decline is due to the other families who do live in rural areas but do not produce agricultural products.

Rural income is lower than for metropolitan areas. In 1978 the median income for nonmetropolitan families was $3,019 lower than metropolitan families (US Bureau of the Census, 1981). There are several reasons for this: some rural areas have a high concentration of retired people whose incomes have been reduced to retirement benefits; most employment available is at low wages; and rural people who do not live on farms, especially Native Americans, have high rates of unemployment (Henderson & Primeaux, 1981).

Some members of the rural population who are young adults have moved to urban areas to find employment with higher wages. This statement is most true of Southern blacks (Copp, 1976). This outmigration lowers rural unemployment (Murphree, 1976), although underemployment and low salaries are characteristic of the jobs available to rural family members (Reynolds, 1976).

Since the 1960s, changes in technology, transportation, and communication have made it possible for manufacturing or large construction and industrial projects to move to rural areas such as laying the oil pipeline in Alaska and producing shale oil in Wyoming and Colorado. The move of manufacturing and these large projects changed the work force in rural areas in two ways—bringing in both new professionals and workers (Dolphin, 1984; Rosenblatt & Moscovice, 1982). The increased manufacturing population caused demands for goods and services that could be provided by the original population, however.

The attraction of rural areas is demonstrated in the 1980 census. Small-town populations have increased 30 percent since 1970, while city dwellers have increased only 1.9 percent (US Bureau of the Census, 1983). Migrants from urban areas may be searching for a community where they feel they have more political control and a greater voice in decision making (Associated Press, 1983b). The migrants can use their newfound political power either to unite with the rural values present in the community or create pressures for urban types and levels of services (Ford, 1978).

Changing values in relation to sex roles, economic need, increased job opportunities, and smaller families have made it possible (or necessary) for more rural women to work outside the home. Unfortunately, their employment is clustered in low-paying jobs (LaGodna, 1981).

Tax Base The second rural economic characteristic is the general tax base of the area. In addition to the economic constraint of reduced employment opportunities in some rural areas, the property tax base may be poor. Open land is often government owned and therefore not taxable. For example, Idaho—with 82.6 percent nonmetropolitan population—has federal ownership of 63.7 percent of the land. Wyoming, which is 100 percent nonmetropolitan, has 48.6 percent federal land ownership (US Bureau of the Census, 1980). Other land may be state owned. While federal income tax does not equal state tax, it does give some indication of ability to pay. In the 1979 tax year, the six poorest states had an average per capita federal tax below $600. Five of the six were more than 50 percent rural. Of the ten richest states, which had IRS per capita taxes about $1000, eight were over 50 percent urban (US Bureau of the Census, 1981).

With the small amount of public monies for use, there are fewer funds available for services. Rural areas have a special problem because they have more miles of road per taxpayer to pave and maintain. Of the 3,885 thousand miles of highways in the United States in 1980, 3,190 thousand were in rural areas. Of that amount nearly two-thirds were under county control (US Bureau of the Census, 1980). Long school bus routes add to the cost of rural education. Low income and high cost leave little county money to fund the community nurse or the rest of the county health department. Additionally the inclination to commit funds to increase nurses' salaries in rural areas may be low because nurses are often among the best paid people in the community (Fletcher, 1981).

Another government service that in unlikely to be funded is the provision of buses for public transportation. Due to low income, some rural families cannot afford a car or truck. In urban areas, buses can be used to meet transportation needs of the poor. Few rural communities provide bus service at all, and bus service along county roads is usually only for schoolchildren. This lack of transportation further reduces access of poor rural families to health care services (Dolphin, 1984).

Cost of Goods and Services The final economic characteristic is the cost of goods and services. Costs may be both higher and lower in rural areas. Goods that must be transported into the rural area cost the retail merchant more. If low demand or low population eliminates volume sales, cost to the merchant also increases. These merchants' costs usually are passed on to the consumer. Thus a can of soup is likely to cost more at a general store at a rural crossroads than in an urban supermarket. At the same time, the cost for rural residents to go into urban areas and obtain goods and services not available in rural areas also increases those costs to rural families.

On the other hand, the absence of transportation costs may lower the price of local produce or crafts to rural families. Urban families must pay the cost to transport these goods to the city. Roadside produce stands are an example of a way costs are lowered for rural families. When items are purchased directly from the producer, wholesaler and distributor costs are eliminated. Since rural residents are well acquainted with the talents of their neighbors, a lively trade may exist without paid advertising or other formal organizers of trade.

Cost of many services in the immediate area are actually lower in rural areas. As stated earlier, wages are likely to be lower in rural areas. Likewise costs for services of tradespeople (plumbers, carpenters) and professionals (physicians, lawyers) are lower. The author suggests that perhaps these costs are lower because the providers realize there is a decreased ability to pay. Perhaps there is also community pressure to keep these costs low. A final factor could be the low number of trade unions in rural areas.

Social

The two social elements of the rural culture that are most noticeable are the family and community support networks and the slower pace of life.

Family and Community Support Systems
Rural residents are generally well interconnected. Rural families often operate as extended family networks that are not necessarily organized along kinship lines (Valenzuela & Hallamore, 1979). Such networks constitute a support system for their members. It is true that an urban observer of a small community may hear the frequent explanation, "You know, we *are* all just about related." Other examples of extended families do not involve actual kinship, but do include a family type of involvement. This involvement includes such activities as having people who "look in" on neighbors, transport them to town, prepare extra food for others in time of their need, and feel comfortable making judgments on the positive and negative aspects of the behavior of each member of the community (Ford, 1978). These extended family relationships may increase the number of human resources available to the rural family. (See Figure 21-2.)

Hanton (1980) calls these extended family relationships the *primary helping system* in rural areas. Hanton further states that this system is not open to all rural residents, but is only accessible to those residents who have community approval. Additionally, informal helping systems exist. The informal systems are those institutions that are not pri-

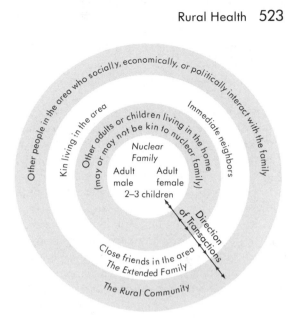

Figure 21-2 The extended family relationships of the "typical" rural family.

marily established to meet health and social service needs—most commonly schools and churches. Only the *formal helping systems* are relatively free to serve those people needing help without the community judgment of being "worthy." The formal helping system consists of those organizations whose primary purposes are health and social service and that are staffed by professionals, such as welfare departments and county health departments.

The community commentary or judgment on the affairs of community members leads to a feeling that "my business is everybody's business." This feeling decreases privacy (Stuart-Burchardt, 1982) and increases conformity to community standards as people in the area feel free to condemn any deviation (Dolphin, 1984).

Family and community networks often serve crime prevention functions for community residents. The community watchfulness characteristic of extended families helps to prevent and control crime. For example, since each car and person can be identified, if a rural resident sees a strange car driving slowly in the neighborhood, he or she is likely to call the sheriff. Generally, crimes are not expected in rural areas; therefore, houses are often left unlocked and keys left in auto ignitions (Stuart-Burchardt, 1982). However, this may be a false perception, since property crime rates have climbed in rural areas to near urban levels while rural violent crime rates have remained low. The reasons proposed by Carter, Donnemeyer, and Wurschmidt (1982) for the property crime rise are: (1) better roads, especially the interstate system, allow easy access and speedy getaway; (2) rural families are away from home for longer hours with husband and wife commuting to urban areas for work and shopping and with children on long bus rides to consolidated schools; (3) houses are widely spaced so it may not be possible to watch one house from a neighbor's; (4) better roads bring recreational travelers into the area so all cars and people are no longer recognizable; (5) there are fewer law officers in rural areas; and (6) fewer security measures such as deadbolt locks and burglary alarms are installed in rural homes.

When members of a rural community perceive there is a crime problem, trust among neighbors decreases (Ford, 1978). This hampers the extended family system. The neighbor assumes that the burglary was committed by a local person. More often the property was taken by a teenage male from another rural community in the general area (Carter, Donnemeyer, & Wurschmidt, 1982). In addition to being destructive of social relationships, reaction to an increased crime rate may increase stress in the rural family. For example, the family may fear loss of property, and they may be concerned that their children could become involved in committing such crimes.

Pace of Life　The pace of life in rural areas is usually slower than in urban areas. Being more in tune with the land and weather seems to bring a sense that "tomorrow will come—there's no rush to do everything today." While this attitude is helpful in reducing stress, it may be exasperating when a plumber is needed for a frozen water pipe. Lack of choice also slows the pace of life, for example, in the area of entertainment. There may be out-

door recreational areas nearby, but multiple movie theaters, the opera, rock concerts, night clubs, and live theater are usually missing. Church activities and school sports events are the usual group entertainment. For that reason, individuals and families in rural areas need to be able to create their own entertainment (Rolshoven, 1982).

Environmental

The environmental influences on the rural community may be the strongest molders of the culture.

Environmental Isolation　The travel difficulties created by distance, rough terrain, and/or severe weather conditions create isolation in rural areas. Help is less easily obtained due to difficult travel (Singh, 1980). Distance between residences limits the number of home visits a nurse can make in one day. Difficult travel also influences the way services are obtained. When a trip to town is only made weekly or monthly to conserve time and gasoline cost, then self-reliance is a necessity. The rural inhabitant must be able to repair, improvise, or do without material items. These requirements for material things spread to values. In most rural families the frontier spirit of independence and self-reliance is very much alive.

Occupational Stress　Other elements in the environment also influence the health needs of rural families. Farming, mining, and lumbering industries are all centered in rural areas since the raw materials are part of that environment. These three occupations are high in occupational hazards; so work injuries may be more frequent and serious (Califano, 1978). Farmers report high levels of stress due to uncertainties about growing conditions, crop prices, and government programs. Another stressor is the high level of debt of many farmers as they borrow in the spring against crop prices in the fall. If the crop fails, the debt is still due. These stresses plus the lack of vacation or sick time lead to high rates of divorce, suicide, and mental illness (Associated Press, 1984b). A physical stressor to farm

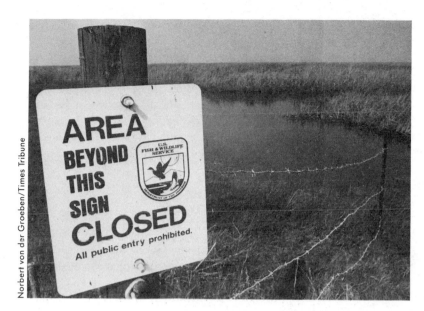

Norbert von der Groeben/Times Tribune

Pollution, most commonly associated with urban areas, is a health hazard in rural areas too. End products of mining operations, waste from dump sites, and chemicals used in farming can contaminate soil, water, and air.

workers is the repeated exposure to concentrated doses of herbicides and insecticides.

Pollution   Another rural environmental health hazard is pollution not found in urban areas. For example, the end products of mining operations present special problems. The remaining products after the ore has been extracted pollute above-ground water supplies. Strip mines that are not returned to former contours remove land from productive use and pollute water runoff. Uranium mining produces radioactive waste products. Residents of rural Nevada and Utah from 1951 to 1962 were exposed to radiation. This exposure, from nuclear bomb tests, increased cancer rates by 50 percent in the fallout area (Anderson, 1984).

Waste products from urban areas that are not burned are usually carried to rural dump sites. If improperly maintained, these sites can be breeding areas for disease-carrying rodents and insects. Dump sites for hazardous chemicals or radioactive materials can become health hazards in air or water if leakage occurs.

While auto exhaust is not usually an air pollution problem in rural areas, smoke from coal or wood fires is a respiratory irritant. This is partic-

ularly a problem in mountain areas, because the air movement is restricted by the geography of the hollows and valleys. In high mountains there is a permanent heat inversion created by upper air warmth from thin atmosphere and increased heat from the sun. These inversions hold any air pollutant close to the ground.

A final source of pollution is inadequate sewage disposal, which contaminates the water supply. In rural communities this contamination may come from inadequate sewage treatment prior to the effluent reaching the community water supply. Away from town, families probably have their own wells or cisterns. These wells can be contaminated by improperly located outhouses or septic tanks. Wells can also be contaminated by underground seepage of waste dumps. One-third of all field workers have an additional sanitary concern as toilets, hand washing to remove pesticides, and clean drinking water are not provided in the fields in the areas of the country where these field workers are employed (Associated Press, 1984c).

The rural community health nurse may have the resource of a sanitarian to help identify sources of environmental pollution. However, it is more likely that the nurse will have to identify possible sources of contamination, send samples for testing, help the community become aware of any problems, and be a change agent for improvement without colleague assistance, since few rural health departments can afford to hire an environmental specialist.

Natural Hazards   Hazards of nature may have great effect on health, economics, and life activities. Flood damage and beach erosion are likely to be greater in rural areas. Washed-out bridges can cut off a family from sources of needed supplies. Drought has a more direct economic effect in rural areas. Snow and mud slides close rural roads longer. Brush and forest fires destroy home and livelihood. House fires are likely to be more destructive in rural areas due to longer arrival time for volunteer firefighters and their equipment. Volcanic damage in Washington and Hawaii has been primarily in rural areas. It is difficult or impossible to prevent physical danger and disruption in life-style from these types of natural environmental factors.

Religious and Other Values

Rural areas tend to have conservative political and moral views. Church attendance is high and traditional religious values are espoused by many rural people. Since citizens usually do not have a chance to interact with people with other thoughts, views, or cultures, change comes slowly. Rural people also seem to prefer the sameness of culture, traditions, and old ways of doing things. While the nonconformity of the town "character" is accepted (Reynolds, 1976), newcomers to the area who challenge the dominant viewpoints and press strongly for change are usually ostracized by the community (Wodarski, 1983).

Religious groups such as the Amish, Mennonites, and other Anabaptists who find their religious values challenged by urbanization have chosen to settle in rural communities. These groups choose a simple life with varying degrees of deemphasis on material things. The Anabaptists also tend to reject violence and emphasize service to others (*Mennonite*, n.d.).

Just as in an urban setting, the rural community health nurse must be aware of the religious values of the family. The nurse should also assess how those values impact the health practices of the family. Finally, the nurse needs to be aware of the impact of conflicts between prevailing rural and religious values and the values, needs, and practices of the individual.

Ethnic

As with the general population, various subcultural and ethnic groups are present in rural communities. Such groups tend to add their unique flavor to the community in which they reside. Examples of subcultural and ethnic groups found in rural communities are described here.

Native Americans   Forty-nine percent of Native Americans, including Eskimos and Aleut populations, live in rural areas (US Bureau of the Census, 1983). Many Native Americans, particularly those who live on reservations, preserve their traditional values and life-styles. The isolation of rural communities make it easier for them to "keep the old ways."

Hispanics   Hispanics have rural population concentrations in the Southwest. In 1980, 10 percent of the total Hispanic population lived in rural areas (US Bureau of the Census, 1983). These families may keep their traditional ways or become thoroughly acculturated (Henderson & Primeaux, 1981). For example, disease may be described by one Hispanic family as being caused by "mal ojo," while another family may no longer speak Spanish.

Blacks   Blacks are found in rural areas predominantly in the South and southeastern United States. Multigenerational family units are common. These families may include elders who have worked in the northern states but who return to the South to be close to family and friends (Osborne, 1978), and other elders who have never emigrated from the South but remained there while their children left for northern cities.

Appalachian Whites   Appalachian Whites are heavily represented in rural America. This group is found from north to south along the Appalachian Mountains in east-central United States with migration outward in all directions. Geography isolated the Appalachian culture for many years, and travel is still difficult in many areas. Suspicion of strangers, particularly government representatives, is common in this subculture. The Frontier Nursing Service (FNS) founded in 1925 by Mary Breckenridge is famous for the community nursing provided in the southeastern Kentucky part of Appalachia. This nursing service began with nurse-midwives on horseback who visited isolated families. The nurse-midwives were successful in lowering the infant and maternal mortality rates and improving family planning practices. Current services include other types of nursing practitioners, clinics, a forty-bed hospital, and a school for nurse-practitioners. FNS now provides comprehensive health care (American Medical Association, 1976). News of the most recent developments in the Frontier Nursing Service can be found in the *Frontier Nursing Service Quarterly Bulletin*.

Other cultural or ethnic groups are located in rural America. All of the factors that isolate rural communities help continue special cultures. For example, Swedish- and German-speaking families are still found from Pennsylvania to the Great Plains. Twenty-five percent of the people in northeast Vermont speak French as a primary language (Christian Science Monitor, 1984). Another example is Asian families. Three to fourteen percent of the various Asian subcultures live in rural areas (Lum, 1983). In the West these families are influential onion and truck farmers. Many of the western families are descendents of the people who came to build the railroad or during the Gold Rush. Recent immigrants from Laos, Cambodia, and Vietnam have settled primarily in urban areas. Other Indo-Chinese families may modify their farming and fishing skills for use in the rural areas.

The language barrier creates problems for the rural community nurses. Hispanics, Germans, Swedes, or French may not speak English, but finding an English translator is usually not too difficult. On the other hand, knowledge of Southeast Asian languages in the general population is rare. The need for communication has led one health department in the tobacco-raising area of rural western Kentucky to request federal funds to hire a translator for their large Cambodian population (Dolphin, 1984).

As can be seen from this discussion, there are many and varied ethnic and cultural groups in rural areas. It is important that community health nurses understand and respect the culture of the people for whom they care. In rural areas this is even more important because the isolation of the rural area probably has slowed the integration of the diverse group into the mainstream of American culture.

Health Care in the Rural Community

Health care in rural communities is likely to be provided by government bodies as part of the political structure. Understanding how politics can affect the funding of health care services will help you see why a particular pattern of services exists.

Types and Organization of Health Services

A county or group of counties is likely to own or provide finances for a small hospital of under 100 beds. In 1978 there were 346 general hospitals with 6 to 24 beds and 2,013 with 24 to 74 beds (US Bureau of the Census, 1980). The area hospital affects the finances of the rural family through a hospital levy or other local tax support. The services of the hospital for the family depend on the skills of the area physicians. General adult and child medical care, simple surgical procedures, general obstetrical and newborn services (perhaps under the care of a nurse-midwife), and emergency care are the most likely services. The hospital may also furnish nursing home services (Dolphin, 1984).

While the county may have ownership, the hospital is also affected by federal government funds. The hospital building may have been constructed or improved through the Hill-Burton Act of 1946. Medicare funds are likely to pay hospital bills for some area residents. Medicare payments are less in rural areas for the same diagnoses, because rural costs have been historically lower, and payment is based on local economics (Piper, 1983).

State control also affects the hospital in three ways. First, Medicaid funding is shared between state and federal tax sources. In states that are predominantly rural, the tax income is often lower (Bacrach, 1981). The lack of resources for taxation means monies for a level of Medicaid payment that would meet actual costs of health care are less available. This again lowers income for hospitals and other providers of rural health care. Second, the department of health at the state level may also have an inspection system for hospitals, particularly those that are not accredited by the Joint Commission for Accreditation of Hospitals (Merrell & Avery, 1983). Third, the National Health Planning and Resources Development Act of 1974 required states to develop regional health planning councils within the state to allocate state and federal funds (Roemer, 1976). The hospital must have any changes in services, particularly expansion, approved by this body.

Health care professionals are also affected by government policy. The low numbers of rural physicians, nurses, and dentists have prompted federal intervention. Since the description of the practice of the various professionals in state practice describes the physician as the director of health care, the supply of rural physicians has been of particular concern to the government.

Because the nineteenth-century development of medical specialties created physicians who needed a large population to support individual practices, the number of physicians in rural areas began to decrease in the late 1800s. The decline was particularly noticeable during the mid-1900s. There were fewer and fewer new physicians choosing general practice (GP) to replace those GPs in rural practice who died or retired. Federal legislation attempted to reverse this trend with the greatest activity during the time of the Great Society of the 1970s. Health legislation was directed at attracting physicians to rural areas through clinic construction, guaranteed salaries, scholarship payback, and substitution for military service during the time of the draft. The specialty area of family practice was also encouraged through grants to medical schools.

The National Health Service Corporation, created in 1970 and administered by the U.S. Public Health Service, provides physicians, dentists, and nurses to underserved rural communities for two-year tours of duty (Rosenblatt & Moscovice, 1982). An example of an area where there was little impact from federal programs to provide physicians is the sixty rural counties that make up the northern two-thirds of Missouri. In that area, the number of physicians began to decrease in the 1960s; by the beginning of the 1980s, thirty-one of the counties reported that 50 percent of their practicing physicians were over the age of fifty-five, with no evidence of increasing replacement rates (Frey, 1981).

The federal government policies and programs also provide payment for health care for specific groups of rural families. The Appalachian Health Program and the Migrant Health Program are two examples. Additionally the U.S. Public Health Service provides care to Native Americans (Rosenblatt & Moscovice, 1982).

Rural nurses have reported that rural families and communities prefer independence to government programs (Dolphin, 1984). These nurses have cooperated with the rural attitude of "we take care of our own" to develop local solutions to locally perceived needs in such areas as emergency care and child-rearing.

Health Care Needs

Before proceeding with specific observations on rural health needs, let's summarize the factors that affect health care:

1. *Availability* of health care is limited due to low numbers of providers. The situation is particularly noticeable with physicians but is also true for dentists and nurses. Nurses may take on more responsibilities due to lack of physicians. Availability is further limited by low government funds to provide health care.
2. *Access* is difficult. Medicare and Medicaid usually do not cover the cost of care. The low wages of rural people make private payment unlikely. Furthermore, the lack of a means of transportation and roads that are impassable at times further interfere with access for some families.
3. *Choice is lacking.* There may be only one hospital and one physician within reasonable travel time. If those care-givers do not meet the needs of the family, alternatives are inconvenient. Families may choose to use folk medicine and other means of self-care to preserve their independent self-reliance in health care and to avoid costly trips to health care providers.
4. *Health hazards* may occur due to stress and accidents at work; environmental contaminants; natural disasters; and the substandard housing, clothing, and nutrition that often accompany poverty.
5. *The helping resource network* available to families should be increased by extended families. Community networks may also limit the aid available to the "unworthy" family.
6. *Religious, racial, and ethnic subcultures* in rural communities flavor the communities. Members of these subcultures may vary from the dominant culture in values and health practices.

Given this background, three health needs predominate in rural communities: (1) the need for prenatal care, (2) the need for self-care among the elderly population, and (3) the need for prevention of automobile accidents and deaths.

Need for Prenatal Care   Problems with obtaining health care can be illustrated in the area of maternal services. Statistics from the *1983 United States Health and Prevention Profile* show that rural southern Blacks are limited in their prenatal health care whether by availability, access or choice (US Public Health Service, 1983). Nationally, infant mortality (death of infants under the age of one) for black babies is twice that for white infants. The national incidence of birth weights below 2,500 grams is also double for Blacks. Since only 57 percent of rural black women receive prenatal care, and rural black women are also the least likely to have fetal monitoring during labor, there does not appear to be a successful program in the rural South to reduce black infant mortality.

The U.S. Public Health Service (1983) reports other concerns about rural prenatal care. They found that rural areas had the greatest incidence of X-ray during pregnancy when ultrasound would have supplied the needed information. Possible explanations for this are: (1) lack of ultrasound equipment or technicians in the rural areas and (2) lack of physician familiarity with the uses of ultrasound. Amniocentesis as an intrauterine diagnostic tool was also less likely to be used in rural areas. Low use may be related to the more conservative style of medicine practiced in many rural areas (Dolphin, 1984). Maternity care is a special concern in rural areas, since the fertility ratio (number of children under the age of five for each 1000 women aged fifteen to forty-nine years) is 313/1000 in rural areas versus 279/1000 for the total United States (US Bureau of the Census, 1980).

Need for Self-Care for the Elderly   At the other end of the age spectrum, two groups of statistics illustrate how self-care needs of the rural elderly are met. The U.S. Public Health Service (1983) reported that of those over sixty-five, twice as many needed help with home management (errands, cleaning, cooking) than needed help with personal care (bathing, dressing). The Service further reported that as age increased, need for help increased; in addition, as family was available to help, need decreased. In 1980, 4.5 percent fewer persons aged sixty and over lived alone in rural areas than urban areas (US Bureau of the Census, 1980). There are at least two possible explanations for this difference: (1) more rural elderly are in nursing homes or, more likely, (2) the rural elderly live with spouse or extended family so home management needs can be met. Because of availability and access problems, it is important that older adults maintain their health as much as possible through institution of self-care measures. Community health nurses can assist by teaching them such measures.

Need to Prevent Automobile Accidents and Deaths Diseases in rural areas are rarely different from urban areas. Some rural areas with high populations of elderly and poor residents may have *more* but not *different* diseases (Rosenblatt & Moscovice, 1980). The one area where there is a significant difference from urban areas is in automobile accidents. Nationally, 70 percent of all automobile deaths occur in rural areas (Califano, 1978). Rural Georgia has 83 percent more auto deaths than urban areas of the state (Did you know, 1983). The difference may be an interaction of several factors: (1) rate of speed is usually higher; (2) roads are more crooked and less clearly marked and maintained; (3) ambulances must travel further; (4) ambulances may have less advanced equipment and more poorly trained/less experienced crews; (5) and rural emergency rooms seldom have trauma specialists on the staff or specialized equipment (Avery & Merrell, 1983; Dolphin, 1984).

In rural areas auto accidents are recognized as a hazard to both residents and visitors. For that reason, rural areas are working hard to improve emergency care. However, Emergency Medical Technicians in rural areas are usually volunteers and may not have ongoing experiences enabling them to deal with certain injuries. There is unlikely to

be a physician at the hospital at the time of ambulance arrival. Rural hospitals are usually short on funds, so purchase of "state-of-the-art" life support equipment is probably not possible, even if someone on the hospital staff knew how to use the equipment. As a partial remedy, helicopter and fixed-wing aircraft services to transport critically ill or injured persons to larger hospitals or trauma centers are rapidly being developed (Rosenblatt & Moscovice, 1982). Air transport is very costly however, which may limit its use.

Resolution of Health Care Problems and Needs

Bacrach (1981) concluded that the problems with meeting health needs of rural populations will be difficult to resolve. Resolution is complicated by intermingling of social, attitudinal, economic, and physical factors. A fifth factor further impedes delivery of rural health services: health planning is usually done for rural areas either in urban areas or by professionals with an urban perspective.

Many areas of need can be met by generalist community nurses, nurse practitioners, and nurse-midwives. Most nurses are sensitive to values and preferences of the people for whom they care. This sensitivity can help capitalize on the strengths of the rural family and community to help them increase their competency in self-care. However, other factors will affect overall health care in rural communities.

Use of Health Services and Health Care Providers

The use of rural health care services is influenced by the definition of illness. Illness is defined differently in rural families. To be considered "sick," one must (1) have symptoms and (2) be unable to do one's daily work (Travel, 1970). Thus someone with hypertension would not be considered "ill" until there had been a CVA ("stroke"). If one is not ill, then one probably does not receive health care. Following the rural definition of illness, only severely psychotic people would be judged to need mental health care (Travel, 1970).

Self-reliance and travel difficulties interact to mold the way rural families use the health care system. Since travel is not easy, many rural families will be sure the family member is *really* sick before visiting a health provider. Since the majority of all illness is self-limiting (goes away without treatment), the habit of waiting is bound to be successful at times (Rosenblatt & Moscovice, 1982). The illness is usually diagnosed by the woman of the family after consultation with relatives and neighbors. The latest TV advertisements and health education are also sources of information. Conjurers, folk medicine, and over-the-counter drugs may be used in the tradition of self-reliance. If this first approach doesn't work, the local community health nurse, pharmacist, or physician will be contacted for "free advice." As a third step, an appointment will be made with a physician or nurse practitioner. Requests for prayer may be forwarded to the church when the symptoms seem serious. If at any time in this sequence the symptoms disappear, the ill person will be considered cured (Murphree, 1976).

Characteristics of the Delivery System

Just as rural definitions of illness vary from urban definitions, the health services delivery system has special characteristics in rural areas. Characteristics of the structure and organization of the rural health services delivery system in rural areas are (Dolphin, 1984):

1. *Simplicity of structure*—The layers of local bureaucracy are fewer and there are fewer people in each layer.
2. *Personalized interactions*—Almost everyone in the area is known to everyone else both professionally and socially. Formal and informal interactions are intertwined. Nurses may help their bankers learn colostomy care. The child of the county commissioner may be a favorite babysitter. The physician may live next door, and both nurse and physician may be regular members of the neighborhood bridge group. Socializing may take place during nursing visits, and nursing care may be given on social occasions.
3. *Low staff turnover and little chance for advancement*—Since there are few community nursing positions in a given rural area, "job hopping" is rarely possible. A nurse who is dissatisfied must leave the area or change the type of nursing position (to a hospital position, for example). Because the nursing staff is small, there are few administrative positions or other chances for advancement without leaving the area. Advanced degrees or on-the-job skills may not enable the nurse to leave the staff nurse role through promotion (Fletcher, 1981).
4. *Twenty-four hours on call*—When the community health nurse is a resident of the area served, the nurse may be considered just as much a community resource as a physician. When that nurse is the primary health resource because there is no physician, this is especially true. The community members ask for help twenty-four hours a day, seven days a week (Fletcher, 1981). One of the jobs of the community nurse is to educate community members about what calls are important and what calls can wait until regular business hours.

Health care facilities may be overextended by the amount of service needed by the population as well as by the limited number of practitioners. In 1980 the rural population contained 4 percent more inhabitants under the age of eighteen than urban areas (US Bureau of the Census, 1983). While the total rural population had 1.5 percent fewer people over sixty-five than urban areas, in some rural areas the elderly population was as high as 20 percent (Frey, 1981; US Bureau of the Census, 1983). The proportion of these two age groups is important because they need a disproportionately larger amount of care than the eighteen to sixty-five age group. For example, the 11 percent of the U.S. population over sixty-five years made 31 percent of the health care expenditures (U.S. Public Health Service, 1983). Furthermore, in geographic areas with reduced population aged eighteen to sixty-five, there is a reduced work force to pay for health services (Singh, 1980). Another rural characteristic that may also overextend rural health services are the new immigrants from the city that expand the population (Bacrach, 1981).

Nursing in Rural Communities

Skills and strategies that result in interventions in a rural setting come from a broad base of nursing knowledge. Rural community health nurses report they deliver holistic care, which is more people-oriented than task-oriented (Goodwill, 1984). These nurses think leadership, change agent skills, and health teaching are as important as technical skills (Biegel, 1983; Fletcher, 1981). In rural settings, nursing creativity is needed to adapt available equipment to the situation and to the preferences of the person receiving care (Dolphin, 1984).

Generalist Role

There are two reasons that the practice of community health nursing in the rural setting is of a broad-based, generalist nature. First, there is likely to be an underdeveloped health service in the area. Duplicate services from various providers are unusual, thus limiting alternatives for care. Services the rural family may want, both illness- and wellness-centered, may be either oversubscribed (for example, too large a population for each physician) or unavailable (for example, no social welfare workers who have special training to help violent families) (Hanton, 1980). These unmet needs lead nurses to incorporate knowledge and skills from other health disciplines into rural nursing practice to better assist rural families (Dolphin, 1984).

The second reason practice is broad-based is that community health nursing in rural areas has a short history. By 1940 a few public health departments had begun to develop in rural areas—more than fifty years after the first visiting nurses and public health nurses began to practice in urban areas. The Red Cross was the first supplier of community nurses to rural areas (Rosenblatt & Moscovice, 1982). This short history may mean expectations of what the nurse "ought" to do are from current expectations rather than from how community nursing has "always been done." The lack of historic expectations may mean the rural community nurse is free to try unusual approaches to problems that borrow from other disciplines or from nursing practice outside community health.

The technical skills needed by the community health nurse in a rural setting are not that different from the community health nurse in an urban setting. Skills in all aspects of the field of community health nursing are needed, because each day in a rural setting includes having to perform parts of the jobs of many types of urban community health nurses and includes all age groups and types of health problems. The one necessary technical skill mentioned by rural nurses as different for their geographic area of practice is skill in car maintenance, especially the ability to change a tire (Dolphin, 1984).

To function most effectively, nurses live and work in the same rural community. Nurses who commute to rural areas from a nearby community miss important opportunities to give nursing care in informal settings. It is also harder for them to become a trusted community member (Dolphin, 1984).

Management Role

Because there may be few nurses in rural settings and because community representatives and other health professionals work together to meet the health needs of rural families, the community health nurse may assume a leadership role and function as manager of the community health team as opposed to the nursing team. For example, one of the physicians in town is the medical director of the county health department, but private practice responsibilities leave little time for functioning in this capacity. In fact, the health department *is* the team of nurses. They function as an independent committee with a thorough understanding of community values and physician preferences (Dolphin, 1984). They provide the care that is needed, expanding their practice to fill the less specialized aspects of the roles of the dieticians, health educators, mental health workers, social workers, and occupational and physical therapists who are missing from the community (Stuart-Burchardt, 1982). The nurses also lobby with the county commissioners for funding. The nurses use their knowledge base, telephone consultations with nursing specialists, conferences with local physicians and other local resource persons, and available printed materials to fill the health needs of the area's population (Dolphin, 1984).

Leadership also is displayed by rural community nurses when they help develop community resources (Tulga & Rohrer, 1980). Families helping each other may be the easiest resource to develop because the dollar cost is low. The nurse may be able to search out family members or extended family with special skills and talents who can provide ancillary services. For example, church groups may be willing to make or collect layettes for families without funds. Folded newspaper pads may be supplied by the same group to a family who is caring for an elderly incontinent relative. Neighbors may be willing to "sit for a spell" with the same person so care-givers can do errands or just have some time alone. The community spirit that leads to barn raisings and help with crops for an ill farmer can be used in more expanded kinds of sharing (Fletcher, 1981).

Two examples of formal rural programs based on neighbor helping neighbor are reported in the literature. In both programs rural family members who were already looked to by others for aid participated in training sessions to broaden their ability to help. Valenzuela and Hallamore (1979) reported on a program in New Hampshire in which mental health workers developed a program called Good Neighbor Network. The members of the community sought out by their neighbors for immediate help received information from professionals. The program included: how to help in prevention of mental illness, how to act in crisis intervention, how to give help to people discharged from psychiatric inpatient units, and how to assist in referrals. Hatch and Lovelace (1980) focused on health education information and ways to encourage treatment compliance as they worked with leaders from rural black churches in the South. Hypertension, diabetes, maternal and child health, alcoholism, and child abuse were the topics covered.

Partnership Role

At other times the nurse is a partner in providing health care rather than a leader. Nurses and physicians are one type of partners. The nurse-physician partnership is usually described as more collegial in rural settings than in urban. However, there are also rural physicians who expect unthinking obedience by nurses (Dolphin, 1984). As part of the partnership, most rural physicians will expect nurses to move from assessment to intervention with less physician-nurse consultation than is usual in urban settings. Standing orders from the physician are likely to cover many more situations in rural areas than in urban areas. The freedom and latitude the nurse experiences in the physician-nurse partnership may be possible because a working relationship and an understanding of "what the doctor wants" and "what the nurse can do well" rapidly develops when there are few nurses and fewer physicians (Dolphin, 1984). However, the nurse must always function within the legal mandates that govern the nursing profession in the state in which he or she works: the rural nurse is at legal risk when carrying out unsigned orders that are not standing orders (see Chapter 24).

Community and nurse are also partners. The community health nurse must understand the needs and resources of the community. Therefore, community assessment is an important tool for the rural nurse. A complete community assessment may be easier to obtain in rural areas, because the factors to assess are fewer in number or less complex. Community assessment is needed as the first step in any change process by the community nurse. The nurse needs to know the extent of the problem or potential problem, level of recognition of the problem by the citizens, resources and potential resources to address the problem, and the most effective means of change in the community.

Statistical data may be available to the nurse from the state. How else can data be collected? A community assessment in rural New York state included data collected through interviews with key informers and through a community forum, in addition to statistical data (Hanson, Matheson, & Reed, 1983). A fourth source of community data is observations by the nurse in the course of daily activities.

Families in rural areas generally have a good understanding of community health needs and problems. They are likely to understand both how area problems and potential solutions will affect them. Because there are so many interrelationships in the rural setting, there is rarely a situation that leaves any family member untouched. Informal community discussions keep everyone informed and serve as a round robin forum. This same method of communication, however, can also be responsible for large amounts of misinformation (Dolphin, 1984).

The final type of nurse partnership is with available nursing colleagues. One of the problems in rural nursing is that since there are few other nurses, supportive relationships are lacking. In urban areas a nurse might interact with visiting nurses, community health nurses, nurses from a division of the public health department, and nurses from home health care agencies. In a rural area, there are likely to be only the community nurses employed by the county health department. In very sparsely populated areas, there may be only one nurse and no physician or hospital in the entire county (Dolphin, 1984).

A formal nursing partnership may occur in a nursing clinic. Nurse-based clinics are developing as the "new" thing for cost control in urban areas (Selby, 1984). Such clinics have been useful in rural areas for some time. The major staffing for such a clinic may be provided by a nurse practitioner (Brooks et al, 1981). Nurse-midwives are effective in rural areas as well. For example, in one rural town, a government-funded clinic staffed by nurse-midwives had so many requests for service by women able to pay for services that an income level had to be set so women unable to afford private care could receive the midwifery services available. Unfortunately, not enough midwives were willing to work there to service all requests (Dolphin, 1984).

Rural community health nurses may find local nurse colleagues and role models in the hospital, nursing home, physician's office, mines or other industry, schools, or large recreation areas. However, not all these institutions may exist in a given rural area and not all of them will employ nurses. Partnership with such people as county extension agents with their skills in nutrition and farm safety may offer a partial substitute for nurse colleagues.

The lack of colleagues is the basic cause of feelings of isolation in rural nurses. This isolation can be either challenging or overwhelming (Dolphin, 1984). To cope with the isolation, the nurse needs to develop a support system with other people who understand the exhaustion that can occur when there are many needs and too few people to meet them (Fletcher, 1981). Written material on prevention of burnout or workshops on the topic may also be useful.

Finally, as a result of professional and geographic isolation, the rural nurse must be self-motivated. Other resources to cope with isolation are: self-confidence, independent judgment, and ability to create opportunities for continuing education (Rolshoven, 1982).

Marketing Role

Families in rural areas are less likely to consider noninstitutional nursing a health care resource than in urban areas. Therefore, the nurse needs to engage in marketing activities to create and maintain a caseload. Furthermore, rural physicians may view nursing as something that only takes place within hospitals and nursing homes. When a family member is discharged from the hospital, the physician may think the family can continue any kind of care without nursing assistance. Word-of-mouth referrals from one family to another help create requests for home visits (Dolphin, 1984).

Nurse-run clinics have the same need for marketing. When people are accustomed to driving a longer distance for health care, they may continue to do so even though a closer clinic has opened. When the planning and operating process includes citizen advisory boards and other community involvement, a feeling of community "ownership" develops (Reaching, 1983). With "ownership" comes increased usage (O'Leary & Barton, 1977). Satisfied customers, community visibility, and printed publicity are also helpful marketing tools for a clinic.

Perceptions of Rural Nursing Practice

Nurses may have both personal and professional reasons for choosing a rural setting for their practice, and it may therefore be useful to discuss the feelings of some rural nurses concerning their own experiences. Since the advantages and disadvantages listed by rural nurses did not vary by area of practice (for example, community, nursing home, or hospital), the following discussion of advantages and disadvantages relates to the practice of nursing in rural areas in general, not just in relationship to community health nursing.

Advantages   The overwhelming majority of the nurses interviewed said the ability to give holistic care, to know everyone well, and to develop close relationships with the community and with coworkers was the best thing about rural nursing. These nurses had all practiced nursing in urban areas as well, but they did not find the closeness there that exists in most rural settings. The second most frequently mentioned advantage was the variety of nursing challenges and the independence of practice; to describe this advantage, nurses used such words and phrases as challenge, responsibility, variety, independence, creativity, using abilities to the fullest, and working in many areas. The final advantage was the reward in being certain to have made a contribution—to see the results of nursing care, to make a difference, to become self-confident, and to be certain of the competence of rural care through personal observations and practice (Dolphin, 1984).

Disadvantages   Two themes emerged to answer the question, What would you like to change about rural nursing? The themes were the problems of isolation and problems within health care institutions. Isolation was the most common problem. Nurses wished that they were not so isolated from peers or from continuing education programs and opportunities. Distances to travel for home visits and the need to be able to provide many different types of nursing were other disadvantages of isolation. Problems within the institutions that employ nurses were poor salaries (this was true only in some areas, in other areas rural pay equaled urban pay), lack of professional respect, slowness to change, poor staffing and inflexible scheduling, being on call twenty-four hours a day, decreased chance for advancement or to obtain noninstitutional jobs, and having to work hard and fast one day then having nothing to do the next day (Dolphin, 1984). All but 3 percent of the 115 nurses interviewed found the advantages outweighed the disadvantages (Dolphin, 1984).

Ethical and Legal Considerations

Community health nurses are often faced with ethical and legal problems in rural communities. One legal problem is the pressure on the nurse to practice medicine without a license (Hodgson, 1982). Rural citizens often want the nurse to substitute as physician to increase their access to health care. Rural physicians appreciate nurses taking on some medical practice activities to lighten their load. When the nurse is the only one on the scene and physician help is far away in time and miles, there is a strong temptation to "do what you can" even when it is outside the nurse practice act (Dolphin, 1984).

"Doing what you can" also leads to the first ethical dilemma—negligence versus abandonment. When the nurse is not sure exactly what to do or how to do it, should care be attempted? Help may not be available even by telephone. Does the nurse give the best care possible with the inadequate knowledge available? Or does the nurse refuse to give care that could possibly be negligent, even when this means abandoning the person needing care because there is no other care-giver available for referral? Abandonment in this case refers to abandoning attempts to give care rather than physically leaving the scene.

Potentially conflicting relationships constitute the second, and likely more common, ethical dilemma. Because relationships in rural settings are so intertwined, it is difficult to know when the nurse should respond as a friend or family member and when as a professional (Bischoff, 1982). It is difficult to maintain the detachment needed for sound judgment when the person needing care is someone near and dear (Thobaden & Weingard, 1983). An example for which the resolution is legally prescribed is the neighbor who is also a child abuser. When the nurse has evidence that abuse is occurring, the law says it must be reported. But what if there are suspicions rather than evidence? How much easier not to ask and to try to counsel the family on discipline techniques! This is a simple example in which the responsibilities of the nurse are quite clear, but testifying for the prosecution at the trial of a very special friend will never be easy.

Confidentiality presents the third ethical problem in rural settings. When everyone is interested in everyone else's business, it is hard to keep information out of the "pipeline" (Stuart-Burchardt, 1982). Friends inquire about one another. It is difficult for the nurse to avoid answering questions without offending the questioner (Dolphin, 1984).

Information sharing may also affect a fourth ethical area—the peoples' right to control their own treatment. When multiple requests and suggestions are made by extended family and other community members for and about the care of a person in both formal and informal settings, the nurse may have trouble remembering if the person receiving care wanted things a certain way or if that was someone else's idea.

Other ethical and legal questions will arise that are similar to those in urban settings—for example, abortion, death with dignity, and informed consent. When there are few other professionals around to observe practice and discuss alternatives, identifying and resolving ethical and legal dilemmas increases in difficulty. Chapter 24 looks at these issues in more depth.

Strategies for Health Promotion

Rural nurses, like urban nurses, use the three levels of prevention to meet health needs of the family. However, the special needs of the rural community as well as rural values modify the skills and strategies from those used in the urban setting. Additionally, primary, secondary, and tertiary prevention are influenced by rural poverty, long distances that must be traveled to give or receive care, isolation from potential helpers and from newer developments in the field, and the values and practices of members of subcultures residing in the area. Since rural families are usually extended families, the skills and strategies used by the rural community nurse may extend beyond the nuclear family to the neighborhood or community.

Primary Prevention

Primary prevention (disease prevention) is difficult in rural settings. Rural populations are oriented to a greater degree than urban populations toward acute care rather than toward health maintenance (Stuart-Burchardt, 1982). Classes such as cardiovascular conditioning, nutrition, coping skills, parenting, or child safety will be poorly attended, especially if there is a cost in dollars, travel, or time lost from work. Classes in preparation for childbirth seem to be an exception to this trend (Dolphin, 1984). Another exception took place in Maine, where a thorough community assessment was done prior to a series of self-care classes. The inclusion of what the rural family members thought they needed to know may explain why the classes were well attended (Irish & Taylor, 1980).

Planning   Just as assessment is universally useful, the process of nursing planning to prevent disease is no different in rural areas than urban. The resources available to the nurse to meet health needs, however, are likely to be more limited in scope and availability. Economic resources of the family may also limit possibilities. The creativity of the rural nurse and the networks of information developed by the nurse are useful in the planning process. Other useful resources are the extended family, community togetherness, and independence in the rural area. "We take care of our own" is a theme encouraging arrangements between neighbors whereby an experienced mother "naturally" comes by to help a first-time parent learn infant care. To avoid passing on "old wives tales" or other misinformation, the rural nurse can form an alliance with these experienced mothers to provide them with a current knowledge base. Teaching with the new mother may also be needed to counteract misinformation. As a second example, the desire to avoid "government meddling" can lead rural families to gather in community action groups. For example, if the community sees child abuse as an area problem, the formation of a telephone hotline for potentially abusive parents may be chosen as an appropriate solution (Dolphin, 1984).

Intervention   In the intervention phase of primary prevention the rural nurse can be creative in providing health education. By placing emphasis on self-care, education programs will be better received (Dolphin, 1984). Schools are a source of ready clientele. With proper planning even sex education may be approved by conservative rural communities (Gumermen, Jacknick, & Sipko, 1980). Another ready audience is found in clinics and doctors' offices. With the shortage of physicians, there may be long waits and a number of people in the waiting room. Carousels with slide-tapes and earphones may effectively fill the waiting time with health teaching.

One-to-one teaching is another way rural nurses can help rural families improve health in the course of the family's daily activities. For example, the nurse might suggest to a farm family that a walk in the fields, rather than checking crop progress by truck, would increase exercise as part of the work day.

Since educational levels of adults are lower in rural areas than in the city, the rural nurse particularly needs to check the reading level of the person involved before written material is left for future use (Copp, 1976). Great tact needs to be used in this assessment since most people are embarrassed if they cannot read well. Another basic consideration in teaching material is the level of English comprehension of the person for whom it is targeted. Some teaching materials are also available in Spanish or other languages. The nurse needs to be aware, however, that some rural residents cannot read in any language.

Health education may be provided to larger groups through posters displayed in areas where there is frequent community traffic—churches, stores, and schools. The nurse may also be asked to speak to community organizations such as women's county extension clubs or just to share with an informal group such as the young mothers who live in the same area. The nurse needs to be alert to expressed and implied needs for health teaching. Teaching opportunities may be more likely to happen when the nurse volunteers her expertise rather than waits for invitations. For example, the nurse may ask community residents, "Would you like for me to come talk to you about (a particular subject)?" or "There's a movie out about (a topic), do you suppose Ann's Sunday school class would like to see it some evening?"

In another mode of primary prevention, the nurse may work closely with health department environmental health workers to reduce or eliminate environmental exposures. In still another primary prevention mode, the rural nurse may provide immunizations in the schools.

Secondary Prevention

Secondary prevention (early case finding) uses the highly developed and broad-based physical and mental assessment skills of the rural nurse. Rural nurses usually know everyone they come in contact with during the day. Watching community members' gaits, listening to speech and thought patterns, and observing family discipline methods can all happen in many settings. Checking on someone who "feels poorly" according to the report of a friend, and observing work habits and energy of schoolchildren may all give clues to possible problems that the nurse will follow up with more detailed assessment. A formalized means of secondary prevention provided to children by the nurse is screening for vision, hearing, or development problems, which are part of the school health program.

Community gatherings may also provide opportunities for screening of groups of rural families. Taking blood pressures after church or checking food choices and chewing habits at a community supper are examples. The nurse must always be vigilant because there are so few professionals in rural areas assessing peoples' health. Furthermore, visits to providers at time of early symptoms are unusual without nursing encouragement due to the

cost of health care and problems in obtaining care (Dolphin, 1984).

Due to the isolating distances and limited number of professionals, nursing assessments must be accurate. There may be no other professional available to validate assessment data. Furthermore, assessment skills are needed across the life span. There is no special nurse in the community for pediatric, maternity, or geriatric care. The rural nurse does it all. Because the family being assessed is usually previously known to the rural nurse, assessment can be more holistic, covering physiological, psychological, social, and spiritual areas. Information about economic conditions, community standing, employment conditions, and other family and extended family members is already known by the nurse from earlier contacts with the family (Dolphin, 1984).

Good assessment skills are important for another reason. The rural nurse can lighten the caseload for the busy rural physician. Assessment data provided verbally or in a written report may be the only information available to the physician for decision making as time and distance complicate a personal trip. The data supplied by the nurse becomes particularly crucial in an emergency or change in condition (Dolphin, 1984).

Interviewing skills are an important part of any nurse's assessment. They become particularly important with rural populations, because some members of the population conceal or minimize health problems. There seem to be multiple reasons for this concealment. The most common reason is that the problem is not severe enough to stop daily activities, so it is judged "not worth mentioning." A second reason may be to reduce health care costs by asking for help for only the most serious problems (Dolphin, 1984). The nurse needs to be alert for hints that problems exist that have been omitted or only received casual reference. Secondary disease prevention will be enhanced by development of these skills.

Early case finding is important in mental health as well as for physical disease. Nurses in rural areas report they observe a high rate of alcoholism, mental illness (especially depression and suicide), and

Case Example 21-1: Integrating Primary, Secondary, and Tertiary Skills

Mrs. Jones, a rural community nurse, arrives at the forty-bed local hospital at 7 A.M. to share breakfast and morning report with the hospital staff of three nurses. She shares information on new hospital admissions and helps complete planning for eighty-four-year-old Mabel Taylor. Mrs. Taylor is a widow who is due to be discharged following hospitalization to regulate her medications that control heart problems.

Rural nurse as a partner

Tertiary prevention

Mrs. Jones then stops at the local health department to pick up messages and plan who will be seen today. She then goes to the school to check on any returnees from illness absences and to consult with Sandra Taylor, Mabel's daughter-in-law, about a classroom teaching plan to help control the chicken pox epidemic in the first-grade class Sandra teaches.

Secondary and tertiary prevention

Kin relations

Mrs. Jones drives to a nearby village to conduct a general health care clinic. A quick stop on the way to change a dressing on a diabetic farmer turns into a longer visit because his wife seems depressed.

Secondary and tertiary prevention

At the clinic, mothers, children, and several elderly are given care. Assessment and teaching take up most of the clinic time. The postmistress stops by with news on the health of several residents. Mrs. Jones and the postmistress have a working relationship that helps with case finding and messages on follow-up care.

Rural nurse as generalist

Primary prevention
Rural nurse as community partner; use of local "grapevine"

After lunch, Mrs. Jones stops by to see Jim Williams, Sandra's neighbor, whom the postmistress mentioned. Jim had some TIAs (Transient Ischemic Attacks) last year. After careful assessment, a call to the physician gives the permission necessary for Medicare reimbursement when Mrs. Jones provides teaching about hypertension medication and low sodium, low cholesterol nutrition.

Partner with physician

Tertiary prevention

The afternoon is filled with scheduled home visits and charting. Mrs. Jones hurries home for dinner, because the elementary school's PTA has asked for a speech that evening on caring for children with chicken pox. Mrs. Jones plans to expand the program to talk about general sick care for children, emphasizing when to seek care from a health professional and how to use isolation methods in the home. Mrs. Jones plans to talk with Sandra about the arrangements to return Mabel home from the hospital and how her recovery will be supervised. This will save Mrs. Jones a phone call tomorrow. By the end of the day, Mrs. Jones has driven 150 miles.

Secondary and tertiary prevention

Effect of distance on amount of care available

family violence (Taylor, 1982). These reports are particularly troublesome since there are fewer mental health services in rural areas (Stuart-Burchardt, 1982). Those services present are not used by the local population due to rural stigmas against "mental problems" (Rosenblatt & Moscovice, 1982).

Problems of confidentiality in the presence of the active community "grapevine" are another concern of those needing counseling (Lieske, 1981). The unwillingness to publicly seek mental health care may mean that it is the community nurse with appropriate skills who gives counsel as part of other family contacts (Dolphin, 1984). Local ministers and educators also often fill this void (Lieske, 1981).

Psychiatric nurse specialists may practice in rural settings in private practice or, more commonly, as employees of the county mental health clinic. These nurses, too, must be generalists because they will see all ages of people and types of mental health problems from crisis intervention to chronic care. Mental health education will also be a part of the job. Rural psychiatric nurses report they can sometimes spot problems from medication or physical disease that had been thought to be emotional problems instead (Dolphin, 1984). This is another example of the need for all health care providers to be alert in assessment since there are too few observers.

Tertiary Prevention

Tertiary prevention (prevention of complications and long-term effect of disease) will be the service that the family most often requests of the rural community nurse (Dolphin, 1984). These requests are congruent with rural acute care orientation (Rural, 1983). At the same time, the lack of return visits to health care providers, missed appointments due to intervening priorities or transportation problems, and shortage of social service providers and occupational, physical, respiratory, speech, or other therapists make tertiary prevention difficult in rural settings (Dolphin, 1984). Compensating for these difficulties, in the course of such daily activities as shopping or attending school sports events the nurse encounters people

previously served (Stuart-Burchardt, 1982). These encounters provide opportunities for brief follow-up assessments. Unfortunately, the assessments are during "time off" and for no pay (Dolphin, 1984).

Since the rural community nurse may both run clinics and make home visits, more complete tertiary care may be given in both settings. Home visits are often most useful because the nurse gets a clearer understanding of how the disease has affected life-style, what resources are available to the family to prevent further disruption, and how much the prevention activities will conflict with usual family activities and values. If preventive measures conflict, they probably will not be carried out. Also the rural nurse needs to be creative in making inexpensive or free referrals and "jerry rigging" equipment to conserve costs for those people with low incomes (Dolphin, 1984).

Another tertiary prevention skill is crisis intervention. Crisis intervention skills in both emotional and physical situations are important in rural areas because there are likely to be no other professionals quickly available (Dolphin, 1984). See Chapter 16 for additional information on crisis intervention.

The last tertiary prevention skill is education. Teaching to prevent long-term effects of disease is enhanced by the knowledge of the community health nurse of what education was provided in the hospital. This information is easy to obtain when the person was hospitalized locally but difficult when urban care has been obtained (Dolphin, 1984). The community health nurse's role at all three levels of prevention is illustrated in Case Example 21-1.

Summary

Community health nursing in a rural setting is constrained and molded by its isolated setting. Few health professionals, few services, long distances to travel, and low funding make the delivery of quality care a challenge. The federal government has been increasingly involved in the planning and provision of rural care since the Great Depression. However, the programs have not resolved the problems.

The nurse who practices community health nursing in a rural setting has a much more general practice than the urban nurse. Rural practice is more independent, requiring excellent assessment skills and judgment. Because there are fewer other health professionals, the rural nurse is likely to use expanded and extended roles, and is also more likely to provide holistic, personalized care.

The extended family and close community found in rural settings give opportunities for nonnurses to give support and assistance to persons needing care. These opportunities are not often available in urban settings. The same closeness provides encounters between the nurse and people needing care in a variety of settings. These encounters can be used for assessment, the three levels of prevention, and evaluation. The encounters also make confidentiality and division of social and professional relationships difficult.

The rural community health nurse has the opportunity to use a broad base of nursing knowledge. The nurse can use leadership skills to improve health care by organizing community resources and by educating and encouraging individuals and families to use nursing services.

Topics for Nursing Research

• Can specific methods for political influences in rural areas be identified? Do these methods vary by community size, geographic area? Does the female gender of a community health nurse affect her political influence in a male-dominated rural system?
• Do the health needs of single rural women vary by geography, income, presence of other family members, or other factors?
• What are the support systems and other helping systems in existence in rural communities? What other helping systems are needed to augment these existing systems, and what changes are needed in current systems?
• How can the effects of the rural environment on health status best be measured?

• What are the common themes in health beliefs and practices among rural subcultures?
• What information is most needed to improve health self-care in rural families?
• How can maternal care be improved in rural areas?
• Can the skills and strategies peculiar to rural nursing be documented? Can rural community nursing be demonstrated to be a nursing specialty?
• Develop a procedure for a nurse to make a community assessment in a rural area.
• Do standards for ethical decision making vary between rural and urban community health nurses?

Study Questions

1. Rural families are different from urban families in that *in rural areas* (choose from answers a through d):
   (1) The families more often have a female head of family.
   (2) The family members are more likely to have traditional sex roles.
   (3) The families are more likely to be poor.
   (4) The families are more likely to be middle class.
   (5) The families are likely to have fewer children.
   (6) The families are likely to have more children.
   (7) The nuclear families are more likely to be closely involved with kin and other community members.

(8) The families are less likely to be traditional Protestants.
   a. 1, 3, 6, 8
   b. 1, 4, 5, 7
   c. 2, 3, 6, 7
   d. 2, 4, 5, 8

2. Which of the following statements is true about the effects of the political, economic, social, environmental, religious, and ethnic characteristics of the rural area on the health care of the rural family?
   a. Because Native Americans have a high level of employment and are, therefore, able to pay for services, many private physicians are attracted to reservation areas.
   b. Because residents of rural areas enjoy trying new ways of doing things, they demand the most up-to-date technical equipment in their local health care institutions.
   c. The county commissioners invest the majority of tax revenue in the county health department to control the many environmental hazards in rural areas.
   d. The extended family provides ancillary health services to families who have community acceptance and approval.

3. Which of the following contributions of a community health nurse would be most useful in improving health of residents in a rural community?
   a. Write letters frequently to the county commissioners to encourage them to upgrade ambulance service
   b. Collaborate with the local physician who has established a private practice in the area
   c. Help individuals and families to improve and use their self-care skills
   d. Establish a health clinic in the most remote area so that residents of that area will have access to health care

4. Which of the following activities is most illustrative of a primary prevention strategy by a community health nurse?
   a. Routinely test urine for glucose for anyone over fifty who attends the nurse's clinic
   b. Set up a vaporizing system for a baby recovering from croup
   c. Refer a person with an alcoholic problem

to the local chapter of Alcoholics Anonymous
   d. Sponsor an elementary art project to prepare posters on the need for handwashing after handling pesticides and before eating

References

American Medical Association: *Health Care Delivery in Rural Areas.* American Medical Association, 1976.

Anderson K: Atomic test case. *Time* (May 21) 1984; 123 (21):41.

Associated Press: Migrants seek basic sanitation. *Greeley (Co.) Tribune* (May 26) 1984c; 76 (220):A1.

Associated Press: Farmer: Rural counseling needed. *Greeley (Co.) Tribune* (January 24) 1984b; 76 (97):C3.

Associated Press: Block backs rural "partners." *Greeley (Co.) Tribune* (May 1) 1984a; 76 (193):C6.

Associated Press: One in 41 lives on farm: Report. *Greeley (Co.) Tribune* (December 27) 1983a; :B3.

Associated Press: Rural towns have a special quality. *Greeley (Co.) Tribune* (October 9) 1983b; 75 (355):A10.

Avery P, Merrill GP: Ambulance service falters in rural areas. *Rocky Mountain News* (August 23) 1983; 125 (123):21.

Bacrach LL: *Human Services in a Rural Area: An Analytical Review.* Human services monograph series No. 22. US Department of Agriculture, Washington, DC, 1981.

Biegel A: Toward a definition of rural nursing. *Home Healthcare Nurse* (September–October) 1983; 1 (1):45–46.

Bischoff HG: Rural settings: A new frontier in mental health. In: Babich KS (editor), *Mental Health Issues in Rural Nursing.* Boulder, Colo.: Western Interstate Commission for Higher Education, 1982, p. 14.

Brooks EF et al: New health practitioners in rural satellite health centers: The past and future. *J Community Health* (Summer) 1981; 6 (4):246–256.

Califano, JA: Rural health: A crisis of our time. *Biosciences Communication* (January–February) 1978; 4 (1):5–8.

Carter TJ, Donnemeyer JF, Wurschmidt TN: *Rural Crime.* Totowa, N.J.: Allanhed, Osmun and Co. Publishers, 1982.

Christian Science Monitor Wire Service: Female farmers. *Greeley (Co.) Tribune* (May 1) 1984; 76 (196):C5.

Copp JH: Diversity of rural society and health needs. In: Whiting L, Hassinger E (editors), *Rural Health Ser-*

vices: Organization, Delivery and Use. Ames, Iowa: Iowa State University Press, 1976, pp. 26–37.

Did you know? Rural Health Newsletter (Ga.) (November) 1983; 2 (3):8.

Dolphin N: Interviews with 115 Rural Community Nurses. Unpublished data. Greeley, Colo., 1984.

Fletcher, D: Report on Rural Nursing. Denver, Colo.: Office of Rural Health, 1981.

Ford TR: Rural USA: Persistence and Change. Ames, Iowa: Iowa State University Press, 1978.

Frey DC: Health Care at the Crossroads. Moberly, Mo.: Area II Health Systems Agency, 1981.

Goodwill J: Nursing Canada's indigenous people. Canadian Nurse (January) 1984; 80 (1):6.

Gumermen S, Jacknick M, Sipko R: Sex education in a rural high school. J Sch Health (October) 1980; 50 (8):478–480.

Hanson P, Matheson G, Reed PA: A tri-county needs assessment for the purpose of rural health promotion program development. Home Healthcare Nurse (September–October) 1983; 1 (1):22–28.

Hanton S: Rural helping systems and family typology. Child Welfare (July–August) 1980; 59 (7):419–421.

Hatch JW, Lovelace KA: Involving the Southern rural church and students of health professions in health education. Public Health Reports (January–February) 1980; 95 (1):23–25.

Henderson G, Primeaux M: Transcultural Health Care. Menlo Park, Calif.: Addison-Wesley, 1981.

Hodgson C: Ambiguity and paradox in outpost nursing. Int Nurs Rev (July–August) 1982, 29 (4).108–111.

Irish EM, Taylor JM: A course in self-care for rural residents. Nurs Outlook (July) 1980; 28:421–423.

LaGodna G: The single rural woman: Invisible struggles. Adv Nurs Sci 1981; 3 (2):17–23.

Lieske AM: Rural community mental health center: Adaptation of a conceptual framework. J Psychosoc Nurs Men Health Serv (November) 1981; 19 (11):18–20.

Lum JLJ: Asian Americans in the United States. In: Bessent H (editor), Nurse Researchers: Selected Abstracts, Vol. 1. Kansas City, Mo.: American Nurses Association, 1983, pp. 10–26.

Mennonite, The. Crockett, Ky.: Rod and Staff Publishers, Inc. n.d.

Merrell GP, Avery P: Colorado officials have failed to respond as rural health care system deteriorates. Rocky Mountain News (August 26) 1983; 125 (126):34.

Murphree AH: The anatomy and physiology of a rural county. In: Reynolds RC, Banks SA, Murphree AH (editors), The Health of a Rural County: Perspectives and Problems. Gainesville, Fla.: University Presses of Florida, 1976a, pp. 12–28.

Murphree AH: Folk beliefs; Understanding, health, ill-ness, and treatment. In: Reynolds RC, Banks SA, Murphree AH (editors), The Health of a Rural County: Perspectives and Problems. Gainesville, Fla.: University Presses of Florida, 1976b, pp. 111–123.

O'Leary JB, Barton, SN: Health cooperatives in rural communities. Biosciences Communication (May–June) 1977; 3 (3):218–230.

Osborne O: Aging and the black diaspora. In: Leininger M (editor), Transcultural Nursing: Concepts, Theories and Practice. New York: Wiley, 1978, pp. 317–334.

Piper LR: Accounting for nursing functions in DRGs. Nursing Management (November) 1983; 14 (11):47.

Reaching into the community—CHC. Frontier Nursing Service Quarterly Bulletin (Spring) 1983; 58 (4):1–7.

Reynolds RC: Rural America and health care. In: Reynolds RC, Banks SA, Murphree AH (editors), The Health of a Rural County: Perspectives and Problems. Gainesville, Fla.: University Presses of Florida, 1976, pp. 5–11.

Roemer, MI: Rural Health Care. St. Louis: Mosby, 1976.

Rolshoven R: Rural nursing: A challenge . . . not for everyone. Nursing Careers (January–February) 1982; 3:10.

Rosenblatt RA, Moscovice IS: Rural Health Care. New York: Wiley, 1982.

Rural clinics try out patient education in four demo projects. Health Care Education (February–March) 1980; 9 (1):1.

Selby TL: Nurse managed centers show potential. The American Nurse (May) 1984; 16 (5):1.

Singh SP: Rural health and health care delivery. Human Services in the Rural Environment (July–August) 1980; 5 (1):3–11.

Stuart-Burchardt S: Rural nursing. Am J Nurs (March) 1982: 82 (3):616–618.

Taylor J: Viewing health and health needs through many eyes: The ethnocentric approach. In: Babich KS (editor), Mental Health Issues in Rural Nursing. Boulder, Colo.: Western Interstate Commission for Higher Education, 1982, pp. 85–94.

Thobaden M, Weingard M: Rural nursing. Home Healthcare Nurse (November–December) 1983; 1 (2):9–13.

Travel N: Rural program development. In: Grunebaum H (editor), The Practice of Community Mental Health. Little, Brown, 1970, pp. 413–438.

Tulga G, Rohrer HH: Developing home health care services in rural areas: A case study of decision points. Home Health Review (December) 1980; 3 (4):5–11.

US Bureau of the Census: Money, Income and Poverty Status of Persons in the United States (Advanced Data). Washington, DC: Government Printing Office, 1981.

US Bureau of the Census: Number of Inhabitants, United States summary, 1980 census of population. Washington, DC: Government Printing Office, 1983.

US Bureau of the Census: *Statistical Abstracts of the United States: 1980*. Washington, DC: Government Printing Office, 1980.

US Public Health Service: *1983 United States Health and Prevention Profile*. Washington, DC: Government Printing Office, 1983.

Valenzuela WG, Hallamore AG: The "Good Neighbor Network": Gate-keepers to rural mental health support system. *Psychosocial Rehabilitation Journal* 1979; 3 (3):20–24.

Wodarski JS: *Rural Community Mental Health Practice*. Baltimore, Md.: University Park Press, 1983.

Chapter 22

Women's Health

Alice J. Dan, Linda A. Bernhard, and
Denise Webster

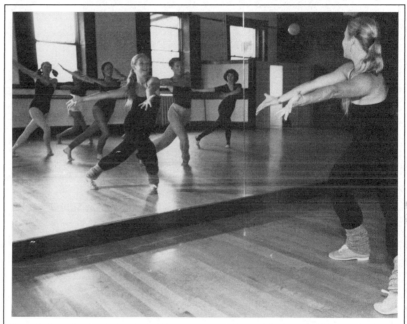

© John J. Krieger/The Picture Cube

Women's health means much more than obstetric-gynecologic care. It also encompasses the physical, mental, and social wellbeing of women in the context of their whole lives.

Chapter Objectives

After completing this chapter, the reader will be able to:

- Describe the relationship between women's health and women's status in the community
- Identify health needs and problems of women at different ages and in various community settings
- Describe settings where community health nurses might find women in need of health care
- Discuss strategies community health nurses can use to meet health needs of women

As women have become more articulate in voicing their viewpoints, needs, and desires, the field of women's health has become a defined area for nursing research, practice, and education. This chapter provides the reader with an overview of women's health in the community. We also offer a perspective for viewing health needs and concerns of women and strategies for meeting those needs.

What Is Women's Health?

The purpose of women's health practice is to meet the needs of women both as consumers and as providers of health care. Sometimes the term *women's health* is used to refer only to ambulatory obstetric-gynecologic care, but such a definition, like traditional medical views of women, limits the scope of women's health to just reproductive concerns. A more comprehensive definition, adapted from the definition used by the Women's Health Group at the University of Illinois at Chicago, addresses the full range of roles and interests in women's lives:

Women's Health refers to a non-traditional approach to the health care of women. Women are viewed holistically within the context of their lives. Women's physical, mental, and social statuses are interdependent, and together determine health or illness. Women's Health deals with women's life experiences from multiple perspectives: historical, political, cultural, developmental, and socio-economic. An awareness of the variability of women's experiences provides the background a practitioner uses to understand a client's view of her situation. To this end, the provision of health care and the formulation of research questions that benefit women are those which arise from women's lived experiences.

Women's Health is concerned with women both as consumers and providers of health care—in multiple settings and while assuming changing roles. As women's life experiences change, so will education, nursing care, and research in Women's Health (*Graduate Nursing*, n.d.).

This definition emphasizes understanding women's health from the point of view of women. Most health research and medical care have been conducted from male perspectives. Not only have the researchers and practitioners been generally men,

but many studies have used primarily male subjects (Dan & Beekman, 1972). Nevertheless, the results have been applied to women as well as men. While there is much that is useful and positive in past work, it is limited in addressing women's concerns, and the additional information gained from women's perspectives must be taken into account. Several elements have emerged as significant aspects of a women's health approach:

1. *The recognition of women's experience in many health-related roles.* Women have many different kinds of responsibility for health and nurturance of themselves and of others. As consumers, women obtain health care for family members. They provide care at home and need information and resources to support this role. As workers, women constitute greater than 80 percent of the health-care work force in the United States; however, their perspectives as women are underrepresented in the way the health system operates (Marieskind, 1980). As the largest health profession, nursing must address the special concerns of women as health care providers.

2. *A developmental emphasis on health throughout the life span.* Women of all ages have particular health needs. Throughout the life span, women are constantly being socialized into different roles, and their physical and mental health must be viewed in relation to their developmental changes. When femininity is defined as weakness or dependency, social pressure to be feminine is not healthy for women.

   Female babies are treated differently than male babies. Studies have shown that parents verbalize more to girl babies and handle boy babies with more physical vigor (Block, 1979). Little girls are socialized to be sweet, polite, and neat, while little boys are socialized to be rough and tough. These differences can affect women's health. For example, many adult women are hospitalized for depression as a result of their socialization to be dependent (Gordon & Ledray, 1985; Williams, 1979).

Menarche and menopause are developmental changes that all women experience, but their experiences vary greatly. Women's reproductive capacities are a significant aspect of their lives; care and support for whatever decisions women make about their reproductive roles are important aspects of women's health. However, these concerns are not central to all women throughout their lives. That is, some women choose *not* to bear children, and their only concern about their reproductive ability is to control it. Others, who do wish to have children, are concerned with that aspect of their lives only for a few years.

Adolescent women and older women especially have not received the attention given to women in their peak reproductive years. Adolescent women may have health concerns related to their first pelvic examination or to their first sexual intercourse. Older women are often widows and have special needs as a result of that experience, as well as problems such as osteoporosis, related to the aging process in women. A women's health approach concerns itself with all of these kinds of developmental changes and related health matters among women of all ages.

3. *Orientation to health, rather than disease.* Traditional approaches based on disease-oriented models are often inappropriate to meet the needs of women. For instance, women live longer than men and bear children. These two facts are not illnesses to be eradicated, but they do indicate areas of vulnerability to health problems. Rather than a narrow focus on caring for illness, women's health looks broadly at health-maintaining strategies.

Issues such as occupational health and safety, nutrition and eating behavior, unnecessary surgery, or incest and rape are representative of the broad range of women's health concerns. These issues have psychosocial, as well as physical, health implications. For example, poor women who desired sterilization have been used as "guinea pigs" for medical students and residents who needed to learn to perform hysterectomies (Corea, 1985; Scully, 1980). In addition, social and political factors in women's lives, such as safety and violence, pornography, and media images of women are being examined for their physical and mental health consequences.

An emphasis on health maintenance requires education for promotion of health and prevention of disease. Such an approach enables clients to be more self-reliant in health care. This self-care orientation equalizes responsibility for health between consumer and provider, and maximizes the efficient use of available health care resources.

4. *The nurse as health care provider.* Women are seeking new kinds of health care, and the field of women's health is attempting to address this demand. The elements of a women's health approach are more compatible with models of nursing care (in which the nurse functions as a consultant in health matters) than they are with the more hierarchical medical model (where the client is expected to do what the physician says). Nursing is concerned with the total person in the context of family and community and the nurse as health care provider to women can fill many roles, including that of advocate, consultant, and ally in self-care.

In recent years, the women's health movement has challenged the ability of the American health care system to be responsive to women's needs and concerns. Among the issues raised are (1) unwarranted assumptions, often based on stereotypes, about what clients want; (2) power differences in health care relationships, such that clients feel deprived of their rights to make decisions about their own care; and (3) lack of access to clear and helpful information, free of mystifying jargon, on which to base health decisions (Mulligan, 1983).

Stereotypes about women are distorted images based on uninformed cultural beliefs. A classic study of psychotherapists revealed how stereotypes about women can influence health professionals and affect the care women receive. Broverman and her associates (1970) asked psychologists, psychiatrists, and psychiatric social workers to describe a mature healthy adult, a mature healthy male, and a mature healthy female. They found that the adjectives used to describe the adult were similar to those describing the male, including "independent," "active," and "aggressive," while the female was described as "dependent," "passive," and "submissive." How can women be treated as adults when those caring for them hold views of women that exclude normal adult behavior? Fortunately, the impact of the women's movement has begun to change many of these ideas, but the process is slow and uneven.

Some stereotypes are so internalized by women themselves, either from women's earliest years of socialization or from the social values placed on these stereotypes, that even when women begin to question them, it is difficult to move beyond them. Two examples of this are the value of being thin and the wearing of makeup. Social support is extremely important in helping women to change their understanding of themselves and to enable them to function as autonomous adults. Health care providers can be a source of support, but groups of women themselves are especially effective in helping women realize that they are not alone in finding that the stereotypes do not fit. "Consciousness raising" groups provide an atmosphere of mutual support where women can work together to make sense of their experiences and to identify obstacles to their control over their lives.

Women have been at the forefront of the consumer health and self-help movements. The consumer movement focused on increasing consumers' control of their own care. Avoiding unnecessary costs and gaining access to information were important goals of the consumer health movement. One recommendation that has been useful to women is to obtain a second opinion before undertaking a major treatment, such as surgery. This strategy has been successful enough in saving money that some insurance companies now require it.

Another branch of activity leading to present-day women's health approaches is the self-help movement, which focuses on the sharing of skills. Egalitarian in its outlook, self-help philosophy emphasizes the demystification of knowledge—that is, avoiding technical jargon and speaking to people in terms they will find useful and empowering. Although there has been a thread of antiprofessional attitude in some self-help groups, the self-help movement in general is primarily directed against hierarchical relationships. When professionals acknowledge that health care is an exchange between equals, rather than a one-way transaction, then their expertise can be used in ways that strengthen rather than demean women.

A concern of women's health advocates is that self-help and self-care not be allowed to become a substitute for professional care for women who do not have access to professional services because of their economic, social, or cultural situations. Self-care philosophy can improve professional care for all persons.

Another concern of the women's health movement is poverty. Recent statistics show that poverty among women is rapidly increasing worldwide (Anand, 1983), a trend referred to as "the feminization of poverty." Pearce (1982) notes that two-thirds of all poor adults in the United States are women. The numbers of female-headed households are increasing, while their incomes relative to other families are decreasing (Pearce, 1982). These conditions are more marked in minority communities, where social, political, and cultural factors can additionally hinder access to traditional medical care. For example, some traditional Hispanic people view the hospital as a "last ditch effort" and as a place to die, so they do not go to a hospital when they need care. Rural women, too, face poverty and, particularly, they lack access to adequate health care (Kasper & Soldinger, 1983).

Although women's mortality rates are lower than men's, their morbidity is higher. Women report more illness than men, and experience more days of restricted activity and higher rates of inpatient and outpatient care than men do (Moore, 1980). However, why sex differences exist in types of diseases and disabilities experienced by women and men has not been adequately studied.

The World Health Organization has recognized women's health needs as a priority because women constitute half of the world's population and because women's health will influence health of future generations (World Health Organization, 1980). Women have always provided care for their family members. Women's responsibilities and concerns for the health of others are an important aspect of an emphasis on women's health.

While women's health clearly includes reproductive care and concerns, much of the existing research in this area concerns the fetus or the baby—not the woman. A women's health focus places priority on the study of the woman and her experience as a woman, wage-earner, wife, and mother.

Resources for maintaining and promoting health must be available to women. Women's health implies the need for not only medical care, but for a broad range of sociocultural and environmental approaches to health care. Nursing approaches are particularly well suited to the task of community leadership in women's health, and nurses can therefore contribute greatly to improving health care for women.

Women's Health Needs Across the Life Span

This section highlights special needs of women throughout the life span. The examples here have been chosen to illustrate some of the important decision points and interpersonal dynamics of women's lives. How these occasions are resolved depends on the contexts in which they happen. In this section, positive aspects of female development and opportunities for growth, as well as particular vulnerabilities, will be discussed.

Early Childhood

Early socialization in families often emphasizes sex differences. Children learn early that "boys can do more than girls" and many girls internalize the idea that it is better to be a boy. The low self-esteem of many women is likely to be based on their early childhood feelings that girls are not valued. In some groups this devaluation actually results in limiting opportunities for growth or even for food (Guttentag & Secord, 1983). Such behavior should be recognized as child neglect. Of course, not all women have low self-esteem, but nurses should be aware of the risks.

Girls need to learn that they are capable individuals and can participate in many activities, such as sports, traditionally reserved for boys. However, a truly nonsexist approach to child-rearing also values being female. The environment beyond the home often influences the way children express these values (see Case Example 22-1).

The case example demonstrates the importance of valuing female choices, not just the freedom for girls or women to be like males. Gender identity, the knowledge that one is female or male, is established by age three (Money & Ehrhardt, 1972). Over the next several years, cognitive developmental processes elaborate gender and other aspects of identity formation. When it is understood that girls and boys of this age are learning to differentiate maleness and femaleness, their attachment to cultural trappings of gender can be seen as a stage in this development.

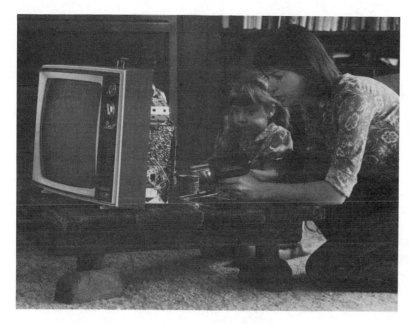

Socialization into the female role begins at birth. Some parents consciously avoid modeling stereotyped behaviors for their daughters, promoting the notions of individual skill and value regardless of gender.

Some researchers (Chodorow, 1978) maintain that social arrangements calling for female care of young children result in additional differences in male and female identity. Since masculinity becomes defined in separation from mother, males are thought to be more threatened by intimacy, while girls are more relationship-oriented (Gilligan, 1982).

School Age

Differences between girls' and boys' identity may help to explain the variations in their school experiences. Girls, who tend to be more sensitive to approval from teachers, adjust well in the early school years. But by fourth grade, boys' style of individuation begins to result in greater self-confidence, and by eighth grade, these differences in self-assurance are marked (Gold, Brush, & Sprotzer, 1980).

The pluralistic nature of society means that many girls can find support for being as bright and as skilled as they can be, even if teachers and parents try to channel them into stereotypically female roles and activities. Being a positive role model and encouraging girls to aspire and achieve is an impor-

---

Case Example 22-1: Environmental Influence on Socialization into Gender Roles

Ron and Carol were both feminists who wanted their firstborn daughter, Leigh, to be free and nonsexist. While they provided nonsexist toys and all kinds of clothing, and were good examples themselves of nonsexist behavior and dress, Leigh, age four, preferred to wear dresses, always chose pink, and regularly spoke about "my favorite pink." She needed to identify herself as a girl, not a boy.

At this stage in development, daughter strongly identifies with female role despite nonsexist child-rearing.

---

tant function for female health care professionals in their contacts with children.

Girls in minority families may have particular difficulty establishing a positive self-concept in situations where discrimination is a problem (Reid, 1982). Society's devaluing of women, blacks, and other groups may be internalized as part of a self-concept with negative aspects. For minority children, establishing a positive self-concept could be difficult if they live in a family where the expectations are different from those of the white dominant culture. Even if the family has adopted the norms of white society, they are still apt to be discriminated against because of their minority status (Reid, 1982). Black daughters traditionally do receive a great deal of support from their families, and this support is very important in their development of self-esteem.

Puberty and Adolescence

A significant period of development for the young girl is the time of her menarche. Often young girls "compete" to see who will be first to become a woman. The way she learns about her menstrual cycle, and even from whom, can have an important effect on how she manages her menstrual cycle throughout her life (Brooks-Gunn & Ruble, 1984). For example, if she is taught to call her menses "the curse," it may very well become such. On the other hand, if she is taught that menstruation is a normal, significant, and important part of her life, she may accept it as nonproblematic.

Adolescent women, experiencing body changes and trying to become more independent, are especially vulnerable to social pressure. Society's views of women result in mixed messages that can have serious consequences for teenagers' health. Female beauty, for example, is seldom portrayed in all the diverse shapes, sizes, and colors of the real population of women. Instead, slimness is emphasized as absolutely necessary for an attractive body.

The fear of being too fat, reinforced by fad diets and diet pill advertisements, can result in eating disorders, such an anorexia nervosa or bulimia. Anorexics refuse food, sometimes to the point of life-threatening starvation, yet in their distorted body image, they may still see themselves as fat. Bulimics engage in binge-eating and vomiting to rid themselves of the food before it is used in their bodies. Less extreme behaviors include compulsive eating and cycles of dieting and binging, which are characteristic of some women throughout their lives (Bruch, 1978).

A second area of socially pressured behavior in adolescence is substance abuse. Offering a quick and easy sophistication, alcohol use and smoking have increased dramatically among teenaged women (Gritz, 1984; Young Drinkers, 1982). It is now estimated that over 70 percent of adolescent women drink alcohol, and that 15 percent are problem drinkers. Teenaged women are the most rapidly increasing group of smokers, and if present rates continue, they will soon outnumber young male smokers (Kasper & Soldinger, 1983). (See Chapter 26 for a detailed discussion of substance abuse.)

Another high risk, high pressure topic for teenagers is sexuality. Social changes over the last twenty years have included the sexual "revolution," the Gay Liberation Movement, and increased availability of contraceptives and abortion. Although these changes provide more choices for adolescents, they do not make the decisions any easier.

The double standard of sexual behavior still exists: girls should look sexy, but may not act sexually; while boys can be sexually active. At the same time, the availability of contraceptives and abortion can be used by boys to pressure their girlfriends into having sex when the girls are not ready. (See Case Example 22-2 and see Chapter 25 for a detailed discussion of adolescent pregnancy.)

The road to independent adulthood contains many hurdles of special significance for women. In some groups a woman is not considered adult until she marries (Rubin, 1979). Some traditional urban Catholic families may allow a daughter to go away to college, but when she finishes college, she is expected to return to live in her parents' home if she is not married. On the other hand, some families may regard college as a bridge to indepen-

Case Example 22-2: Pressure to Become Sexually Active

At fifteen, both Karen and Don were experiencing the excitement of a close boy-girl friendship for the first time. Although they enjoyed being physically close, Karen was not ready for more than holding and kissing. She told Don that she wanted to wait for more intimacy. She felt shocked and hurt when Don tried to engage in more intimate petting. Chagrined, Don explained that his older brother had told him that "girls really want it, they just pretend not to, so you have to push them."

It is hard for girls to say what they mean when society says that women do not know what they mean.

dence, and college graduates are expected to become launched from the family and establish families of their own.

Marriage

For some women the decision to marry also involves a decision about what to call herself. Will she use her birth name, her husband's name, or a new version combining both names? Sometimes it is appropriate to use one name professionally and another for informal occasions. Guidance for these decisions is available from places such as the Center for A Woman's Own Name in Barrington, Illinois, or from some local chapters of the National Organization for Women.

People bring many expectations with them when they enter new relationships such as marriage. A recent study of college students noted interesting differences between races and sexes in attitudes toward family roles and personal achievement for women (Crovitz & Steinmann, 1980). Black students saw the ideal woman as significantly more independent than white students did. Furthermore, the attitudes of black men and women were more similar than were those of white men and women. Women of both races tended to believe that men want a more traditionally oriented wife than men claimed to want, but this difference was particularly marked for the white students. This study suggests that both men and women are ready for independence and achievement in their relationships, but that they are still influenced by tra-

Case Example 22-3: Discrepancy Between Social Expectations and a Woman's Actual Experience

Louise, age twenty-eight, is a recovering alcoholic, describing the events leading to her drinking problem: Married at nineteen, she delivered her first child at age twenty-two. "I was raised to believe that it was normal for women to marry and have babies early but it was not at all what I expected. Suddenly I felt housebound, isolated from friends who didn't have children, and very unhappy. The worst part was that I wasn't *supposed* to feel this way. I felt there was something wrong with me, and alcohol seemed to help me feel OK about myself."

Early marriage and child-rearing leads to isolation and alcohol as a coping mechanism

ditional stereotypes. The conflicts that can arise may lead to health problems, as illustrated in Case Example 22-3.

Childbearing

The past twenty years have seen rapid changes in family life cycle patterns for women including a decline in the number of children women expect to have (actual family size also decreased from an average of 3 children in the 1960s to 2.4 children in 1975); a decreased in unwanted births, from one in five in 1966 to one in twelve in 1976; and a reduced time frame of active mothering. More women are having children later in life, and there is an increase in single-parent families, particularly among black women. Other changes include alternative structures for mothering, including cohabitation, communal arrangements, lesbian couples, stepfamilies, joint custody, and various arrangements with adolescent mothers (Gerson, Alpert, & Richardson, 1984).

On the whole, although the outcomes of these changes is unknown, it would appear that fewer, more wanted children are being raised by better prepared mothers. However, the stresses of parenting are also better documented than ever before. These begin with the decision whether or not to have a child.

Four possibilities exist: a woman wants children and is able to become pregnant; she wants children, but, for some reason, is unable to become, or remain, pregnant; she does not want children but is able to become pregnant; and she does not want children and is unable to become pregnant. Of course, not all women know which of these situations exists for them. Some women use contraceptives for years, but then when they choose to become pregnant, find they have difficulty doing so. Even the woman who wants to have children probably does not want to have as many as she biologically could have (theoretically about one each year from puberty until menopause), so stress can arise from trying to avoid pregnancy.

Even before conception, decisions made by parents can affect the lives and health of women. Pref-

erences for sons, especially firstborn sons, has been found among both women and men across many cultures (Williamson, 1976b). This means that girls are less likely to be wanted, and parental disappointment when a girl is born can cast a shadow over a girl's early life.

Another implication of the preference for sons is the potentially disastrous consequences of newly developed techniques for sex control and sex preselection (Rorvik & Shettles, 1970; Williamson, 1976a). In the long run, if and when sex preselection becomes widely available, males may be chosen to such a disproportionate extent that females become rare. Even more likely, males will be selected as firstborn, with all the apparent advantages in ambition and achievement of firstborn children. If most girls are selected as secondborn children, their second-class status will be reinforced. Ethical issues of sex preselection and control are a major concern for those who value women and women's contributions to society (Holmes, Hoskins, & Gross, 1980).

Related to the issue of childbearing and non-childbearing is the issue of safe and effective contraception. Most contraceptive methods are designed to be used by women, and all available contraceptives have certain hazards associated with their use. Heterosexually active women are put at risk by using, or not using, contraceptive methods. Women face conflicts about abortion as a birth control method or as a backup for method failure. Furthermore, abortion is still viewed by many as stigmatizing, and is still not readily available to all women who need or want it.

Child-rearing

Once children are present, the issues surrounding child-rearing arise. In most families women continue to have the major responsibility for child care. Child-rearing gives many women a sense of pride and happiness, and makes them feel needed and worthwhile. However, the constancy of child care can cause women to become fatigued and vulnerable to illness. Women who are constantly around young children (including full-time mothers, daycare personnel, elementary school teachers, and pediatric and community health nurses) are routinely exposed to the frequent communicable diseases of children.

Most of the popular literature on parenting consists of "how-to" advice, rather than accounts of actual parenting experiences, so most new parents are poorly prepared for the stress of parenthood. There is evidence that marital satisfaction is negatively affected by the addition of a child, that role conflict ensues, and that parents need support for coping with the strains of their new roles (Gerson, Alpert, & Richardson, 1984; Lewittes, 1982). Most parents have legal responsibility for their children for at least eighteen years, and women bear most of the burdens of caring for them during those years.

Women are very aware of the amount of care that infants require, of the "terrible twos," and of the rebellion normal among adolescents. Studies show that the periods of child development with the highest stress for parents (mothers) are toddlerhood and adolescence (Gerson, Alpert, & Richardson, 1984).

The main problem that makes both toddlers and adolescents stressful to care for is the amount of supervision they require. Toddlers must be watched constantly, because their investigative nature can easily put them at risk for injury. Adolescents too must be supervised, but the problem for the mother is the stress of making, or helping the adolescent make, decisions for what is appropriate behavior, which may be in conflict with the adolescent's peers' demands. Additionally, mothers are often at the stage of midlife when their children are at the stage of adolescence. Thus the mother has her own developmental crises to face, as well as helping her children to manage theirs.

Adulthood and the World of Work

In addition to family expectations, women face difficulties in preparing for and entering the job market. Although the majority of adult women work outside the home, and the majority of young women intend to obtain paid employment for most of their adult lives, opportunities for women are still limited by the male breadwinner–female homemaker–nuclear family stereotype (Blaxall & Reagan, 1976).

Choosing a job and/or career involves another series of choices for women. When a woman decides to take a job or must work to support herself, she must first decide what she wants to do. It may be that she will "do anything" just to have an income. Other women can make choices—whether it will be a career or temporary employment, and whether it will be in a "traditional women's occupation" (e.g., nurse, teacher, stewardess), or in a nontraditional occupation (e.g., carpenter, lawyer, pilot).

Women are suspected of inadequate work motivation, because they value family roles. Young women may be discouraged from attaining high levels of education, or from committing themselves to a career, because they will "just get married." Jobs for women are disproportionate in teaching, health, or service fields, with lower pay (60 percent of the male average) and fewer opportunities for advancement. These differences restrict women's financial resources and negatively affect women's self-esteem, since such differences indicate to women that their work is less valuable than men's work.

There are many books giving advice to young women today on how to make it in a male work world—for example, *Dress for Success* and *Games Your Mother Never Taught You*. While it is encouraging to see women's aspirations raised, it is questionable to assume that a majority of wage-earning women can, or would choose to, fit into a male work model.

Women's lives seem to require a different structuring of work to accommodate the family life cycle. More than a fourth of women wage-earners are employed part-time, for example, and they tend to be more poorly paid and to have inadequate health insurance coverage and other benefits (Kasper & Soldinger, 1983). In the long run, making the system of work responsive to women's needs will require many women organizing to support each other and to bring about change.

Many factors affect the levels of stress and satisfaction of working women. In addition to adequate pay, benefits, and promotions, two important factors are sexual harassment and occupational health hazards. Sexual harassment is defined as the unwanted imposition of sexual requirements in the context of a social relationship where there is unequal power (MacKinnon, 1979). Under this definition sexual harassment is illegal and is considered sex discrimination. If a supervisor expects sexual favors for advancement, a working woman has grounds for a sex discrimination suite.

Other instances of sexual harassment, such as lewd comments by coworkers, are unfortunately more common and harder to prosecute. However, employers do have a responsibility to provide a working environment free from discriminatory practices. Publicizing company policies against sexual harassment can be an effective way of stopping unpleasant incidents. Providing social support for women coping with sexual harassment is also an important function.

Health Hazards of Work   Health hazards in the workplace are another concern for women. Until recently, hazards affecting women's reproductive potential were the major focus, with employers excluding women from jobs where exposure to hazardous substances might cause birth defects. New information on hazards in women's jobs is regularly available from the Women's Occupational Health Resource Center at Columbia University.

Examples of other health hazards affecting women in the work place include noise (e.g., cannery workers), temperature extremes (e.g., laundry workers), required shift rotation (e.g., nurses), and machine design (e.g., factory workers). Women coal miners (and other female workers in traditionally male jobs) suffer health problems resulting from having to wear men's shoes, clothing, and hard hats, simply because garments designed for women are not available (White & Bales, 1983).

Women working in the home also face many health hazards from substances such as detergents, bleach, cleaners, and microwave radiation. Furthermore, they are subject to burns, cuts, falls, and other "minor injuries." Women working both in and out of the home have become more involved

in sports, exercise, and recreation, and consequently are experiencing sports injuries previously seen primarily in men.

Combining Employment and Children   Regardless of the occupation she has, the woman who manages both a job *and* a family is subject to a great deal of role conflict. Her family expects her to care for her children and the home, yet she may need or prefer to pursue her job. She is pulled in both directions, and may find herself doing neither job well, making her stress even more intense.

Having multiple roles can be beneficial to women, however. Their self-esteem can be enhanced as they achieve job satisfaction, have greater economic security, and accrue other personal benefits. They learn to use their time effectively, and their stress may actually be decreased, resulting in better health status (Verbrugge, 1982).

Older research implied that children of mothers who worked outside the home might have more developmental problems than children whose mothers were always present in the home. Current research suggests that children are *not* impaired by having their mothers work outside the home, and in fact, that children—and mothers—do best when the mother is doing what she *wants* to do, whether that is in or out of the home. Children of wage-earning mothers seem to be advantaged in that they have to learn to be independent at an early age. For young girls, having a mother who works outside the home can be an important role model (Hoffman, 1974).

However, women continue to have concerns for flexibility in their work schedules, because, if a child is sick, it is usually the mother who must stay home from her job to care for the child. Women also have concerns about losing their work benefits if they must take a leave of absence for pregnancy reasons.

Housework   Housework is also a source of stress for many women. While modern conveniences have decreased the amount of heavy lifting, housework still requires time and energy, and it does not go away. Research shows that most married women do the regular daily housework, whether they work outside the home or not (Vanek, 1974). Women not employed outside the home spend over fifty hours per week on housework, and women who are employed outside the home still spend over thirty hours per week on housework. Their husbands spend approximately eleven hours per week on housework. In addition, when there are children, the amount of housework increases substantially, and it is the woman's hours of work that increase to meet the demand, not the husband's (Hartman, 1981).

Women who work only in the home have a greater tendency toward various health care problems, including obesity, alcoholism, and depression (Gove, 1972). Women who view themselves as "just a housewife" are at particular risk for mental health problems. If their identity comes only from their husband and children, they cannot develop the independent potential that they have as women.

Midlife

Midlife women face many changes and decisions. A common assumption has been that midlife is the time of the "empty nest" and menopause. Some women look on this time with anxiety and concern; they may worry about the changes that they think will happen to them and they may fear being lonely.

Other women view midlife as a time of renewed vigor and activity. Some will enter the labor force after not being in it for many years. The proportion of women in the labor force is highest at age forty-seven (Gelein & Heiple, 1981). Self-esteem and health in these women may be enhanced.

The leading cause of death for women between the ages of thirty and fifty-four is cancer (Kasper & Soldinger, 1983). Nonwhite women are at greater risk for death from breast cancer, while invasive cervical cancer rates are twice as high among black women as among white women (Kasper & Soldinger, 1983). Many of these deaths could be prevented with screening and early detection programs. Health insurance, unfortunately, may not cover preventive care, such as Pap smears, mammograms, or chest X-rays, so even women who have insurance may not seek regular health checkups. Other women may simply have no insurance or may not understand the importance of checkups. It is important to teach women how to monitor their bodies, so they will be able to identify changes that should be checked further with a health care professional.

Breast self-examination, which should be performed by all women, becomes particularly important for midlife women since the risk for developing breast cancer increases with age. Some ethnic groups, such as Hispanic women may be sensitive or embarrassed about touching their own breasts, so it is helpful to know that explanations are available in Spanish (e.g., *Nuestros Cuerpos, Nuestras Vidas*).

Hypertension is another major health problem for midlife women, especially for black women. Hypertension problems are related to diet, overweight, stress, toxemia of pregnancy, and the use of birth control pills. It is particularly important for women at risk for hypertension to control their salt intake and to avoid smoking (Richmond, 1983).

Older Women

Health problems for midlife and older women include diabetes, gall bladder disease, osteoporosis, and coronary heart disease. Controversies still rage over the advisability of hysterectomy and/or estrogen replacement therapy (ERT) for menopausal women. Although many unnecessary hysterectomies seem to have been performed (Scully, 1980), many women also have reported improved well-being following hysterectomy, especially if bleeding was a problem prior to the operation (Webb & Wilson-Barnett, 1983).

Some women's health advocates continue to oppose the use of ERT (Seidler, 1984), but recent claims about the usefulness of estrogen in preventing osteoporosis have renewed its popularity. Osteoporosis is a condition found in many older women in which a gradually severe reduction in bone mineral content results in fragile, easily broken bones. Black women are at lower risk for osteoporosis than white women (Peck, 1984).

Women over sixty-five are the fastest growing low income group in the United States (Kasper & Soldinger, 1983). Poverty contributes to many of their health problems through inadequate nutrition, housing, and transportation.

Almost two-thirds of women over sixty-five are widows, and many live alone (McElmurry, Glass, & Egan, 1981). Widowhood is a difficult adjustment for some women; those with activities outside the home adjust better than those with a very traditional role. Strong kinship ties help black women survive this crisis (Lewittes, 1982).

Because women live longer than men, they are subject to many chronic illnesses, and need to consider the issues of long-term care. Nursing homes are one alternative, but adult care homes, home health care, and adult daycare are also options. Medicare and private insurance may not cover all of these costs (Rourke, 1984).

Drug use is another major problem for older women. Some physicians prescribe "combination pills" containing tranquilizers and other drugs to treat pain, stomach problems, or headaches. Even ERT is sometimes combined with tranquilizers without the knowledge of the woman. Older women may be exploited physically, mentally, and economically by physicians who prescribe unnecessary drugs for them.

Since women are often underrepresented in clinical trials of drugs, some side effects may be unexpected (Seidler, 1984). Multiple drug use may result in interactions among drugs. Disorientation and depression can be the consequence of overmedication.

For many older women, emotional problems or depression are more a result of social isolation than of aging per se. Friendship networks are important sources of support to women of all ages, but especially critical for older women. Helping women visit friends, stay in touch, or make new friends is

a meaningful contribution to their health. See Chapter 23 for additional information on health problems of older adults, including women.

Settings Where Women's Health Needs Can Be Identified

Women's health needs occur everywhere women are. Traditional community settings where any health care provider ought to be aware of women's health needs and problems include homes, schools, industrial sites, prisons, well-baby clinics, church and other community groups, and senior citizens' residences and centers.

Other alternative settings for women's health now can be found in many areas. Practitioners may assist women in battered women's shelters, women's health centers, nurse-managed clinics, self-help groups and other community organizations, hotlines, and services for homeless women. Some women's health practitioners are in independent practice or work with nurses in a practice; others practice with alternative health care practitioners utilizing acupuncture or holistic health centers.

Women's health practitioners may consider working at camps for children and adolescents, or working with employees at such camps. Women's health practice with female children is especially important and can be extremely valuable in socializing female children to be assertive and empowered. Some camps are for girls only, while others have children of both sexes. Specialty camps for children (and occasionally for adults) who have asthma, cystic fibrosis, diabetes, or epilepsy, or who are physically or mentally disabled may be very good settings for women's health practitioners who want to help women feel better about themselves.

Providers may also be involved with groups of women at women's bookstores. Many female owned and operated women's bookstores now provide classes, discussion groups, and other networking services for women.

Delivery of Women's Health Care in the Community

Identifying the stress points in women's lives is an important step in building new knowledge to improve women's health. Breaking away from stereotyped ideas can help women to recognize what it is in their lives that truly strengthens them, and where the problems are. But knowing that each woman is a different individual means that each health care interaction must involve full participation of both consumer and provider. Toward this end, women's health practitioners envision a change in the traditional role relationships of health care provider and patient. To create a system that strengthens women requires a variety of strategies to help transform traditional medical care into a participative process, and to reconceptualize the nature of nursing practice to support this process.

Several philosophical points of view concerning women's issues and women's health exist. Each emphasizes different problems and suggests different solutions for making the health care system more responsive to women's needs and concerns. Fee (1983) delineates the liberal, socialist feminist, and radical feminist philosophies. The liberal approach focuses on equality of access and of equal opportunities for women. Without attempting to change the basic system, liberal feminists try to counter sex discrimination by increasing the number of women in medicine, for example, or by changing the education of health professionals to eliminate sexist ideas and practices.

Socialist feminist strategy aims to change the present system of health-care-for-profit. Starting from the belief that capitalist social organization is the basis for both class and sex oppression, socialist feminists argue that working class and Third World women have different problems than middle- and upper-class white women, and that health care providers need to be sensitive to the particular concerns of poor women.

The radical feminist philosophy is woman-centered and criticizes the oppressive effects of basic cultural institutions, including the traditional nuclear family and compulsory heterosexuality. Radical feminists are responsible for creating many of the alternative institutions caring for women, such as women's shelters, rape crisis centers, and women's health centers.

Although their emphases and tactics may differ, women who care about women's health, regardless of their philosophy, can work together to create and maintain better systems of health care for women. Some problems can be managed in a variety of ways, and women working together can find the best and most efficient strategies for each problem.

Self-Care Model for Women

One approach to women's health care that can be used by women's health providers, regardless of their philosophy, is the use of a self-care model in fostering women's health. The components of a self-care focus include: (1) equalizing responsibility for health care between the client and the care-giver, (2) providing information that will empower the client, and (3) respecting the experience of the client.

Equalizing responsibility between the provider and the client implies that each has information and expertise that are needed to maintain the client's health. A collaborative, nonhierarchical relationship is established in which both persons share in the process of health care. The contributions of each are valued and used.

Providing information for the client is a very important part of a self-care model, but it implies a very different approach to education than what has come to be called patient or health education (Levin, 1978). Patient education implies that the client is sick or has a disease for which education is needed; education in a self-care model implies education for health and prevention of disease. Additionally, patient education begins with objectives that the provider has for the client, while self-care education begins with objectives that the client identifies for herself.

Respect by the care-giver for the experiences of the client suggests the importance of supporting women and helping them to validate their own experience. Women's health providers recognize the importance of providing health care to women in ways that give women power and that build their self-esteem and self-reliance. By focusing on the woman's lived experience (McBride & McBride, 1982) and accepting it for what it is, the woman's self-esteem is supported, and she is made to feel worthwhile.

These three components of a self-care focus clearly overlap. That is, equalizing responsibility for health care includes identifying needs and objectives for education; providing information cannot effectively be done without considering and respecting each woman's individual experiences. Each component is as necessary as the others for maintaining a woman-oriented health care approach.

Needs Assessment

Studies of women's health needs and concerns indicate that many of the needs that women express are within the realm of nursing. Women need access to information, assistance with self-care, and advocacy in negotiating the health care system.

Using Orem's (1985) self-care framework, nurses can assess health needs in the areas of preventive concerns associated with universal needs, such as nutrition and exercise, occupational health and safety, or community supports to provide women with personal safety from physical and psychological abuse.

Developmental needs such as family planning, parenting, and changing self-image over the life span must be identified in women at the times they are relevant to each woman. Health deviation needs, such as information about surgery for cancer or prescription drugs for depression must also be assessed. Both self-care practices and self-care deficits must be identified so that nursing systems can be developed to meet the needs.

A "Women's Health Needs Assessment Guide," developed by members of the Women's Health Group at the University of Illinois at Chicago is presented in Table 22-1. The needs assessment is divided into the three general areas of self-care requisites as defined by Orem (1985), and in addition, a section related to needs in the area of health care has been added.

Women's health providers can use the needs assessment with clients as a method for identifying specific concerns of individual women or of groups of women. The guide can be used in whatever ways are useful for the provider and client.

A Look to the Future

The future of women's health care rests on the establishment and use of a body of knowledge that is women's health. That body of knowledge will be developed through the integration of research, theory development, and women's health practice. Community health nurses and all nurses must be involved in all phases of this important work.

A group of faculty from a number of midwestern nursing schools has identified the following needs specifically related to research in the area of women's health:

1. Research priorities related to Women's Health care concerns throughout the life cycle, and to women as clients in the health care system
2. Educational programs for scholars who are developing or implementing research in Women's Health
3. State-of-the-art conferences on Women's Health which disseminate research information to clients and providers

Table 22-1   Women's Health Needs Assessment

	Need for information	Need for service	No need
Universal			
Nutrition and diet	___	___	___
Exercise and rest	___	___	___
Self-esteem	___	___	___
Personal safety, protection from violence	___	___	___
Sexuality	___	___	___
Stress management	___	___	___
Environmental health hazards (home, work, school)	___	___	___
First aid, accident prevention	___	___	___
Developmental			
Pregnancy and birth	___	___	___
Prenatal care, birth preparation	___	___	___
Breast-feeding	___	___	___
Genetic counselling	___	___	___
Birth alternatives (midwifery, birthing centers, home birth)	___	___	___
Childhood	___	___	___
Child care arrangements	___	___	___
Parenting support	___	___	___
Incest, child abuse	___	___	___
Menstrual education	___	___	___
Adolescence	___	___	___
Acne, skin care	___	___	___
Dysmenorrhea	___	___	___
Sexually transmitted diseases	___	___	___
Contraception	___	___	___
Abortion	___	___	___
Substance abuse	___	___	___
Young adulthood	___	___	___
Breast self-examination	___	___	___
Infertility	___	___	___
Premenstrual syndrome	___	___	___
Midlife	___	___	___
Osteoporosis prevention	___	___	___
Obesity	___	___	___
Menopause	___	___	___
Role changes	___	___	___
Aging	___	___	___
Widowhood	___	___	___
Poverty	___	___	___
Isolation	___	___	___
Long-term care	___	___	___

(continued)

Table 22-1 *(continued)*

	Need for information	Need for service	No need
Health Deviation			
Cancer	___	___	___
Surgery	___	___	___
Mastectomy	___	___	___
Hysterectomy, oophorectomy	___	___	___
Depression	___	___	___
Anorexia Nervosa	___	___	___
Alcoholism	___	___	___
Endometriosis	___	___	___
Hypertension	___	___	___
Woman abuse	___	___	___
Sexual assault	___	___	___
Cystitis	___	___	___
Vaginitis	___	___	___
Toxic shock syndrome	___	___	___
General health care needs			
Prescription and nonprescription drugs	___	___	___
Medical devices	___	___	___
Sanitary products	___	___	___
Relationship with health professionals	___	___	___
Finding health care	___	___	___
Affording health care	___	___	___
Providing health care at home	___	___	___
Other needs			
_____			
_____	___	___	___

4. Communication networks among scholars working in the area of Women's Health research
5. Use of research findings on women and health in legislative and administrative policy decisions
6. Use of women's experiences as the base for building research, service, and educational initiatives in Women's Health

(McElmurry et al, 1980)

Some of these goals are beginning to be achieved, and exciting things are happening. Major conferences related to women's health, such as "Women,

Health, and Healing," sponsored by the University of California, San Francisco, have been held. A new interdisciplinary organization, the International Council for Women's Health Issues, was established at the First International Congress on Women's Health Issues, in Halifax, Nova Scotia, Canada, in October, 1984. And the Public Health Service Task Force on Women's Health Issues has published its report of recommendations (Report, 1985). However, the field of women's health is still very young and is wide open for nurses to become involved.

Strategies for Health Promotion

With a focus on women's health, rather than illness, women will be seeking health care in different ways than they have previously. Community health nurses can respond to this need with primary, secondary, and tertiary prevention strategies.

Primary Prevention

Primary prevention strategies are those specific and identifiable measures that protect against disease or injury. They are based on knowledge of potential threats, risks, and measures of control. This is the major focus for community health nurses in women's health care. Primary prevention in women's health means the community health nurse must identify women's health needs and concerns and work with women to develop self-care strategies for managing their individual needs.

Women have always been health care givers to their families and themselves. Unfortunately, many times their families came first, and women had little time, money, food, or energy to spend on their own health. Recently, as society has become more health-oriented in general, and with the influence of the self-care movement, women are becoming more concerned for their own health. Nurses must help women realize that being healthy themselves and providing their own self-care is essential to their ability to care for all the other persons in their lives.

Educating Women About Health Issues

Women are interested in living health life-styles. They recognize the importance of a nutritious diet, adequate rest, fitness, and exercise. Community health nurses should foster this interest and teach women about health habits, the importance of sleep, minimizing the use of alcohol, and stopping smoking.

Community health nurses can provide education regarding the needs of women at various age groups. For example, older women might be encouraged to obtain flu shots to decrease the possibility of developing an illness that could be quite harmful to their health.

As girls embark on adolescence, they need specific kinds of information about their developing bodies. Sex and menstrual education must go beyond the usual school hygiene programs on how babies are made. New information on toxic shock syndrome and treatment for dysmenorrhea needs to be made available (see Boxes 22-1 and 22-2). Perhaps more important is the opportunity for the community health school nurse to prepare young women for self-care, by informing them about routine gynecologic procedures. The first pelvic examination will be less traumatic or unpleasant if a girl has been taught what to expect. This knowledge can begin to help her feel more secure in health care relationships. In some cities, Feminist Women's Health Centers offer instruction in self-examination techniques, so women can become better acquainted with their bodies (Federation of Feminist Women's Health Centers, 1981).

Nurses may also help women by educating them about accidents at home, at work, and at leisure. For example, elderly women living alone often have throw rugs in their homes, which, on highly waxed or polished floors, may easily move and cause the woman to fall. Little girls who want to imitate and "help Mommy" could easily be injured in the kitchen by being burned or by pulling something down on their heads from a countertop.

Community health nurses can teach women how to keep useful health records for themselves and their families. For example, women can record their menstrual cycles, or when they or their children received immunizations or had diseases. In addition, they should keep records of their parents' health problems. This information may be invaluable to them when they have a health problem.

Nurses can teach women to become aware of the risk factors in their lives and to work to minimize or reduce them. For example, if a woman knows that her father had diabetes and heart dis-

Box 22-1 Toxic Shock Syndrome (TSS)

Although rare, TSS can be fatal, and young women (aged fifteen to nineteen) are somewhat more susceptible than other groups. Therefore, all girls should be familiar with the symptoms and know what to do if they occur during menstruation.

- *Cause* Source unknown. Bacterial infection. Associated with tampon use.
- *Symptoms* High fever, sunburnlike rash, hypotension (dizziness, fainting), and peeling skin—especially on palms and soles of feet.

- *Treatment* Remove tampon immediately, go to physician at once for diagnosis and treatment.
- *Prevention* Minimize use of superabsorbent tampons, reduce risk by using tampons interspersed with sanitary pads during menstruation, change tampons frequently, practice good hygiene—especially hand-washing (Institute of Medicine, 1982).

---

ease, she could be taught active measures, such as maintaining her normal body weight and limiting her salt intake, to decrease her risk of acquiring those diseases herself.

Some states require a home visit by a community health nurse for every newborn. These visits represent an entree to assessing health care needs for the mother or for other women in the family. They also provide an opportunity for teaching women about keeping health records for their infant, as well as for themselves, and other members of the family. Particularly important in this context is to address the stress of the postpartum period and to determine that there is enough support for the mother.

Community health nurses should be as concerned about women's mental health as they are about women's physical health. Women can improve their mental health by taking time for themselves. Just taking twenty minutes a day for herself in which to relax can have great benefit for a woman. Benson (1975) describes a variety of techniques that can be used for relaxation and stress management. Exercise, yoga, meditation, or self-defense or tai chi classes can be beneficial. Nurses can help women arrange their schedules so they can find the time to take for themselves.

The consciousness raising groups of the early women's movement have helped women value each other as women and appreciate networking with other women. Organizations such as the National Organization for Women, National Women's Health Network, and Feminist Women's Health Centers help women to come together for support or to receive printed information about topics of interest and concern to them.

Many of these organizations provide resource centers where women may come to read or where they can call or write to receive materials on a particular topic. Some of these places such as the Women's Health Exchange at the University of Illinois or Women's Health Resources at Illinois Masonic Medical Center (both in Chicago) provide materials for both professional and lay women. The Boston Women's Health Book Collective has become recognized as an international resource for women's health. These resource centers can be an important service for community health nurses themselves, as well as for client referrals.

Women who have been able to join with other women have learned ways to foster their health by working and learning together. Women's clinics and self-help groups have been developed across the country. Mostly middle-class white women developed these self-care clinics; poor white women and minority women have been underrepresented. Many of these clinics provide their services free of charge or on a sliding scale basis, so that poor women could be helped, but more must be done to get women to the clinics.

Box 22-2   Dysmenorrhea (Menstrual Cramps)

- *Cause* Currently thought to be related to excess uterine prostaglandins.
- *Symptoms* Abdominal cramps, usually beginning within hours of onset of menstruation. Pain typically decreases after twenty-four hours. Nausea, vomiting, diarrhea, headache, chills, flushes, and fatigue, due to other prostaglandin-related symptoms that are sometimes experienced.
- *Treatment* Self-care treatments include heating pad to abdomen, exercise, and knee-chest position. For severe symptoms, current treatment of choice is a prostaglandin inhibitor. One type (Ibuprofen) is available without a prescription. Others (Motrin, Postel, Anaprox) are prescription drugs. Contraindications include allergic sensitivity to aspirin or other prostaglandin inhibitors, and chronic stomach or intestinal problems, such as ulcers or colitis (Budoff, 1981).

Women's clinics are not available everywhere, particularly in rural areas. Community health nurses can work with community women to organize and operate such clinics (Milio, 1970), but one must not underestimate the time, energy, and skill that it takes to organize such a clinic with community women.

Female nurses are in a unique position whereby they can become regular members of women's groups and clinics—as women and as health professionals. Feminists have reacted against medicine and physicians, but often they do not have the same negative feelings against nurses (Boston Women's Health Book Collective, 1984). Nurses have much to offer such groups, but they must approach cautiously and find ways to help them equalize their power with the women in the groups. Nurses can also work to find ways to involve minority and poor women in these clinics and groups, and facilitate their membership. This may require community outreach and education.

Community health nurses can help women in choosing modes of health care. Many health care methods and approaches are used by women. Nurses can assist women in learning about both traditional and nontraditional methods of healing and health care. Many alternatives, such as acupressure, naprapathy, and rolfing, can be used alone or as adjuncts to traditional medical care (Weiss, 1984). The nurse should help the woman to consider her reasons for choosing an alternative, as well as the legal and ethical issues related to alternate forms of health care.

Nurses must be health advocates for women. In the community, advocacy can involve direct services such as helping a woman who wants to deliver her baby at home to explore the benefits and risks of this choice and to find certified nurse-midwives who can provide that service. Teaching breast self-examination to a women's group at a church is another type of direct community advocacy that a community health nurse can provide. Nurses might suggest that a woman seeking health care take a friend with her, so that if she feels afraid or becomes threatened, her friend can be prepared to advocate for her and ask the questions that she would if she were able. The nurse might also suggest preparing in advance a list of questions to ask.

Programs in some areas teach local community women to be health advocates for their peers. Community health nurses may be educators in these programs, and even more importantly, they can refer women to participate in such programs. Once the advocates are trained, nurses can use them in seeking out women who need more in-depth health care services than the advocates can give.

Health advocacy for women can also be indirect, political action. Nurses may lobby for women's concerns and health care issues in the political arena, and they can let it be known that they are nurses when they do. They may work for passage of legislation, such as health insurance and rape laws that will improve the health of women.

Other political activity for nurses includes being elected or appointed to the board of directors of agencies and other groups that are involved in the care of women, such as battered women's shelters. It is critical to bring a nurse's and a health perspective to many of these boards, which have very often consisted of physicians and other executives, who often are illness or disease oriented. Visibility of nurses and women is important in furthering the cause of Women's Health care.

A Women's Health Program In this section we'll discuss several approaches used in the development of the women's health program at the University of Illinois, and we'll show how these projects lead to new models of practice in women's health nursing. Each of the projects represents an approach to identifying and meeting health needs of women, using innovative models for nursing practice. They are examples of what a group of nursing faculty, students, and practitioners can create by working together and pooling their energies and expertise. They indicate directions for a new model of nursing practice that would emphasize the experiences of community women; communication among researchers, providers, and lay women; promotion of self-care; and mutual support among women in communities. The ultimate goal of all of these activities is promotion of health among women.

1. *Community Workshops.* Most basic to an effective program of services to women is the integration of research, theory, and practice. Recognizing the interdependence of these three functions, the group articulated a philosophy, stating that research in women's health should be based on concrete concerns expressed by consumers and providers in the community (Webster & Dan, 1984). It is equally important that results of research be available to community women for their evaluation and subsequent use. Thus, a strategy used by the Women's Health Group that may be useful for other women's health practitioners is the creation of forums for the exchange of ideas among researchers, practitioners, and consumers of women's health care.

Community workshops are an important way to begin such a dialogue. The subject matter may range from general women's health issues (Mackey, 1980b) to more specific topics, like breast cancer, menstrual problems, or coping with violence against women. Or they may address a more specific group of women such as high school women, black women, or older women. It is useful to provide time not only for sharing of information, but also for feedback, processing, and building on ideas and information presented.

A successful workshop in Chicago invited representatives from over 100 community groups to an all-day conference about research needs in women's health. The morning speakers focused on research issues for women and the uses of research in policy development and legislative decisions. The afternoon sessions provided small group discussions on a variety of women's health topics and were planned to identify research questions evolving from the ideas and concerns of community women. The proceedings of this workshop, which were published and distributed to participants, continue to provide information on woman-defined concerns that nurses should be addressing in practice and research (see Table 22-2).

2. *Consultation Sessions.* It is also worthwhile to make special efforts to gain views of practicing nurses in the community who are interested in women's health. A series of consultation sessions was held with the Women's Health Group and small groups of nurse clinical specialists whose interests included public health, midwifery, psychiatric nursing, breast cancer, parenting, and substance abuse (Mackey, 1980a). These discussions yielded significant insights on women's health needs in the community.

Table 22-2   Research Questions Generated by Community Women

Topics	Questions
Abused women, rape, and incest	1. How do socialization practices teach men a sense of entitlement? 2. Do parents who have incestuous relationships have children who repeat the pattern? 3. What is the context of husband abuse? Are women abusing men in self-defense? 4. Is pornography related to violence against women?
Aging (menopause and other issues)	1. What are the primary reasons of overmedication of the elderly? 2. What are the myths about aging? How do we effectively dispel myths about aging?
Birth experience	1. What criteria should consumers use in selecting a birth attendant? 2. What is continuity in maternity care? How is it measured and provided, and what is its outcome?
Cancer	1. How effective are alternative cancer treatments such as biofeedback and imagery? 2. How do practitioners' attitudes contribute to patients' development of guilt feelings about cancer diagnosis?
Parenting	1. What is the most effective way to teach birth control to teenagers? 2. Support systems (grandparents, friends, relatives) contribute to effective parenting. How is parenting affected by divorce or moving to a new area?
Preventive health (nutrition, occupational health hazards)	1. Women may be exposed to chemicals during their pregnancy. How long are these retained by the body in breast milk? 2. No one has identified the needs of pregnant women in industry. How much can they lift and carry? How long a break should they have? Are there dangers in eating machine food? (For example, is some food contaminated?)
Sexuality	1. How can we best respond to the active sexuality of twelve- and thirteen-year-olds? 2. How can we increase knowledge among health professionals about gay and lesbian life?
Teenage health issues	1. What meaning do adolescents attribute to structural educational experiences concerning birth control? 2. What are cultural attitudes concerning birth control? 3. How do cultural attitudes concerning birth control affect behavior?
Holistic health: alternative healing systems	1. What are ways of getting women involved in their own healing? 2. What are the outcomes when the healer involves the woman in the healing process?

The clinical specialists emphasized the community's need for accessible health care that is adapted to women's needs and nonjudgmental about their life-styles. Single or working mothers, for example, are sometimes made uncomfortable by health professionals' insensitivity to problems of arranging child care, or they may have difficulty scheduling visits to pediatricians during their nonworking hours. Other groups who may suffer from a lack of good health care include adolescents, lesbians, minority women, prostitutes, or other occupational groups, such as stewardesses.

A second emphasis of the clinical specialists was the need for education about prevention of disease, maintenance of health, and early case finding, rather than crisis intervention. Information and support are necessary in many areas, like breast self-examination, alcoholism, alternatives to traditional hospital births, coping with postpartum stress, and sexually transmitted diseases.

Finally, the clinical specialists stressed the importance of teaching women to be responsible consumers of health care. Effective self-help means that each woman knows what is normal for her, and when she needs professional help. Specific areas for self-care education include nutrition, relaxation and other ways of coping with stress, and first aid for children.

3.   *Health Advocacy and Career Awareness for Community Women.* Another project involved the development of a health advocacy training program. Recognizing the lack of access to health care for young, urban, minority, and low income women, the group designed a short-term program to present women's health care, health advocacy, and health career awareness. The purpose of the program was to increase the effective use of health services by training community women as health advocates. Participants were taught basic practices for health promotion and illness prevention. The concept of advocacy emphasized the knowledge and skills needed to function in that role. The

focus on career awareness introduced the trainees to the multiple positions and educational options available in health care.

Twenty-six trainees, between the ages of seventeen and twenty-one, completed the two-month program. The 145-hour training program included classroom sessions, field placements, group counselling, field trips, and independent assignments. The content and experiences in women's health included basic health practices, child and substance abuse, aging, mental health, rape, community resources, advocacy skills, assertiveness training, health skills for parents, self-defense, self-help, and health teaching and promotion. Each trainee was provided a physical assessment by a nurse practitioner, and each completed a computerized life-style and life expectancy index. The counselling sessions covered developing self and other awareness, communication skills, evaluating personal preferences, employment capabilities, planning for future health career training, and enhancing job-seeking skills.

Data gathered from trainees, project staff, and placement site staff indicated that the program provided a positive experience. The subject matter, reference materials, and resource networking provided a beginning level of knowledge and skill in women's health advocacy.

It is hoped that these three projects or approaches to women's health will stimulate community health nurses to use their creative energies and find other new and helpful approaches to the health care of women.

Secondary Prevention

Secondary prevention strategies involve early diagnosis and treatment to limit or stop the progression of already established diseases or injuries, preventing complications and sequelae, and limiting disability. While most of women's health care involves primary prevention, there are some secondary prevention strategies that community health nurses can use.

One of the most important secondary prevention strategies for community health nurses is health screening and case finding. Blood pressure screening is becoming a very popular procedure, and many community groups, as well as community health nurses, are providing this service in shopping malls, churches, and at health fairs. Blood pressure screening is a simple approach to preventing unnecessary deaths due to stroke. Black women are particularly at risk for hypertension, and nurses should always check blood pressures in these women (Richmond, 1983).

Teaching women to do breast self-examination is also a method of health screening, with the goal of early diagnosis and treatment for identified breast disease. Community health nurses should help women to view breast self-examination as an important self-care strategy that gives women control over their bodies.

Since stress is always present, and can become a health problem if a woman experiences too much stress or is unable to deal with it, community health nurses can help women by helping them learn ways to manage stress. Women can improve their health by avoiding undue stress and by learning to manage the normal stresses in their lives. They must become aware of their own tolerance level for stress and try to stay below that level. Women can use techniques such as biofeedback and self-hypnosis to help them in stress management (Weiss, 1984).

Women considering therapy should be helped to seek out nonsexist therapists. Some women may benefit most from feminist therapy (Johnson, 1980). Community health nurses can be helpful to women who desire therapy by making referrals to appropriate therapists.

Community services to help women include schools for adolescents who are pregnant or are new mothers. Such schools often have classes in health and care for the mothers, as well as classes in baby care. Other schools exist only for adolescents who have babies; in these schools daycare is provided for the babies, and child care classes are held for the mothers. Community health nurses can play a tremendous role in these schools in promoting the health of women and children.

A serious health problem of white middle- or upper-class adolescent women is anorexia nervosa. Community health nurses in schools, or other settings, may identify young women who have this problem and can refer them to appropriate facilities. Adolescents are apt to deny the problem, so identifying the problem may be difficult, but early diagnosis and treatment is critical to the future health of these young women. Community health nurses can educate school teachers and parents about prevention and early diagnosis of anorexia (Neuman & Halvorson, 1983).

Nurses are always neighbors, and as such, they are often called on to help neighbors in times of crisis. Nurses need not wait for crises, but can provide health education to their friends, neighbors, and families by being a good example of health and by providing resources about health for them. When a crisis does occur, and a nurse is called, he or she can later use the event as a health teaching example about first aid and/or use of emergency services. Nurses must decide, however, how available as professionals they wish to be without receiving remuneration for their services.

Nurses must work to change and improve the existing health care delivery system so that it better serves the needs of women. Nurses can help women be less afraid of the health care delivery system by educating and empowering them with self-care approaches and with ways to manage the system, thus demystifying it. Nurses should insist on sensitive, appropriate care for women—in the places and in the ways that women want and need.

One problem with the health care delivery system for women is access. There are many reasons why a "9 to 5" health care system does not meet the needs of many women. Women who work during those hours sometimes cannot afford to take time off from work; it may be difficult or impossible to make child care arrangements; or they may not have transportation to go at those times. Women's clinics try to meet these needs by being open during the evenings and on weekends when women may be more able to come.

Most of the situations in which community health nurses intervene are complex—involving issues of physical health and illness along with developmental and psychosocial concerns. Case Example 22-4 illustrates a community health nurse's involvement with a family over developmental and psychosocial concerns. In the course of providing ongoing care (secondary prevention), the nurse uses opportunities for health education, support for positive development and improved communication (primary prevention).

Tertiary Prevention

Tertiary prevention strategies are rehabilitative and are used to maintain an optimal level of health and functioning in a person with an irreversible health problem and to prevent unnecessary suffering or disability. Community health nurses are most likely to encounter these situations in home care for a woman with a chronic health problem.

Disabled women (for example, women who have had spinal cord injuries) may be found in all the settings where community health nurses work. Community health nurses should work with disabled women to make their situation more comfortable. Nurses can provide resources to disabled women and inform them about clinics where their unique needs can be met. Community health nurses can also work politically to help achieve a totally barrier-free environment, so that the lives of disabled women (and men) will be easier.

Certain chronic diseases, such as asthma, rheumatoid arthritis, thyroid conditions, and systemic lupus erythematosis are more common in women than in men. Community health nurses can work with women who have these diseases in ways that will help them maintain their health at the highest level possible.

Self-help groups may work at the level of tertiary prevention. Community health nurses may become involved as consultants in some of these groups such as postmastectomy groups, rape and incest victims, or mothers who abuse their children. They may also work in halfway houses for women who have been released from mental institutions. The challenge with these groups is to support them in their own self-enhancing efforts.

Community health nurses may become involved in helping families transfer an elderly member to a nursing home or a long-term facility. The nurse can help the family by teaching them about factors to consider when choosing the facility (Wallace, 1982). The nurse may also help both the family and the elderly woman by supporting them through the stress, grief, and guilt that may be involved in the process of such a move. Alternately, the nurse may provide support in helping families to keep an elderly member in the home.

Some hospice programs are managed by community health nurses who provide care to a dying person, as well as to the family members of that person. While hospice care is unique, the community health nurse may also have dying patients in a regular caseload. Providing sensitive, competent care to the entire family may provide access to the female members of the family for further women's health support and education.

Finally, some women who are full-time caregivers can use "respite services," which provide supervision and health care for the elderly and disabled. Such services are usually available during the day or continuously for short periods of time, such as while the women are on a vacation. Women can take their dependent elderly relatives or sick and disabled children to these respite centers. The persons will be well cared for and will benefit from the social stimulation they experience, while the women benefit from the "respite" and break they get from the continual responsibility of care. Although this is primary or secondary prevention for the women, it is tertiary prevention for the dependent person who is brought to the respite service.

Case Example 22-4: Assessment and Health Teaching with Three Generations of Women

Sarah, a community health nurse, is visiting Lydia, a thirty-five-year-old single mother. Lydia is raising her three children in her mother, Jo's, home while she works in a factory and goes to school to finish her GED. Lydia was just discharged from the hospital after having a cholecystectomy.

Community health nurse makes home visit with post-surgery patient.

Lydia is recovering well, but Sarah learns that she is worried about her twelve-year-old daughter, Lisa, because of her moodiness around home and her irritability with her younger siblings. Lisa has recently begun to be concerned about changes in her body and has been refusing to join the family for dinner because she is on a "diet."

Assessment: Nurse obtains information on family members.

Sarah discovers that Lydia has not discussed with Lisa the significance of her body changes and the sexuality issues that accompany early adolescence, such as breast changes and menstruation.

Nurse identifies need for open communication between mother and daughter.

Sarah encourages Lydia to discuss her own ideas about pubertal changes and the ways she learned about her sexuality. Lydia always felt uncomfortable talking with her own mother about such things and does not want Lisa to get incorrect information. Sarah discusses the myths and realities of menstruation with Lydia and encourages her to ask Lisa what she has heard about "becoming a woman." She also leaves some educational pamphlets about menstruation and sexuality for both Lydia and Lisa to read and discuss.

Nurse encourages and facilitates open communication and provides information.

On her next visit to Lydia's family, Sarah learns that Lydia and her daughter have had several conversations about menstruation, and since the last visit, Lisa has begun to menstruate. Her periods, however, have not been regular, and Lydia is not sure whether to believe her mother who insists that irregular periods are a sign that Lisa is sexually active with boys. She is also unsure about advising Lisa on the use of tampons since her mother believes such use will predispose her to early sexual activity as a result of taking away her "virginity." Lisa has responded to these accusations with anger and withdrawal.

Nurse identifies misunderstanding about menstruation.

Sarah takes this opportunity to discuss with Lydia her own sexual history and the relationship she has with her mother. Lydia asks many questions about normal anatomy and physiology and choices of birth control for herself. Jo and Lisa are invited to join in the discussion; Sarah asks them questions about their beliefs and values related to sexuality.

Implementation: Nurse teaches women about physical development, sexuality, contraception, and menstruation, and facilitates open discussion among them.

Sarah visits the family several months later and learns from Lydia that, although Lisa is having many of the usual concerns about being an adolescent, they are now able to talk with each other about problems. Sarah supports the open communication that had developed among the women. She determines that Lydia knows where to obtain additional information on sexuality, as well as resources for her own contraceptive needs.

Because of the effective preventive measures used earlier, the nurse observes optimal functioning and lack of additional problems among family members.

Sarah also checks Lydia's mother's blood pressure for hypertension screening and Lydia's continued progress of recovery from cholecystectomy surgery.

Secondary prevention: Nurse conducts monitoring and follow-up.

Summary

Women's health has traditionally referred to obstetric and gynecologic medical practice. A contemporary women's health perspective is very broad and places nurses in a primary position to assist women with promoting and maintaining their health. A majority of clients seen by community health nurses are women, and thus community health nurses must be especially sensitive to and knowledgeable about the special health needs and concerns that women have. This chapter has presented many of those concerns as well as strategies for community health nurses to use in providing women's health care.

The nursing profession is in an excellent position to coordinate efforts of many different groups, both professional and lay, such as nursing alumni associations, businesswomen's groups, and support groups for young mothers, who have an interest in women's health. As a profession composed primarily of women, nurses are also major consumers of health care who understand the problems of female clients. The field of women's health presents a unique potential for nursing to demonstrate leadership in the community.

Topics for Nursing Research

• Compare the health needs of midlife women with those of older women from the perspective of women themselves.
• Explore the concept of networking as it is implemented between professionals and lay-women consumers in a health center designed for women.
• What support systems are needed by wife-mothers who work outside the home?
• What is the relationship between stress, poverty, and physical illness among adult women?
• What do preadolescent females ten to four-teen years old know about their bodies including sexual development and menstruation?

Study Questions

1. Which of the following is *not* a significant aspect of a women's health approach?
   a. Primary concern is for women's reproductive health.
   b. Women's experience involves a variety of health-related roles.
   c. Women of all ages are included.
   d. An emphasis is on health maintenance.
2. A community health nurse involved with sharing information about self-examination, nutrition, and exercise at a feminist women's health center is most likely to subscribe to which of these political strategies?
   a. Liberal feminist
   b. Socialist feminist
   c. Radical feminist
   d. A combination of the three
3. A self-care approach to women's health care is primarily based on the conceptual framework of which nursing theorist?
   a. Martha Rogers
   b. Dorothea Orem
   c. Betty Neuman
   d. Sister Callista Roy
4. A community health nurse conducts an aerobic exercise class at a senior citizen's center. This would be an example of which level of prevention?
   a. Primary
   b. Secondary
   c. Tertiary
   d. Could include all levels of prevention for various women in the class
5. How can community health nurses become women's health practitioners with a feminist perspective?
   a. By identifying themselves as feminists
   b. By recognizing the significance of women's experiences and special health care concerns and working with women to help achieve them
   c. By becoming members of boards of directors of women's organizations

d. By lobbying state and federal legislators about issues and bills of importance to health care delivery

6. Why is research important for women's health care?

   a. Because it is important for all nursing practice to be research-based

   b. To provide a basis for developing nursing curricula

   c. To help women learn about and maintain their own health

   d. All of the above

References

Anand A: Reshaping the economy: Can women afford to stay out? Paper presented at National Women's Studies Association. Columbus, Ohio, June 1983.

Benson H: *The Relaxation Response.* New York: Avon, 1975.

Blaxall M, Reagan B (editors): *Women and the Workplace: The Implications of Occupational Segregation.* Chicago: University of Chicago Press, 1976.

Block JH: Socialization influences on personality development in males and females. Paper presented at American Psychological Association Master Lecture Series on Issues of Sex and Gender in Psychology. New York, September 1979.

Boston Women's Health Book Collective: *The New Our Bodies, Ourselves.* New York: Simon and Schuster, 1984.

Brooks-Gunn J, Ruble D: Menarche: The interaction of physiological, cultural, and social factors In: Dan AJ, Graham EA, Beecher CP (editors), *The Menstrual Cycle,* Vol. 1. New York: Springer, 1980.

Broverman IK et al: Sex-role stereotypes and clinical judgments of mental health. *J Consult Clin Psychol* 1970; 34 (1): 1–7.

Bruch H: *The Golden Cage.* Cambridge, Mass.: Harvard University Press, 1978.

Budoff PW: *No More Menstrual Cramps and Other Good News.* New York: Penguin, 1981.

Calderone MS, Johnson EW: *The Family Book about Sexuality.* New York: Harper & Row, 1981.

Chodorow N: *The Reproduction of Mothering.* Berkeley: University of California Press, 1978.

Corea G: *The Hidden Malpractice,* Updated ed. New York: Harper & Row, 1985.

Crovitz E, Steinmann A: A decade later: Black-white attitudes toward women's familial role. *Psychology of Women Quarterly* 1980; 5 (2): 170–176.

Dan AJ: Abortion and women's health: Responsibility of nurses. In: McCloskey JC, Grace HK (editors), *Current Issues in Nursing.* Boston: Blackwell Scientific Publications, 1981.

Dan AJ, Beekman S: Male versus female representation in psychological research. *Am Psychol* 1978; 27: 1972.

Federation of Feminist Women's Health Centers: *A New View of a Woman's Body.* New York: Touchstone, 1981.

Fee E: Women and health care: A comparison of theories. In: Fee E (editor), *Women and Health: The Politics of Sex in Medicine.* Farmingdale, N.Y.: Baywood, 1983.

Fleming J: Sex differences in the educational and occupational goals of black college students: Continued inquiry into the black matriarchy theory In: Horner M, Nadelson CC, Notman MT (editors), *The Challenge of Change.* New York: Plenum, 1983.

Gelein JL, Heiple P: Aging. In: Fogel CI, Woods NF (editors), *Health Care of Women: A Nursing Perspective.* St. Louis: Mosby, 1981.

Gerson MJ, Alpert JL, Richardson MS: Mothering: The view from psychological research. *Signs: Journal of Women in Culture and Society* 1984; 9(3): 434–453.

Gilligan C: *In a Different Voice: Psychological Theory and Women's Development.* Cambridge, Mass.: Harvard University Press, 1982.

Gold AR, Brush LR, Sprotzer ER: Developmental changes in self-perceptions of intelligence and self-confidence. *Psychology of Women Quarterly* 1980; 5 (2): 231–239.

Gordon VC, Ledray LE: Depression in Women. *J Psychosoc Nurs* 1985; 23 (1): 26–34.

Gove WR: Sex roles, marital roles, and mental illness. *Social Forces* 1972; 51 (1): 34–44.

Graduate Nursing Concentration in Women's Health (mimeograph). Women's Health Exchange, University of Illinois at Chicago, n.d.

Gritz ER: Cigarette smoking by adolescent females: Implications for health and behavior. *Women and Health* 1984; 9 (2/3): 103–115.

Guttentag M, Secord PF: *Too Many Women?* Beverly Hills, Calif.: Sage, 1983.

Hartman HI: The family as the locus of gender, class, and political struggle: The example of housework. *Signs: Journal of Women in Culture and Society* 1981; 6 (3): 366–394.

Hoffman LW, Nye FI: *Working Mothers.* San Francisco: Jossey-Bass, 1974.

Holmes HB, Hoskins B, Gross M: *Custom-made Child.* Boston: Humana, 1980.

Institute of Medicine: *Toxic Shock Syndrome.* Washington, DC: National Academy Press, 1982.

Johnson M: Mental Illness and psychiatric treatment among women: A response. *Psychology of Women Quarterly* 1980; 4 (3): 363–371.

Kasper AS, Soldinger E: Falling between the cracks: How health insurance discriminates against women. *Women and Health* 1983; 8 (4): 77–93.

Levin LS: Patient education and self-care: How do they differ? *Nurs Outlook* 1978; 26 (3): 170–175.

Lewittes H: Women's development in adulthood and old age: A review and critique. *International Journal of Mental Health* 1982; 11 (1–2): 115–134.

Mackey M: Nurse consultation to the Women's Health Research Group on the topic of the Women's Health Exchange. Unpublished manuscript. Chicago: University of Illinois, 1980a.

Mackey M (editor): *Women's Health Research: An Exchange of Ideas.* Proceedings of a conference. Chicago: University of Illinois, June 1980b.

MacKinnon CA: *Sexual Harassment of Working Women.* New Haven, Conn.: Yale University Press, 1979.

Mangold MM (editor): *La causa Chicana.* New York: Family Service Association of America, 1972.

Marieskind HI: *Women in the Health System: Patients, Providers, and Programs.* St. Louis: Mosby, 1980.

McBride AB, McBride WL: Theoretical underpinnings for women's health. *Women and Health* 1982; 6 (1/2): 37–55.

McElmurry BJ et al: Proposal: Institute for research on women's health. Unpublished manuscript, Chicago, 1980.

McElmurry BJ, Glass L, Egan E: Health assessment of older women using self-report data. Paper presented at American Nurses' Association Council of Nurse Researchers. Washington, DC, September 1981.

Money J, Ehrhardt AA: *Man and Woman, Boy and Girl.* Baltimore: Johns Hopkins University Press, 1972.

Moore EC (editor): Women and health, United States 1980. *Public Health Reports* 1980; 95 (Supplement to the September-October issues): 1–85.

Mulligan JE: Some effects of the women's health movement. *Topics in Clinical Nursing* 1983; 4 (4): 1–9.

Neuman PA, Halvorson PA: *Anorexia Nervosa and Bulemia.* New York: Van Nostrand Reinhold, 1983.

Orem DE: *Nursing: Concepts of Practice,* 3rd ed. New York: McGraw-Hill, 1985.

Pearce D: The feminization of poverty. Paper presented to Women In Poverty Conference. Chicago, May 1982.

Peck WA: National Institutes of Health Consensus Development Conference Statement: Osteoporosis. Bethesda, Md., April 1984.

Reid PT: Socialization of black female children. In: Berman PW, Ramey ER (editors), *Women: A Developmental Perspective.* NIH Publication No. 82-2298. Washington, DC: US Department of Health and Human Services, 1982.

Report of the Public Health Service Task Force on Women's Health Issues. *Public Health Reports* 1985; 100: 73–106.

Richmond J: The silent killer: High blood pressure. *National Women's Health Network News* 1983; 8 (3): 3.

Rorvik DM, Shettles LB: *Your Baby's Sex: Now You Can Choose.* New York: Dodd, Mead, 1970.

Rourke S: How to choose a nursing home. *National Women's Health Network News* 1984; 9 (2): 11.

Rubin LB: *Women of a Certain Age.* New York: Harper, 1979.

Schuster I: Review article: Recent research on women in development. *Journal of Development Studies* 1982; 18 (4): 511–535.

Scully D: *Men Who Control Women's Bodies.* Boston: Houghton Mifflin, 1980.

Seidler S: ERT: Drug company sales vs. women's health. *National Women's Health Network News* 1984; 9 (2): 7.

Stack C: *All Our Kin.* New York: Harper, 1974.

Staples R, Mirande A: Racial and cultural variations among American families: A decennial review of the literature on minority families. *Journal of Marriage and the Family* 1980; 12 (1): 887–903.

Vanek J: Time spent in housework. *Sci Am* 1974; 231 (5): 116–120.

Verbrugge LM: Women's social roles and health. In: Berman PW, Ramey ER (editors), *Women: A Developmental Perspective.* NIH Publication No. 82-2298. Washington, DC: US Department of Health and Human Services, 1982.

Wallace MT: Before you consider a nursing home. *Network News* 1982; 7 (5): 9.

Webb C, Wilson-Barnett J: Self-concept, social support and hysterectomy. *Int J Nurs Stud* 1983; 20 (2): 97–107.

Webster D, Dan AJ: Development of a graduate concentration in women's health nursing, or "what is women's health and what does it have to do with nursing?" Unpublished manuscript. Chicago: University of Illinois, 1984.

Weiss K (editor): *Women's Health Care: A Guide to Alternatives.* Reston, Va: Reston, 1984.

White C, Bales J: Coal miners say lives are threatened. *Network News* 1983; 8 (1): 3.

Williams JH: *Psychology of Women: Selected Readings.* New York: Norton, 1979.

Williamson NE: Sex preferences, sex control, and the status of women. *Signs: Journal of Women in Culture and Society* 1976a; 1 (4): 847–862.

Williamson NE: *Sons or Daughters? A Cross-Cultural Study of Parental Preferences.* Beverly Hills, Calif.: Sage, 1976b.

World Health Organization: Health and the status of women. Paper prepared for the World Conference of the United Nations Decade for Women: Equality, Development, and Peace. Copenhagen, Denmark, July 1980.

Young drinkers: New survey on alcoholics. *Network News* 1982; 7 (5): 5.

Chapter 23

Health of Older Adults

Lucille Davis

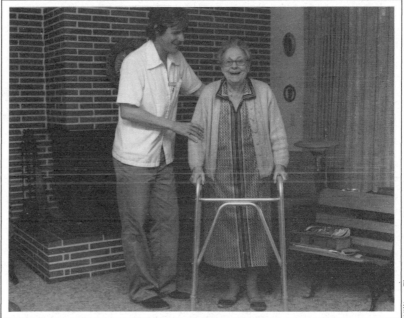

William Thompson

In working with elderly clients, the goals of community health include preventing unnecessary physical and psychosocial decline and facilitating social interaction, wellness, and dignity.

Chapter Outline

Chapter Objectives

After completing this chapter, the reader will be able to:

- Describe demographic trends of the aging population and their relationship to health needs and health care of the elderly
- Discuss and compare biological and psychosocial theories of aging
- Identify health care policies that affect health of the elderly
- Explain the importance of ethnic group identity in older adults
- Describe developmental tasks of the elderly
- Discuss the community health nurse's role in promoting health and wellness among the elderly
- Identify and describe common health problems of older adults
- Outline the family's role in health promotion of older family members
- Give examples of primary, secondary, and tertiary prevention strategies community health nurses can use in care of older adults

Our society is undergoing a demographic revolution precipitated by a dramatic increase in the older population. As a separate demographic group, the aged are becoming a visible majority instead of an invisible minority. The number and proportion of individuals past sixty will have a major impact on social and health systems well into the next century (Sommers & Fabian, 1981, p. 1).

Aging and Society

The changing demographic picture becomes clear when analyzed historically. The first American census in 1870 indicated that fewer than 20 percent of the population lived to reach the age of seventy. Currently more than 80 percent can expect to do so. It is predicted that the older population will probably approach 30 million by the year 2000. Increased life expectancy has occurred gradually over the last century in the United States. Life expectancy can be differentiated from life span, which refers to the greatest number of years any species has been known to survive. The life span of humans is between 110 and 120 years. Over the past century, the life expectancy of many persons appears to be drawing closer to the current human life span (Quadango, 1981).

The increase in longevity has influenced definitions and perceptions of old age. Neugarten (1974) indicates that later life can be divided into two distinct age categories: the young-old (fifty-five to seventy-five) and the old-old (seventy-five and over). She viewed each age category as having different needs and perspectives. As the health status of the aged improves and longevity increases, the latter half of the cycle may be further redefined according to the following age categories: very young old, fifty-one to sixty; young-old, sixty-one to seventy; middle-aged old, seventy-one to eighty; very old-old, ninety-one to one hundred; and elite-old, one hundred and over (Kelly, 1985). Regardless of the names given to each category, it is important to remember that aging is a continuous, complex process that begins with conception.

It is interesting to note that stereotypes of the aged are primarily based on images of the old-old, although this age group currently does not consti-tute the majority of older individuals. The young-old constitute about 15 percent (31 million) of the aged population. According to Neugarten, the young-old are relatively healthy, well educated, and politically active, and they perform traditional responsibilities for work and family. In contrast, the old-old constitute less than 4 percent of the aged population. In the old-old group, the probability of illness, especially health problems of a chronic nature, increases, and many of them require supportive social services and special features in the physical environment to facilitate maximum functioning. For all people there is a need for preventive care to prevent unnecessary physical and psychosocial decline and to facilitate social interaction and feelings of dignity.

Definitions of Aging

We live in an era characterized by rapid changes in technology and knowledge. Therefore, the norms and definitions of old age have undergone significant change. As a result, society's current treatment of, and programs for, the aged are based on outmoded definitions and false assumptions. For example, the use of the chronological age of sixty-five as the beginning of "old age" is patterned after Bismarck, the chancellor of Germany in 1880, who tried to promote social programs for the working class and demonstrate the government's concern for the aged through old-age pensions. Our Social Security system was based on Bismarck's plan and was instituted during the Depression as a means of assisting the poor and those unable to work. At the time, the selection of sixty-five as the beginning of old age was appropriate since individuals in the majority of western countries did not survive beyond this age. From a historical perspective, programs for the aged such as Social Security were politically functional or expedient because only a minority of persons would survive long enough to take full advantage of these social programs. This is in contrast to the present social scene where longevity has become a reality for more people; as a result, there is a current economic crisis where the viability of programs for the aged such as Social Security and Medicare is threatened.

A program such as our Social Security system reinforces a static definition of old age and views the aged as a homogeneous group. However, the aged, like other age groups, are characterized by considerable variability in health status and life experience. A more accurate measure of age might be the adage "you are as old as you feel." Some individuals are "old" at fifty, others are not "old" at ninety. As Kelly suggests, "physiology, not chronology—how one feels—not what the calendar says, is the true measure of age" (Kelly, 1985, p. 159). The focus on chronological age does not allow one to identify and appreciate the impact of changing social cultural factors on older persons. Ebersole and Hess (1981, p. 9) suggest, "Perhaps the greatest change has been the rapidity of change. Older persons have been catapulted through numerous socioscientific periods—the Victorian Age, an agrarian age, the atomic age, and into the space age and the microelectronic age—in a single life span." It is also useful to identify events that occur throughout life and influence the aging process. For example, the interaction of individual events such as disease and trauma, which occur randomly but accumulate with longer life, impact on how individuals age. It is also necessary to separate the effect of age per se on conditions related to age-disease interactions.

Nurses who provide health care for the aged need to understand the complex nature of aging in order to address issues pertinent to normal aging, as well as problems associated with age-related diseases such as chronic illness. For example, there is an association between cancers and environmental factors such as pollution and radiation to which people of all ages are exposed. It is obvious, however, that older persons have been exposed to these environmental hazards longer. This greater exposure, coupled with biological changes in older people, such as the breakdown of the immune system, makes them more vulnerable. Therefore, we can see that old age alone does not cause cancer, but that such diseases can be considered age-related (Engelhardt, 1977).

Aging and Health Policy

The most important factor shaping health policy for the aged is the future demographic profile in the United States. Ball (1981) presents the following facts: (1) In the next twenty-five years the ratio of the number of persons sixty-five and over to those between twenty and sixty-four is expected to increase only slightly and (2) in the years 2005 to 2030, the number of persons sixty-five and over will increase significantly from about 35 million to over 60 million. Therefore it seems that the dependency ratio will increase so that each productive worker may need to support more and more nonworkers, resulting in a shift of resources toward the nonworkers. The dilemma society must face is related to the number of retired elderly, the number of workers and their productivity versus the number of nonworkers, and how much of our national resources we wish to allocate to health care for all age groups in general, and the aged specifically (Ball, 1981).

The nation's early response to health care of the aged was the passage of Medicare in 1965. A goal of this program was to provide major protection against the cost of medical care for the aged. In the words of President Johnson: "Never again would older people have to go without medical care; nor would they or their children be bankrupt in the process of obtaining that care" (Ball, 1981, p. 21). Although Medicare as a national health insurance for the elderly succeeded in protecting older persons against expensive hospital care, it created more problems than it solved. The total plan was much more expensive than anticipated. For example, "the inflation of medical care costs and gaps in the program resulted in older people spending twice as much for medical care in 1977 as they spent in 1966 before Medicare took effect" (Ball, 1981, p. 22).

Furthermore, Medicare focused only on acute *medical* care rather than *health* care. The medical system that is supported by Medicare is based on "sick care" rather than health care. Thus, it perpetuates the stereotype of aged persons as "sick." Although Medicare pays for medical care including doctors, hospitalization, and drugs, it is only partially effective, because the areas paid for are not primary determinants of health for the elderly. Most people over sixty-five are in good health; only 15 percent require assistance with activities of daily living and only about 5 percent are institutionalized. Therefore a primary goal of a national health policy for the aged should be to promote and maintain physical and psychosocial health.

From a preventive perspective, a health policy for the aged needs to encompass the younger ages and be a part of a broad plan to promote health for the nation. Health in the later years is contingent upon health habits and behaviors individuals practice before the age of sixty-five. Factors such as a safe work environment, healthful life-styles including adequate nutrition and exercise, and an ability to cope with life stressors are important in promoting health throughout life. Health care for the aged should also include a mechanism for ensuring adequate income to provide essential resources basic to health such as adequate nutrition, housing, and clothing. More importantly, a secure income is important for mental health. Retired aged persons who may have little savings or opportunity to replenish depleted resources may lose self-esteem and independence. Furthermore, current policy may force older people into poverty since they are not eligible for assistance until they "spend down" or use all of their financial resources such as savings or their homes.

Health care policies that would broaden health care for the aged to include support for nursing and social services are needed. Planning for long-term health care of aged persons must consider available choices that are congruent with individuals' needs. In addition health care strategies must take into account both the social and health dimensions of long-term care since these aspects are inseparable.

A classic example is provided in the area of homemaker services. Such services are not paid for by Medicare if the person has not been hospitalized; people are eligible for such services only if they are part of a physician-approved plan that is linked to skilled nursing care or some type of therapy such as physical or speech therapy. This represents a major problem, since in many cases someone to assist with chores or activities of daily living can actually *prevent* institutionalization of many older persons, which is a more expensive form of care.

Although we have elements of a long-term care policy in place, we have not put the pieces together in a coordinated way. We do not have the range or continuum of coordinated programs for the aged, which should range from home-based to institutional care. For example, long-term institutional care can range in practice from group or communal living with availability of backup medical, nursing-social services for those who can largely care for themselves through a variety of more individual arrangements designed for persons with different degrees of functional ability. An ideal plan for aged persons should be based on a consideration for all options—institutional and noninstitutional—depending upon the needs of the person. Moreover, people should be able to move from setting to setting as their level of need changes. Unfortunately, current planning usually involves making a choice between institutionalization and home or community which may not always be a very pleasant choice. Regardless of the setting or care options, emphasis should be on intervention and prevention. Intervention is direct care in response to an actual problem. In contrast, prevention occurs without the belief that something is wrong. In this case, there is an attempt to delay or prevent illness. A comprehensive health care policy for the aged would support both types of care inside and outside institutions.

Although there are settings providing the full range of services at a specific location, the usual procedure is for persons to be grouped together in skilled homes and/or intermediate facilities. Adequate support for coordinated services for the aged will become even more important in the future, especially for persons seventy-five years old and older, since this group is increasing more rapidly than the younger aged population (sixty-five to seventy-five). According to Ball, (1981, p. 27), "We need to increase the availability of social and medical services that help elderly people maintain their own private living arrangements as long as they can and want to, and we also need to provide more and better group residences and long term nursing homes, both intermediate and skilled."

Advances in medical technology have extended the length of life but have, at the same time, raised questions about the quality of life in old age. A large part of medical expenditures are spent for services rendered to older persons in the last few days of life in a hospital. Although these expenditures may be worthwhile in terms of returning some people to useful functioning, in many cases it may simply prolong a painful death. Therefore, a complex question that has ethical and legal ramifications is, "How much of what we are doing for older people in the last year of life really contributes to a life that is worthwhile, or is it simply a small extension of an entirely unsatisfactory existence?" (Ball, 1981, p. 33). We need a policy that supports services that provide humane and sensitive services to older persons regardless of their needs and conditions. Unfortunately, care provided outside acute medical settings is defined as "custodial care," because "a cure" is not possible. Prevention and psychosocial or rehabilitative care may be seen by governmental and private insurers as undeserving of health care resources. This view needs to be changed if the quality of life for aged persons is to improve.

Changes in policy for the aged will need to be addressed in relation to costs. Several social changes may potentially control costs and enhance the quality of life for the aged at the same time. It is predicted that future cohorts of older people will be healthier and more educated. In addition, there is greater support for persons who may wish to work beyond sixty-five years old. These factors will not only be good for the economy but will make it possible to support better programs for social services, health, and income security for increasing numbers of aged people. Cost containment concerns are pushing providers and institutions to consider alternatives and options for older people such as home care, daycare, and the use of informal networks of friends, neighbors, and volunteers to support and enhance resources for the aged.

The cost of long-term care and how to pay for it remains a central issue. Currently, the reimbursement system determines the philosophy and delivery of care. This view must be reversed so that reimbursements can be based on definitions of care as well as cost analysis. Moreover, the issue of need versus age must be addressed in restructuring policies and programs so as to avoid programs that are based solely on age. If benefits are targeted for those who have the greatest need, regardless of age, the quality and quantity of health service can increase for everyone.

Theories of Aging

Although gerontology is a relatively new field, a variety of theories have emerged to explain the phenomenon of aging. While there is no single explanation for the human aging process, models or frameworks of aging are based on biological and psychosocial theories. A brief overview of both types of theories are presented. The discussion of psychosocial theories is more detailed because such theories are most useful to understanding life-style and nursing care of the older adult in the family and community.

Biological Theories

There are a variety of theories about why and how the body ages. Examples of two popular biological theories are the Wear and Tear and Autoimmune theories.

Wear and Tear Theory The Wear and Tear theory asserts that the body, like a machine, eventually wears out. This approach has been used to understand various degenerative aspects of aging as well as the multiple rates of deterioration. This explanation is based on the idea that the essential ingredients of the life process essentially "run out"; thus the body eventually dies (Hickey, 1980).

Autoimmune Theory The basic premise of this theory is that, as age increases, there is an increase in mutations in cell divisions and that the body responds to those mutations as foreign matter. In an attempt to neutralize the mutations, antibodies are produced, resulting in an autoimmune response. Although autoimmune responses are intended to be adaptive (self-protecting), in the process of producing these responses the body essentially destroys itself (Crandall, 1980).

Another aspect of this theory is related to the notion that the body's immune system, which consists of the white blood cells and antibodies, declines as the body ages. Thus with increasing age, the person's immunity to disease also decreases (Hickey, 1980).

Psychosocial Theories

Four types of psychosocial theories are disengagement, activity, continuity, and socioenvironmental. As we will see, no one theory can stand alone to explain aging.

Disengagement Theory The most persistent and controversial theory is disengagement theory. The theory postulates that the aging process is a period of inevitable withdrawal, characterized by decreased interaction between the aging person and others in his or her social environment. This withdrawal (or disengagement) allows the individual to prepare for incapacitating diseases or even death (Cox, 1984). A major assumption of this theory is that the disengagement is mutually beneficial to the individual as well as to society. As health and energy decline, the individual is allowed to withdraw from previous work roles, the pressures of social life, and high level performance and productivity. Society benefits from the higher productivity of younger, energetic, recently trained persons who can assume the critical roles once held by older, presumably less capable persons (Cox, 1984).

Disengagement theory has four basic characteristics (Crandall, 1980):

1. Disengagement does not happen suddenly. It is a gradual process, reflected by the decline in the number and intensity of roles that occur with increasing age.
2. Disengagement is an inevitable, universal process—a normal part of the social structure of society.
3. Disengagement is mutually satisfying for the individual and society in that the individual is able to relinquish selected social roles and society can prepare others to fill these roles.
4. Disengagement as a normative process is reinforced by laws and policies, such as mandatory retirement.

To date, findings from testing of this theory have been contradictory. For example, some research suggests that it is not age itself, but age-related losses such as poor health and loss of friends and income, that bring about disengagement. Critics also argue that there is no proof that withdrawal of older people from vital social roles is good for society, because there is always the danger that the most knowledgeable, capable, and experienced people are removed from vital roles involuntarily.

Second, if disengagement is abrupt (for example, mandatory retirement), older people may be left with no substitute roles, a loss of self-esteem, and undue preoccupation with self and even death (Cox, 1984).

Although many older adults experience declining health and energy levels and decrease their life spaces as they become less mobile, many aged persons remain healthy and active to their deaths. Thus the theory explains only a limited aspect of the aging experience.

Activity Theory To a great extent, activity theory is the antithesis of disengagement theory since it maintains that the relationship between the social system and the individual remains fairly stable as the individual moves from middle to old age (Cox, 1984). This theory emphasizes the stability of the personality system as an individual moves into old age. Thus there is no need to compensate for loss, such as retirement from social roles, as a person moves into old age. In fact, except for biological changes, the elderly are considered essentially the same as middle-aged people and should maintain as long as possible the activities and attitudes of the middle years. Their social and psychological needs are essentially the same, and consequently, older people can and should find substitutes for activities they are forced to give up.

Proponents of activity theory contend that old age is a continuation of life, and people who age successfully are those who remain engaged, active, and productive and retain a viable social network and a positive orientation toward work and social responsibilities. They "wear out rather than rust out" (Cox, 1984). As with disengagement theory, this theory is limited in that it does not explain the variation of activity and life satisfaction observed among the aged.

Continuity Theory This theory takes the perspective that, as they age, people attempt to maintain continuity in their habits, commitments, and preferences consistent with their personalities. This theory integrates the intrapsychic develop-

mental changes expressed in disengagement theory as well as the assumption that activity enhances the well-being of many aged persons.

In contrast to disengagement and activity theory, however, continuity theory emphasizes the unique and personal factors within the individual's biography that impact on adaptive patterns, or the way the person ages. The focus of this theory is on diversity and the various ways persons adjust and cope with age-related changes.

Socioenvironmental Theory In response to the limitations of disengagement and activity theories, Gubrium (1973) developed the socioenvironmental theory of aging. This theory has three components:

1. *Normative* component, which involves behavior expectations shared by persons in social situations
2. *Individual* component based on the amount of behavioral flexibility people have in terms of their resources such as health and money
3. *Personal* component in which persons consider the meanings that norms and their individual activities have for themselves and their interactions with others

This theory is holistic because it integrates both individual (aged persons) and social (environmental) contexts. Morale or coping of aged persons is viewed as related to the person's activity resources (health, financial solvency, and social support) and the activity norms in the environment. Problems result when an aged person's resources are not congruent with the norms or expectations of their environments.

This brief discussion of theories (biological and psychosocial) does not adequately explain the multifactorial and dynamic nature of aging. To capture the reality of aging persons it is necessary to view them from their unique and personal histories, and also to look at the influences of other factors such as ethnicity.

Ethnicity and Aging

An appreciation of the cultural diversity of the aged is a relatively new phenomenon. Prior to 1950, emphasis was placed on the aged as a homogeneous group with common needs. There was little attempt to distinguish the aged in terms of race, ethnic group membership, religion, social class, level of education, gender, or other factors that influence adaptation or responses to aging (Crandall, 1980). It was not until the early 1960s that the aged were recognized in the gerontological literature as a culturally heterogeneous group. Since the 1960s more effort has been made to identify and analyze various subgroups within the elderly population. There has been a proliferation of literature on various ethnic groups such as Black Americans, Native Americans, Asian Americans, and Hispanic Americans. (See also Chapter 5 of this text.) Therefore this section will not discuss these cultural groups, but will present some concepts important for understanding ethnicity and aging.

We live in a pluralistic society. There are currently over 100 different ethnic groups within this country. Eleven million people living in America are foreign born, and about one-third still prefer their native language (Place, 1981). Since the way individuals experience and define aging is inextricably linked to cultural heritage, it is important to understand the ethnic background of aged persons as well as the culture in which they were socialized. Ethnicity, which encompasses culture, provides a basis for understanding behavior and attitudes of ethnic aged through identifying the culturally conditional beliefs, values, and attitudes of their heritage (Yurick, Robb, & Ebert, 1984). As discussed in Chapter 5, ethnicity refers to a shared history, a sense of group consciousness, and distinct customs transmitted from older to younger generations, which provides a focus for identity and group activity. Thus ethnicity is a source of identity and history for aged persons (Place, 1981).

Which has the greatest impact on aging—ethnic origins or other social factors? One approach argues that the consequences of growing old are so significant that they overshadow other types of status that have been important throughout life such as class, socioeconomic status, and education. A second, more accepted view suggests that there are multiple factors influencing the lives of aged persons, and other factors, such as social class, may be confounded with ethnicity. Some processes (such as some physiological changes) are normal and universal and unaffected by ethnicity. However, the importance of learning and the environment increase the likelihood that ethnicity is also a meaningful variable (Place, 1981). Although older persons are inclined to maintain ethnic patterns, they are able to be flexible in crossing ethnic boundaries if necessary to satisfy certain needs such as friendship and social activities. Some aged persons have been discriminated against throughout their lives because of their race and, therefore, arrive at old age disadvantaged in terms of income, education, and access to health care. These people are in a kind of "double jeopardy" as a result of race and age discrimination. Some aged persons are considered to be in triple or quadruple jeopardy if they are old, poor, minority group members, and female (Yurick, Robb, & Ebert, 1984).

Although ethnic identity may increase with age, it is necessary to appreciate similarities as well as the cultural differences that exist between and within aged ethnic groups. Nurses need to know the meaning of ethnicity from each person's perspective. Ethnic age peers become significant for the aged as they seek order, meaning, and definitions in their lives. Therefore, ethnic group identity can be seen as a resource for the aged, whether it is through churches or other social and voluntary associations. Furthermore, these organizations support coping mechanisms that enable ethnic aged persons to deal with their minority status (Yurick, Robb, & Ebert, 1984).

Aging and Health

Given the changing age demography, it is clear that in the future the health care system will include greater numbers of aged persons. In fact, when current nursing students reach the prime in their careers, they will be spending as much as 75 percent of their practice with older people (Sommers & Fabian, 1981). Community health nurses encounter the aged and their families at different points on the health continuum and have a pivotal role in promoting health for the well aged and the frail aged. The nurse collaborates with the aged and the family in maintaining health, adapting to health losses, and lending support through the dying process.

Health of the Elderly: A Holistic Perspective

As compared with the traditional medical model, which views health as the absence of disease, a holistic model of health focuses on wellness—the individual's well-being in the physical, mental, and social domains. As discussed in Chapters 13 and 16, wellness is a process that is not static but is constantly developing. To achieve wellness, the older adult must be capable of performing at an optimum level of functioning (Gress & Bahr, 1984). In essence wellness is a growth and development process throughout life and people with a wellness personality are able to:

be informed about principles of general hygiene

sleep sufficiently to restore their energy

exercise to keep fit

maintain a level of morale or "spirit" that produces a challenging and satisfying life (Gress & Bahr, 1984, p. 11)

In contrast to the holistic model of health, the traditional medical model does not encompass the concept of wellness, since it defines health as the absence of disease and since it does not include the potential for self-actualization or well-being (see Figure 23-1). The traditional health continuum progresses in only one direction—toward greater dependency and eventually institutionalization and death.

Throughout the health-illness continuum, the nurse who utilizes a holistic approach emphasizes wellness or well-being. According to Ebersole and Hess (1981), "Wellness is a balance between one's environment (internal and external), and one's emotional, social, cultural and physical processes." The authors further identify five dimensions of wellness: (1) self-responsibility; (2) nutritional awareness; (3) physical fitness; (4) environmental awareness; and (5) stress management. This perspective is significant for the aged because a state of wellness can be achieved even if the person has a chronic condition. Despite a chronic condition, this person can be encouraged, or taught, to function at the maximum state of health at which he or she is capable.

Erikson (1963) describes middle adulthood as a period when the individual faces the conflict of generativity versus stagnation (see Chapter 16). Consistent with the wellness perspective, the following developmental tasks must be achieved during middle adulthood:

1. Accepting the aging of self and others
2. Coping with pressures of social and occupational responsibilities and mobility
3. Recognizing the importance of good health habits and practices
4. Completing a periodic personal reassessment of life goals (Gress & Bahr, 1984, p. 11)

According to Erikson, during the later years the individual confronts the conflict of ego integrity versus despair (see Chapter 16). Additionally, older adults face developmental tasks of:

1. Becoming aware of the risk to health, and adjusting life-style and habits to cope with risks

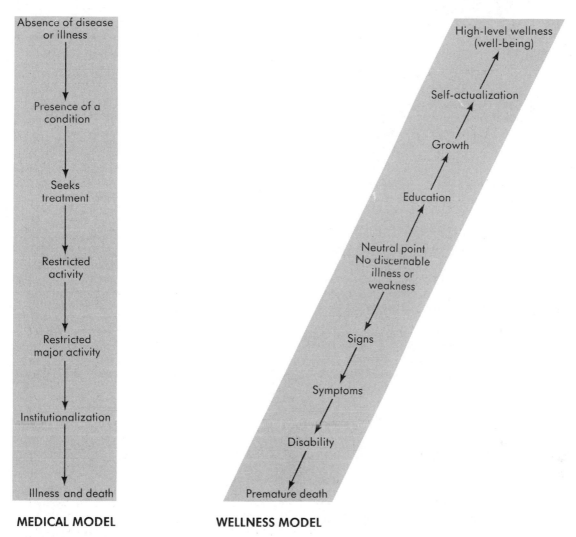

Figure 23-1 Traditional wellness and health continuums.

2. Adjusting to loss of a job, income, and family and friends through death
3. Redefining self-concept
4. Adjusting to changes in personal and new physical environment
5. Adjusting previous health habits to current physical and mental capacities (Gress & Bahr, 1984)

The older adult's ability to meet developmental tasks successfully and to make satisfactory adjust-

ments in later life depends on a number of factors including individual resources—what the individual brings to the situation—and social resources—what society contributes (Yurick, Robb, & Ebert, 1984). Good health, financial resources, good relationships with significant others, an ability to adapt to stress, and a sense of purpose in life are examples of individual resources, all of which can contribute to satisfaction with life in the later years and the achievement of wellness or a sense of well-being. Social resources that can help to achieve the same goal are money, health care, housing, home help, food, and transportation (Yurick, Robb, & Ebert, 1984).

The existence of social service in communities does not mean that all elderly people who need such services receive them. Constraints such as age, sex, race, and location of residence may hinder or prevent the use of services by people who need them the most. Community health nurses are in excellent positions to assist families in overcoming barriers and utilizing health and social services. Through their roles of education, coordination, and linking, they can educate elderly adults about available community services, coordinate such services, and link individuals and families to specific services.

Not all elderly adults need social service, and later life is not necessarily a period of poor health. Many older adults remain healthy and continue to enjoy healthy and satisfying lives until their deaths. However, community health nurses can work with all older adults and their families, assisting them to maintain and promote their own health, whatever their state of health or wherever they are located on the health-illness continuum.

Promoting Wellness among the Elderly

The community health nurse's role is to emphasize positive health attitudes and habits and to strengthen the ability of older adults to take the initiative and assume self-responsibility for their own health, and to work with them to achieve the maximum level of wellness of which they are capable. Nurses can concentrate their efforts in the following areas known to be essential in health promotion: self-responsibility, nutritional awareness, physical fitness, environmental awareness, and stress management.

Self-Responsibility Community health nurses can support and encourage older adults to accept responsibility for their own health. They can teach them about body structure and function, how to institute good health practices and health measures, and how to detect early signs of disease or health problems. The more informed older adults are about their bodies and how to take care of them, the more confident they can feel in assuming responsibility for their own health. The nurse can teach, encourage, and perform other functions on behalf of families and individuals, but ultimately, individuals and families are responsible for making their own health and wellness decisions.

Accepting responsibility for health and wellness means that older adults institute self-care measures that can improve their physical and psychological health and that can allow them to function at their maximum capacity with competence and self-confidence. Community health nurses should be sensitive to the degree of self-responsibility older adults are willing or are capable of accepting. While some may accept total responsibility, particularly if this has been their pattern in the past, others may need strong support and encouragement to assume minimum levels of self-responsibility, particularly if their self-confidence or ability for self-care has been lowered by situational factors such as a serious illness.

Nutritional Awareness Adequate nutrition, including proper hydration, is essential to the health and well-being of older adults. The amounts and types of calories and nutrients that are required in old age vary, depending on each individual's age, level of activity, and energy expended. Some illnesses that are more prevalent among the elderly than among other groups such as atherosclerosis, osteoporosis, diabetes, and diverticulitis are considered to be diet related (Yurick, Robb, & Ebert, 1984). Other health problems such as arthritis and heart disease can be complicated by inadequate nutrition such as overweight, which stems from an overconsumption of carbohydrates. Lack of fiber in the diet coupled with dehydration can aggravate conditions common among the elderly such as constipation and hemorrhoids.

Community health nurses have an important role in teaching older adults about proper nutrition, including the need for fresh fruits, vegetables, whole grain, lean meats, and legumes. A regular schedule of fluid intake is also essential to prevent dehydration. Nutrition centers or feeding programs available throughout the United States as a result of government funding are excellent sites for teaching adequate nutrition to the elderly. Even if elderly adults are knowledgeable about proper foods and nutritional intake, other factors that may indirectly and negatively affect their nutritional states include limited income; lack of transportation and/or fear of crime limiting where they can shop for food; lifelong food habits of under- or overnutrition; cultural and ethnic food preferences; and depression or other physical and emotional states that result in loss of appetite. (See Box 23-1.)

In addition to teaching elderly adults about proper diet and nutrition, community health nurses have an important role in assessing the dietary status of their elderly clients. A variety of assessment guides can be used. One is the diet recall discussed in Chapter 8 of this text.

Physical Fitness   Physical fitness through exercise and other physical activity can improve health and well-being in older adulthood. People of any age who are physically fit look, feel, and function better. Engaging in a group fitness program is not only an excellent way for older adults to increase body functions, but it also gives them the opportunity to meet and share ideas with others, thus increasing their level of social interaction. Group fitness activities such as dance, exercise, and yoga classes can achieve these goals. Other physical activities such as walking, swimming, and mild stretching done on a regular basis can be tailored to meet individual needs and also achieve similar goals.

Community health nurses are in excellent positions to organize physical fitness programs for older adults in a community. For example, a community health nurse can consult with a senior citizen housing complex. After assessing each resident to determine his or her ability to participate in exercise, health programs are recommended according to each person's physical capacity and personal interest. Programs can include dance classes, yoga sessions, nutrition awareness groups, and other such activities. Before as well as during the management of physical fitness programs for older adults, it is important that the following be considered: their baseline activity tolerance, the body movements necessary for the exercises, their pulmonary function, the amount of effort to be expended and the person's cardiovascular status. It is important that the exercise program be tailored to the condition and unique needs of each person participating.

Environmental Awareness   In order for older Americans to remain healthy it is essential that they remain safe. Visual and hearing impairments make them particularly vulnerable to accidents.

Box 23-1   Nutrition Program for Older Americans

The Nutrition Program for Older Americans, which is known as Title III and is administered by the Department of Health and Human Services, provides to people over sixty years old community-based noon meals at a nominal fee that is often optional. The largest component of this program is the congregate meals served at senior citizen centers, churches, schools, and other locations. These meals are designed to provide one-third of the RDAs; health and welfare counseling and nutrition education are also provided regularly (Roe, 1983). Another benefit to participants is the regular social interaction.

For the elderly who cannot leave their homes, local organizations help them meet their nutritional needs in various ways. Often using a combination of federal and local funds, some deliver ready-to-eat meals; others supply frozen dinners; and others provide grocery service to people in their homes.

SOURCE: Christian JL, Greger JL: *Nutrition for Living*. Menlo Park, Calif.: Benjamin-Cummings, 1985, pp. 506–507.

They are subject to falls, bumping into walls, and driving accidents due to inability to see adequately or hearing car horns. They may also fail to hear certain alarms such as smoke detectors.

Community health nurses can teach older adults about environmental hazards and how to reduce such hazards and keep their environment safe. Possible safety modifications of their environment include adequate lighting, particularly in hallways and at the top of stairways; handrails, particularly in bathrooms; bathtub mats; and easy-to-reach kitchen cabinets. Falls resulting in serious injuries are so common at this time that the elderly adult should be alert to wet and slippery floors, throw rugs, and small pets that can easily trip the unwary walker.

Stress Management   Older adults can be subject to physical, psychological, and social stress brought about by loss of income resulting in poverty or near poverty; bereavement resulting from loss of a spouse, particularly a lifelong spouse or other loved one; loss of role and status as a result of retirement; and loss of cognitive functioning (Cox, 1984). Managing stress effectively is crucial to maintaining wellness. Community health nurses can assist older adults with stress management techniques such as relaxation and biofeedback, and can identify and strengthen coping mechanisms including family relationships and the family's ability to be supportive to its members and to manage stress.

Aging and the Family

Personal and social changes associated with later life create unique needs for the aged and their families. Each decade of life beyond sixty-five years increases the probability of a person having a crisis associated with physical, psychological, or social loss.

Individuals are usually labelled as "aged" when they are unable to function independently and the family is required to respond to the person's physical or psychosocial dependency needs. Consequently, knowledge about the family system of the aged is a prerequisite for understanding the context of the aged person's circumstances. Contrary to popular myth suggesting that the aged are abandoned by their families, about 80 percent of the care of the aged is provided by the family (Eliopoulos, 1984). In addition, the aged person is usually living with a family member before institutionalization. Even though families use external resources, such as clinics, in care of the aged, frequently families are the primary providers of direct support, physical care, and financial assistance as well as being advocates in the care-giving system (Stuart & Snope, 1981). More and more, families with older people need education and counseling to anticipate age-related changes and the expected transitions of old age.

The older family must meet unique challenges in regard to role changes:

Many families have a hard time accepting the progressive signs of physical and the psychologic decline of an aging member. Loss of hearing, sight, short term memory and physical mobility can usually be accepted . . . but the high probability of chronic disease, the need for extended care involving high medical costs, and the certain prospect of progressive debilitation constitute a specter that haunts everyone (Stuart & Snope, 1981, p. 138).

Furthermore, many middle-aged children continue to support their children and may not have the financial or psychological resources to also contribute to the care of their aging parents. The crisis is related to the multiple needs inherent in the total family system, where the middle-aged children are "sandwiched" between their children and parents:

At the time that aged parents are reaching senescence, adult children are generally at a stressful time in their lives. Daughters are at the age of menopause, and grandchildren are entering college or being married, or perhaps being divorced and coming home with a child. How problems are handled depends on the history of the relationship and also on what is happening in the lives of all individuals in the family (Stuart & Snope, 1981, p. 138).

Another factor affecting aging families is the changing role of women, the traditional caregivers. As women become more involved in expanded career roles outside the family, they can no longer be counted on as providers of care. In other words, working family members are becoming less able to provide the resources needed to support aging relatives. This makes it important for community health nurses and other health professionals to address the health needs of aging families as a whole, not just of individuals.

Developmental Crises of Aging Families

Some developmental crises where support may be required for aging families include: (1) child launching, (2) retirement, and (3) death of a spouse. The family and the aged person's responses to these crises can be negative and defeating or positive and growth producing.

Child Launching Women whose identity is primarily related to their family roles are the most vulnerable to the crisis of children leaving home. These individuals may suffer depression because of the limited number of role options they perceive open to them. However, in other instances women may welcome the freedom and the chance to explore new opportunities. In fact in a recent national survey, it was found that "women in the post-parental stage experience higher levels of morale than do those with children still at home" (Kuypers &

Bengtson, 1983, p. 215). Men may also grieve for children who leave home and experience role loss associated with the father role. Also, they may need to relate to their wives on a different level due to a return to the couple relationship.

The community health nurse who encounters isolated older women and men can assist them in identifying other roles and opportunities outside the family such as employment opportunities and resources or networks composed of older peers who could serve as peer counselors and positive role models.

Retirement In our society individuals' self-esteem is closely linked to their work role. In a society where high value is placed on production, the question of "what you do" is significant for older individuals who cannot or choose not to be employed. Although responses to retirement have focused primarily on men, with a greater number of women in the work force, issues related to retirement will also apply to them. The concept of retirement is a relatively new phenomenon. In the past only the rich and powerful could afford to retire; retirement was made possible for the masses by the modern industrial society. Creation of retirement was facilitated by four major factors: (1) the increased longevity of more people who could work beyond middle age; (2) society's ability to support a large nonworking population; (3) very little demand for the labor of the aged and the rapid obsolescence of their skills and knowledge; and (4) the availability of governmental or private pension plans that made retirement financially possible (Crandall, 1980). Some older persons adapt successfully to retirement, while others may experience physical and psychosocial difficulties related to this event.

Successful adaptation to retirement is related to numerous factors such as the person's health, amount of self-esteem gained from work, and quality and quantity of support systems. More importantly, the retirement event per se does not appear to be as traumatic as the potential decreased roles available for the person after the retirement event. According to Crandall (1980), "If individuals consider themselves to be retired, they will generally act out their concept of a retiree. If individuals are considered by others in the society to be retired because of age or health limitations, the role of retiree will often be forced on them since it will be the only available role option" (p. 344).

Until recently, the laws and norms related to retirement were fixed—decisions about retirement were based on chronological age (usually sixty-five). However, the laws are changing; in 1970 a law was passed that permits private and public employees to stay on the job until seventy, unless they are in high risk situations. Retirement cannot be seen as an old-age event anymore, since the norms have become more flexible. Some persons will opt for early retirement, while others will remain employed. However, regardless of when the decision to retire is made, it precipitates significant changes such as reordering of schedules, interpersonal contacts, networks, and sense of self. The family is frequently the setting of negotiating role changes related to retirement. Usually, if the retiree's family and friends accept other roles such as leisure roles, the person will also do so (Crandall, 1980).

The meaning of retirement to the individual and family is linked to factors such as economics and health. For example, it was found that living in a family situation is conducive to higher life satisfaction among the retired aged. However, when the income variable was controlled, there were no differences between those living in a family setting and those not living in this type of situation. Therefore, it is clear that income may be a more significant factor than the family setting. When providing care to a family where retirement of an older person is anticipated, the community health nurse can help the person and the family to explore the meaning of retirement and alterations of lifestyle and roles that may be necessary as the result of changed economic resources, loss of friends at work, or how previous skills can be used in new roles such as working as a volunteer or a part-time employee.

Death of a Spouse Living alone as a result of losing a spouse is another expectable transition associated with old age. Since women continue to outlive men, widowhood is more likely than widowerhood. As Kuypers & Bengtson (1983) indicate, "By age 65, three out of five women in America are without spouses, and by age 75 the figure is more than four out of five." About one in three men over 75 is a widower (Kuypers & Bengtson, 1983, p. 216). Adapting to this type of loss is influenced by many factors. For women, the economic factor is particularly important, since widows as a group constitute the poorest of the population with the average annual income less than $2,000.

The responses to single status for both men and women are based not only on the significant loss, but also on many of the concomitant changes. For example, with widowhood there may be not only a loss of income but also a loss of social status, particularly if the woman has primarily married friends, who are reluctant to socialize with her. Also, there is a loss of self-esteem if the woman's identity came primarily from the husband. Men's economic and social status may not change, especially if there is no loss of income. Therefore, men may experience problems of a different nature when they lose their spouse. The impact of the loss of the wife may be more severe for men, because they may experience almost simultaneously several role losses, such as loss of job, health, and a wife. In addition, widowerhood can be more stressful because men may be confronted with new domestic roles, such as cooking and cleaning, which are unfamiliar.

The nurse can assist aged individuals and their families adapt to the loss of a spouse and the related changes by providing support during the bereavement process. The normal bereavement process includes anger, guilt, depression, and quiet. It may be of short duration, or it may linger and become chronic. Kuypers refers to Lopata's study of widows where 48 percent indicate they were adjusted to their husband's death by the end of the first year, while 20 percent reported that they had not resolved their grief and did not expect to (Kuypers & Bengtson, 1983). Other longitudinal studies of bereavement indicated that those who responded by becoming depressed were more likely than others to report poor health during that year. Since unresolved bereavement or grief is associated with physical and/or psychological illnesses, the nurse can assist in preventing such complications by helping families recognize that it is a family process, by providing counseling and support to grieving individuals, and by referring them whenever necessary to other resources such as mental health professionals.

Family Support

The family unit is an important support system for older persons. At this stage the family is multigenerational with lengthy family histories, so there is that history and experience, as well as the new inputs from younger generations, to draw from.

Family members, including siblings, can offer support in several ways: regular communications, household maintenance, food preparation, trans-portation, financial resources, and affection. Family members can help one another to deal with family crises, and they can also influence and reinforce one another to practice healthy life-styles and to reinforce preventive measures such as good eating habits. When working with older families, community health nurses need to be sensitive to the special needs of adult children who provide care or constitute the major support systems of elderly parents. Community health nurses can also provide direct and indirect support for families as they care for their aging parents. For example, organizing self-help groups for families in the community may be useful for encouraging mutual problem solving (Cicitelli, 1983). The nurse can serve as a positive role model as well as provide information particularly when physical illness or chronic disability is present.

Health Problems of the Elderly

The community health nurse must have a thorough understanding of the kinds of health problems older adults may experience. Not all of these problems are physical; psychological disorders can also occur.

Physical Problems

Although physical problems may affect persons at any age, advancing age beyond sixty-five increases one's susceptibility to chronic health problems. In fact, as people become older (over seventy-five), the greater is the likelihood that they will have multiple chronic problems that are interrelated.

The simultaneous presence of several conditions calls for a holistic approach, which leads to more appropriate planning, intervention, and preventive strategies. The majority of aged persons adapt successfully to crises associated with chronicity, especially those still living with a spouse or family. However, in some cases, one severe illness such as a heart attack or a stroke can interfere with successful individual family coping. Although chronic illnesses are not considered curable, they can be treated to minimize their effects on the daily lives of families and aged persons. Consequently, it is important to consider not only the immediate crisis, but also the broader socioenvironmental context of aged persons and their family and individual strengths. Sommers and Fabian (1981) discuss the "chicken and egg" relationship between physical problems and economic and psychosocial problems.

The sequential relation between loneliness, depression, impaired nutrition, physical inactivity and illness has been repeatedly demonstrated . . . the major obstacle to returning the patient to his own home may be architectural rather than his physical or mental condition. Also housing arrangements, group or sheltered, may be more significant to healthy independent living than any types of medical intervention (Sommers & Fabian, 1981, p. 3).

The following description of various chronic problems are intended to provide an overview of some of the important long-term health care needs of aged persons. The reader is referred to other comprehensive medical and nursing books that address these problems in more detail.

Cardiovascular problems   The general category of cardiovascular problems refers to numerous diseases of the circulatory system including the heart and blood vessels. The treatment of aged persons with "heart problems" comprises a large part of long-term care (Hickey, 1980). The variety of age-related physiological changes in the muscular structure of the heart tends to reduce its general strength and efficiency as a pump, although such changes do not typically lead to disability or the need for treatment. Pathological changes can occur if they are associated with cardiovascular conditions such as hypertension, atherosclerosis, or congestive heart failure.

Hypertension   Hypertension is not typically considered an "old age disease" since only one out of eight aged persons has high blood pressure. It should be noted that these persons can be survivors, since many of them probably had hypertension when they were younger and lived into old age. At any rate, when combined with other problems, hypertension can be a serious concern in late life. When treating hypertension in the aged, nurses should give attention to the combined effects of age-related changes and diseases, because they may complicate treatment and increase mortality risks (Hickey, 1980).

Although specific treatments for hypertension such as anti-hypertension drugs are available, the effectiveness of treatment is highly dependent upon the person's cooperation and requires considerable self-discipline and change in life-style. For example, it may be necessary for the individual to limit salt intake, change diet, or lose weight. These changes are frequently more problematic for older persons who are coping with other life changes such as loss of family and friends and declining physical functions. Support from friends and caregivers is necessary for interventions to be successful.

Atherosclerosis   A disease in which the normal blood flow is obstructed by a collection of fatty plaques, atherosclerosis is a common condition in older persons. If coronary arteries become obstructed, it may lead to symptoms of angina pectoris or to a myocardial infarction, commonly called a heart attack. Cerebral thrombosis or cerebral vascular accidents (strokes) can result from compromised blood flow to the brain.

The treatment for heart attack and strokes is similar to that of hypertension. Changes in diet, exercise, and drugs are the important components in the medical regime. During the acute stage, hospitalization may be necessary. After a severe stroke there may be a lengthy recovery period in an extended care facility and additional rehabilitation care at home. According to Hickey (1980, p. 105) "Recovery from a stroke is a slow and sometimes frustrating process which undoubtedly places emotional strain on the patient, family, friends and providers regardless of the setting (institutional or non-institutional)." Frequent and thorough monitoring following cardiovascular illness is also necessary to prevent complications.

Respiratory Problems   Similar to the impact of aging on the cardiovascular system, there are also normal age-related changes in the respiratory system. The incidence of chronic obstructive pulmonary disease (COPD), which includes chronic bronchitis and emphysema, increases with age. Chronic bronchitis is an inflammation of the bronchi from excessive mucus secretion, which interferes with the normal air flow from the lungs and causes shortness of breath and recurrent coughing (Hickey, 1980). Treatment involves medication, diet management, and respiratory therapy. In contrast to bronchitis, emphysema results in anatomical deterioration and disease in the lungs such that the air spaces distal to the terminal bronchioles become enlarged. The result is a loss of elasticity in the tissue so that air is trapped in the lungs and

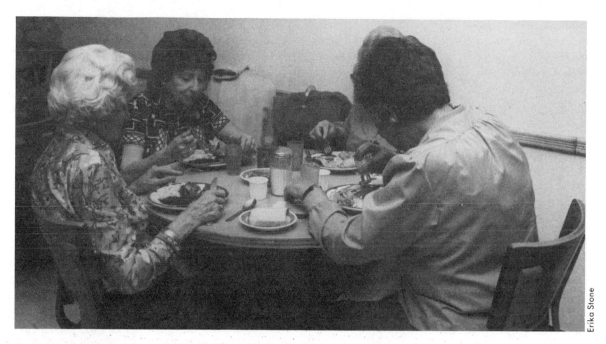

Erika Stone

Congregate meals, sponsored by community agencies or other organizations, provide not only a nutritious diet but also opportunities for
social interaction.

there is difficulty in expelling the air. Treatment
consists of the use of expectorant drugs, antibiot-
ics, and intermittent positive pressure breathing
(IPPB) machines to control and regulate the flow
of oxygen. Also, as with other chronic conditions,
changes in life-style may be necessary because energy
is limited.

Arthritis   Arthritis is a common problem in
the aged and refers to inflammation and degenerative changes of the bones and joints. Rheumatoid
arthritis, a chronic inflammatory disease, results in
swelling, limitation of motion, and stiffness on
arising in the morning. Rheumatoid arthritis is not
necessarily related to old age, but its associated
pain is frequently more severe in late life.

Treatment consists primarily of symptomatic
relief, rather than cure. Energy-saving measures such
as frequent rest periods and the use of canes and
crutches to reduce stress on affected weight-bear-

ing joints may be helpful. From a preventive
approach, the use of monitored physical therapy
and special exercises can aid in the preservation
and strengthening of unaffected muscles and joints.

Digestive Problems   Problems in digestion,
including continuing gastrointestinal distress, are
frequent occurrences in older persons. The aging
process results in tissue changes in the gastrointestinal system such as muscular rigidity, decreased
absorption rates, and biochemical changes related
to aging.

Equally important as these physiological and
biological changes is the impact of environmental
and behavioral factors. These include change in
the dietary habits of older persons, which in turn
affect bowel patterns. Furthermore, poor dentition
coupled with limited transportation and finances
may lead to elimination of foods, such as meat and
high fiber foods, necessary for a nutritious diet.

Additional psychosocial factors like eating alone can result in poor motivation to prepare and eat nutritionally balanced meals. Therefore, interventions such as congregate and mobile meals and others discussed earlier in this chapter can play a useful role in nutritional care for the aged.

Visual Problems   A steady decrease in visual efficiency is common in most people as they age. It is estimated that about 7 percent of those sixty-five to seventy-four and 16 percent of those over seventy-five experience physical changes within the eye. The rate and amount of change are influenced by heredity and environmental factors. If there are pathological changes, these can be related to tissue change in other parts of the body. All aspects of visual functioning activity accommodation, light sensitivity, and spatial ability are important, since a decrease in any of these abilities may be the primary cause for decreased functioning or may affect other aspects of living such as social interaction, mobility, and orientation. Two eye conditions most commonly seen in older persons are cataracts and glaucoma.

Cataracts occur to some degree in more than 95 percent of persons over sixty-five. However, they can be treated and remedied. Medical treatment consists of removal of the lens. Aphakia results from removal of the cataract and occurs because the eye has no focusing mechanism, even though vision may be 20/20. Glasses designed for the person with aphakia may limit the visual field and cause magnification of images, which can be confusing for the aged person. Sensitivity to the person's status and adjustment before and after cataract removal is important to assess in order to determine type of support and assistance required.

Glaucoma, another cause of visual impairment among the aged, can occur without warning. Glaucoma is very dangerous because it is irreversible. The underlying pathology is related to the production of an elevated intraocular pressure, which leads to optic nerve damage. Although the types and causes of glaucoma are different, all forms involve impairment in the outflow of aqueous humor from the eye. A decrease in peripheral vision and blurred vision not corrected by eyeglasses are early symptoms. If untreated, tunnel vision followed by blindness occurs. The best treatment is prevention, which should consist of frequent eye examinations, including intraocular pressure testing and prompt treatment.

Hearing Problems   A decline in hearing also occurs with increasing age. Approximately 13 percent of the young-old (sixty-five to seventy-four) and 26 percent of the old-old (over seventy-five) have serious hearing problems (Crandall, 1980). Atrophy of nerve tissue in the ear is a primary cause of hearing loss; reduction of blood flow to the auditory nerve caused by hardening of the artery leads to degeneration of the nerve. Other causes of hearing problems include calcification of the bones in the inner ear.

The two types of hearing loss are (1) loss of volume and intensity of a sound and (2) loss of pitch or level of a sound. In contrast to what is commonly believed, more elderly people suffer loss of the ability to hear high-pitched sounds rather than loss of volume. Therefore, raising the volume of one's voice is not successful in helping an older person to hear. In fact, the louder one shouts, the less likely the person is to hear; on the other hand, whispering may enable the person to hear better since it decreases the pitch of one's voice.

It is important to assess the hearing ability of aged persons, because hard-of-hearing persons may be labeled "senile." Hearing problems can also be related to depression or social isolation. Also, hearing loss interferes with accurate interpretation of sounds, thus creating situations where persons may not be able to assess dangerous situations. For example, a person with impaired hearing may not hear a fire alarm. Interventions to improve hearing problems include having a quiet environment, simple verbal communication, face-to-face interaction, and the use of hearing aids.

Organic Brain Disorders   In organic brain disorders there has been physical damage to the brain or physical impairment of the brain's functioning. This type of impairment usually involves a pro-

Box 23-2   Alzheimer's Disease

Alzheimer's disease is a specific type of organic brain disease, first described by a German neurologist, Alois Alzheimer in 1906. It includes symptoms and physiological abnormalities characteristic of presenile (before age sixty) and senile dementia (onset after age sixty). Both are now combined together as Alzheimer's disease.

It is estimated that at least 60 to 70 percent of the aged who present symptoms of gradual memory impairment and intellectual decline have Alzheimer's disease. The incidence of the disease is 5 to 6 percent of persons sixty-five and over. Nationally, this accounts for about 1½ million people (Pratt et al, 1985). Although the disease is not the consequence of aging, incidence increases with age; by the age of eighty the incidence is 15 to 20 percent of the elderly population (Mortimer & Schuman, 1981). There is a definite decrease in life expectancy depending on the age of onset of symptoms. The range of the course of the disease is two to twenty years, with the terminal stage taking place on the average of five years after the onset of the first symptoms.

Although there are a variety of theories that attempt to explain the disease, presently there is little understanding of the disease and there is no specific treatment. The impact of the disease is immense to the afflicted individual, the family, and the larger community. It exacts tremendous emotional costs due to the gradual and total loss of physical, psychological, and social functions. Consequently, patients and their families need a great deal of support from care-givers such as community health nurses, even if institutionalization in a nursing home becomes the family's only alternative. Family support groups (particularly for spouses and daughters, the usual family care-givers) can be an effective medium for providing the support families need. Increasing their confidence in problem-solving and helping them to redefine difficult situations and marshal social support have been found to be helpful (Pratt et al, 1985).

gressive process of deterioration and noticeable changes in memory, orientation, and judgment. In earlier stages of the illness, some individuals, with the provision of support services, can continue to live at home. For others, as the illness progresses, hospitalization or institutionalization may be necessary. Organic brain syndrome is irreversible in about 10 to 20 percent of older adults who have this condition (Crandall, 1980). Acute brain syndromes are caused by a metabolic malfunctioning, which may be related to the presence of other physical conditions such as infections or high temperatures. In other cases it may involve drug or alcohol intoxication, cerebrovascular accidents, head injuries, or other psychosocial traumas. The major distinction between an acute brain disorder or confusional state and a chronic brain disorder is the sudden onset of the former as contrasted with the steady progression of the latter. (See Box 23-2.)

Affective and Functional Disorders

The most prevalent affective and functional disorders of the elderly are anxiety and depression, which in many ways resemble confusional states and organic brain disorders. These and other mental health problems in the aged are often difficult to diagnose because they are often symptomatic of many other conditions including physical disorders and various chronic illnesses. Physical and mental health are so frequently interrelated among older adults that it is sometimes difficult to identify problems that are purely in the realm of mental health. For example, a chronic physical condition such as arthritis can lead to depression, a psychological problem; and depression can further lead to isolation, a social problem. Also, crises associated with age-related events may result in psychological problems. Hickey (1980, p. 23) reports, "A nonspecific form of anxiety or depression may result from a generalized state of dissatisfaction and frustration with the aging process, with age related health problems, and with the various vicissitudes of being an old person, such as a loss of one's major roles in life, social isolation and limited autonomy."

Depression can manifest itself by physical and psychological symptoms such as withdrawn and hostile behaviors, insomnia, loss of appetite, and weight gain or loss. These symptoms frequently intensify the condition and, if left untreated, can lead to chronic depression and suicide. Early interventions that can reverse the condition include family, group, and/or individual counseling and environmental stimulation.

The complexity of mental health problems in the elderly makes treatment difficult and challenging. However, treatment intervention for one condition such as a physical problem may result in dramatic improvement in other areas like mental or social functioning.

Misuse and Abuse of Drugs

Drugs are frequently prescribed for the multiple health problems among the elderly. However, for a variety of reasons, the drug intended for treatment may create other problems.

Misuse and abuse of drugs, whether intentional or not, is a common problem among the elderly population (Roe, 1983). The potential for misuse and abuse exists among this group for the following reasons:

- Older adults are prescribed a high percentage of drugs by their physicians. Over 25 percent of all prescribed drugs are consumed by persons sixty-five years and over (Roe, 1983). This population tends to have varying chronic conditions for which multiple drugs are prescribed.
- Older adults tend to be involved with many different physicians, who may each prescribe drugs for them without a full inquiry into their drug history or into the amounts and types of drugs they currently have in their possession.

- Older adults tend to medicate themselves with a variety of over-the-counter drugs, the most common being laxatives, analgesics, antacids, and sedatives. Laxatives are frequently taken for constipation, analgesics such as aspirin for arthritis, antacids for gastric distress, and sedatives for sleep.
- Over-the-counter drugs are often taken in addition to prescription drugs.
- Older adults have peers who also take a variety of prescription and nonprescription drugs. This may influence them in their own drug-taking behavior. In addition they may exchange drugs with relatives and friends.
- Older adults may develop a pattern of reliance on drugs to help them problem-solve or to cope with stress. Stress may be related to chronic physical disability, loss of loved ones, alterations in work and home environments, and changing roles (Futrell et al, 1980; Roe, 1983).

The potential for abuse and misuse of drugs among the elderly population exists not only for prescription and over-the-counter drugs but for substances such as caffeine and alcohol as well. Indeed alcohol problems among the elderly may well be hidden and understated (Futrell et al, 1980). Different types or patterns of drug misuse and abuse have been identified:

- *Overuse*—intentional or accidental overdosage
- *Underuse*—taking less dosage because of forgetfulness or cost (expense) of drugs
- *Erratic use*—omitting a dose and then compensating or making up the missed dose (Caroselli-Karinja, 1985)

In addition to the general negative effects of drug abuse, this group is particularly susceptible to adverse and toxic effects of medication because of impaired drug absorption capacity (Caroselli-Karinja, 1985).

Adverse nutritional effects of drugs and drug-food incompatibilities occur when:
1. The drug is an antinutrient

2. The drug, which has adverse nutritional effects, is taken for a long time
3. The patient is on a multidrug regime
4. The diet is nutritionally inadequate
5. There is excessive drug use or abuse of prescription or over-the-counter drugs
6. Disease-related malabsorption is present
7. The patient is malnourished
8. The patient is not given special diet instructions
9. Physicians and nutritionists are unaware of the risks (Roe, 1983, p. 171).

The potential for abuse is highest among older adults who are already in the condition of marginal mental compensation (Caroselli-Karinja, 1985) and also people who have misused or abused drugs in their earlier lives or who have obtained secondary gains from medications.

Community health nurses have a role in assessment and monitoring of drug use and in educating and counseling older adults about the potential for misuse and abuse of drugs at the individual, family, and community levels. In assessment the nurse should obtain a thorough history of the client's drug use including prescription and nonprescription drugs and such substances as coffee, tea, and vitamins. The nurse should be alert to signs and symptoms of drug abuse and misuse. Community health nurses can monitor the amount and types of drugs older clients take, side effects, and therapeutic effects. They also have the responsibility to teach elderly individuals and families about the effects of drugs (both therapeutic and nontherapeutic) on the body, and on health and wellness in general.

Strategies for Health Promotion

The primary objective of health promotion is to encourage aged persons and their families to assume maximum involvement, control, and responsibility by utilizing their own strengths and resources. The community health nurse encounters aged persons and their families at various positions on the health continuum, with different values, thus requiring different amounts and intensity of assistance. If the family does not have the strength or ability, the nurse may need to act promptly with minimal input from the family. At other times, aged individuals and their families have adequate resources and skills but need support to implement formulated plans independently.

Wherever the person and the family are on the health-illness continuum the goal of nursing intervention activities is to facilitate independence, growth, and optimum wellness. When assisting the family, the nurse should be sensitive to current and past relationships that are unique to the family. The nurse focuses on what the family can do instead of hypothetical solutions. Also the community

health nurse needs to know what community resources exist and how to mobilize them in planning care that is uniquely suited to meet the needs of older individuals and their families.

To promote health and wellness of the aged and their families, nursing interventions encompass primary, secondary, and tertiary prevention, and often operate on more than one level. The community health nurse should be prepared to offer primary, secondary, and tertiary prevention strategies along the continuum of services as described by Tobin and Liebermann in Table 23-1 (Tobin & Liebermann, 1976, p. 26).

Primary Prevention

Many programs and services for aged persons focus on remedial or maintenance care rather than on prevention. This is unfortunate since there is considerable variability in the capacities of older persons biologically, psychologically, and socially.

Table 23-1 Alternative Ways of Structuring the Delivery of Services

A Continuum of Service:	Individually Delivered	Congregate Delivered	
	Home-Based	Congregate Organized	Congregate Residence
From services for the comparatively well elderly	Out-Reach Information and referral Telephone reassurance Friendly visiting Work at home Senior Wheels to shopping, doctor, dentist, and social functions	Adult education Recreational senior center Nutrition sites (Wheels to Meals) Sheltered workshop	Senior housing (includes retirement hotels) Senior housing with recreation Senior housing with recreation and social services
Through services that provide alternatives for preventing premature institutionalization	Escort service Homemaker service (housekeeping, handyman, and so forth)	Multipurpose senior center (all of the above plus outreach, and health and social follow-up)	Sheltered care
To services for those whose needs may demand institutional care or its equivalents	Meals on Wheels Home health care (visiting nurse, rehabilitation, speech therapy, dentist, and doctor) Foster home care (complete social and health care for bedridden person in a home)	Outpatient day or hospital care	Halfway house Mental hospital Institutional care (nursing home and home for the aged) Intermediate nursing care Skilled nursing care Short-term crisis care Vacation plan Terminal care

SOURCE:
Tobin S, Liebermann L: *Last Home for the Aged.* San Francisco: Jossey-Bass, 1976.

Consequently, there are numerous areas of functioning where aged persons can improve physical, mental, and social functions within very broad parameters (Fries, 1981).

Emphasis in primary prevention includes the reduction of environmental stressors. Environmental needs of the aged include availability and accessibility of health and social services (including transportation), adequate social and economic resources, and the opportunity for social interaction with significant others such as family, friends, and neighbors.

Other types of programs designed for primary preventive care are educational programs that provide information and anticipatory guidance about potential problems with aging family members. Examples of primary prevention programs include support groups for families who have aged parents, as well as anticipatory guidance for groups of older people who are anticipating life-style changes such as living alone or going to a nursing home. Adult daycare facilities, senior centers and well-elderly clinics are other locations where primary prevention programs can be implemented.

Another aspect of primary prevention is the role modeling that occurs for individuals and their older families as they see other families with similar problems cope successfully with crises associated with transitions of aging. According to Kuypers & Bengtson (1983, p. 228), "The efforts, struggles and successes of one family can be shared and understood so to speak beyond the family. In going beyond the family, all involved will apply these new experiences to future crisis." Case Example 23-1 illustrates a primary prevention strategy by a community health nurse.

In some cases the community health nurse intervenes to reduce family problems associated with transitions of aging such as retirement and widowhood. Specific interventions may include providing information to individuals and families and reinforcing support networks the family has identified. Family stress can be caused by a lack of basic information as family members confront a disabling event. For example, by providing information about Alzheimer's disease and responding to family members' questions about the condition, community health nurses can assist families to better cope with the problem. They can also help families reduce stress and cope more with chronic and disabling conditions by linking them to community support systems and other resources that can reinforce and strengthen their own coping mechanism and thus promote health.

Secondary Prevention

Secondary prevention is focused on early diagnosis and treatment of older persons with physical or psychosocial illnesses. Health assessment is an important aspect of secondary prevention, since assessment provides information essential for prompt treatment.

Community health nurses are in excellent positions to conduct health assessment of older adults because they have access to this population in their homes and in the community. Health assessment is a holistic process, permitting the community health nurse to obtain data related to the functioning of the various body systems as well as to the status of the person within the family, community, and society. The nurse uses these data to provide individualized care to the person.

Through health assessment the community health nurse is able to participate in early case finding, apply early treatment, and encourage self-care measures that prevent further physical or psychological disability (Eliopoulos, 1984).

Assessment is a dynamic process that involves the use of multiple techniques including interviewing, observation and physical examination (see Chapter 7). The reader is referred to Eliopoulos (1984) for a comprehensive assessment guide specific for older adults.

Since community health nurses frequently are the first persons to see aged persons and their families, they can facilitate early and appropriate diagnosis and treatment during a time when treatment can be most effective. In addition to assessment, other approaches important to secondary prevention include health screening programs, which evaluate the functioning of aged persons by detecting early signs of disease, and referrals. Early referral to appropriate treatment can help to initiate treatment promptly, thereby preventing further disability.

Screening programs are more likely to succeed if they are part of an already existing system such as a senior housing project, a church, or a daycare center. Such settings permit the nurse to conduct educational programs that provide information about signs and symptoms of physical and psychosocial age-related problems, as well as where and how to obtain effective treatment. Case Example 23-2 illustrates a community health nurse's role in sec-

Case Example 23-1: Primary Prevention Strategy for Elderly Client

Mrs. Hannah, a sixty-nine-year-old widow and regular participant at a local seniors' center, was absent for a few weeks. Mrs. Jones, a community health nurse and health consultant to the center, was concerned and made a home visit to assess what had happened to Mrs. Hannah.

Community health nurse makes home visit to assess situation of older adult.

A distraught Mrs. Hannah, who was most happy to see Mrs. Jones, told her the following: A new family with teenage boys who had started a music rock group had recently moved next door to Mrs. Hannah. Mrs. Hannah became increasingly upset when the group began playing music "all during the day and night," and when different types of "strangely dressed" young people began crossing her lawn to visit the family next door. The environmental pressure exceeded Mrs. Hannah's limit, and she retreated, hardly leaving her home, and frequently calling the police for various misdemeanors she observed.

Nurse listens with acceptance as client recounts her difficulties.

Prior to this incident, Mrs. Hannah was quite comfortable in her home. Her home was quiet and orderly, and she seemed to require little stimuli or seek for new experiences. Young mothers invited her to neighborhood gatherings and occasionally prevailed on her for babysitting services. She responded to these increased demands with a bright affect and seemingly high morale. However, the rock group's increased activities affected her negatively. Mrs. Jones assessed that she (Mrs. Hannah) was getting increasingly agitated and depressed, and was in potential crisis.

Nursing diagnosis is formulated.

Mrs. Jones recognized the need for Mrs. Hannah to evaluate her current living situation, to identify her strengths and resources as well as alternatives and to devise a plan of action. Mrs. Jones assisted Mrs. Hannah with these needs activities to prevent a full-blown crisis from occurring, to prevent deterioration of Mrs. Hannah's psychological health, and to help her preserve her current life-style in her home, and consequently prevent institutionalization.

Nursing action is based on anticipatory guidance.

With assistance from Mrs. Jones, Mrs. Hannah mobilized her resources—community residents from the seniors' center and from the neighborhood families for whom she babysat. A delegation from this group met with the family next door and a solution was reached. The rock group was to use a hall in a nearby community center for practice. Mrs. Hannah was satisfied with the resolution. She was able to remain in her home and continue the regular activities and contacts she previously enjoyed. The environmental stress removed, her physical and mental health remained intact.

The problem resolution is an example of primary prevention.

SOURCE:
The case materials were obtained from Elaine Blake who worked with these clients as part of her clinical practicum while a graduate student in gerontological nursing at Northwestern University.

Case Example 23-2: Secondary Prevention for Elderly Client

Mr. Austin, a seventy-year-old male, had a stroke last year, which left him paralyzed on his left side. His wife, who is sixty-nine years old, has poor eyesight and is hard of hearing. However, she manages to take care of Mr. Austin, who has started to stay in bed more and more during the last few months. Due to inadequate fluid and food intake, along with inactivity, he had become dehydrated and developed a fecal impaction. Mr. Austin continued to require frequent hospitalization because of generalized weakness and severe dehydration. Following his last hospitalization, a home health nurse was assigned to him.

Mr. Jones, the home health nurse, assessed Mr. Austin's family situation during his first visit. He determined that Mr. Austin had low self-esteem as a result of his condition and accompanying limitations, and that his physical condition, including his nutrition and mobility, would improve if he felt better about himself. Assessment data also revealed that although Mr. and Mrs. Austin had been close, their increased dependency needs, particularly that of Mr. Austin, placed a new constraint on their relationship such that they had difficulty relating to one another.

Nurse's assessment shows client's physical and emotional well-being are interrelated.

Key problems are identified.

Working with Mr. and Mrs. Austin, Mr. Jones devised and implemented a plan that included the following: a homemaker service to assist Mrs. Austin with shopping and cooking; a physical therapist to work with Mr. Austin weekly for rehabilitation; and a diet plan for fluid and food intake that the homemaker and Mrs. Austin would develop and Mr. Jones would monitor. Mr. Jones made the appropriate referrals and initial appointments and planned for follow-up. Plans were implemented, and with this assistance the couple felt relieved. Since their dependency on each other decreased, they could manage their daily routines with less stress. After a year, Mr. Austin had not been hospitalized. Improvement of his socio-emotional environment prevented further deterioration of his physical condition.

Planning involves client and his wife.

Plan is implemented.

The problem resolution is an example of secondary prevention.

---

ondary prevention. Note the type of assessment strategies and other intervention skills the nurse uses.

Tertiary Prevention

Tertiary prevention emphasizes restorative care that enables the aged person to achieve optimum function after an acute illness or crisis. Although it may be necessary for the person to enter a hospital to obtain medical intervention, the community health nurse works with the hospital staff to facilitate the aged person's transition back to the community. This may mean supporting the patient and his or her family while the patient is recovering. For example, if the older person returns home after a stroke and needs assistance with activities of daily living, the nurse will need to educate the family regarding the best way to assist the person.

Moreover, if the aged person has experienced a crisis due to a loss and does not receive appropriate support during the crisis, the family may compound the problem as noted in Case Example 23-3.

Tertiary prevention becomes important when considering the aged population who reside in

Case Example 23-3: Educating the Family

Mrs. Brown, a seventy-five-year-old woman, was referred to the nurse because of confusion. She had lived with her son and daughter-in-law since her husband died a year ago. The family told the nurse that Mrs. Brown constantly talked about "fixing supper for papa" and kept saying that "he would be home soon." The family did not test this reality with her—they did not discuss that "papa" had been dead for a year. They sent flowers weekly and the card was signed "papa." The community health nurse talked with the son and daughter-in-law, explaining that Mrs. Brown needed to grieve for her husband, as the first step toward accepting the reality of his death. The nurse also reinforces the need for the family to help Mrs. Brown to participate in activities that will enable her to interact with her environment. Social interaction is important in supporting reality orientation.

Lack of family honesty causes confusion in client.

Community health nurse provides needed teaching to family members.

Table 23-2 Nursing Roles in Three Levels of Prevention

Primary Prevention	*Secondary Prevention*	*Tertiary Prevention*
1. Promote health through clinic and home contacts	1. Report case findings and make appropriate referrals	1. Initiate rehabilitation strategies during illness phase
2. Provide appropriate resources	2. Assess response to illness and compliance with treatments	2. Maintain communication with social networks
3. Make clients and families aware of options and resources	3. Provide information about medication and treatments	3. Assist with follow-up services
4. Involve clients in citizens' councils and political action groups	4. Counsel clients and family members	4. Provide consultation and educational programs to those responsible for providing care to the aged
5. Educate clients to self-responsibility for health	5. Identify existing or impending illness	5. Support legislation and policies that impact on the aged

nursing homes. Demographically, most nursing home residents are older (over seventy-five), female, and have no family. In many cases, social and behavioral problems, rather than physical illness are the primary reasons given for nursing home admission. Whatever the reason, over 50 percent of nursing home residents have chronic health problems (Hickey, 1980). The challenge of nursing home care is to provide care that is congruent with the capability of the residents and to rehabilitate them to their highest potential. The community health nurse is frequently the health professional who provides the link between the nursing home and the community. Unfortunately, there may not be a great deal of reversibility and flexibility between institutional and community health services. The community health nurse works collaboratively with aged persons and their families as well as other health professionals in assessing when nursing home care is required or when the home situation is appropriate for the person to live in the community. Specialized health care services for the aged such as daycare, home health care, or hospice care have different requirements and provide different levels of care. Therefore, the nurse may be in the best position to assess the needs and resources of the client and make recommendations regarding the appropriate environment.

Through a multiplicity of roles, the community health nurse has the opportunity to participate in all three levels of prevention. These roles may be traditional such as neighborhood clinic nurse consultant or they may be more unusual such as serving on health planning councils on the local, state, or national level. Examples of how community health nurses can function at each level are listed in Table 23-2.

Summary

The most significant fact about aging is that in the future there will be larger numbers of older people. Consequently, greater numbers will live long enough to experience the process of aging, and this changing age demography will have a profound social, political, and economic impact on our society.

As new information is gained on all the issues addressed in this chapter, new perspectives and solutions will be developed related to aging. For example, the growing number of extended families with three to four generations has yet to be incorporated into our policies and programs for the aged. As Hickey (1980) suggested, "We may be overestimating the incidence of such phenomena as dependence and isolation of family support networks in which both the children and the parents are elderly" (p. 168).

Furthermore, an aging society will necessitate a greater demand for health care that encompasses a continuum of health care services for aged individuals and aging families during the later years. As the largest group of health professionals, nurses will play pivotal roles in providing the quantity and quality of health care needed for an increasingly diverse aged population.

The community health nurse will continue to be involved in activities that focus on improvement of quality of life rather than chronological age as reflected in the following:

Let us never know what old age is
Let us know the happiness time brings
Not count the years (Hickey, 1980, p. 173).

Topics for Nursing Research

• Develop a research protocol to evaluate institutional care of the aged, including the nursing milieu.

• Develop a research plan to evaluate nursing care provided by home health and other community services for the elderly.

• Identify the health needs of black, Hispanic, and white elderly adults in a multiethnic community.

• Compare and evaluate nursing care needs of older adults across ethnic and socioeconomic groups.

• Identify the outcome of teaching elderly adults self-care methods. Explore the extent of

utilization of self-care measures among older adults.

• Explore the role of the community health nurse between the family and an elderly institutionalized family member.

• Compare the differences in the health care needs of the young-old and old-old person.

• Identify the effects of a regular exercise and diet program on the health of older adults.

• Evaluate the effectiveness of the community health nurse's networking and collaborating roles with senior citizens in a specified community or communities.

Study Questions

1. Which of the following statements is true regarding demographic trends of the aging populations?
   a. Life expectancy of the older population is expected to increase dramatically in the future.
   b. Life expectancy of older adults is expected to decrease dramatically in the future.
   c. Life expectancy of older adults will remain the same in the future.
   d. Life expectancy of the young-old will decrease but that of the old-old will increase.

2. An explanation of aging as a process characterized by decreased interaction between the aging person and others in the environment and by withdrawal of the aged person from social roles is associated with which of the following theories of aging?
   a. Autoimmune theory
   b. Disengagement theory
   c. Activity theory
   d. Socioenvironmental theory

3. Which of the following statements have been used as arguments to explain the relationship between ethnicity and aging?
   a. The consequences of growing old are so

significant that they overshadow other influences such as ethnicity.
   b. The influences of ethnicity are relevant given the importance of learning and environmental factors.
   c. Neither of these statements is a relevant explanation.
   d. Both of these statements are relevant explanations.

4. The need to change current health care policies that affect older adults is based on which of the following rationalizations?
   a. Current health care policies are based on the medical model, are disease oriented, and support illness care, while most older adults are healthy.
   b. Current health care policies support primary prevention measures, while most elderly people have chronic conditions requiring tertiary care.
   c. Current health care policies support ambulatory adults, while most older adults are in institutions.
   d. Current health care policies are family oriented, while most older adults have no family.

5. Which of the following are important strategies to maintain wellness among older adults?
   a. Promotion of self-responsibility

b. Adequate nutrition
c. Physical fitness
d. Environmental safety
e. Stress management
f. All of the above
g. None of the above

6. Which of the following statements would be helpful to community health nurses in assessing mental health problems of elderly adults?
   a. Symptoms of mental illness are often masked by confusional states or other physical conditions.
   b. Symptoms of mental illness are often profound when they occur in old age.
   c. Mental health symptoms are common among the elderly.
   d. None of the above.

References

Ball R: Rethinking national policy on health care for the elderly. In: Sommers A, Fabian D (editors), *The Geriatric Imperative.* New York: Appleton-Century-Crofts, 1981.

Caroselli-Karinja M: Drug abuse and the elderly. *J Psychosoc Nurs Ment Health Serv* 1985; 23 (6): 25–30.

Christian JL, Greger JL: *Nutrition for Living.* Menlo Park, Calif.: Benjamin-Cummings, 1985; 506–507.

Cicitelli V: Adult children and their elderly parents. In: Brubaker T (editor), *Family Relationships in Later Life.* Beverly Hills, Calif.: Sage, 1983, pp. 31–46.

Cox H: *Later Life: The Realities of Aging.* Englewood Cliffs, N.J.: Prentice-Hall, 1984.

Crandall RC: *Gerontology: A Behavioral Science Approach.* Reading, Mass.: Addison-Wesley, 1980.

Ebersole P, Hess P: *Toward Healthy Aging.* St. Louis: Mosby, 1981.

Eliopoulos C: *Health Assessment of the Older Adult.* Menlo Park, Calif.: Addison-Wesley, 1984.

Engelhardt H: Treating aging: Restructuring the human condition. In: Neugarten B, Havighurst T (editors), *Extending the Human Life Span: Social Policy and Social Ethics.* Chicago: U. of Chicago Press, 1977.

Erikson E: *Childhood and Society,* 2nd ed. New York: Norton, 1963.

Fries J, Crapo L: *Vitality and Aging.* San Francisco: W. H. Freeman, 1984.

Futrell M et al: *Primary Health Care of Older Adults.* Duxbury, Mass.: Duxbury Press, 1980.

Gress L, Bahr RT: *The Aging Person: A Holistic Perspective.* St. Louis: Mosby, 1984.

Gubrium JF: *The Myths of the Golden Years.* Springfield, Ill.: Charles C Thomas, 1973.

Hickey T: *Health and Aging.* Monterey, Calif.: Brooks-Cole, 1980.

Kelly C: An old person is not an old person is not an old person. *Geriatric Nursing,* 1985; 3 (3): 159.

Kuypers JA, Bengtson U: Toward competence in the older family. In: Brubaker T (editor), *Family Relationships In Later Life.* Beverly Hills, Calif.: Sage, 1983.

Mortimer J, Schuman L (editors): *The Epidemiology of Dementia.* New York: Oxford University Press, 1981.

Neugarten B: Age groups in American society and the rise of young-old. *The Annals of the American Academy of Political Science* 1974; 415: 187–198.

Place LF: The ethnic factor. In: Berghorn FJ, Schafer DE (editors), *The Dynamics of Aging.* Boulder, Colo.: Westview Press, 1981.

Pratt GC, Schmall VL, Wright S, Cleland M: Burden and coping strategies of caregivers to Alzheimer's patients. *Family Relations* 1985; 34 (1): 27–33.

Quadango J: Who are the elderly? A demographic inquiry. In: Berghorn F, Schafer D (editors), *The Dynamics of Aging.* Boulder, Colo.: Westview Press, 1981.

Roe D: *Geriatric Nutrition.* Englewood Cliffs, N.J.: Prentice-Hall, 1983.

Sommers A, Fabian D (editors): *The Geriatric Imperative.* New York: Appleton-Century-Crofts, 1981.

Stuart M, Snope F: Family structure, family dynamics and the elderly. In: Sommers A, Fabian R (editors), *The Geriatric Imperative.* Appleton-Century-Crofts, 1981.

Tobin S, Liebermann M: *Last Home for the Aged.* San Francisco: Jossey-Bass, 1976.

Yurick A, Robb S, Ebert N: *The Aged Person and the Nursing Process.* Norwalk, Conn.: Appleton-Century-Crofts, 1984.

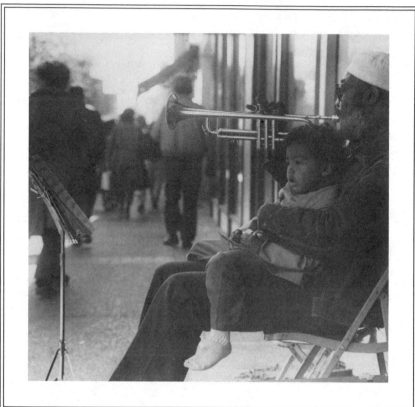

Laura K. Hawkins

"Community health nurses should be active in the policy arena not because nurses are numerous and not just because nursing needs resources in order to continue to serve the public, but primarily because this is a crucial modality for influencing the health of defined populations. . . . Such a posture is good ethics, good politics, and good community health practice." (Williams CA: Making things happen: Community health nursing and the policy arena. Nursing Outlook *(Jul/Aug) 1983; 31(4):228.)*

4 Contemporary Issues and Problems in Community Health Nursing

Chapter 24

Legal and Ethical Issues in Family and Community Health Nursing

Nancy J. Brent

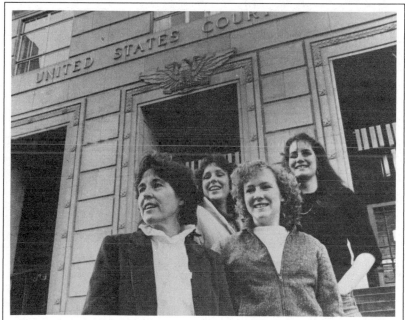

Bill Murphy/The Oregonian

While legal and ethical matters are encountered in everyday nursing practice, standards and laws are set in the political and governmental arena. Participation in the political process is one avenue of leadership and change for community health nurses.

Chapter Outline

Chapter Objectives

After completing this chapter, the reader will be able to:

- List some of the legal and ethical issues confronting community health nurses
- Compare and contrast the legal and ethical issues
- Identify ways in which community health nurses can protect their own and their clients' legal rights
- Identify possible solutions to the ethical issues

Community health nurses' role in the delivery of health care has always been to provide holistic nursing care to individuals, groups, and families (American Nurses' Association, 1980). Inherent in this role is the premise that the consumers of community health nurses' services actively participate in their care and the decision making that must take place in relation to that care (American Nurses' Association, 1980). The legal issues impacting upon the community health nurses' role, and the rights of their clients, are legion. Most importantly, community health nurses' function, like that of their colleagues, has changed radically. At one time, nurses were considered to be exten-

sions of physicians, their employers. As a result, nurses were rarely, if ever, sued because it was clear that no money could be obtained if a judgment were entered against them. Instead, the physician and/or the hospital were named as defendants, because they were obviously in a better financial position than the nurse. Today, however, with the nurses' role expanding to include autonomous practice and with salaries for nurses beginning to reflect the skill and education required for these new duties, nurses are no longer able to sit back and be legally "protected" by physicians and employers. With autonomy has come legal accountability.

Legal Aspects of Community Health Nursing

Legal accountability obviously demands that community health nurses be constantly aware of the latest developments in the law that affect their practice, their rights as health professionals, and the rights of their clients. They must realize that a right is a claim to which an individual is entitled and which can be enforced by law. In addition, they must understand what duties—obligations they owe to their patients by law—they must carry out. To do so, they must attend continuing education programs, seminars, and workshops dealing with nursing and the law in order to keep abreast of such developments. In addition, attending professional meetings and conventions where programs are offered and/or nursing leaders discuss these developments is vital. Many nursing journals contain featured articles dealing with legal issues in nursing, and community health nurses should subscribe to as many of these as possible. Also, contacting their state legislator concerning state statutes and regulations that affect nursing practice can also be a source of information for community health nurses. Last, an attorney can also be consulted concerning current court deci-

sions and state and federal laws that affect nursing practice.

Legal accountability includes more than knowledge about laws that have ramifications for their nursing practice. Accountability also includes taking responsibility for one's actions. Thus, the importance of carrying one's own malpractice insurance is vital for the community health nurse. By purchasing this insurance, community health nurses are attesting to the fact that they can no longer rely on someone or something else to protect their legal interests. Rather, they must take the responsibility for doing so themselves.

By becoming knowledgeable about the legal issues in community health nursing, community health nurses can incorporate this information into each step of the nursing process. As described by Murchison, Nichols, and Hanson (1982), this incorporation will lead to responsible decision making by nurses (Davis & Aroskar, 1978).

This chapter is not intended to be a source of specific legal advice in specific situations, nor is it a substitute for legal advice. The reader is encouraged to seek competent legal advice when required.

Ethical Aspects of Community Health Nursing

Keeping abreast of the latest developments in the legal arena will be helpful to community health nurses, but it will not provide all of the answers to situations that they will confront when providing care to clients. In fact, situations often arise when community health nurses must balance the patient's legal rights with that client's own contrary wishes and/or values. In addition, the nurse is often confronted with clients' legal rights, wishes, and values that are contrary to the nurse's *own* values. When a situation like this involves "moral claims" that conflict with one another, an ethical dilemma occurs (Murchison, Nichols, & Hanson, 1982). Since community health nurses are likely to face ethical dilemmas daily, we'll take a brief look here at some guidelines for resolving these dilemmas.

One way in which to establish guidelines concerning ethical dilemmas is to be familiar with the many factors that are involved when dealing with an ethical issue. We also need to understand the definitions of those factors.

<u>Ethics</u> itself has been defined as principles and rules that dictate one's conduct in a given situation or situations (Davis & Aroskar, 1978). Ethics includes "morality" or "moral duty." Thus, when talking about ethical solutions to problems, we are concerned about what is "good" and what is "bad," the concept of "obligation," and the concepts of "right" and "wrong" (Davis & Aroskar, 1978). It is important to note that although the individual selects to act in a certain way based on his or her concept of "morality," the latter is developed from society's existing system of laws, ethical codes, and mores (Frankena, 1973).

In addition to these factors, which influence the individual when dealing with an ethical dilemma, another factor that the individual brings into the situation is his or her personal values. A *value* is something of importance or significance. A value can, of course, be something material or a "set of personal beliefs and attitudes about the truth, beauty, worth of any thought, object, or behavior. They are action oriented and give direction and meaning

to one's life" (Simon, Howe, & Kirschenbaum, 1972, p. 44). In addition to personal values, social values may be incorporated into the individual's own set of personal values. Regardless of whether an individual's values are personal, social, or a combination, the values are acquired during the development of the individual and his or her parents, friends, schooling, and religious training, and clearly influence, consciously or unconsciously, any decision made by the individual.

Because all of the factors discussed thus far can impact on the community health nurse's decisions when faced with an ethical dilemma, it is helpful for the nurse to participate in the *values clarification process*. Values clarification is defined as the process of assessing, exploring, and determining what one's own personal values are and what priority they have when making personal decisions (Fenner, 1980). The clarification process involves three major groups: prizing, choosing, and acting. Prizing involves the processes of holding one's own beliefs and behaviors in high esteem and then sharing them with others when the opportunity arises. Choosing, on the other hand, involves knowledge of alternatives, knowledge of the consequences of selecting one alternative over another, and then selecting freely from the alternatives. The acting step in this process is composed of incorporating the value into one's behavior consistently.

The values clarification process can help community health nurses to grow on a professional and personal basis. By consciously identifying those values that impact upon their actions, they will be better able to understand themselves. In addition, they will be able to provide better patient care to clients because their own values will not unconsciously stand in the way of providing that care.

Solutions to ethical dilemmas are rarely easily identified (see Box 24-1). In addition, there are no clear-cut answers to such dilemmas. Nevertheless, community health nurses can attempt to resolve the dilemmas they face by possessing adequate self-knowledge concerning their own values and their

Box 24-1   Resolving Ethical Dilemmas

One method of analyzing an ethical dilemma is to answer the following six questions:

1. Who are the relevant actors in the situation?
2. What is the required action?
3. What are the probable and possible consequences of the action?
4. What is the range of alternative actions or choices?
5. What is the intent or purpose of the action?
6. What is the context of the action? (Wilson & Kneisl, 1983, p. 86)

The answers to these questions can be obtained through the utilization of one of the many ethical theories that have been developed by ethicists in an attempt to understand why certain decisions are made (Davis & Aroskar, 1978). One such theory, *Egoism*, states that an individual makes a decision based on what is best for him or her with little or no regard for another. *Deontology*, on the other hand, focuses on the importance of the moral significance of the values of the actor and on obligations and duties derived from specific rules and principles (Davis & Aroskar, 1978). *Utilitarianism* supports the idea that decisions should be based on the "greatest good for the

greatest number." The *Ideal Observer Theory* supports decision making based on an objective and unemotional approach. The *Obligation Theory* states that two basic principles, the importance of doing good and the idea that justice means equality, should govern one's actions. The *Justice as Fairness* theory takes the position that decisions should be based on the viewpoint of the least advantaged population in society.

Another framework that may help in attempting to resolve ethical dilemmas is the Bioethics Approach formulated by Anne J. Davis. Davis (1981) identifies six principles that can serve as guidelines in decision making when dealing with ethical dilemmas:

1. Autonomy—the right to make one's own decisions
2. Nonmaleficence—the intention to do no wrong
3. Beneficence—the principle of attempting to do things to benefit others
4. Justice—the distribution, as fairly as possible, of benefits and burdens
5. Veracity—the intention to tell the truth
6. Confidentiality—the social contract guaranteeing another's privacy

own ethical framework, and then utilizing that knowledge to help their client participate in the same process. In so doing, clients are able to make their own decisions about the care to be under-taken, and community health nurses, having resolved their own ethical issues, can provide optimal care, as free as possible from any of their own personal biases.

Professional Ethics in Community Health Nursing

As we have seen, community health nurses, like all other individuals, do not live in a vacuum. Rather, their approach to their personal and professional life and the decisions they must make in both spheres of experiences are a culmination of personal and societal values, norms, principles, and ethics. In addition to the personal and societal influences, community health nurses' decisions are also affected by professional ethics.

Professional ethics are usually developed into a

code that identifies standards of practice that become formal guidelines for professional practice (Kozier & Erb, 1983). In addition, such codes provide a frame of reference for the professional when making complex decisions (Kozier & Erb, 1983). Professional ethics highlight the issue of what is "right" or should be done in a health care situation that requires a moral decision (Davis & Aroskar, 1978).

Most health professionals have developed their own code of ethics, and the nursing profession is no exception. Historically, nursing was closely aligned with religion and "social reform" movements (Dolan, 1978; Griffin, 1969). As a result, its ethical development evolved from these two foundations. The first example of a professional code for nurses was the Nightingale Pledge (Griffin & Griffin, 1969), which is still utilized today by many schools of nursing. In 1950, the American Nurses Association formally adopted the *Code for Nurses* to provide nurses with a "framework to make ethical decisions and discharge responsibilities to the public, to other members of the health team, and to the profession (American Nurses' Association, 1968).

The code cannot and does not presume to provide answers to all of the ethical dilemmas the nurse may face in the profession. It does, however, provide a guideline as to the minimum that is expected of members of the profession. As such, the code can provide a basis for censure, suspension, expulsion, or reprimand of any members of the American Nurses Association if any of the code principles are violated. It is important to note that the code may exceed the law, but it is never less than what the law requires of the individual nurse (American Nurses' Association, 1968).

The code also contains interpretive statements for each of the eleven code requirements. These interpretive statements clarify and discuss at length the eleven requirements.

In addition to knowing and understanding their own code of ethics, community health nurses must also be cognizant of other health professionals' codes. Likewise, they must be familiar with other documents affecting their ethical practice such as the American Hospital Association's Patient Bill of Rights, the Nuremberg Code, and the results of the President's Commission for the Study of Ethical Problems in Medicine and Biomedical and Behavioral Research published in 1983.

Although there are no easy answers to ethical dilemmas, community health nurses must be aware of the potential for problematic situations to occur and be clear about their own values in order to provide ethical care without forcing their values on the client.

Reporting: Confidentiality and Privacy

Community health nurses must be constant protectors of their clients' privacy and confidentiality rights. Clients must know that the information they share with the nurse will not be discussed indiscriminately. If the nurse-client relationship is to thrive, it must be based on trust and honest disclosure. In order to ensure that information given to nurses (and other health professionals) is not shared with others than those directly involved in their care, the law has developed protections for such information and affords a legal remedy to clients if confidential information is disclosed without their authorization.

The civil remedy of invasion of privacy allows individuals to sue if information shared about them interferes with their right to be free from unreasonable interferences into their personal life. There are several types of invasion of privacy actions. Some include publicly disclosing private facts concerning the individual, and intruding upon the individual's private affairs or seclusion. Because community health nurses will often be in the position of receiving and having access to information highly personal to their clients, they should seek client consent before disclosing that information to anyone other than those directly involved in that client's care.

A second legal remedy afforded an individual if confidential information is disclosed without permission is a breach of confidentiality action. This legal remedy is most often codified in a state's privileged communication statute which says that certain professionals, such as doctors, attorneys, and priests cannot reveal information obtained during the course of their professional relationship with an individual unless the individual consents to the release of information. The statutes, of course, include exceptions; for example, if a doctor is sued for malpractice by a client, the privilege no longer applies to that client. If it were to continue to apply, doctors could not defend themselves against a client's charges because doctors would have difficulty obtaining that client's permission to release information perhaps vital to the doctor's defense in such an event.

Although nurses are rarely, if ever, named in privileged communication statutes, nurses working in psychiatric nursing often have the mandate to protect from disclosure information about their clients found in mental health records. This mandate derives from state confidentiality statutes, which provide additional safeguards for clients receiving mental health services (Ill. Rev. Stat., 1979).

The legal duty to protect the client's privacy and confidentiality rights also extends into the judicial system. In fact, most privileged communication statutes mandate that the health professional not disclose in court information received during the professional relationship unless the situation is included in one of the exceptions listed in the statute.

In addition to the legal protections afforded a client's privacy and confidentiality rights, ethical protections provide additional support. The American Nurses' Association Code for Nurses mandates that nurses protect the client's right to privacy by "judiciously" protecting information of a confidential nature, and mandates disclosing information

in a court of law only after permission is obtained by the client or when required by law (American Nurses' Association, 1968, pp. 6–7).

In addition to being familiar with the legal and ethical protections afforded a client's privacy and confidentiality generally and in relation to court testimony, community health nurses must also be aware of those situations in which they are legally required to disclose information about a client, both inside and outside a courtroom. Those situations are spelled out in reporting statutes and include the presence of child abuse, communicable diseases, and in circumstances of sudden or accidental death.

It is beyond the scope of this chapter to discuss all the mandatory reporting statutes that may be present in a particular state. However, the statute dealing with child abuse and neglect bears discussing because it concerns a situation with which many community health nurses may come in contact.

Although it is not a new problem, child abuse and neglect has recently caught the attention of society and the legal system, and both have taken an active role in protecting children who are abused or neglected. In 1973, the Child Abuse and Treatment Act (88 Stat. 4(1973)) was passed in an attempt to help health care institutions develop programs to identify, prevent, and report child abuse. After this act was passed and programs set up pursuant to its mandate, many states enacted child abuse statutes. Although the statutes vary from state to state, many similarities exist. One consistent feature of most statutes is the granting of a social service agency (for example, the department of children and family services) and a law enforcement agency (for example, the local police department) the power and authority to act, pursuant to the statute, in protecting the abused or neglected child (Hemelt & Mackert, 1982). A second consistent feature of these statutes is the identification of those individuals who are *required* to report the presence of child abuse and neglect and—in the case of health professionals such as physicians, psychologists, and nurses—dissolves the "privileged quality of communications" between that health professional and the client as a basis for not reporting the child abuse (Ill. Ann. Stat., 1975). A third characteristic feature of the child abuse statutes is the civil and criminal immunity afforded individuals for good faith participation pursuant to the mandates of the act. In some statutes, a presumption of good faith is prescribed for those individuals who are required to report incidents of child abuse or neglect (Ill. Ann. Stat., 1975).

Community health nurses must be familiar with their state's child abuse and neglect statute. In particular, the nurses must understand the definitions of *abuse* and *neglect* in the statute and must be aware of their own responsibilities for reporting child abuse and neglect as well as the reporting procedures to be followed. If community health nurses do not report known or suspected cases of child abuse as required, they are not protecting the health or, in some instances, the life of that child. In addition, an opportunity may be missed to help a dysfunctional family learn healthier, more successful ways of dealing with the frustrations they are experiencing. Finally, nurses who do not follow the mandate of the child abuse statute may create further legal liability for themselves. If the abuse statute contains provisions for individuals who do not report known or suspected cases as they are required to do, then penalties can be imposed on the community health nurse according to those provisions. In addition, community health nurses may be subjecting themselves to additional criminal or civil liability by not intervening on behalf of the child who is abused or neglected.

Despite the existence of mandatory reporting statutes, this legal duty to report a particular situation might present an ethical dilemma for community health nurses. For example, do they have a right to interfere with a family in which a child is being abused? What right, if any, do community health nurses have in making a judgment that abuse and/or neglect is taking place? By reporting their suspicions, the child may be removed from the home. Should nurses "break up the family" like this when perhaps another alternative may be just as helpful to the family? And, of course, there is the ever-haunting possibility that no abuse or neglect ever took place; the injury, for example, *was* an accident. Clearly there is no *legal* liability for a "good faith reporting." But what about an ethical misjudgment?

These questions are not easy to answer. Community health nurses must, however, find answers to be comfortable with their ethical decision. They can reach a decision by being certain that all the data necessary to make the decision are present, identifying the conflicts presented by the dilemma, identifying alternatives and outcomes to a proposed course of action, determining ownership of the dilemma, identifying the appropriate decision-maker, and clarifying the nurse's obligation (Kozier & Erb, 1983).

As they seek to define their legal and ethical role in protecting clients' privacy and confidentiality, community health nurses might keep in mind a basic rule of thumb: information cannot, and should not, be given about a client, either inside or outside of a courtroom, unless that client has given permission to release the information, or unless the nurse is under a mandate to provide that information.

Consent

Like all other nurses, community health nurses must be concerned about making sure that consent for treatment is properly obtained by the physician before initiating treatment. Individuals must fully understand the procedures for treatment before informed consent can be given.

Guidelines for Obtaining Consent

With minor clients (usually defined as under a certain age in each state) the consent of the minor's parent(s) or guardian is essential before treatment can begin. Thus, when caring for a minor client, the community health nurse must be certain that the parent having custody of the client is also the guardian of the minor, especially where the parents are divorced. Likewise, when minor clients are staying with relatives other than their parents, unless these relatives have been appointed as guardians, their consent to any treatment of the minor may be invalid unless a successful argument can be raised that they were acting *in loco parentis*—that is, in the place of the parents. This type of situation arises, for example, when Johnny is left with his grandmother for the summer while his parents are in Europe. Johnny continues to have sore throats while at his grandmother's. Grandmother takes him to the doctor, and the doctor suggests that Johnny have his tonsils out. The grandmother consents, but unfortunately, when the parents return from vacation, they are angry that the surgery was done because they do not believe in surgery. The parents sue the hospital, alleging that their consent was not obtained. The hospital would probably assert that consent was obtained by the grandmother who was acting *as a parent* for Johnny while his real parents were out of the country.

These are certain exceptions to the general legal principle that the parent(s) or legal guardian must consent for treatment to the minor, and these exceptions are often codified in state statutes, which vary from state to state. Some of the more common exceptions include an emergency situation or treatment involving a married minor. When the exceptions exist, the permission of the minor's parent(s) or legal guardian is not needed to institute treatment. In an emergency situation, consent for treatment is "inferred." If the minor is married, he or she can give consent for treatment himself or herself.

Adult clients' consent must be obtained only from that client himself or herself. The substituted consent of another family member, spouse, or other relative is not legally valid consent unless a state statute permits such substituted consent, or one of those individuals has been appointed as a personal guardian of a client who has been adjudicated disabled (the term *incompetent* is retained in many statutes) and therefore unable to make responsible decisions concerning care.

Because disability is not always readily apparent to the community health nurse, it is vitally important that the nurse specifically ask family members whether or not such a determination has ever been made and, if so, to see the order appointing the guardian. The nurse should determine the type of guardianship, any limitations on the length of the appointment, and other specifics. Because family members may not be clear about these specifics, especially if the guardian appointed was someone other than those family members, the attorney who represented the guardian should be consulted. If a guardian has been appointed, then that individual must be consulted concerning consent for treatment of the client.

Community health nurses who work with mentally ill clients must remember that the existence of mental illness does not, in and of itself, give rise to disability. Rather, there must be an adjudication of disability by a court. Many mental health statutes, such as the one in Illinois, reinforce this point by stating that there is a presumption of competency for the mentally ill (Ill. Rev. Stat., 1979).

Consent for Research or Experimentation

Community health nurses may be involved in caring for patients and/or families who are participating in research or experimentation with new drugs or treatments. Thus, concern about the legal issues involved in research and experimentation is vital. The most important legal issue involves that of the informed consent of the patient or individual who is participating in the research or experimentation.

The importance of informed consent with experimentation and research is not unique to those situations alone. The informed consent of all individuals receiving health care is and must be obtained in order to avoid charges of "battery"—an unpermitted touching—or lack of informed consent being brought against the health professional, the institution, and/or the physician. However, with experimentation and research, the issue of informed consent becomes even more important, because its presence is mandated by federal regulations. The following information is required to be given to all subjects involved in research and/or experimentation:

1. Research's purpose, expected duration, procedures involved, and which procedures are experimental
2. Foreseeable risks and discomforts
3. Alternative procedures that might be of benefit to the participant
4. Benefits to the subject or others
5. Description of compensation and/or medical treatment when injury occurs if the research involves "more than minimal risk"
6. Voluntary nature of participation—if individuals refuse to consent, no penalty will be assessed against them; if they decide to participate, they can quit at any time
7. Extent of confidentiality of records involved in research
8. Guidelines detailing who to contact concerning questions about the research or if injury occurs (45 CFR 116, promulgated in 46 *Fed. Reg.* 8366, 8386, January 26, 1981)

The preceding information is required, except for prescribed circumstances, to be on a consent form, and the consent of the participant must appear in writing on that form.

Because the obtaining of the individual's consent is an important step in the process of human experimentation and research, many authorities believe that the consent should be obtained by the researcher himself or herself (Annas & Katz, 1981).

As a result, individual health professionals who are not members of the research team or who are not participating in conducting the research should not obtain this consent. Community health nurses or other health professionals can act as witnesses to the consent obtained from the individual, so long as they have been present to observe the information given the individual pursuant to federal regulations. If community health nurses are placed in a position of not observing that process but are asked to obtain the signature of the individual on the consent form, they can refuse to do so, or, alternatively, sign the form as a "witness to signature only."

When providing care to individuals or families who are involved in research or experimentation, community health nurses should be certain that the consent of their patients has been obtained, and obtained properly. In addition, because they work so closely with patients, they must be constantly aware of any indications that patients may give concerning their desire to revoke their consent. They must also monitor patients' physical and mental status and report any adverse side effects of the treatment or experimentation.

Community health nurses must also be certain that they themselves adhere to the legal requirements concerning research. As part of the research team, they must follow the research protocol, and be certain that their documentation of the research and their patients' involvement is accurate, clear, and factual.

In addition to these legal concerns, the ethical issues in research and experimentation involve using human subjects for such treatment and research (1) when it is not clear that either is entirely without harmful consequences to the human subjects; (2) when it is done to obtain new scientific knowledge about a particular approach and *does not* involve "treatment" to a control group; (3) when there is a question of how "voluntary" the experimental group really is; and (4) when the rights of the individual may be in conflict with the betterment of society. Despite regulations and guidelines protecting individuals involved in research and experimentation, these issues still survive.

Family Concerns

When working with families, community health nurses may confront problems related to the legal aspects of family structure and family function. To help the family and individual members work their way through these problems, nurses rely on a concrete understanding of the issues involved and of ready sources for further information, if the family requires it. Issues that the nurse may be most likely to face revolve around legal responsibility for the care of children, such as guardianship and adoption, or around reproductive issues such as abortion, birth control, and genetic counseling.

Guardianship

Due to the nature of the community health nurse's role with families, individuals, and groups, community health nurses may be in positions to recognize the need for a guardian to be appointed for a certain client. For example, they may care for an elderly client who insists on living alone but whose organic brain condition prevents her from managing her funds and her personal care. The availability of guardianship protection for such clients should be brought to the attention of caring family members. If family members are not willing or interested in providing guardianship services for their family member, nurses can contact the Office of the Public Guardian in their state or other individuals or agencies who may be willing to take this responsibility.

In order to understand the process and procedure of appointing a guardian, community health nurses must be familiar with the state guardianship statutes. These statutes vary from state to state, but there are certain similarities.

First, guardianship provisions for minors are included. The law views minors, except in certain circumstances, as unable or incompetent to make decisions concerning their care, education, and other matters requiring consent due to their age, lack of experience, and undeveloped ability to rea-

son. As a result, the parents, biological or adoptive, are considered to be the legal guardians of their minor children and thus have the legal authority to make decisions for the child until the child reaches the age of majority. When the parents cannot undertake this responsibility for whatever reason(s) and another individual or individuals must fulfill this role, guardianship statutes enumerate the qualifications and the procedure(s) to appoint a guardian for a minor. As is the case when a guardian is appointed for an adult, guardianship for a minor can be appointed for the person and/or the estate. The guardianship can be temporary or permanent, limited or plenary.

Guardianship for adults who are adjudicated disabled must also be done in accordance to the procedures established in the state guardianship statute. What is defined as disability varies, but in Illinois, for example, adults are disabled if because of mental deterioration or physical incapacity, or mental illness or developmental disability, they cannot manage their person or estate, or because of "gambling, idleness, debauchery or excessive use of intoxicants or drugs" spend their estate in a way that exposes themselves or their family to want or suffering (Ill. Ann. Stat., 1979). Guardianship statutes provide procedural safeguards for the individual who is alleged to be disabled; for example, a petition must be filed, and the individual must receive a copy of the petition and notice of the hearing to be held, and how and under what circumstances the guardianship can be terminated.

In addition to the judicial procedures for appointing a guardian for a minor or disabled adult, another type of guardian is known as the *guardian ad litem*. A *guardian ad litem* is an individual, oftentimes a lawyer but not necessarily so, who is appointed by the court to protect the interests of an individual during the pendency of a legal proceeding before the court. *Guardian ad litems* are often used during disability proceedings to ensure that the alleged disabled person's interests are being fully protected. *Guardian ad litems* are also used in adoption proceedings. The judge in any of these proceedings has the power to appoint a *guardian ad litem*; no special judicial procedures are usually required. The *guardian ad litem*'s duties include meeting with the individual whose interests he or she is protecting, discussing that individual's medical and/or psychological responses to treatment with the community health nurse and/or doctor, submitting his or her recommendations to the court, and attending all court proceedings in relation to the issue before the court.

If community health nurses are caring for a client who has a guardian appointed, or for whom a *guardian ad litem* has been appointed, they will need that individual's cooperation. Upon verification that the individual is whom he or she claims to be (asking to see the Letters of Administration and/or order appointing the person to his respective position), nurses should share whatever information they have concerning the client's medical care with the guardian or *guardian ad litem*. Of course, they should be sure to let their client know that they have done so, and in the case of a *guardian ad litem*, obtain the client's permission to share that information beforehand. Also, if community health nurses are working with psychiatric clients, they must be certain to adhere to any statutory restrictions concerning the release of information about their client before doing so.

Even when community health nurses adhere to the legal requirements surrounding guardianship, they still face ethical dilemmas. For example, what about that elderly client whose organic impairment makes it difficult and dangerous for her to live alone, but who is very clear about the fact that she never wants to go to a nursing home or have someone else make decisions for her? And, perhaps even more difficult, what about the client whose family does not care and doesn't want to get involved?

What do community health nurses do when a client's guardian does not see a medical procedure as "necessary" for the client but which the nurse sees as vital to the client's well-being?

The concerns of the client are clear: the importance to the individual in making his or her own decision, the need for a safe environment in which to live, the right to privacy, and an interest in possessing a life-style that is more than just physical survival. What is less clear is what the community health nurse's role will be when he or she is faced with balancing these ethical concerns.

Adoption

Community health nurses may also work with an individual or family who is interested in adopting a child. State statutes concerning adoption vary, but most contain specific provisions concerning who may adopt a child, the procedural requirements for adoption, consent and notice provisions, and the mandate of the confidentiality of adoption records and files (Ill. Rev. Stat., 1960). In addition, many states prohibit the payment of money or the exchange of things of value for placing a child in adoption (Ill. Rev. Stat., 1960).

The adoption of a child is usually a happy event, and community health nurses may face few difficulties when this process occurs. However, nurses may be faced with a family in which they observe that a child or children are not being cared for properly, are sexually abused, or need medical care to which the parent or parents refuse to consent.

In such a situation, community health nurses must, of course, know their legal responsibilities in reporting the existence of child abuse and/or neglect. This legal responsibility will be discussed at length in the later section "Domestic Violence." Community health nurses must also deal with the ethical dilemmas presented in this type of situation. Is it their place to report what they believe to be "poor parenting" when it is possible that the report may result in the parent or parent(s) being declared as unfit and their parental rights terminated? Whose values are nurses using to judge the family's "good parenting"—their own or the family's? And what about the children who oftentimes demand that they be allowed to stay with the parent who may be neglecting, abusing, or being otherwise indifferent to them? Such ethical issues are not easily resolved, but must be grappled with when nurses are faced with a decision to report child abuse and/or neglect.

Reproductive Issues

Another area that community health nurses should be aware of is that of reproductive issues. Many families are often faced with decisions about abortion, birth control, or genetic counseling, and it is important for community health nurses to be familiar with the legal and ethical concerns for each of these issues.

Abortion

The controversy surrounding abortion is not a recent one. In fact, legal and ethical debates concerning this procedure took place as far back as the fourth century A.D. Despite its long history and recent decisions that have legally protected a woman's right to obtain an abortion, abortion continues to be an issue of legal and ethical concern. Prior to 1973, abortions in the United States were done cautiously and under strict guidelines (Davis & Aroskar, 1978, p. 96). However, in 1973, *Roe v. Wade* (410 U.S. 113 (1973)) and its companion case *Doe v. Bolton* (410 U.S. 113 (1973)) were decided by the U.S. Supreme Court. In both cases, the Court declared Texas and Georgia abortion statutes unconstitutional because both had placed restrictions on a woman's right to obtain an abortion. The Court then delineated the rights of a woman seeking an abortion. During the first trimester of pregnancy, a woman and her licensed physician have the right to decide whether or not an abortion will take place. At this point in the pregnancy, the state has no "compelling interest" in placing any restrictions on this right of privacy. Thus, the abortion can occur without any outside intervention. During the second trimester of pregnancy, the Court reasoned that the state has an interest in the health of the mother because, during this period of pregnancy, an increased risk to the mother can occur if an abortion is performed during that time. Thus, the state can pass regulations which "promote(ing) its interest in the health of the mother . . . in ways that are reasonably related to maternal health" (410 U.S. 113, 163 (1973)).

In the third trimester of pregnancy, the Court held that the state could regulate and "even proscribe" abortions except those necessary to "preserve the life or health of the mother" because the state, at this stage of the pregnancy, has a compelling interest in the mother's health and that of the "potential(ity) (of) human life" of the unborn child (410 U.S. 179, 175 (1973)).

In 1976, in *Planned Parenthood of Central Missouri v. Danforth* (96 S. Ct. 2831 (1976)) the Supreme Court decided that the definition of "viability" of a Missouri abortion statute was upheld. That definition defined viability as that point when the unborn's life can be continued outside the mother's womb naturally or by artificial support systems. The Court held that since the determination of viability rests on the judgment of the physician, the definition in the statute was adequate and did not need to specify the number of weeks after which viability occurred.

In addition to protecting the privacy rights of women who seek abortions by striking down regulations that unreasonably restrict that right, the Supreme Court also dealt with the issue of whose consent was necessary before an abortion could be done. In the *Planned Parenthood v. Danforth* decision the Court held that obtaining the informed consent of the pregnant (adult) woman prior to the abortion was permissible, but struck down the consent requirements of parents of pregnant minors under eighteen years of age and of husbands of the pregnant woman as violations of those pregnant individuals' privacy rights. And in *Belloti v. Baird* (96 S. Ct. 2857 (1976)), the Court asked the Federal District Court in Massachusetts to interpret the consent requirements of a Massachusetts abortion statute that required a judicial consent for an abortion for unmarried minors when the parents of that minor refused to consent to the abortion. The Massachusetts Federal Court (428 F. Supp. 854 (1977)) declared the statute unconstitutional because it allowed the parents unlimited veto power over the decision to abort, placed the pregnant minor in a position of having to present her case in a court of law, and did not provide for the possibility that a minor could consent to an abortion under certain conditions—for example, if the minor was a "mature minor."

Although the decisions discussed thus far clearly underlined the right of a woman to seek an abortion, the Supreme Court has decided a number of cases in which it held that states are not required to pay for those elective abortions. As a result of those decisions, many state and federal statutes prohibit the funding of abortions by Medicaid and by the programs funded by the Public Health Service and the Department of Health and Human Services.

The controversy over the right of a woman to obtain an abortion is not yet over. This area continues to be one of constant legal turmoil and debate. Pro- and antiabortion forces are continually protecting and challenging the legality of the abortion question. As a result, community health nurses must keep abreast of the latest developments concerning these decisions. This includes a thorough knowledge of the state regulations concerning abortion. Despite the fact that presently the decision to abort is a protected one that legally remains with the woman and her licensed doctor during the first three months of pregnancy, the decision is often not an easy one for the client to make. The pregnant woman may have conflicts about the decision to abort. Allowing her to ventilate her feelings, positive and negative, will be helpful. Exploring alternatives to abortion, including adoption, may also be helpful.

It is clear that community health nurses cannot help their clients with this decision until they are clear about their own thoughts and feelings concerning abortion. If they are able to balance their own values concerning abortion with those of the client's, even though the two viewpoints may be totally different, nurses can probably work with the client without creating an ethical dilemma for either of them. If some working solution to the dilemma is not possible, then community health nurses can decide not to work with the client who is thinking of an abortion. This right has been codified in federal and state statutes, and are called "Conscience Clauses." The Federal Clause, located at 42 U.S.C. S 300a-7, states that employees who work in agencies receiving a loan, loan guarantee, contract, or grant from the federal government under the Community Mental Health Centers Act, the Developmental Disabilities Services and Facilities Construction Act, the Public Health Service Act or from the Department of Health and Human Services cannot be required to perform or assist in abortion or sterilization procedures if such procedures are contrary to their moral or religious beliefs. In addition, these agencies are not required to perform abortions if contrary to their philosophy.

State conscience clauses are similar to the federal clause, but many provide a wider base of protection by allowing a health professional to refuse to participate in *any* act contrary to their ethical or religious beliefs in providing or refusing to provide medical care. In these types of conscience clauses, "medical care" is defined as including advice or procedures dealing with sterilization, contraception, or abortion. In addition, many state criminal abortion statutes offer a provision allowing health professionals to refuse to participate in abortions and provide immunity from civil, administrative, disciplinary, and criminal proceedings, penalties, or punishment (Ill. Ann. Stat., 1975).

If community health nurses elect not to work with a client because they personally object to abortion, the nurses should, of course, discuss this decision with the client and make arrangements for continued nursing care of the client.

Birth Control

Perhaps as controversial as the issue of abortion, birth control has created legal and ethical debates throughout history. Despite this debate, the legal right of adults to utilize contraceptive measures was underscored in several decisions based on the constitutional right of privacy (381 U.S. 479 (1965)) (405 U.S. 438 (1972)) (410 U.S. 113 (1973)). In addition, a minor's right to obtain birth control information and devices has been supported (428 U.S. 52 (1976)) (431 U.S. 678 (1977)) (96 S. Ct.

2857 (1976)). Prior to this support, and in some instances, *after* the support, many states enacted statutes restricting the right by imposing time frames before the information or devices could be given or by requiring parental notification by the agency that their child was seeking birth control information. However, recently the trend is to provide birth control information and contraceptives to minors (Ill. Rev. Stat., 1969).

This trend is based on the growing awareness that adolescent sexual activity occurs despite the availability of birth control services, and that providing these services may contribute to a decrease in unwanted pregnancies and venereal disease. (For a detailed discussion of adolescent pregnancies, see Chapter 25.)

Despite the legal protections that birth control services possess, the ethical concerns it generates are not easily resolved. For the adult woman, utilizing birth control may be contrary to her religious and moral beliefs. In addition, she and her spouse may disagree as to whether or not she should be using birth control. In addition, financial, career growth, and other factors may influence the decision to have (more) children.

For the minor female, birth control services generate additional ethical dilemmas—not only for the minors themselves but possibly for parents and community health nurses. The knowledge that a minor female is or may be sexually active cannot be ignored. Yet, providing information concerning birth control is often seen by the parent as approving of that activity. On the other hand, the possibility of an unwanted pregnancy creates additional ethical dilemmas—adoption and abortion.

Community health nurses, whether working with an adult client or a minor family member, must resolve their own feelings concerning birth control. When so doing, they can help the client(s) explore their own respective concerns, feelings, and fears surrounding this area of family concern.

Genetic Counseling

Community health nurses may be asked by clients if genetic counseling is a wise undertaking before making the decision to have a family. Many years ago, the availability of this service was scarce. However, with the many advances in medicine and research, this process is more readily available to couples who choose to undertake it.

The legal underpinnings for genetic counseling took place in two cases (227 A.2d 689 (1967)) (519 S.W.2d 846 (1965)). In both cases, the parents were not told that the Down's syndrome and polycystic kidney disease, respectively, could have been detected early in the pregnancy. In addition, the parents of the child born with the kidney disease were told incorrectly that this second child's chance of having the disease was "nil" despite the fact that their first child died of the same disease.

As a result of these cases, the courts held that a cause of action against a physician for malpractice could lie, that the physician has a duty to give accurate information to their patients, and that material information—such as the existence of a diagnostic test (in these cases, amniocentesis)—can't be withheld from them.

Since these two cases, additional cases have been decided that have expanded the scope of legal remedies afforded individuals who were not given proper information concerning genetic counseling, pregnancy, and birth defects. Also, some states have passed "wrongful death" and "wrongful life" statutes, which allow for recovery of certain expenses incurred in the birth process and for moneys spent for the care and treatment of the child.

Perhaps the ethical dilemmas associated with the decision to undertake genetic counseling *prior* to pregnancy are not as severe as those that may arise once pregnancy has occurred and counseling and diagnostic tests reveal that a congenital abnormality exists. Yet prior to pregnancy, many dilemmas arise, and community health nurses may be faced with such issues as the couple who want children very badly and really don't want to know for a fact that there may be some reason that they should not have children. This is clearly a dilemma if the potential biological mother's or father's family, for example, has a history of congenital abnormalities present at birth. Or, the potential biological mother may clearly see the need for genetic counseling, but her spouse sees it as a threat to his "good name and reputation."

Discovering a genetic difficulty after pregnancy raises ethical dilemmas already discussed. Should the couple consider abortion? Can the adoption of a child satisfy the couple's yearning for children of their own? If the couple decides to have the child, can they afford and withstand the financial and emotional strain of caring for a handicapped child?

The community health nurse's role in these dilemmas will most likely be as a facilitator and listener for the couple as they attempt to resolve these different issues. Likewise, teaching may become an additional role for the nurse if the couple decides to keep the child. Should the child be kept at home? Would an institutional placement be better? What kind of nursing care will be needed in either setting?

How community health nurses intervene in these ethical dilemmas with the family will certainly affect the couple's decision in working through this area.

Death and Dying

Death, euthanasia, and the issues of "quality of life" and the "right to die" are emotionally laden topics. The difficulty for professional nurses in resolving the complex legal, ethical, and moral issues surrounding death stems, in part, from the focus of the health professions on preserving life, preventing disease, and promoting health. At one time, this focus was a relatively uncomplicated one, because advances in medical science had not progressed to the point they have today. However, with the recent technological advancements in medical science, health professionals are having to cope with patients whose lives can be artificially maintained indefinitely. These strides have created new legal and ethical dilemmas that must be considered in determining (1) the "quality of life" that is being maintained, (2) that individual's "right to die" with dignity, and (3) which definition of death will be utilized in determining when death has taken place.

At one time, the determination of when an individual died was a relatively simple one for the physician. The doctor made the determination based on accepted medical criteria. The utilization of the common law "heart and lungs" standard, which was exclusively relied on until recently, dictated that an individual was dead when the heart and lungs no longer functioned spontaneously. This relatively simple standard was not useful to the phy-

sician when advances in medical science provided a means of keeping body organs functioning with the use of sophisticated machinery, not by spontaneous action. Thus, in addition to the heart and lungs standard, a brain death standard developed by the Ad Hoc Committee of the Harvard Medical School in 1968 (Ad Hoc Committee, 1968) was added to the determination of death criteria. The criteria has been widely accepted (*Dying*, 1982) for determining whether or not brain death has occurred and, if so, provides a new standard of medical criteria upon which the decision to terminate life support systems can be based. The criteria includes testing for awareness and responsiveness; turning off the respirator for short, regular intervals to determine if the patient can breathe spontaneously; testing reflexes; thoroughly going through the medical record to determine if any drugs might be causing clinical signs and symptoms observed. The tests are to be made at least twenty-four hours after they are first done, and perhaps again after another twenty-four hours have passed. If there is no change in the results after these time periods, then a determination can be made. In addition to the aforementioned criteria, diagnostic tests such as EEG (electroencephalogram) or CAT scan can be helpful in supporting or negating the test results (McCabe, 1981).

By July 1982 the Harvard Criteria had resulted

in the codification of the brain death standard in thirteen states and the District of Columbia under the Uniform Determination of Death Act. The act defines death as: "An individual who has sustained either (1) irreversible cessation of circulatory and respiratory function, or (2) irreversible cessation of all functions of the entire brain, including the brain stem, is dead. A determination of death must be made in accordance with accepted medical standards" (*Uniform Laws Annotated*, 1983, pp. 15–16).

Other states have adopted the brain death standard by case law. Still others, such as Kansas, have codified a brain death standard in separate legislation (Kans. Ann. Stat., 1971).

Thus the brain death standard is gaining in use across the country in one form or another for determining when death occurs, yet controversy surrounds the definition of death and the means for determining its presence. Moreover, legal, ethical, and moral dilemmas also exist about acting on that determination.

The existence of this controversy is clouded even further by the difficulty in defining euthanasia and its relationship with death determination, whether utilizing a brain death or heart and lungs standard as examples of acts of euthanasia. Clearly, the issue of whether or not one is dead and the subsequent decision to terminate life support systems is an important issue legally, but it should not raise the same issues that the concept of euthanasia does. Euthanasia involves deciding to withdraw or terminate life support systems care, or actively participating in "mercy-killing" of patients who are not clinically dead, either from a brain death or heart and lungs standard, but who are clinically "alive."

Perhaps the most complete definition of euthanasia is that of Joseph Fletcher (1974), whose definition includes four ways of dying based on choice, responsible freedom, and purpose:

1. *Voluntary and direct euthanasia*—This form is usually carried out by the patient. Suicide would be an example of this form.

2. *Voluntary but indirect euthanasia*—This form is characterized by the patient giving the power to others to make the decision to end his or her life. The use of a Living Will is an example of this type of euthanasia (see Box 24-2).

3. *Direct but involuntary euthanasia*—With this type of euthanasia, the patient has no say in the decision to terminate his or her life.

4. *Indirect and involuntary euthanasia*—This form includes simply the utilization of care aimed at providing comfort and supportive measures only (Fletcher, 1974, pp. 113–122).

The second type of euthanasia, as defined by Fletcher, is perhaps the least troublesome for health professionals. There has been a recent trend, from at least a philosophical vantage point, of accepting an individual's decision to terminate his or her own life, especially when a chronic debilitating illness or fatal illness is the motivating factor behind such a decision. The law has begun to protect those types of decisions as well, and this is evidenced by the codification of right-to-die statutes, natural death statutes, case law upholding the right of competent adults to refuse life-sustaining treatment, and the development of legally protected substituted consent to withhold treatment for individuals who cannot consent themselves (President's Commission, 1983).

Suicide, on the other hand, can be a more troublesome issue for the health professional, because it is viewed as a much more "active" decision to terminate life (as opposed to the more passive or indirect decision to not consent to further medically necessary hospitalization, for example), and the health professional's legal duty is somewhat different. For example, when an elderly client tells the community health nurse that living alone without family and enough money to pay for all the care he or she needs due to chronic illness, is more than he or she can handle, and that the only solution is death by one's own hand, the nurse is faced with very different legal and ethical issues than if that same elderly client handed the nurse a duly executed Living Will indicating that further

Box 24-2 Example of a "Living Will"

TO MY FAMILY, MY PHYSICIAN, MY LAWYER, MY CLERGYMAN
TO ANY MEDICAL FACILITY IN WHOSE CARE I HAPPEN TO BE
TO ANY INDIVIDUAL WHO MAY BECOME RESPONSIBLE FOR MY HEALTH, WELFARE OR
AFFAIRS

Death is as much a reality as birth, growth, maturity and old age—it is the one certainty of life. If the time comes when I, _____, can no longer take part in decisions for my own future, let this statement stand as an expression of my wishes, while I am still of sound mind.

If the situation should arise in which there is no reasonable expectation of my recovery from physical or mental disability, I request that I be allowed to die and not be kept alive by artificial means or "heroic measures." I do not fear death itself as much as the indignities of deterioration, dependence and hopeless pain. I, therefore, ask that medication be mercifully administered to me to alleviate suffering even though this may hasten the moment of death.

This request is made after careful consideration. I hope you who care for me will feel morally bound to follow its mandate. I recognize that this appears to place a heavy responsibility upon you, but it is with the intention of relieving you of such responsibility and of placing it upon myself in accordance with my strong convictions, that this statement is made.

Signed _____

Date _____

Witness _____

Witness _____

Copies of this request have been given to _____

_____

_____

_____

_____

chemotherapy treatments will not be consented to. At the very least, the nurse in the former situation must explore the client's verbalizations and determine if the verbalizations are rational and well thought out and then assess whether hospitalization, medication, or other interventions may be necessary. Ethically, however, the nurse's views might conflict with or be in agreement with the patient's decision to terminate life. What, then, is the nurse to do? Should the nurse quietly agree with the client that no one will be told of the decision? Or, should the nurse immediately intervene and prevent the individual from carrying out the decision? (See Case Example 24-1.)

The latter two types of euthanasia, which involve direct or indirect action on the part of the health professional, create other ethical, legal, and moral dilemmas. Ethically and morally, for example, the fact that the patient may not make the decision concerning death and the reason for the decision become paramount.

Legally, all types of euthanasia have significance. There have been some suits filed against various health professionals alleging murder, negligence, malpractice, and wrongful death (*State v. Robaczynski*, 1979 in Criminal Court of Baltimore, No. 578-23001; *Tucker v. Lower*, 1972 in Richmond, Va. Land Eq. Court). Until the laws in this

Case Example 24-1: Death and Dying Issues

Mary Jones, a community mental health nurse, has been seeing John Smith, a sixty-year-old retired judge, for about three weeks since his discharge from the city's psychiatric unit. He had been hospitalized for a month for depression. Mr. Smith linked the onset of the depression with the death of his wife, Mildred, after an extended illness. John and Mildred never had children, so he has no one at home with him. The only relative John has is a distant cousin on his wife's side of the family who lives in Cleveland, Ohio.

When Mary sees John for his weekly visit at the mental health clinic, John tells Mary he is thinking of not returning to the clinic for any further visits because "I won't be around much longer." He also gives her several books she had indicated an interest in reading, saying that she "might as well have them."

Assessment of client's potential for suicide

Mary is concerned about these verbalizations and attempts to clarify their meaning further with John. He finally does admit that "I am going to do myself in. I have nothing further to live for. I want to be with Mildred." He begs Mary not to tell anyone about this revelation and not to intervene in an attempt to save him.

Ethical and legal dilemma

Mary reminds John about the contract they had made when they began their relationship concerning the fact that there were certain times when confidentiality could not be adhered to, as when a serious risk of harm or death confronted the patient. Mary states that the possibility of suicide is one such situation in which confidentiality could not be kept, and one in which she feels ethically and legally bound to intervene.

Restatement of nurse-client relationship

John appears to be somewhat relieved by her response, and asks what could be done for him. "I'm just so lonely," he says. "I'm not really sure I want to die. I just don't see any other alternative."

Client responds to discussion

Mary suggests several things to John including the fact that she will contact his physician to see if the medication he is taking for depression might need to be increased. In addition, she suggests they meet more regularly until he is feeling less depressed and suicidal. After John expresses an interest in doing something "useful," she suggests they visit the Retired Citizen's Organization in the city. Its purpose, she explains to John, is to utilize the skills and expertise of retired citizens as consultants to business and industry. John seems very interested, and a visit is set up by Mary for the following day.

Suggested interventions

Acceptance of strategies

---

area become clarified, it is certain that these types of cases will continue to be filed in the future, and their outcomes will determine what role, if any, health professionals can have in participating in euthanasia, and under what circumstances those role(s) will be legally acceptable. Because community health nurses are not immune to the difficulties and controversies surrounding euthanasia,

the determination of why death occurs, and the possibility of inclusion in a legal suit for their participation in caring for a dying patient, nurses must be familiar with any state and federal statutes and case law impacting on death and the care of the dying patient. In addition, they should become involved in committee work in their agency that develops policies and guidelines for nursing judgment in these situations. Political activism is also essential for community health nurses. Communicating with state and federal legislators, participation on state nurses' association committees, and belonging to N-CAP are ways in which community health nurses can help make (needed) changes in this area.

Community health nurses must also be aware of their own feelings concerning death, dying, and euthanasia. Until they come to some decision concerning their own feelings, help cannot be given to the individual patient *or* his or her family.

Finally, the documentation of the care given the dying patient by the community health nurse is vitally important. That documentation, including what was done for the patient, what the patient said or did, written orders by the doctor concerning treatment to be withheld, and the existence of a legal document such as a Living Will may provide the nurse with the necessary defense to allegations against her by the family, the estate of the individual, or the individual himself.

Domestic Violence

Domestic violence is an area of increasing concern not only to the legal profession but to the health professional as well. Since legal and ethical issues in family violence are likely to confront the community health nurse at some time, this section discusses some basic statutes concerning domestic violence.

Violence Against Adult Family Members

Family violence has become such a problem that many states have enacted domestic violence acts to protect family members, especially women and the elderly, from acts of physical abuse, sexual abuse, harassment, and restrictions on personal freedom (Ill. Rev. Stat., 1982). Under these acts, an order of protection can be sought by the victim of the violence or any person on behalf of another. The order may include any of the following remedies: order the abuser to refrain from any physical or psychological harming of the victim; grant exclusive possession of the residence or household to the victim (under certain conditions); and require psychological counseling for the abuser (Ill. Rev. Stat., 1982). Many statutes have specific provisions tying

in the state's office of law enforcement to arrest the abuser if necessary, and to provide transportation to a medical facility for treatment or to a shelter for temporary housing (Ill. Rev. Stat., 1982).

Of course, the Domestic Violence Act is not the only remedy an individual has against family violence. Criminal proceedings can be initiated, or an order of protection can be sought in an already pending criminal action.

If community health nurses are confronted with domestic violence when caring for a client, they may want to discuss these options with that client, and suggest that the client consult an attorney to clarify his or her rights. However, ethical issues are immediately raised. Should nurses attempt to discuss the possibility of domestic violence with the client? Is it presumptuous to assume, for example, that the client is the "victim"? Could he or she be the instigator? And, what about the elderly family member living with a "friend" who is physically abusing her, but by seeking an order of protection will effectively no longer have a place to live once the abuser receives notice of the action filed against him?

These ethical dilemmas are not easy to answer but must be confronted by community health nurses before intervening, or deciding not to intervene, with the client's apparent family violence.

Child Abuse and Neglect

The topic of child abuse and neglect, and the nurse's mandatory duty to report suspected cases, has been discussed in the earlier section "Reporting." It is important for nurses to keep in mind, however, that there are other meanings in addition to the more traditional definitions of child abuse and neglect. For example, there is physical abuse or neglecting to provide adequate food (see Chapter 28). Most child abuse statutes include in the definition of abuse any type of sexual abuse. Usually, sexual abuse of children in families takes two forms. One form, rape, is the less common of the two forms (Wells, 1983). When it occurs, the child victim often suffers physical injury or death as a result of the violence of the incident. The abuser or attacker is most often criminally prosecuted under the state's various sexual offenses statutes.

The second form of sexual abuse of children is more insidious and takes place over a period of time. Here the sexual contacts (which may or may not include intercourse) with the child and the abuser are spread out over a period of time. The abuser, such as the father, uncle, or the stepfather, have easy access to the child in the child's home.

Either because of a fear on the part of the child to tell someone about these contacts, or being threatened by the abuser that if he or she tells anyone, something will happen, these contacts can go undetected for long periods of time. In fact, it is rarely the child-victim who does disclose the contacts (Wells, 1983).

Because the latter form of sexual abuse is less obvious and because child victims are usually hesitant to disclose it, community health nurses must be constantly attuned to the communications and behavior of any children or adolescents they may be seeing as clients. If sexual abuse is suspected, suspicions must be reported so that an investigation by the appropriate agency can be undertaken.

Whatever the form family violence takes, community health nurses are in a unique position for providing assistance to the victim of that violence. That assistance may take the form of providing information concerning the availability of help, which can include suggesting a consultation with an attorney. Or, as has been discussed, that assistance may take the form of nurses fulfilling their legal duty to report their reasonable suspicions so that help can be given to the apparent victim of sexual abuse.

Participation in the Legal and Political Process

Community health nurses cannot practice their profession in isolation. As has been discussed in this chapter, many factors infringe on their practice. In addition, factors such as the expanding role of the nurse, new developments in medicine, and new diseases require not only increasing their skills and expertise but also increased accountability for those skills and expertise.

Consumers of health care are requiring more accountability for the care they receive, and nurses are not immune to that requirement of accountability. This increased legal accountability has resulted in nurses being involved in lawsuits and

will continue to do so. For example, figures released by the National Association of Insurance Commissioners indicate that in 1978, the number of registered nurses named in lawsuits was 3,775 compared to 834 lawsuits in 1976 (Crane, 1983).

Legal Process

Because of the increased participation of professional nurses in lawsuits, it is important for community health nurses to familiarize themselves with the potential roles they may participate in during a lawsuit. As defendants, community health nurses will be defending their actions against a charge of negligence—that is, that their nursing care in some way contributed to the injury of the patient (plaintiff). If community health nurses are called upon to testify in court about certain facts at issue in the case of which they have personal knowledge, then their role becomes that of a witness. For example, community health nurses may be asked to testify about their observations of a client's emotional state on the day on which that client decided that he or she would not accept further treatment for a chronic illness.

Community health nurses may also be involved in a lawsuit as an expert witness. In this role nurses are asked for their opinion as to whether the nursing care given by the defendant in a given situation met the standard required of the professional nurse by law. In this role the expert witness is usually asked to render the opinion based on a hypothetical question, which is composed of the facts in the case at trial.

As discussed earlier in this chapter, in addition to familiarizing themselves with the potential roles they may participate in if involved in a lawsuit, community health nurses should also have knowledge of the judicial system itself. Attending continuing education programs dealing with law and nursing issues is one way in which this goal can be achieved by community health nurses. Community health nurses should also carry their own malpractice insurance to ensure direct collaboration with the insurance company concerning the progress of the case.

Political Process

Nurses' participation in the political process is not a new concept, but its position as a leader in developing and establishing legislation affecting health care is difficult to document (Bostrom & White, 1981). Whatever the historical participation of the profession in relation to health care, today's nurse is faced with the dilemma of participation (with all of its ramifications) or nonparticipation that clearly can result in someone else or another agency, organization, or other interest group defining the nurse's practice.

The debate over whether or not the nurse's participation in the political process is of any consequence is a hotly contested one. Some believe that even when nurses or nursing organizations, such as the ANA, have been involved in the political arena, the influence exerted has been weak at best (Bostrom & White, 1981). Others point to the impact the ANA, for example, has had in obtaining economic security for nurses through its support for collective bargaining and through its role as a labor organization for nurses.

Another debate centers on whether or not the nurses should be participating in the various political processes. Is it ethical for nurses to go on strike, for example? Is it legal? What if patients cannot get the care they need because the nursing staff is out picketing for better staff-patient ratios and higher pay? And what about lobbying for or against certain state or federal legislation? Can and should the nursing profession "pick and choose" which bills it will support and which it will ignore?

A third area of debate centers on the cutbacks in funding for nursing education. If no monies are available, fewer and fewer individuals will be able to study nursing. As a result, the nursing shortage already in existence in some geographic areas of the country will become more profound.

Finally there is the concern over being able to control one's profession. Proposed state and federal laws that influence the practice of nursing must be examined by nurses. Nurses cannot sit back and "let someone else worry about" a bill that, if passed, would allow nonnurses to pass medications without any RN supervision. Another issue of concern to community health nurses is their overall responsibility for the quality of care provided for the general public.

There are no easy answers. However, if an informed decision is not made, and policy, laws, and regulations affecting the practice of nursing become effective, nurses cannot later complain and decry the state of affairs.

Summary

The discussion of the selected legal and ethical issues presented in this chapter has been brief. It is clear, though, that community health nurses, like their colleagues in other specialties of nursing, must keep up with the many legal issues that confront their practice. It is also clear that new ethical and legal issues will continue to develop, and community health nurses cannot be satisfied that they know all there is to know about how these issues affect clients. In addition, community health nurses will need to continue their role as "client advocates" in order to ensure that the rights of clients are not eroded away and, at the same time, encourage clients to take action to ensure the safety of their *own* rights and responsibilities concerning health care. These are not simple tasks, but in doing them, personal and professional growth will result.

Topics for Nursing Research

• How has the community health nurse's role changed due to the recent changes in the delivery of health care, such as DRGs, and the resulting legal implications of those changes?

• What are the similarities and differences of the ethical issues confronting the community health nurse in the past ten years and the resulting legal implications?

• How do community health nurses perceive their role in relation to participation in the political process?

• How do community health nurses, compared with consumers, perceive their role in relation to the protection of clients' legal rights?

Study Questions

1. When community health nurses are faced with a client they believe may be unable to make decisions for himself or herself due to an organic brain condition, which of the following would be an *in*appropriate response?
   a. They should not force their own values on the patient.
   b. They should attempt to discuss their concerns with the client and get his or her input.
   c. They should contact the family after discussing their concerns with the client.
   d. They should begin guardianship proceedings for the client.

2. If community health nurses are subpoenaed to testify concerning a client, they should:
   a. Ignore the subpoena and not show up on the day they are asked to, since patient confidentiality must be protected at any cost
   b. Discuss the subpoena with the client and determine what the client would like them to do
   c. Contact an attorney concerning the subpoena
   d. Go to court on the day subpoenaed and raise patient confidentiality as the reason they will not testify

3. One of the community health nurse's clients, a fourteen-year-old female, asks what a diaphragm is. The nurse is upset and embarrassed by the question. The nurse should:
   a. Tell the girl to talk with her mother about the question
   b. Tell the girl what a diaphragm is and then discuss with her the disadvantages of getting involved in a sexual relationship too early
   c. Ask the girl to explain why she is asking about a diaphragm before asking further questions or giving any advice
   d. Send the girl to the community's birth control center

4. Before purchasing malpractice insurance, community health nurses should inquire into all of the following except:

a. The cost of the policy
b. What it specifically does and does not cover
c. What role, if any, the nurse would have in determining if a case were settled or went to trial if he or she were sued under the policy
d. If their employer carries malpractice insurance for them

5. Community health nurses' ethical perspectives on the situations they confront on a daily basis can come from which of the following sources?
   a. Their own religious views
   b. The profession's code of ethics
   c. Their own values, ideals, and guidelines
   d. All of the above

References

Ad Hoc Committee of the Harvard Medical School to Examine the Definition of Brain Death: A definition of irreversible coma. *Journal of the American Medical Association* 1968; 285: 337.

American Nurses' Association: Code for nurses with interpretive statements. New York, 1968. (Prepared by the ANA Committee on Ethical, Legal, and Professional Standards).

American Nurses' Association, Division on Community Health Nursing: *A Conceptual Model of Community Health Nursing.* Kansas City, Mo.: American Nurses' Association, 1980.

Annas J, Katz B: *The Rights of Doctors, Nurses, and Allied Health Professionals.* New York: Avon Books, 1981, pp. 136–137.

Bostrom C, White J: Nursing's role in the governance of health care. In: McCloskey J, Grace H (editors), *Current Issues in Nursing.* Boston: Blackwell Scientific Publications, 1981, p. 389.

Crane, NB: How to reduce your risk of a lawsuit. *Nursing Life* (January/February) 1983: 17.

Davis AJ: Ethical dilemmas in nursing, JONA and Nurse Educator's 1981 Joint Leadership Conference, 1981. Cited in Wilson HS & Kneisl (editors), *Psychiatric Nursing,* 2nd ed. Menlo Park, Calif.: Addison-Wesley, 1983.

Davis J, Aroskar A: *Ethical Dilemmas and Nursing Practice.* New York: Appleton-Century-Crofts, 1978.

Dolan J: *Nursing in Society: A Historical Perspective,* 14th ed. Philadelphia: Saunders, 1978.

Dying, Death and Dead Bodies in Hospital Law Manual, Vol. II. Gaithersburg, Md.: Aspen Systems Corporation, June 1982, pp. 39–41.

Fenner KM: *Ethics and Law in Nursing: Professional Perspectives.* New York: Van Nostrand, 1980.

Fletcher J: Ethics and Euthanasia. In: Williams RH (editor), *To Live and Die: When, Why, and How.* New York: Springer-Verlag, 1974.

Frankena WK: *Ethics,* 2nd ed. Englewood Cliffs, N.J.: Prentice-Hall, 1973.

Griffin G, Griffin J: *Jensen's History and Trends of Professional Nursing.* 6th ed. St. Louis: Mosby, 1969.

Hemelt MD, Mackert ME: Child abuse. In: *Dynamics of Law in Nursing and Health Care,* 2nd ed. Reston, Va.: Reston, 1982.

Kozier B, Erb G: Values, rights and ethics. In: *Fundamentals of Nursing,* 2nd ed. Menlo Park, Calif.: Addison-Wesley, 1983.

McCabe JM: The new determination of death act. *American Bar Association Journal* (November) 1981; 67: 1476.

Murchison I, Nichols T, Hanson R: *Legal Accountability in the Nursing Process.* 2nd ed. St. Louis: Mosby, 1982.

President's Commission for the Study of Ethical Problems in Medicine and Biomedical and Behavioral Research: *Deciding to Forego Life-Sustaining Treatment: A Report on the Ethical, Medical, and Legal Issues in Treatment Decisions, and Defining Death: A Report on the Ethical, Legal, and Medical Issues in Treatment Decisions.* Washington, DC: Government Printing Office, 1983.

Simon SB, Howe LW, Kirschenbaum H: *Values Clarification: A Handbook of Practical Strategies for Teachers and Students.* New York: Hart Publishing Company, 1972.

Uniform Laws Annotated, master ed. Vol. 12. St. Paul, Minn.: West Publishing Company, 1983.

Wells DM: Child abuse sexual syndrome: Expert testimony: To admit or not admit. *Florida Bar Journal* (December) 1983; 12: 673.

Wilson HS, Kneisl CR: Ethical Reflectiveness. In: *Psychiatric Nursing,* 2nd ed. Menlo Park, Calif.: Addison-Wesley, 1983.

Chapter 25

Adolescent Pregnancy

Barbara Bryan Logan

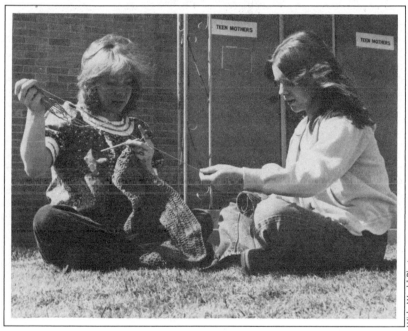

Adolescent pregnancy is an event with implications reaching into family structure, developmental pressures, peer influence, and social conditions. Care for the pregnant teen involves showing sensitivity to the dilemma, helping with appropriate choices, supporting decisions, and meeting physical needs.

Chapter Outline

Chapter Objectives

After completing this chapter, the reader will be able to:

- Describe the scope of adolescent pregnancy
- Provide theoretical explanations for why adolescents become pregnant
- Outline and discuss consequences of adolescent pregnancy
- Explain how adolescent pregnancy affects the family system
- List and describe primary, secondary, and tertiary prevention strategies community health nurses can employ in adolescent pregnancy

Adolescent pregnancy has become a prevalent phenomenon and one of society's great health and social concerns. Increasing numbers of teenagers are sexually active (Zelnik & Kantner, 1980) and become pregnant, resulting in a dramatic rise in children born to and living with unwed teenage mothers (Alan Guttmacher Institute, 1981). Many authors (for example, Burden & Klerman, 1984; Chilman, 1980; Furstenberg, 1976) have addressed the serious negative consequences of adolescent pregnancy for teenage mothers, their children, and for society in general. This phenomenon, which cuts across all socioeconomic and racial lines, has received increasing national attention in the last decade.

This chapter presents an overview of the problem of adolescent pregnancy, beginning with a description of its scope in contemporary society. We'll analyze adolescent pregnancy and its consequences against the background of the developmental issues of adolescence. By exploring the impact of adolescent pregnancy on the family and community, we'll also develop the basis for health promotion strategies that community health nurses can use in working effectively with this population at risk.

The Scope of Adolescent Pregnancy

The epidemic of adolescent pregnancy has become a public issue. A well-publicized report, *Eleven Million Teenagers*, published by the Alan Guttmacher Institute (1976), and substantiated by research findings and population data, dramatized the problems of adolescent sexuality and childbearing. It received extensive press coverage and was instrumental in calling the public's attention to the problems related to increased sexual activity, pregnancy and parenting among adolescents. The grassroots community, government officials, private foundations, and health professionals all became interested in the problem and collectively viewed it as an epidemic.

The Adolescent Health Services, Pregnancy Prevention and Care Act of 1978, sponsored by Senator Edward Kennedy, made it possible for the government to fund public and private agencies and organizations to conduct research and to establish programs designed to prevent adolescent pregnancies or provide services to adolescent parents. The extent of adolescent pregnancy is evident by the statistics compiled by the Alan Guttmacher Institute (1981) and summarized by Neinstein and Stewart (1984) as follows:

1. Of the 10 million females in the United States between the ages of fifteen and nineteen, 1.1 million become pregnant each year. In addition, 30,000 girls younger than fifteen become pregnant each year.

2. Of these pregnancies, 50 percent go to delivery, 74 percent are unintended pregnancies, and 66⅔ percent are among unmarried adolescents.

3. Of the 1.1 million adolescent pregnancies each year:
   - 27 percent result in birth to married couples
   - 22 percent result in out-of-wedlock births
   - 13 percent terminate in spontaneous abortion
   - 38 percent terminate in induced abortion

4. The United States has the seventh highest adolescent childbearing rate among industrialized countries.

5. One-third of all abortions are obtained by teenagers; one-fifth of all births are among teenagers; and 46 percent of all births to unmarried females are among teenagers.

6. The fertility rate among U.S. females has declined among females eighteen years and older but continues to rise for teenagers eighteen years and younger.

7. More than one-third of those who are sexually active premaritally have a premarital pregnancy before age nineteen.

8. One of five female teenagers becomes preg-

nant within one month of her first sexual contact; 50 percent become pregnant within six months of their first sexual contact.

9. The number of pregnant teenagers has increased 13 percent from 1973 to 1978, and the pregnancy rate per 1,000 females has increased from 10 percent to 11 percent (p. 387).

The upward trend in adolescent pregnancies became evident in the 1950s. In the 1970s, such pregnancies escalated (Allison-Tomlinson, 1982; Chilman, 1979; Zelnik & Kantner, 1980). Statistical reports for the early 1980s indicate that the out-of-wedlock adolescent fertility rate is still increasing but at a much slower rate than in previous years (Zelnik & Shah, 1983). This change may be attributed to a decline in the number of adolescents in the population, or it may mean that teenagers are becoming more effective contraceptors.

Despite effective use of contraceptives among many teenagers, a sizeable number of them who are sexually active use contraceptives sporadically or not at all (Zabin & Clark, 1983). Some depend on chance (Freemen & Rickels, 1979) and as a result are saddled with unplanned, unintended, and often unwanted pregnancies. Current trends indicate that most adolescents who become pregnant out-of-wedlock keep and parent their babies (Alan Guttmacher Institute, 1981; Resnick, 1984; Sklar & Berkov, 1974). Consequently, adolescent pregnancy and parenthood presents a serious challenge to health professionals, among them community health nurses, who are responsible for planning and providing health services to pregnant adolescents and their families.

Concepts of Adolescence

The adolescent who finds herself unexpectedly pregnant takes on a major adult task when she is only on her way to becoming an adult. She is in the process of relinquishing childish ways at the same time she is adopting more adult behaviors and responsibilities. The crisis of pregnancy creates uncertainties concerning the adolescent's self-concept, her self-identity, and her outlook for the future. She is faced with immediate questions such as What will I do? Who will I turn to? What will happen to me? and Who will I tell first?

The adolescent may think she has done something wrong in becoming pregnant and experience feelings of shame and guilt. These feelings may affect her more than the adolescent father for a number of reasons. While societal attitudes may be more accepting of premarital sex among teenagers, it is the young woman who actually shows the physical signs of the behavior by becoming pregnant. Men are encouraged to engage in sexual activity as

a measure of their manhood, but are not strongly encouraged to accept responsibility for their actions.

If shame and guilt do damage the pregnant teenager's self-concept, she may conceal the pregnancy in its beginning stages. This can complicate the problem in the long run, since effective resolution of the pregnancy crisis requires early intervention by significant adults. For instance, if the adolescent wishes to terminate the pregnancy through a legal abortion, this action may require parental consent and involvement and the intervention of health care professionals early in the pregnancy. If the adolescent waits too long to acknowledge the pregnancy, it may be too late to resolve it through such an option.

Pregnancy alone causes many physical and emotional changes in the female, but when it occurs in adolescence, it is compounded by changes normal to adolescence itself; the resulting triple developmental crisis can be overwhelming to the young woman (Lippert, 1984). As a result of the preg-nancy, the adolescent simultaneously faces the cri-sis of adolescence, the crisis of pregnancy, and the crisis of establishing a relationship with a member of the opposite sex. Caught between childhood and adulthood, the adolescent has performed an adult act, with serious adult consequences, but must depend on others, mostly adults to make important decisions and answer important questions. Having sought independence, the pregnant adolescent may find herself even more dependent on the adults in her life.

Adolescent pregnancy is discussed and pre-sented in the literature as if it were entirely a female issue, as if the young woman were solely responsible for the situation. The event of pregnancy, how-ever, can certainly present a crisis for the adoles-cent male as well. How each individual handles this crisis depends on a variety of circumstances, such as the adolescent's age, the family, environ-mental factors, and the particular decisions that have to be made concerning the pregnancy. To better understand the impact of pregnancy in ado-lescence, it is important to view the event within the context of adolescence itself.

Theoretical Perspectives on Adolescence

No single description of adolescence adequately characterizes all aspects of this developmental period. However, most theorists agree that adolescence is a period of transition (or a bridge) from childhood to adulthood. During this period all adolescents must at some time resolve issues related to:

- Self-image or sense of identity
- Self-esteem
- Acceptance of change in self
- Independence
- Peer relationships
- Relationship with the opposite sex
- Cognitive and vocational achievement
- Mood swings or depression
- Desire to act out (White, 1972)

In a physical sense adolescence has been described as a period that signifies that the body is capable of reproduction. A boy becomes a man since his body can produce sperm capable of fertilizing an ovum to produce new life, and a girl becomes a woman since her body can produce ova capable of fertilization by a male, also to produce new life (Draper, Ganong, & Goodell, 1980). During this time the body undergoes significant changes. For example, there is dramatic physical growth spurred on by hormonal changes in every part of the body. Arms, legs, and trunk lengthen, and the sex organs become much more developed. There is a new awakening of sexual feelings, and the adolescent must find socially acceptable ways to express these feelings. The struggle to discover such ways could leave the adolescent in conflict, confused or ambivalent.

Lidz (1968) describes the ambivalence and con-flicts of the adolescent period as:

A time of physical and emotional metamorphosis during which the youth feels estranged from the self the child had known. It is a time of seeking: a seeking inward to find who one is, a searching outward to find one's place in life, a longing for another with whom to satisfy crav-ings for intimacy and fulfillment. It is a time of turbulent awakening to love and beauty and also of days darkened with despair. It is a time of the care-free wandering of the spirit through the realms of fantasy and in pursuit of idealistic visions, but also of disillusionment and disgust with the world and the self (p. 298).

Whereas Lidz describes the period of adoles-cence in general, some theorists focus on the spe-cific tasks adolescents are expected to accomplish. Havighurst (1972) develops a list of eight such tasks. The adolescent is expected to: (1) accept one's own physique and use the body effectively; (2) achieve appropriate sex-role formation; (3) achieve new and more mature relationships with peers of both sexes; (4) achieve emotional independence from parents and other adults; (5) prepare for a voca-tion; (6) prepare for marriage and family life; (7) desire and achieve socially responsible behav-ior; (8) acquire a set of values and an ethical system as a guide to behavior. The adolescent woman who is faced with an unwanted, unplanned pregnancy may become preoccupied with feelings of guilt and shame or a sense of failure. She may develop a negative body image (although temporarily) as she gains weight and her figure changes as a result of the pregnancy. She may become more dependent on, rather than independent of, parents. This situation would undoubtedly inhibit her ability to accomplish the tasks outlined by Havighurst.

As discussed in Chapter 16, Erikson (1950) defines adolescence as one of eight stages of ego development. This stage classified as "identity vs. role confusion" is one in which the adolescent developmental task is to develop a sense of identity. Thus, like Havighurst, Erikson focuses on the task the adolescent is expected to accomplish. In this stage the young person seeks to answer the question, "Who am I?" Young adulthood, the next stage in Erikson's schema, is successfully entered when ego identity and role integration are established. Lack of resolution of these issues can lead to role confusion and identity crisis.

Adolescence also has been defined in terms of egocentrism and narcissism (Elkind, 1967, 1970, and 1978). Elkind (1967) contends that the adolescent, like the toddler, is preoccupied with self and, as a result, creates his or her own personal reality to go along with the ordinary reality of everyday life. He also suggests that adolescents' sensitivity to the physical and sexual changes they are experiencing makes them self-conscious. They begin to assume that people around them are as obsessed with their behavior and appearance as they are, and that they are always the center of attention (Elkind, 1967). They judge themselves as if from the point of view of other people. This imaginary audience that they have created can often be highly critical, constantly pointing out physical and personality deficits. This increases adolescents' self-consciousness and causes them to vacillate between self-admiration and self-criticism. Elkind explains that their exaggerated sense of uniqueness, a belief that they are totally different from other people, sometimes leads them to feel that they are immune to events that happen to ordinary

people. Elkind's theory provides partial understanding of why some adolescents may engage in sexual intercourse without birth control. It is possible that they magically feel invincible—that they cannot get pregnant.

From all theoretical perspectives adolescence is a critical time when the child integrates the personality and moves toward becoming a mature adult. The adolescent peer group can play an influential role in this process.

Peer Influences in Adolescence

As adolescents progress toward adulthood, they seek more independence and autonomy in making their own decisions. In their decision-making process, the opinions of their peers are often more valued than those of their parents.

During adolescence there is great tendency to exert peer pressure to coerce others to comply or conform to the needs and desires of the peer group. Often this pressure is more perceived than real (Newman, 1984)—that is, teenagers perceive that their peers have certain expectations of them and behave in ways to meet those expectations. In a study of the influence of peer pressure on adolescent smoking, Newman (1984) discovered that pressure to smoke was less related to desire to smoke than it was to (1) pressure to appear independent; (2) pressure for recognition; (3) pressure to appear grown-up; and (4) pressure to have fun. These same pressures can result in behaviors that ultimately lead to pregnancy in adolescence.

For instance, adolescents who refrain from dating and engaging in sexual intercourse may feel that they are not as grown-up or having as much fun as friends who are dating and who are sexually active. Such adolescents may feel, and may actually be, very unpopular. Since teenagers are concerned about the impression they make on their peers and want to be recognized and accepted by the peer group, the decisions they make and their behaviors are likely to reflect those of the majority of the group.

The peer group can also serve as a testing ground for adolescents. They typically confide in their friends before confiding in others. Thus, adolescents are prime sources of help for one another, but they are not always equipped to provide the kind of help that may be needed, particularly when situations such as pregnancy are involved. For such matters the support of peers and the need for independence from parents must be balanced by firm guidance from parents and other significant adults such as community health nurses. The peer group is an excellent target group with which community health nurses can work to bring about positive health and responsible decision geared toward prevention of adolescent pregnancies.

Sexuality in Adolescence

Sexual behavior among adolescents has been changing over the last decades. All reports indicate that premarital sexual intercourse has become relatively common among young men and women. For example, a nationwide survey of thirteen- to nineteen-year-olds indicated that 45 percent of girls and 59 percent of boys reported having experienced sexual intercourse at least once (Sorenson, 1973). The percentages continue to increase (Zelnik & Shah, 1983).

Whereas premarital sex had been fairly common and generally accepted for men (Kinsey, 1948), the increasing numbers and acceptance of premarital sex for women are more recent phenomena. Zelnick and Kantner (1980) report that the proportion of women aged fifteen to nineteen who had experienced premarital sexual intercourse increased from 30 percent in 1971 to 43 percent in 1976 and then to 50 percent in 1979. Reporting from the same data, a national probability sample survey of young men and women in the United States carried out in 1979, Zelnick and Shah (1983) state that the average age at which women had their first intercourse was 16.2 compared to 15.7 for men. The authors

found some differences between men and women regarding their first sexual experience. Whereas more than six out of ten young women felt a commitment to their first sexual partner and said they were either going steady or engaged to them, most men reported having a casual relationship with the woman. The initiation of sex appeared to be a "spur of the moment" decision for most young women. Only 17 percent of them, compared to 25 percent of men, planned their first sexual intercourse.

Sexuality in adolescence, however, encompasses more than sexual intercourse. It involves the awareness and expression of oneself as a sexual person, and includes the feelings, attitudes, and behaviors that accompany this awareness. In achieving a sense of sex-role identity, adolescents become aware of themselves as sexual persons and must come to grips with their sexuality. They experience increase in sexual drives and feelings and may have a tremendous task of controlling these sexual urges, especially since they are bombarded with sexual stimuli from various sources, particularly the media.

The messages about teenage sex-roles and responsibilities are often confusing and contradictory. On the one hand, our society encourages and accepts teenage sex (as evidenced by explicit and implicit messages encouraging sexual activity in many newspaper and TV ads and pop songs). On the other hand, pregnancy and birth out-of-wedlock are considered highly unacceptable. This is particularly true if the woman is a very young teenager. Some teenagers are ambivalent about their own sexuality. They don't want to become pregnant but fail to use contraceptives. How the adolescent expresses his or her sexuality is influenced by close friends, adolescent peer group, the media, and also by cultural expectations, morals, and religious beliefs.

Part of the reason many adolescents fail to deal with their own sexual responsibility is due to the lack of communication between teenagers and their parents about sexuality. Such communication is often nonexistent or contradictory. Parents are often uncomfortable discussing the subject, and when they do, their words are often contradictory to their actions. This is important because in the socialization process sex-role behavior is learned primarily through observation and imitation of significant others, such as parents. Community health nurses who have contact with parents of adolescents can help these parents communicate openly with their children about adolescent sexual development.

Theoretical Explanations for Adolescent Pregnancy

Many explanations have been offered for why adolescent women become pregnant. Some of these explanations are psychoanalytic or psychological interpretations such as low self-esteem due to absence of feminine identification with a well-regarded mother coupled with a close daughter-father relationship, hostility and distance in the parental marriage, traumatic family events such as the mother having a hysterectomy, and peer pressure to engage in sexual activity (Abernethy, 1976). Others are the adolescents' own simple explanations such as "I made a mistake" or "I just got caught" (Bryan-Logan & Dancy, 1974; Furstenberg, 1976). Other psychological explanations include the adolescents' desire to manipulate their parents or partner, the desire for increased autonomy (Nadelson, Notman, & Gillon, 1980), blind impulsive acting out against parents (Wolf, 1973), acting out against themselves (Miller, 1973), and the subconscious wish for a baby who represents someone for them to love and someone who also needs them and will love them (Epstein, 1980). Psychoanalytic and psychological theories of pregnancy in adolescence explain the occurrence in terms of unconscious motivations resulting from early parent-child dysfunctioning. The assumption is made that pregnancy is consciously or unconsciously wanted.

Newer theories explain adolescent pregnancy as resulting from relevant factors in the social-cultural milieu (Phipps-Yonas, 1980). Such explanations point to social conditions in the environment that lead to ignorance about contraceptive use, lack of access to contraceptives, absence of social sanctions against pregnancy, and economic obstacles to contraceptive use (Hatcher, 1976; Miller, 1976).

Still other views of adolescent pregnancy suggest that there are no essential differences between pregnant and nonpregnant adolescent girls (Phipps-Yonas, 1980).

Lack of adequate information about sex, reproduction, and contraception (particularly effective contraceptive methods such as the pill) and an overwhelming need for privacy about sex and birth control among adolescents (Kisker, 1985) may explain some adolescent pregnancies. Young men and women may believe that they are either too young, or that they engage in sexual intercourse too infrequently to become pregnant. Some may not understand the proper use of contraceptives, and may, for example, take a pill immediately before intercourse, believing that this will prevent pregnancy.

Some teenagers are caught in the confusion of wanting to have sexual intercourse and believing that sex before marriage is wrong. They may rationalize that their reputation for good behavior is not damaged if they have sex secretly and only occasionally. They may, therefore, fail to use contraceptives regularly and before intercourse, because this would signal their premeditated intention to do something wrong.

Biological factors have also been cited as explanations for adolescent pregnancies; menarche and puberty take place earlier now than in previous years. At present, menarche and puberty take place at about ages twelve to thirteen compared to ages sixteen to seventeen in the late nineteenth century. Because of this change teenagers are fertile at younger ages (Neinstein & Stewart, 1984). The effect of this change—coupled with adolescents' newly awakened sexual desires, more relaxed family and school controls, more relaxed sexual attitudes in society, and increased sexual stimulation from the media—is increased freedom and opportunity to have sexual relations.

Clearly, evidence to support explanations for why pregnancy occurs in adolescence is inconclusive. Furthermore, virtually all explanations are focused on the young woman. Research investigations into the male role in adolescent pregnancies are greatly needed.

Whatever the reasons the adolescent woman becomes pregnant, the pregnancy is likely to result in many negative consequences for herself and her family. While some pregnant adolescents encounter little or no unusual difficulties and, with adequate support, arc able to overcome major problems, those who experience negative consequences are of particular concern to community health nurses.

Consequences of Pregnancy in Adolescence

The negative consequences of pregnancy in adolescence have been well documented (Chilman, 1979; Furstenberg, 1976; Phipps-Yonas, 1980; Young, 1967) and can be categorized as (1) physiobiological-medical, (2) psychosocial-cultural, (3) educational, and (4) economic.

Physiobiological-Medical

Plionis (1975) reviewed studies showing that from a medical perspective pregnant adolescents are a high risk group because of high incidence of medical problems for the mother and the baby. Commonly identified problems for the mother are complication of pregnancy such as toxemia, difficult labor and delivery, iron deficiency anemia, and proneness to illness. The younger the teenager, the more likely she and her offspring can suffer serious medical consequences. The Alan Guttmacher Institute (1981) reports of New York data indicate that maternal mortality rate among adolescent mothers is 2½ times higher than for mothers aged twenty to twenty-four (18 compared to 7.1 per 100,000 live births).

Complications for the infants are prematurity and low birthweight. The infants are also more likely to be physically, intellectually, and developmentally impaired, resulting in higher rates of mortality than those associated with infants born to older parents (Bernstein, 1971; Braen & Forbush, 1975; Johnson, 1974; Osofsky, 1968). These infants are at high risk because of maternal problems that can compound their condition, such as poor maternal nutrition, lack of prenatal care, and short postmenarche interval prior to conception.

Reports of infant health indicate that in 1981 the highest proportion of low birthweight babies were born to mothers under age fifteen (14 percent compared to 6 percent of babies born to mothers aged twenty-five to thirty-four) (Digest: Family Planning Perspectives, 1984). In addition, babies born to mothers younger than eighteen had higher morbidity and mortality rates than infants born to other mothers. Furthermore, babies born to young mothers have an increased risk of dying in the first month after birth because of low birthweight and have an increased risk of death and illness throughout the rest of the first year of life because of socioeconomic disadvantages. Overall, medical complications of pregnancy are associated with lack of immediate prenatal care—teenagers tend to seek care late in pregnancy. Evidence shows that when they receive adequate prenatal care, complications diminish.

Psychosocial-Cultural

Becoming pregnant in adolescence can be very stressful for the teenager, predisposing her to many emotional conflicts. Bacon (1974) reports that early motherhood requires an accelerated role transition that is at variance with the socially prescribed sequence of life cycle processes. The stress encountered in the assumption of the adult role of mother, without proper transition and preparation for the role, can lead to conflicts with significant others such as parents, boyfriends, peers, teachers, and neighbors. For example, the young mother may be faced with meeting the demands of self versus those of the child, dealing with loneliness and isolation from peers, and managing feelings of uncertainty and anxiety due to role insecurity (Young, 1967). Herzog (1970) reports that teenage parents of our current society are particularly vulnerable to stress due to loss of cultural guidelines for childbearing. Our culture has no systematic ways of preparing young people to be parents while still adolescents.

Teenage parenting can lead to irritability and depressed feelings when the young parents are deprived of the adolescent social network of which they are an integral part. For the young woman, separation from this peer network into the role of motherhood can lead to feelings that only the mothering role is open to her. Awareness of alternatives to future childbearing becomes restricted. Subsequently, teenage mothers may marry and form unstable, less successful marriages that are prone to disruption (Glick & Norton, 1977) or have subsequent out-of-wedlock pregnancies and ultimately be dependent on welfare. Repeat pregnancies and welfare dependency have been reported to be very common among teenage mothers.

Educational

Early childbearing is associated with decreased educational attainment. Stevens (1980) summarized studies documenting that teenage parents are educationally disadvantaged primarily because they drop out of school as a result of the pregnancy with very slim chances of returning. Some teenagers who remain in school in the initial stages of motherhood eventually drop out because they find the burden of child care so severe that it leaves them little time for schoolwork. Falling behind in their schoolwork, missing school days, and fearing failure can cause them to drop out altogether.

There is some disagreement in the literature as to whether girls who become pregnant are low achievers and less academically capable in the first place, or their lack of educational achievement is a result of the pregnancy. Whatever the specific reason, the results and the impact on the girl and the baby are the same: the interruption of education results in a vicious cycle of limited opportunity to learn marketable skills and compete in society. This can lead to a cycle of poverty, low family income, and more pregnancies. However, although the educational future for many adolescent mothers is dismal, some adolescents who become parents do remain in school and achieve to their academic potential. This is possible through individual resources, flexible school programming, and family support.

Economic

Adolescent pregnancy and childbearing can place a heavy economic toll on teenagers and drain the economic resources of the family (Bacon, 1974; Furstenberg, 1976; Trussell, 1976). These authors report that teenage parents are likely to be single and dependent on their families or public assistance. Early childbearing increases the chances that young mothers will require Aid to Families with Dependent Children (AFDC) (Burden & Klerman, 1984). Almost half of AFDC expenditures go to households in which the woman bore her first child as a teenager (Moore, 1979, 1981).

General lack of skills and experience necessary to obtain well-paying jobs compounds the problem and can lead to prolonged economic dependency. The father of the baby, usually a teenager himself, or young enough so as not to have established himself economically, is typically unable to meet the financial burden of the new baby. The cumulative consequences of interrupted education and lower economic potential are likely to diminish the teenage mother's overall career attainment and serve as barriers to her further achievements.

The family of the pregnant adolescent can play a crucial role in limiting her economic dependency (Burden & Klerman, 1984).

Impact of Adolescent Pregnancy on the Family System

Chapter 2 describes the social systems approach to understanding families. Viewing the family as a set of interacting parts, we realize that whatever affects one part of the family affects the entire family and, likewise, whatever affects the entire family affects each individual member. Consequently, when a teenager becomes pregnant, the pregnancy affects not only her but also her entire family, and the reactions of the entire family to the pregnancy affects the teenager. Thus, if the pregnancy is a crisis for the adolescent, it is likely to be a crisis for the entire family system.

The impact of the pregnancy is felt not only by the pregnant girl's family but also by the adolescent boyfriend's family as well. The pregnant teenager is undoubtedly involved in a complicated network of relationships within and between various subsystems (as illustrated in Figure 25-1), but the relationship she has with her child's father and her own family are likely to be most crucial.

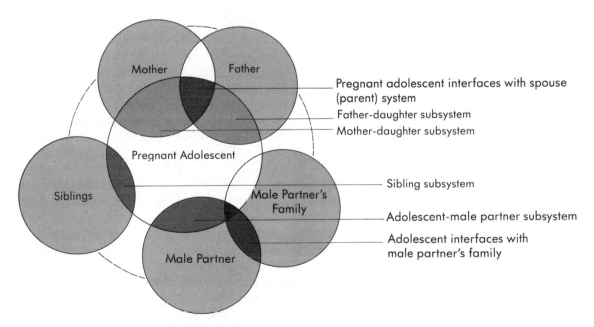

Figure 25-1 Pregnant adolescent relationships with subsystems.

The Adolescent Mother—Male Partner Subsystem

Whether or not the pregnant teenager and her partner decide to marry and live together in the same household or remain single, the male partner's role as the baby's father makes his relationship to the mother and to the rest of her family crucial. Little has been written concerning this role, although it has been reported that 45 to 63 percent of pregnant adolescent girls remain in contact with their male partner throughout pregnancy and after delivery (Furstenberg, 1976; Lorenzi, Klerman, & Kekel, 1977). However, whereas many male partners provided social and economic support and remained in contact with their children for up to five years following the initiation of pregnancy, the frequency of visits and supports declined over time (Furstenberg, 1976; Pressor, 1980). Also, fathers assisted very little in the actual day-to-day demands of raising their out-of-wedlock children (Pressor, 1980).

Many pregnant adolescents' male partners are themselves young teenagers with special concerns and needs. Panzarine and Elster (1982, pp. 21–22) identified the following areas of potential psychosocial stresses for adolescent fathers:

- Role responsibilities of fatherhood (feelings of uncertainty and self-doubt regarding capabilities as father; responsibilities of fatherhood appear overwhelming)
- Relationship with partner (concern with partner's changing body and mood swings and with decision making concerning marriage and their continued relationship)
- Changes in usual sources of support (concern about reactions as well as type and level of support they will continue to receive from family and peers)
- Health of mother and babies (fears of complications of childbirth)
- Anxiety regarding labor and delivery (uncertainty about own role)

Other studies portray the male partner from the young woman's perspective. For example, in an interview study (Logan, 1972), eleven pregnant adolescents freely discussed their babies' fathers as young men with whom they had a special relationship. Most of them reported that their real interest in boys began with this male partner. These findings are consistent with other studies indicating that pregnant adolescent women feel a commitment to their partner. They were either engaged to them or going steady (Zelnik & Shah, 1983). Despite any initial positive feelings and a good relationship, however, many boyfriends were unable to assist the young women in serious decisions concerning the pregnancy because most were young, economically and emotionally dependent on their own families, and unable to make important decisions concerning marriage, abortion, or financial support.

Rosen, Ager, & Martindale (1979) report that men are mostly involved in adolescent pregnancy at the point of resolution of the pregnancy. They strongly influence the adolescent to keep the baby as opposed to terminating the pregnancy. However, when the young woman decides to keep her baby and remain with her family, it is her family, not the baby's father who has the final say in decisions concerning her and the baby. This is because expectant fathers tend to be unemployed (Hendricks, 1981) and are unable to contribute financially to the pregnant teen: limited finances diminish their decision-making power. In some instances the mother of the teenage girl actively intervenes with the teenage father and his family to obtain some level of support for her daughter and the expected baby. The level of support a young father can offer is influenced not only by economic circumstances, but also by his own family's situation, as illustrated by Case Example 25-1.

Families of unmarried adolescent women who keep their baby and remain in their family's household usually have difficulty deciding if and how to incorporate the father of the child as a family member. Some fathers enter their bids to support the child, and if his offer is accepted by the adolescent's family, he is accorded certain rights to call upon

---

Case Example 25-1: Parental Involvement in Adolescent's Pregnancy

This widowed mother had decided that her daughter would keep the baby and deliver at a private hospital. She wanted her daughter to marry the father of the baby, but his mother thought he was too young.

"I told him [the boyfriend] that he was to give me $15.00 every week as long as he was working, commencing with that week. So far he hasn't missed a payday. He even gave a raise of $20.00 without my asking. Last week he brought a money order. I didn't say anything, because I know that's his mother's doing. She told him to get some type of receipt for his money."

Adolescent's mother confronts and negotiates financial arrangements with daughter's boyfriend

"When I talked to her [the boyfriend's mother], she told me she thought her son was too young to get married. I told her that if he is old enough to have sex, he is old enough to assume the responsibilities that go along with it. . . . I told her that I understand that many mothers like to hold on to their sons, but she couldn't hold him forever. You see, Carla is my daughter, and I assume the responsibility for her as long as she lives in my house. . . and I told her the same thing. I told her that I have every intention of taking care of my daughter properly. I made arrangements for Carla to deliver at a private hospital. Her boyfriend came to tell me about a cheaper hospital that his mother had suggested. I told him to tell his mother that so far, he was meeting his obligations, and as long as Carla is my daughter and I was responsible for her, I will make the decisions."

Adolescent's mother confronts and negotiates with boyfriend's mother

Adolescent's mother makes decisions for pregnant daughter

---

the mother in the home, to help in selection of the name of the child, and to visit the child after delivery (Furstenberg, 1981). Some young women find themselves in the difficult position of balancing the claims of their baby's father, who wants to be included, against the demands of their parents, who frequently want to restrict the father's access to the child. Parental attempts to control the expectant mother-father relationship are often based in the parents' belief that the young man is to blame for the pregnancy, and on an underlying hostility toward the expectant father for being unable to support the mother and baby financially.

Adolescent fathers who have good relationships with the adolescent mother throughout and after pregnancy often provide her assistance in areas such as finances, babysitting, caretaking, and transportation of mother and baby to health facilities. These fathers can also provide the love and support the adolescent mother needs as she learns to become

a mother. Ideally, the teen mother and father can share their feelings and support one another as they develop as parents, but psychological counseling may be needed to achieve this. As we'll see later, community health nurses can be instrumental in facilitating this process.

The Adolescent Mother's Own Family System

The pregnant adolescent's own family can be her greatest source of support. The family can provide housing, child care, financial aid, and emotional supports—all of which can be especially important if she remains unmarried and attempts to raise the child without a husband (Pressor, 1980). Such supports can make a significant difference in the young mother's subsequent educational and economic success (Burden & Klerman, 1984).

The family can also be a source of stress to the adolescent, depending upon how they react to the pregnancy. The parents' reactions depend on their rules, goals, and values. While some parents may be very accepting of the pregnancy, other parents may view the pregnancy as evidence that their teenager has challenged the rules they established, causing them to become very hurt, angry, and disappointed. With the pregnancy, they are confronted with their daughter's sexual maturity, and this discovery may have been their first involvement in the sexual behavior of their daughter. It also may have caught them off guard, not knowing how to respond.

Not all parents have this difficulty; some are involved in the sexual development and behavior of their daughters all along. Jessor and Jessor (1975) studied transition of youth from virginity to non-virginity and concluded that parental values, and support and degree of connectedness with the youth distinguished between teenagers who became nonvirgins and teenagers who remained virgins. Other authors suggest that in instances where parents communicate openly with their teenager about sex, their child's involvement in sexual activity was less and the child was less likely to become pregnant in adolescence (Inazu & Fox, 1980). However, many adolescents and parents are often too embarrassed to discuss sexual issues openly (Kisker, 1985), and adolescents may not hear or retain what parents think they are communicating (Newcomer & Udry, 1985).

Several factors may delay open communication about the pregnancy among parents and between parents and their children. For instance, the obvious sexual maturity of the adolescent may precipitate uneasy feelings on the part of the parents about their own sexuality, depending on how parents are managing that area of their lives at that particular time. Second, the pregnancy may have come at a time when the parents are dealing with their own personal issues, such as careers, retirement, chronic illness, or aging parents. Third, the parents may have thought they had come to the end of their parenting responsibilities but perceive the coming of their new grandchild, parented by their dependent adolescent, as partly their responsibility. Thus, instead of completing their parenting responsibilities, they may feel that they are beginning all over again.

Most studies indicate that of all family members the mother of the adolescent girl feels most involved with the teenager and the pregnancy. The mother is likely to be the first to know about the pregnancy. However, if the daughter does not tell her, the mother may not openly acknowledge that she knows. It is as if both mother and daughter enter into an implicit collusion to deny the pregnancy until they come to a point where this denial cannot be maintained. Case Examples 25-2 and 25-3 illustrate the denial process. Case Example 25-2 is a verbatim account from a study by Logan (1972), and Case Example 25-3 is a case reported by Lippert (1982).

It is not clear why mothers participate with their daughters in initial denial of the pregnancy. Most mothers in the Logan (1972) interview study were themselves upset, angry, and ashamed because their daughters became pregnant. Many were extremely disappointed and thought that they had failed to raise their daughters in such ways that their daughters would not become pregnant. Some felt guilty that they may have contributed to the situation in some covert or overt way. Some mothers also wondered what their friends would think of their mothering skills, and if they would consider their pregnant daughters "bad" or negative influences on other young women who were not pregnant. The pregnancy may have reawakened feelings related to the mother's own sexuality such as previous experience with premarital sex and out-of-wedlock pregnancies. Mothers may also be dealing with their own menopause and declining fertility and become threatened by their daughter's pregnancy. Some mothers may envision themselves as the primary caretakers of the grandchildren, which would result in a restriction of their roles and freedom. Mothers may also be ambivalent as to what approach to take with their daughter—whether to act in ways that would increase their daughter's dependence on them, or whether to push their daughter toward more independence and adult responsibilities, and thus allow her to struggle with the pregnancy without

Case Example 25-2: Adolescent Daughter Denies Pregnancy

"Well I knew that Sonia was pregnant all the time, but everytime I would ask her, she would get mad and start to cry. I would say to her, 'Sonia, you are gaining weight, your clothes are getting too small.' Then she would say, 'You just want me to say I'm pregnant and I know I'm not.' This went on every day. [After several weeks] Sonia still didn't tell me she was pregnant. One of my older daughters came over and told me that I was slipping. I said to her, 'You mean because I didn't say anything about Sonia being pregnant?' Sonia was sitting right there. They all acted very surprised that I knew. Sonia of course denied it at first." [Sonia was nearing the end of the first trimester when the pregnancy was openly acknowledged.]

Mother is aware of pregnancy and confronts daughter; daughter denies condition.

Mutual denial continues.

Third person (sibling) intervenes. Pregnancy is openly acknowledged several weeks later.

---

the parents' initial assistance. Definitive answers to these questions are yet to be supplied through further research.

Pregnant adolescents and their mothers are reported to have very close relationships (Pressor, 1980). Therefore, it does appear that once mothers overcome the initial shock of the pregnancy and are able to work through their initial disappointment and angry feelings, they are able to assist their daughter through resolution of the crisis of pregnancy and provide considerable support. Taking time to work through these feelings may have contributed to their initial silence and delay in openly acknowledging the pregnancy. It should be emphasized that in Logan's (1972) study not all mothers initially denied their daughter's pregnancy. Some confronted their daughters and insisted on having the pregnancy confirmed or denied by medical tests as soon as they suspected the situation.

Pregnancy in adolescence may upset the family's equilibrium, causing members to make necessary changes to bring about a new balance. When family members accommodate to the situation, they are able to provide the pregnant adolescent the support necessary to make constructive decisions concerning the pregnancy. How well they arrive at their decisions depends on how well they function as a unit. When resolving the issue of the pregnancy, they may encourage the adolescent toward decisions involving any one of the following options:

1. Abortion (terminating the pregnancy)

Case Example 25-3: Mother and Daughter Deny Pregnancy

A thirteen-year-old girl came to the pediatric emergency room with gastrointestinal discomfort and swollen abdomen. She was accompanied by her concerned and anxious mother. The child was obviously pregnant but denied her pregnancy. The mother was equally certain that her daughter was not pregnant. Examination determined that the girl was twenty-six weeks pregnant. . . . When the mother was asked if she had noted her daughter's condition, she said she had thought her daughter was just getting fat (Lippert, 1982, p. 84).

Denial of pregnancy between mother and daughter

2. Delivery (bringing the pregnancy to term and keeping the baby with the following alternatives)

- Legal marriage (resulting in nuclear type of family structure)
- Common-law marriage (with the father of the baby)
- Living with adolescent's family with baby (creating an extended type of family arrangement)
- Alternative type of family arrangement (with older siblings, boyfriends, other relatives, or friends—creating an augmented type of family style)
- Living alone with child (one-parent family structure; possible but very unlikely because of adolescent's age)
- Adoption (formal or informal)

Most families whose adolescents choose to keep their baby and remain in the household successfully work out a system to accommodate the new baby. This system necessitates a flexible division of labor and sharing of responsibilities that may extend beyond members of the immediate family to other relatives and friends. This system can be very useful to the adolescent, because it allows her to shift some of the burdens of child care tasks and responsibilities to trusted others while she attends to her own adolescent development tasks. On the other hand, this may also create some dilemmas for the adolescent, since the more dependent she becomes on her family, the harder it will be for her to achieve a sense of personal independence. Also, there may be so much overlap in enactment of child care responsibilities that the structure of authority within the family becomes unclear. The adolescent's authority vis-à-vis her child may be undermined, particularly when she disagrees with her mother. This could cause problems of detachment and disengagement between the adolescent and her baby.

Family relationships may change as the baby grows and reaches different developmental stages. Whereas family members may be enthusiastic and helpful initially, their enthusiasm may decrease as they grow accustomed to the baby and must meet its growing demands. It is important for family members to understand that while the grandmother or older sisters can serve as coaches for the adolescent mother and as a system of apprenticeship whereby she can learn and become socialized into the mothering role, their primary goal should be to promote and improve the quality of the mother-child relationship, while fostering healthy communications and interactions among all family members.

Implications for Community Health Nurses

Community health nurses have a significant role to play in adolescent pregnancy at the individual, family, and community levels. In this section we'll discuss general implications for community health nurses at these levels; we'll describe specific recommendations and strategies in the next section.

The Individual Level Community health nurses are in excellent positions to provide appropriate intervention and the health and social services that can minimize the risk of complications in pregnancy and childbirth for the young mother. For instance, community health nurses can use their knowledge of crisis theory and crisis intervention and their skills in counseling and communication techniques to first establish a trusting and meaningful relationship with the teenage mother and then to assist her in resolving the crisis of pregnancy. The nurse's knowledge of physiology of pregnancy and growth and development in adolescence is the basis for a complete assessment of the adolescent's physical and emotional state. The nurse can help the young woman to understand what is happening to her and to make effective decisions concerning the pregnancy. Thus, the nurse can function as the adolescent's advocate—being supportive and understanding while the adolescent resolves the crisis of pregnancy. The community health nurse is also equipped to make referrals and establish linkages on behalf of pregnant adolescents, depending on the choices available and the decisions they make.

The Family Level The community health nurse's primary role with the family is to facilitate open communication among all family members regarding the pregnancy, but in so doing the privacy and self-respect of the pregnant adolescent should be considered. For example, if the adolescent gives the nurse confidential information, it is up to the adolescent to bring that information to the attention of other family members. The nurse can, however, encourage and support the adolescent in sharing the information.

Before open communication and problem resolution can take place, the nurse may have to allow individual family members time for direct expression of their personal feelings and reactions about the pregnancy. If the family is in a state of shock about the pregnancy, the nurse can assist them in developing effective coping strategies that will move them closer toward decision making and resolution of the crisis. This may necessitate open discussion of the family's ideals, cultural beliefs, and values in addition to their feelings.

Working through family members' feelings and relationships as a result of adolescent pregnancy may take time and several meetings. It may well be necessary for community health nurses to collaborate with psychiatric mental health nurses in this process.

The Community Level Community health nurses can use their knowledge of community resources to assist the adolescent and her family to locate the resources they need. Such resources can be in the areas of (1) *health,* particularly comprehensive prenatal and postnatal care; (2) *social service,* such as abortion or adoption agencies; (3) *education,* such as schools or special programs where the adolescent can continue her education with minimum disruption; and (4) *economic assistance* through public agencies. It is important that the adolescent is involved in all the steps of the referral process and understand and agree with all the referrals made on behalf of her and her family. This is crucial, since the adults in her life may be inclined to exert their power and influence to make decisions *for,* instead of *with,* her.

Strategies for Health Promotion

This section includes recommendations and strategies for community health nurses from the perspectives of primary, secondary, and tertiary prevention.

Primary Prevention

The best strategy for community health nurses to employ in adolescent pregnancy prevention is primary prevention, the goal of which is to reduce the incidence of adolescent pregnancies. A good approach to this task is to help young people to realize their life potential, to expose them to other components and facets of life, and to help them make responsible choices and decisions regarding their life goals. Young people should be kept stimulated in supervised activities in the social, athletic, and scholastic areas. Routes to adulthood other than childbearing should be presented to them. Community health nurses can participate in primary prevention of adolescent pregnancy by (1) conducting outreach to adolescents at risk; (2) maintaining a holistic approach to adolescent health; (3) providing sex and family life education; and (4) teaching family planning.

Outreach to Adolescents at Risk Community health nurses can take the initiative to reach out to adolescents at risk of becoming pregnant—those who are sexually active and those who have reached or are nearing puberty. This group should be targeted for pregnancy prevention efforts. Community health nurses can work with other community representatives to meet with adolescents in schools, youth groups, or recreational and community centers.

The community health nurse can collaborate with the school nurse and other professionals and community leaders to convene representatives from local schools, PTAs, or other youth-oriented agencies to increase community awareness of teen problems and issues, as well as to share and develop strategies for pregnancy prevention. Nurses can also reach teens through newspaper ads, radio and TV public service announcements, and appearances on local radio and talk shows. The purpose of reaching out to teens is to provide them with information that can help them to make informed life choices, plan life goals, and make responsible decisions concerning their sexuality.

Holistic Approach to Adolescent Health
Community health nurses can provide leadership in establishing or improving community adolescent health programs. The nurse can help to ensure that a holistic approach is taken and that adolescents are treated in privacy with integrity, respect, and a nonjudgmental attitude. Such programs should be designed specifically for teenagers and be comprehensive in nature so that the adolescents can meet as much of their health care needs as possible in one place. This reduces the need for traveling to different places and the number of health personnel required to attend to adolescents. Special care should be taken that adolescents are treated in confidence, that long waiting periods are avoided, and that adolescents are treated as people in their own rights who know what their needs are. Community health nurses can organize and conduct health surveys or polls of adolescents themselves to obtain their perspective on what they consider to be their own health needs and concerns. Services can then be planned and implemented to meet those needs.

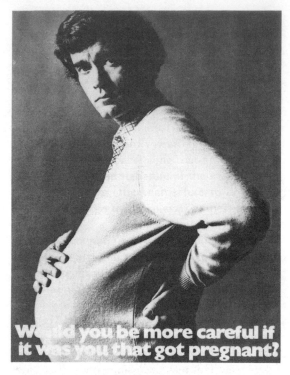

Would you be more careful if it was you that got pregnant?

Community health nurses can be instrumental in providing appropriate and complete information about sexuality and development to teens. School and community youth programs, individual teaching, and visual aids geared toward a teenager's level of understanding are all effective methods of sex education. (Reproduced courtesy of Pharmacists Planning Service, Inc., P.O. Box 1336, Sausalito, CA 94965. Posters are available upon request. © Pharmacists Planning Service, Inc.)

Sex and Family Life Education   The majority of young people obtain their sex education from TV, magazines, and informal sources such as their friends and peer groups. Unfortunately, information from these sources is likely to be inaccurate and one-sided, and to reflect society's double standard for sexual behavior (that is, the male role in assuming responsibility for unwanted pregnancies is underemphasized). Community health nurses and other health professionals have the responsibility

Table 25-1   Suggested Content Areas of Sex and Family Life Education for Adolescents

Growth and Development	Relationships	Health	Self-Management	Social/Cultural
Puberty: changes that occur; hormones' influence on body functions	Communicating with parents and teachers	Self-care	Managing sexual feelings and interactions	Family and community values
Sexual awakening	Communicating with peers	Grooming	Responsible decision making	Religious influences
Pregnancy and childbirth	Developing sexual relationships— dating; commitment and marriage; intercourse and pregnancy possibility	Nutrition	Personal values	Opportunities for youth employment
		Exercise	Developing a positive self-image	Community educational opportunities
		Physical checkups	Choosing a vocation and making life's choices	Family and community expectations
		Family planning— types and sources of contraceptives		Community resources for adolescent growth and development (for example, social, recreational, competitive)
		Abortion		
		Sexual abuse		

to provide accurate sex and family life education to both young women and men. The goal of such education should be to equip young people with the skills, knowledge, and attitudes that will enable them to make intelligent choices and decisions about their sexuality, to examine and clarify their values, to discuss intimacy and their attempts at establishing intimate relationships, to understand the responsibilities of parenthood, and, therefore, to delay pregnancy and parenthood. Specific areas to be included in sex and family life education programs are summarized in Table 25-1.

Although sex education is an important component of family life education, often it is not openly discussed because it can be a sensitive and controversial issue. The controversy primarily centers on responsibility: who should teach sex education— the family, the schools, religious groups, or some other health professional group? Criticisms have also been levied against sex education programs: they are not comprehensive enough, not enough students receive the information, and they rarely provide the kind of information that would help adolescents avoid pregnancy and understand the responsibilities of parenthood (Scales, 1982).

Scales also reports that innovative successful sex education programs have the following characteristics: "involvement of parents and community groups; careful, long range planning focusing on the training of teachers and detailing of curricula; and a conviction that sexuality education, to be adequate, must go beyond the mere provision of facts, and enable students to clarify their values in life and about sexuality" (Scales, 1982, p. 227).

Case Example 25-4: Collaboration with Community Representatives

Mrs. Bendes is a community health nurse who works for the health department in a community with high adolescent pregnancy rates. Recognizing the potential health risks to adolescent mothers and their children, Mrs. Bendes contacted Ms. New, a school nurse for three junior high schools in the community, to discuss possible ways of minimizing adolescent pregnancies. Together Mrs. Bendes and Ms. New devised a family life and sex education program for junior high school students. They presented their ideas to Mrs. Blow, the district superintendent for the schools involved. Mrs. Blow was enthusiastic but felt the idea should be presented to members of the parent-teachers association. Mrs. Bendes and Ms. New gave a well-organized informal presentation to this group but met with great opposition. Parents felt their children would be provided sex education with no moral guidance and that sex education might actually encourage their youth to become sexually active.

Mrs. Bendes and Ms. New sought support from health department officials, local clergy, social service agency representatives, and community leaders, some of whom were parents of adolescents. This group met to discuss the issue of adolescent pregnancies in their community. Convinced that it was a problem to be dealt with, they organized a one-day community conference and open hearings on adolescent pregnancy. At the conference, Ms. New and Mrs. Bendes gave a well-documented presentation on the scope of adolescent pregnancies in the community. Adolescent mothers and fathers and other sexually active teenagers gave frank and open testimonials, and other social service community representatives discussed various aspects of adolescent pregnancies. So successful was the conference that a group of parents emerged to form a task force on sex education for junior high students in the community. They pledged support of Mrs. Bendes's and Ms. New's program and agreed to meet together with the district superintendent, school principals, and the parent-teachers association at regular intervals to work toward having a successful sex and family life education program in three community junior high schools.

Nurse identifies adolescent pregnancy as a community problem.

Community health nurse collaborates with school nurse.

Community health nurse and school nurse devise a health education program.

Community input sought: parents oppose sex education program.
Nurses seek community support.

Nurses collaborate and establish linkages with community leaders, parents, and professionals.

Program implementation: through community support, conference on adolescent pregnancy is held.

Community task force—a support group for community health nurse and school nurse—is established.

Sex and family life education program is implemented with community support.

Community health nurses can participate in developing and implementing sex and family life education programs or seminars for several target groups in the community: (1) adolescents through schools or school based health clinics, churches, or community youth programs; (2) parents through health clinics, churches, PTAs, and other community programs; and (3) other professionals who work with adolescents such as teachers and youth officers. Case Example 25-4 illustrates a collaborative effort.

Family Planning Like sex education, family planning can be a sensitive issue. Yet, adolescents who are sexually active, or planning to become so, need accurate family planning information since effective contraceptive use is an excellent pregnancy prevention measure. Community health nurses have an important role in counseling teenagers about availability and types of contraceptives. Box 25-1 summarizes advantages and disadvantages of popular contraceptive methods. In addition to providing contraceptive information, community health nurses should create opportunities for adolescents to discuss and explore their feelings, attitudes, and values concerning contraceptive use. Special efforts should be made to reach out to teenage men so that they also have accurate information about contraceptives as well as understand the important role they have in pregnancy prevention.

Confidentiality may be an important factor in these discussions. Zabin and Clark (1983) report that the five principal reasons adolescents give for choosing a family planning clinic are (1) confidentiality—the clinic doesn't inform parents; (2) staff cares about teenagers; (3) proximity to their homes; (4) friends come to the clinic; and (5) clinic is the only one they know. Community health nurses can incorporate these findings when they work with adolescents. They should be particularly sensitive to the confidentiality issue and to the realization that adolescents respond best to a caring professional staff.

Secondary Prevention

Secondary prevention is aimed at minimizing the consequences of teenage pregnancy. Strategies for community health nurses to employ in this area relate to (1) early detection and resolution of the pregnancy, (2) adequate prenatal care, and (3) good nutrition. These strategies should result in positive outcomes for the adolescent mother and baby.

Early Detection and Resolution of the Pregnancy Community health nurses can play important roles in the early detection and resolution of pregnancy. First, nurses can participate in community programs to educate community residents and workers about the early signs and symptoms of pregnancy. This education would be particularly useful to teachers, youth officers, parents, and adolescents themselves. When signs and symptoms of pregnancy are recognized and acknowledged early, decisions concerning what to do about the pregnancy can also be made early, thus affording the teenager greater options. Since adolescent women are likely to confide in their boyfriends early in the pregnancy, it is important that teenage men also know how to recognize early signs and symptoms of pregnancy and be encouraged to urge their pregnant girlfriends to seek confirmation and effective resolution of the pregnancy as soon as possible. Community health nurses who are in contact with young males can be instrumental in this endeavor.

Community health nurses can also facilitate the early detection and resolution of pregnancy by making it possible for adolescents who suspect that they are pregnant to obtain pregnancy tests quickly and in confidence. Nurses typically come in contact with such adolescents when they come to a clinic or when they telephone for information. In some instances, community health nurses are approached by a family member who suspects that the adolescent is pregnant. Whatever the setting of the nurse-client encounter, it is of utmost importance to consider the quality of the nurse-client (adolescent) interaction since the latter has been shown to be a very important variable in treatment outcomes and contraceptive compliance among young women (Nathanson & Becker, 1985).

Adequate Prenatal Care As soon as the pregnancy is confirmed, pregnant adolescents should begin prenatal care. Adequate prenatal care is essential in the prevention and early detection of complications of pregnancy. Such care begins with a comprehensive physical examination including the adolescent's health history, and habits and lifestyle such as allergies, food preferences, smoking habits, and use of alcohol and other drugs. The status of the pregnancy is usually evaluated, and the adolescent's family and social environment is assessed. Community health nurses can participate in the following ways:

Box 25-1   Methods of Contraceptives

Method	The Pill	Minipills	Intrauterine Device (IUD)
What is it?	Pills with two hormones, an estrogen and progestin, similar to the hormones a woman makes in her own ovaries.	Pills with just one type of hormone: a progestin, similar to a hormone a woman makes in her own ovaries.	A small piece of plastic with nylon threads attached. Some have copper wire wrapped around them. One IUD gives off a hormone, progesterone.
How does it work?	Prevents egg's release from woman's ovaries, makes cervical mucus thicker, and changes lining of the uterus.	It may prevent egg's release from woman's ovaries, makes cervical mucus thicker and changes lining of uterus, making it harder for a fertilized egg to start growing there.	The IUD is inserted into the uterus. It is not known exactly how the IUD prevents pregnancy.
How reliable or effective is it?	99.7% if used consistently, but much less effective if used carelessly.	97–99% if used perfectly, but less effective if used carelessly.	97–99% if patient checks for string regularly.
How would I use it?	Either of two ways: 1. A pill a day for 3 weeks, stop for one week, then start a new pack. 2. A pill every single day with no stopping between packs.	Take one pill every single day as long as you want to avoid pregnancy.	Check string at least once a month right after the period ends to make sure your IUD is still properly in place.
Are there problems with it?	Must be prescribed by a doctor. All women should have a medical exam before taking the pill, and some women should not take it.	Must be prescribed by a doctor. All women should have a medical exam first.	Must be inserted by a doctor after a pelvic examination. Cannot be used by all women. Sometimes the uterus "pushes" it out.

What are the side effects or complications?	Nausea, weight gain, headaches, missed periods, darkened skin on the face, or depression may occur. More serious and more rare problems are blood clots in the legs, the lungs, or the brain, and heart attacks.	Irregular periods, missed periods, and spotting may occur and are more common problems with minipills than with the regular birth-control pills.	May cause cramps, bleeding, or spotting; infections of the uterus or of the oviducts (tubes) may be serious. See a doctor for pain, bleeding, fever, or a bad discharge.
What are the advantages?	Convenient, extremely effective, does not interfere with sex, and may diminish menstrual cramps.	Convenient, effective, does not interfere with sex, and less serious side effects than with regular birth-control pills.	Effective, always there when needed, but usually not felt by either partner.

Method	Diaphragm with Spermicidal Jelly or Cream	Spermicidal Foam, Jelly, or Cream	Condom ("Rubber")
What is it?	A shallow rubber cup used with a sperm-killing jelly or cream.	Cream and jelly come in tubes; foam comes in aerosol cans or individual applicators and is placed into the vagina.	A sheath of rubber shaped to fit snugly over the erect penis.
How does it work?	Fits inside the vagina. The rubber cup forms a barrier between the uterus and the sperm. The jelly or cream kills the sperm.	Foam, jelly, and cream contain a chemical that kills sperm and acts as a physical barrier between sperm and the uterus.	Prevents sperm from getting inside a woman's vagina during intercourse.
How reliable or effective is it?	About 97% effective if used correctly and consistently, but much less effective if used carelessly.	About 90–97% effective if used correctly and consistently, but much less effective if used carelessly.	About 97% effective if used correctly and consistently, but much less effective if used carelessly.

(continued)

Box 25-1   *(continued)*

Method	Diaphragm with Spermicidal Jelly or Cream	Spermicidal Foam, Jelly, or Cream	Condom ("Rubber")
How would I use it?	Insert the diaphragm and jelly (or cream) before intercourse. Can be inserted up to 6 hours before intercourse. Must stay in at least 6 hours after intercourse.	Put foam, jelly, or cream into your vagina each time you have intercourse, not more than 30 minutes beforehand. No douching for at least 8 hours after intercourse.	The condom should be placed on the erect penis before the penis ever comes into contact with the vagina. After ejaculation, the penis should be removed from the vagina immediately.
Are there problems with it?	Must be fitted by a doctor after a pelvic exam. Some women find it difficult to insert, inconvenient, or messy.	Must be inserted just before intercourse. Some find it inconvenient or messy.	Objectionable to some men and women. Interrupts intercourse. May be messy. Condom may break.
What are the side effects or complications?	Some women find that the jelly or cream irritates the vagina. Try changing brands if this happens.	Some women find that the foam, cream, or jelly irritates the vagina. May irritate the man's penis. Try changing brands if this happens.	Rarely, individuals are allergic to rubber. If this is a problem, condoms called "skins," which are not made out of rubber, are available.
What are the advantages?	Effective and safe.	Effective, safe, a good lubricant, and can be purchased at a drugstore.	Effective, safe, can be purchased at a drugstore; excellent protection against sexually transmitted infections.

Method	Condom and Foam Used Together	Periodic Abstinence (Natural Family Planning)	Sterilization
What is it?		Ways of finding out days each month when you are most likely to get pregnant. Intercourse is avoided at that time.	Vasectomy (male). Tubal ligation (female). Ducts carrying sperm or the egg are tied and cut surgically.

How does it work?	Prevents sperm from getting inside the uterus by killing sperm and preventing sperm from getting out into the vagina.	Techniques include maintaining chart of basal body temperature, checking vaginal secretions, and keeping calendar of menstrual periods, all of which can help predict when you are most likely to release an egg.	Closing of tubes in male prevents sperm from reaching egg; closing tubes in female prevents egg from reaching sperm.
How reliable or effective is it?	Close to 100% effective if both foam and condoms are used with every act of intercourse.	Certain methods are about 90–97% if used consistently. Other methods are less effective. Combining techniques increases effectiveness.	Almost 100% effective and *not* usually reversible.
How would I use it?	Foam must be inserted within 30 minutes before intercourse and condom must be placed onto erect penis prior to contact with vagina.	Careful records must be maintained of several factors: basal body temperature, vaginal secretions and onset of menstrual bleeding. Careful study of these methods will dictate when intercourse should be avoided.	After the decision to have no more children has been well thought through, a brief surgical procedure is performed on the man or the woman.
Are there problems with it?	Requires more effort than some couples like. May be messy or inconvenient. Interrupts intercourse.	Difficult to use method if menstrual cycle is irregular. Sexual intercourse must be avoided for a significant part of each cycle.	Surgical operation has some risk but serious complications are rare. Sterilizations should not be done unless no more children are desired.

(continued)

Box 25-1 *(continued)*

Method	Condom and Foam Used Together	Periodic Abstinence (Natural Family Planning)	Sterilization
What are the side effects or complications?	No serious complications.	No complications.	All surgical operations have some risk, but serious complications are uncommon. Some pain may last for several days. Rarely, the wrong structure is tied off, or the tube grows back together. There is no loss of sexual desire or ability in vast majority of patients.
What are the advantages?	Extremely effective, safe, and both methods may be purchased at a drugstore without a doctor's prescription. Excellent protection against sexually transmitted infections.	Safe, effective if followed carefully; little if any religious objection to method. Teaches women about their menstrual cycles.	The most effective method; low rate of complications; many feel that removing fear of pregnancy improves sexual relations.

SOURCE:
U.S. Public Health Service: *Family Planning Methods of Contraception.* DHEW Publication No. HSA 78-5646. Washington, DC: US Government Printing Office, 1978.

1. Prepare the adolescent for the physical exam by telling her what will be done and who will do it
2. Explain to the adolescent that the exam itself and all the questions asked in it are related to her health and that of the baby's
3. Arrange for a supportive individual to accompany the adolescent during the initial, and subsequent, visits
4. Answer all questions asked by the adolescent to minimize any possible fears or misconceptions

Working in conjunction with maternal and child health nurses, community health nurses can add to the quality of prenatal care available to adoles-cents through health teaching and preparation for childbirth. Films, pamphlets, charts, and other visual aids can be used to help teach adolescents self-care such as good hygiene and good nutrition; management of the physical discomforts of pregnancy such as nausea, skin changes, swollen ankles, and restricted activities; and management of emotional needs, such as how to deal with mood swings and adjust to new body changes as the baby grows. It is also important that the nurse teaches the adolescent about growth and development of the fetus so the adolescent has full understanding of what is happening to the baby before birth, how the fetus changes, and how she can adjust to these changes.

Adolescents need accurate information about

the health care system, pregnancy, and labor and delivery. This can be accomplished through formal or informal childbirth education classes. Films explaining the process of pregnancy and birth can be highly effective, particularly when they are followed by group question-and-answer sessions. The adolescent can benefit from the knowledge of the nurse (group leader) and also from the experience and support of other pregnant adolescents. Preparation for childbirth should also include physical exercises, information on the birth process, and guidance on how to recognize signs and symptoms of labor and what to do about them. In addition, whenever possible, the adolescent should be given a tour of the labor facilities where she will deliver her baby and be allowed to meet some of the personnel who are likely to participate in the delivery process. This will lessen the fears and anxieties many adolescents have concerning the birth process, as will the support of someone close to them such as a boyfriend, mother, or older sister.

Barriers to obtaining adequate prenatal care are long waiting periods in clinics and physicians' offices, inconsistent professional staff, lack of sensitivity to the unique needs of the adolescent population, financial requirements, and long distances to travel to receive care, coupled with lack of transportation (Zabin & Clark, 1983). These barriers should be eliminated at all costs, since adequate prenatal care has been reported to be one of the most important factors for good obstetrical outcome among women of any age, but particularly adolescent women who are likely to be biologically immature.

Good Nutrition Good health during pregnancy depends on good nutrition. Coupled with adequate prenatal care, good nutrition is said to be crucial in minimizing the complications of pregnancy and in producing good outcomes for mother and baby. Both pregnancy and the adolescent growth spurt increase the body's nutritional requirements. The energy demands of the growing fetus and of the growing adolescent increase the body's need for calories, protein, iron, and calcium. When the two events (pregnancy and adolescence) occur together, the mother, the fetus, or both may suffer from nutritional deficiencies. Dietary recommendations are, therefore, increased during pregnancy (Heald & Jacobsen, 1980). See Table 25-2 for recommended requirements.

Although essential, good nutrition is not always easy to achieve among pregnant adolescents. Financial constraints and long established eating patterns, grounded in cultural practices and traditions that are not easily changed, make it difficult for the pregnant adolescent to adequately manage her intake. It may be necessary to enlist the assistance of a nutritionist in managing her diet. Her family and boyfriend should also be included. Attempts to educate the adolescent about nutritional value of foods and management of her diet should be done within her own cultural context. She should be actively involved in management of her nutritional intake, and be allowed to make up diets from acceptable foods she likes. Above all, she should be taught the relationship between her nutritional intake and her own health as well as the health of the baby. She should, for instance, understand that suboptimal nutrition in pregnancy can lead to too much or too little weight gain and complications such as anemia and hypertension for herself and low birthweight for the child.

Tertiary Prevention

Tertiary prevention is aimed at providing adolescent mothers with the resources and support necessary to become adequate parents, helping them adjust to the roles and responsibilities of parenthood while completing adolescent tasks, helping them to prevent repeat pregnancies and to remain in school and, therefore, to avoid prolonged economic and emotional dependence on social welfare agencies and on the family. Specific strategies community health nurses can employ in tertiary prevention are: (1) offering follow-up care, including health assessment and direct services to the new mother and baby; (2) providing psychological counseling and emotional support; (3) facilitating open communication and good relationships in the family system; and (4) establishing links and resources to help adolescents avoid negative consequences of adolescent pregnancy.

Table 25-2   Recommended Requirements for Selected Nutrients during Pregnancy in Adolescents and Most Important Sources of these Nutrients

Nutrient	RDA	Best Sources
Calories	2400	meat, fish, poultry, fats, fruits, grains, legumes, nuts
Protein	78 g	meat, fish, poultry, eggs, milk, milk products, legumes/grains
Calcium	1200 mg	milk (all forms), yogurt, cheese, leafy green vegetables, clams, oysters, almonds
Iron	18 mg[a]	liver, meats, fish, poultry, whole grain and enriched cereals and breads, legumes cooked in an iron pan, leafy green vegetables, dried prunes, apricots, and raisins
Folic Acid	800 mcg[a]	liver, yeast, leafy green vegetables, legumes, whole grains, fruits, and assorted vegetables
Pyridoxine (B$_6$)	2.5 mg[a]	wheat germ, meat, liver, whole grains, peanuts, soybeans, corn

SOURCE:
Morgan B: Nutrition needs of the female adolescent. *Women and Health.* New York: Haworth Press, Vol. 9 Issue 2/3 1984, p. 22.

[a]Supplementation with these nutrients is recommended as follows:
Iron 30–60 mg per day
Folic Acid 400–800 mcg per day
Pyridoxine 3–6 mg per day

Follow-up Care   Through follow-up home visits and adolescent clinic visits community health nurses can assess and monitor the health status of both mother and baby as well as provide them with appropriate health services. Assessment of the mother includes her physical and emotional condition (e.g., vital signs; condition of her breasts, particularly if she is breast-feeding; condition of the uterus, lochia, and perineum; bowel and bladder function; emotional state, including sleep and rest patterns and signs of anxiety or depression; and nature of relationships with significant others). Assessment of the newborn includes areas such as growth and development (e.g., nervous system reflexes; feeding patterns and nutritional status; bowel and bladder function; and sleep and crying patterns). During the assessment process the nurse can identify what services and health information the young mother and her family need.

Much of the direct services community health nurses provide are in the area of health teaching.

New adolescent mothers are often apprehensive about their role of mother and are uncertain about how to take care of their baby. Some adolescents are even afraid to handle the baby. The following passage from the autobiography of novelist Maya Angelou beautifully explains the fears of an adolescent mother after she brings her baby home:

. . . and I was afraid to touch him. Home from the hospital, I sat for hours by his bassinet and absorbed his mysterious perfection. His extremities were so dainty, they appeared unfinished. Mother handled him easily with the casual confidence of a baby nurse, but I dreaded being forced to change his diapers. Wasn't I famous for awkwardness? Suppose I let him slip, or put my fingers on that throbbing pulse on top of his head? (Angelou, 1979, p. 245)

Community health nurses can teach adolescent mothers how to care for their baby so that they can gain confidence in the mother role. This can be done during follow-up home visits to the mothers' homes or at the clinic when they come in for checkups. The following are important content areas to cover in health teaching:

Information pertinent to new baby

- Normal growth and development (rate of development and what to expect at each stage)
- Nutrition (quantity; feeding times; "burping"; breast feeding or bottle feeding; breast milk or formula)
- Infant care (bathing, hair washing; care of umbilicus; skin care)
- Signs and symptoms of illness (colds; fevers; diarrhea and constipation; vomiting; abnormalities)
- Safety (temperatures for bath and formula; carrying the baby; clothing; car seats; crib and bed clothes)
- Emotional status (crying; fretting; sleep pattern)

Information pertinent to self (adolescent mother)

- Self-care (hygiene; rest; exercise)
- Postpartum care (signs of bleeding; condition of lochia)
- Emotional (postpartum "blues"; role strain; stress management)
- Relationships (communicating with significant others—i.e., boyfriends, parents, peers)
- Family planning (contraceptives—types and when to resume)

Resources (phone numbers for)

- Hot lines
- Postpartum units
- Nursery units
- Clinic

(when to call; what constitute emergencies)

In addition to health teaching a vigorous follow-up system of contacting adolescent mothers who have missed postpartum and family planning checkups is of utmost importance in helping to avoid subsequent pregnancies.

Counseling and Emotional Support   In addition to providing adolescent mothers with information about how to care for themselves and their babies, community health nurses should also create avenues for adolescent mothers to express fears and concerns they may have about their role as new parents. Besides feeling overwhelmed by the responsibility of caring for a helpless newborn, adolescents may need even more to engage in activities with their friends to continue their personal and social development. The need to accomplish teenage developmental tasks may thus be in conflict with the desire to care for the baby and be a good mother. In addition to this conflict, some teenagers may also experience difficulties in their relationships with significant others such as their baby's father and members of their family. Community health nurses can function as sympathetic listeners, encourage the teenager to express feelings related to these difficulties and provide her with counseling and support to work through such feelings. Counseling can be done on an individual basis or in small group sessions depending on the needs of the adolescent and the arrangements the community health nurse can make.

Open Communication in the Family System   In families where adolescents continue to live at home with their baby, it is advantageous for community health nurses to approach adolescent parenting from a family systems perspective. Such families often enact a system of shared parenting whereby other family members, particularly the adult women in the family share in parenting the adolescent's child. Community health nurses need to understand this concept in order to provide adequate counseling to the adolescent within the context of the family's sociocultural system. For instance, if the adolescent's mother has power and control over the adolescent and her baby, it is fruitless for the nurse to concentrate intervention efforts solely on the adolescent without obtaining the mother's cooperation and involvement on as many levels as possible. Since there is likely to be entire family participation in child care responsibilities and activities, nurses may need to make a critical assessment of these activities through home visits. Areas that should be evaluated are: family roles and functions, flexibility or rigidity of family boundaries, distribution of power and authority, conflicts and conflict resolution, and family interactions and relationships.

Although it is crucial for grandmothers to support and assist their daughter, it is also equally important that they foster good relationships between their daughter and their daughter's baby. They must be committed to strengthening and developing this subunit within the family. Grandmothers and grandfathers should also understand the importance of fostering the adolescent's continued independence from the family. Community health nurses may consider group counseling sessions for grandmothers, where they can gain support from other grandmothers. Group members can discuss their new grandmother roles and their new child care responsibilities, and can work out effective ways of relating to their daughters and in some cases, their daughter's male partners as well.

Links to Resources   Nurses can play a major role in coordinating services at all levels of prevention: primary, secondary, and tertiary. They can serve as a vital link between the many programs that service adolescents (i.e., AFDC, family planning services; daycare services; Medicaid; schools and education-related programs; nutritional services; maternal and infant programs; neighborhood and primary health care centers; children and youth centers; and child development centers). The community health nurse's roles regarding these gencies may include referral agent, service coordinator or provider, and advocate for the adolescent and family. Acting in these roles can help the teenager and her family receive maximum benefits from the services provided by the community, rather than becoming lost between the cracks as a result of the bureaucratic and fragmented nature of some services. When the nurse enhances the community's capacity to meet the teenager's need for family planning services, good child care facilities, and continued education, the nurse is contributing to minimizing the negative consequences of adolescent pregnancy. It is important, however, that the adolescent and her family remain actively involved in the referral and linking process and that the nurse acts *on behalf of* them rather than *for* them. Otherwise, the family may rely on the nurse as "the expert" to assume all responsibilities.

Summary

Sexual values and patterns have been changing in the United States such that increasing numbers of adolescents are sexually active and are becoming pregnant. Many of these pregnancies are unintended and occur out of wedlock and result in negative consequences such as toxemia of pregnancy, low birthweight, and limited educational and economic potential for the mother coupled with increased dependency. These factors have led to the identification of pregnant adolescents as a high risk group requiring special attention. Community health nurses can play significant roles in minimizing the health risks to adolescents and their infants through direct prenatal and postnatal care, infant care, health education, and psychological counseling. Community health nurses can adopt a family-centered approach in these activities as well as in the primary prevention strategies they develop to help adolescents manage their sexuality and avoid unwanted pregnancies. While the efforts of nurses are useful and necessary, they are limited in preventing adolescent pregnancy and in providing assistance to the adolescent mother and her baby without the infusion of federal funds to support programs and the cooperation and coordinated efforts of national, state and local organizations.

Topics for Nursing Research

• What family life-styles contribute to (or do not contribute to) adolescent pregnancy?

• What explanations do adolescents themselves give for adolescent pregnancies?

• How are the experiences of married pregnant adolescents different from unmarried pregnant adolescents?

• What are the short-term and long-term effects of early parenthood on relations among the adolescent, her siblings, and her parents?

• What are the child-rearing practices of unwed adolescent fathers?

• How do families collaborate to care for the newborn of an adolescent mother, and how do these styles of collaboration affect the parenting skills of (1) the adolescent mother and (2) the adolescent father?

• What factors influence males to become unwed fathers?

• What are the influences of ethnicity or cultural orientation on the likelihood of becoming an unwed adolescent mother or father?

• What social support networks do adolescent parents make use of?

• What role does the adolescent father who marries his partner play in parenting?

• What is the role of the family in resolving an unplanned pregnancy?

• How effective are sex and family life education programs in preventing unwanted pregnancies?

Study Questions

1. Which of the following statements is true about adolescent pregnancy according to 1980 trends?
   a. The rate of pregnancy among older teens has increased while fewer younger teens are becoming pregnant.
   b. Despite widespread availability of contraceptives, many adolescents still experience unplanned, unwanted pregnancies.
   c. Most adolescents who become pregnant out of wedlock give their babies up for adoption.
   d. Interest in adolescent pregnancy has declined over the years.

2. Which of the following have been considered possible explanations for adolescent pregnancy?
   a. Hostility and distance in parental marriage
   b. Peer pressure
   c. Ignorance about contraceptive use
   d. All of the above

3. One of the reasons adolescent mothers are considered a high risk group is:
   a. Both the adolescent mother and the baby are prone to suffer medical complications.
   b. Adolescent mothers generally fail to comply to treatment.
   c. Infants born to adolescent mothers are generally larger than those born to older mothers.
   d. In general, adolescent mothers have few social supports.

4. Which of the following positions should a community health nurse take regarding the unwed adolescent's partner in planning care for pregnant adolescents?
   a. The male partner is on the periphery and cannot be expected to participate in the plan of care for the adolescent mother.
   b. The male partner should be included in the care plan if the adolescent plans to marry him in the near future.
   c. Parental consent is needed if the male partner is to be included in the care plan.
   d. The male partner should be included with consent of adolescent mother.

5. Which of the following are considered primary prevention strategies community health nurses can use in the prevention of unplanned and unwanted pregnancies among adolescents?
   a. Maintaining a holistic approach to adolescent health
   b. Provision of sex and family life education
   c. Outreach to adolescents at risk to unplanned pregnancies
   d. All of the above

References

Abernethy V: Prevention of unwanted pregnancy among teenagers. *Primary Care* 1976; 3 (3): 399–406.

Abernethy V: Illegitimate conception among teenagers. *Am J Public Health* 1974; 64 (7): 662–665.

Alan Guttmacher Institute (AGI): *Eleven Million Teenagers*. New York: Alan Guttmacher Institute, 1976.

Alan Guttmacher Institute (AGI): *Teenage Pregnancy: The Problem That Hasn't Gone Away*. New York: Alan Guttmacher Institute, 1981.

Allison-Tomlinson M: Teenage pregnancies. *Journal of Nursing Care* (April) 1982; 15 (4): 8–12.

Angelou M: *I Know Why the Caged Bird Sings*. New York: Random House, 1970.

Bacon L: Early motherhood, accelerated role transition and social pathologies. *Social Forces* 1974; 52: 333–341.

Berstein R: *Helping Unmarried Mothers*. New York: Associated Press, 1971.

Bierman B, Street R: Adolescent girls as mothers: Problems in parenting. In: Stuart I, Wells C (editors) *Pregnancy in Adolescence: Needs, Problems, and Management*. New York: Van Nostrand Reinhold, 1982.

Braen B, Forbush J: School age parenthood: A national overview. *J Sch Health* 1975; 45: 256–262.

Bryan-Logan B, Dancy B: Unwed pregnant adolescents: Their mother's dilemma. *Nurs Clin North Am* 1974; 9 (1): 57–68.

Burden D, Klerman L: Teenage parenthood: Factors that lessen economic dependence. *Social Work* (January–February) 1984; 29 (1): 11–16.

Chilman C: *Adolescent Sexuality in a Changing Society: Social and Political Perspectives*. Washington, DC: Government Printing Office, 1980.

Chilman C: Teenage pregnancy: A research review. *Social Work* 1979; 24 (6): 492–498.

Digest: Substantially higher morbidity and mortality rates found among infants born to adolescent mothers. *Family Planning Perspective* 1984; 16 (2): 91–92.

Draper T, Ganong M, Goodell V: *See How They Grow: Concepts in Child Development and Parenting*. New York: Butterick Publishing, 1980.

Elkind D: *Children and Adolescents: Interpretive Essays on Jean Piaget*. New York: Oxford University Press, 1970.

Elkind D: Egocentrism in adolescence. *Child Development* 1967; 38: 1025–1037.

Elkind D: Understanding the young adolescent. *Adolescence* 1978; 49: 127–134.

Epstein A: *Assessing the Child Development Information Needed by Adolescent Parents with Very Young Children*. Washington, DC: US Department of Health, Education and Welfare, 1980.

Erikson E: *Childhood and Society*. New York: Norton, 1950.

Freeman E, Rickels K: Adolescent contraceptive use: Current status of practice and research. *Obstet Gynecol* 1979; 23 (3): 388–393.

Furstenberg F: *Unplanned Parenthood: The Social Consequences of Childbearing*. New York: Free Press, 1976.

Furstenberg F, Herceg-Brown R, Jemail J: Bringing in the family: Kinship, support and contraceptive behavior. In: Ooms T (editor), *Teenage Pregnancy in a Family Context: Implications for Policy*. Philadelphia: Temple University Press, 1982.

Glick P, Norton A: *Marrying, Divorcing and Living Together in the U.S. Today*. Washington, DC: Population Reference Bureau, 1977.

Haley J: *Problem Solving Therapy*. San Francisco: Jossey-Boss, 1976.

Hatcher S: Understanding adolescent pregnancy and abortion. *Primary Care* 1976; 3: 407.

Havighurst R: *Developmental Tasks and Education*, 3rd ed. New York: McKay, 1972.

Heald F, Jacobsen M: Nutritional needs of the pregnant adolescent. *Pediatr Ann* 1980; 9: 95–99.

Hendricks L: *Young Fathers—New Stuff* (mimeographed). Washington, DC: Howard University, 1981.

Herzog E: *The Young Family: Some Perspectives in Sharing Supplements: A Report on the National Invitational Conference on Parenthood in Adolescence*. Washington, DC: Consortium on Early Childbearing and Childrearing, 1970.

Jessor S, Jessor R: Transition from virginity to nonvirginity among youth: A social psychological study over time. *Developmental Psychology* 1975; 4: 473–484.

Johnson C: Adolescent pregnancy: Intervention into the poverty cycle. *Adolescence* 1974; 9 (35): 263–271.

Kinsey A: *Sexual Behavior in the Human Male*. Philadelphia: Saunders, 1948.

Kisker E: Teenagers talk about sex, pregnancy and contraception. *Family Planning Perspectives* 1985; 17 (2): 83–90.

Lidz T: *The Person*. New York: Basic Books, 1968.

Lippert P: Adolescent pregnancy in relation to menarche. *Medical Aspects of Human Sexuality* (April) 1982; 416: 84.

Lippert P: The effect of pregnancy on adolescent growth and development. *Women and Health*, (Summer–Fall) 1984; 9 (213): 65–79.

Logan B: Negotiating the mothering role (unpublished master's thesis). Chicago, Ill.: University of Illinois, 1972.

Lorenzi M, Klerman L, Kekil J: School age parents: How permanent a relationship? *Adolescence* (Spring) 1977; 45: 13–22.

Miller W: Psychological vulnerability to unwanted pregnancy. *Family Planning Perspectives* 1973; 5: 199–201.

Miller W: Sexual and contraceptive behavior in young unmarried women. *Primary Care* 1976; 3 (3): 427.

Minuchin S: *Families and Family Therapy.* Cambridge, Mass.: Harvard University Press, 1974.

Moore KA: *Government Policies Related to Teenage Family Formation and Functioning: An Inventory.* Washington, DC: Family Impact Seminar, Urban Institute, 1979.

Moore KA: Teenage childbirth and welfare dependency: Consequences for women, families, and government welfare expenditures. In: Scott KG, Field T, Robertson E (editors), *Teenage Parents and their Offspring.* New York: Grune & Stratton, 1981.

Morgan B: Nutrition needs of the female adolescent. *Women and Health.* New York: Haworth Press, 1984.

Nadelson C, Notman M, Gillon J: Sexual knowledge and attitudes of adolescents: Relationship to contraceptive use. *Obstet Gynecol* 1980; 55 (3): 340–345.

Nathanson C, Becker M: The influence of client-provider relationships on teenage women's subsequent use of contraception. *Am J Public Health* 1984; 75 (1): 33–38.

Neinstein L, Stewart D: *Adolescent Health Care: A Practical Guide.* Baltimore: Urban and Schwarzenberg, 1984.

Newman I: Capturing the energy of peer pressure: Insights from a longitudinal study of cigarette smoking. *J Sch Health* 1984; 54 (4): 146–148.

Newcomer S, Udry R: Parent-child communication and adolescent sexual behaviors. Family Planning Perspectives 1985; 17 (4): 169–176.

Osofsky H: *The Pregnant Teenager.* Springfield, Ill. Charles C Thomas, 1968.

Panzarine S, Elster A: Perspective adolescent fathers: Stresses during pregnancy and implications for nursing interventions. *Journal of Psychosocial Nursing* 1982; 20 (7): 21–24.

Phipps-Yonas S: Teenage pregnancy and motherhood: A review of the literature. *Am J Orthopsychiatry* (July) 1980; 50: 403–431.

Plionis B: Adolescent pregnancy: Review of the literature. *Social Work* 1975; 20 (4): 302–307.

Pressor H: Sally's corner: Coping with unmarried motherhood. *Journal of Social Issues* 1980; 36 (1): 107–128.

Resnick M: Studying adolescent mother's decision-making about adoption and parenting. *Social Work* 1984; 29 (1): 5–10.

Richmond M, Hall F: *Child Marriages.* New York: Russell Sage Foundation, 1926.

Rosen R, Ager J, Martindale L: Contraception, abortion and self-concept. *Journal of Population* 1979; 2: 118–139.

Satir V: *Conjoint Family Therapy.* Palo Alto, Calif.: Science and Behavior Books, 1964.

Scales P: Sex education and the prevention of teenage pregnancy: An overview of policies and programs in the United States. In: Ooms T (editor), *Pregnancy in a Family Context: Implications for Policy.* Philadelphia: Temple University Press, 1982.

Sklar J, Berkov B: Teenage family formation in post-war America. *Family Planning Perspectives* 1974; 6 (2): 80–90.

Sorenson R: *Adolescent Sexuality in Contemporary America.* New York: World, 1973.

Stevens J: The consequences of early childbearing. *Young Children* 1980; 35 (2): 47–55.

Trussell J: Economic consequences of teenage childbearing. *Family Planning Perspectives* 1976; 8: 184–190.

White R: *The enterprise of living: Growth and Organization in Personality.* New York: Holt, Rinehart and Winston, 1972.

Wolf S: Psychosexual problems associated with contraceptive practices of abortion-seeking patients. *Medical Aspects of Human Sexuality* 1973; 7: 169–182.

Young L: Emotional conflicts of young motherhood. In: Farber S, Wilson R. (editors), *Teenage Marriages and Divorce.* Berkeley, Calif.: Diablo Press, 1967.

Zabin L, Clark S: Institutional factors affecting teenager's choice and reasons for delay in attending a family planning clinic. *Family Planning Perspectives* 1983; 15 (1): 25–29.

Zelnik M, Kantner JF: Sexual activity, contraceptive use and pregnancy among metropolitan area teenagers, 1971–1979. *Family Planning Perspectives* 1980; 5 (12): 230–237.

Zelnik M, Shah F: First intercourse among young Americans. *Family Planning Perspectives* 1983; 18 (2): 64–70.

Chapter 26

Substance Abuse

Mary R. Haack

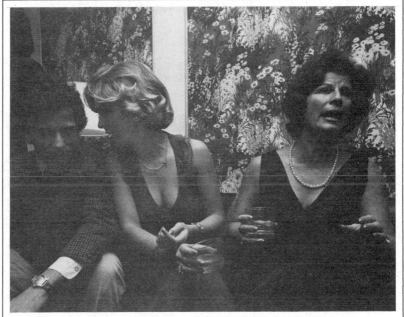

Antonio Mendoza/The Picture Cube

The potential for drug or alcohol abuse exists in every level of society, every occupation, every geographic location. Community health nurses are ideally placed to identify and refer substance abusers.

Chapter Outline

Chapter Objectives

After completing this chapter, the reader will be able to:

- Describe biomedical and social consequences of substance abuse
- Identify issues to be considered when making a treatment referral for an addicted person
- Define the role of the community health nurse in prevention of substance abuse and substance addiction
- Explain the importance of the community health nurse's attitude toward treatment of the substance-addicted client

The use of certain mood-altering substances is so common in our society that it is sometimes difficult to know when it becomes a problem. Such "common" use includes recreational drinking of alcohol by adults and the use of caffeine as a stimulant in the form of coffee, tea, or cola drinks. Certain substances are used medically for the alleviation of pain, relief of tension, or to suppress appetite. Problems arise, however, when the substances are used in an abusive manner, producing physical and behavioral changes that interfere with appropriate functioning.

As these physical and behavioral changes become manifest, they come to the attention of family members, friends, employers, and others. Often the substance-abusing person will come to the attention of community health nurses by virtue of their unique professional role in the community, which provides access to individuals within a well context. Nurses thus become ideal people to make early identification of the substance-abusing or substance-addicted person and to assist in referral, treatment, and after-care. Community health nurses also have an important role in prevention because of their relationship to healthy people.

This chapter is designed to increase community health nurses' confidence and competence in dealing with clients who have substance abuse problems. The topics covered in this chapter include the patterns of substance use in the United States and the extent of the problem and reasons for use; the biomedical and social consequences of use and abuse; the etiology of substance abuse; the diagnosis and early identification of physical and behavioral changes accompanying substance abuse; mechanisms of referral and types of treatment; and strategies for prevention.

Patterns of Substance Use and Abuse

Alcohol as food, euphoriant, or social lubricant continues to be a reality of modern society. Alcoholic beverages in the form of wine, beer, and distilled spirits are widely available in all Western societies. Alcohol consumption varies greatly from person to person, however, depending on individual preferences and social norms. U.S. survey data suggest that one-third of the adult population consists of people who seldom drink or abstain entirely. Another third consists of people who have up to three drinks per week. The remaining third contains people who have four or more drinks per week. About one-third of the last two groups have been defined as problem drinkers. It has been estimated that more than 10 million adults who are eighteen years and older (approximately 11 percent of the adult population) consume about half of all alcoholic beverages sold (Clark & Midanik, 1980).

The United States has the highest level of illicit drug use of any nation in the industrialized world. Roughly two-thirds of all American young people (64 percent) try an illicit drug before they finish high school. More than one-third have used illicit substances (cocaine, stimulants, and sedatives) other than marijuana. At least one in every sixteen high school seniors is actively smoking marijuana on a daily basis. These figures actually reflect a trend toward a decrease in the use of illicit substances among young people in recent years. In the older adult group, however, lifetime prevalence levels for hallucinogens and cocaine have increased, because people who began use of illicit substances as young adults are now moving into the age twenty-six and older category (National Institute on Drug Abuse, 1982).

An estimated 10 million Americans are alcoholics in contrast to 700,000 Americans who are estimated to have a problem with opiates. Almost no addiction is pure, however; most substance abusers use more than one substance or use substances in combination.

Certain reasons may be given for the use of more

than one substance. The most obvious is to enhance the effects of the basic mind-altering substance used. Alcohol is a central nervous system (CNS) depressant. Using other classes of depressants (narcotics, sedatives, minor tranquilizers, or volatile solvents) along with alcohol will, at a minimum, add to the depressant action. Pills are also easier to conceal if drinking is inappropriate. In certain instances the related drugs are supra-additive when used in combination with alcohol—that is, the effect of the two drugs is greater than the sum of their doses.

People sometimes mix addictive prescription drugs without realizing the consequence of mixing these substances. Another reason why more than one agent may be used is to counteract certain undesired effects of the basic psychochemical. Amphetamines make some users too tense and jittery ("wired up"), though euphoric. In such cases alcohol is used to take the edge off the tension state. At times, combinations of drugs are used when the preferred agent is not at hand, of poor quality, or too expensive. When heroin is not available, the user may substitute codeine cough syrup, propoxyphene (Darvon), alcohol, and marijuana alone or in combination. Finally, there is multiple drug use for its own sake. There is still an occasional person who will take anything and everything that is available (Cohen, 1981).

Conventionally, alcohol and drug addicts have been thought to be at risk for sustaining adverse physiological consequences from alcohol and drug use, but this is not consistently true. Some alcoholics never show organ damage from alcohol use, while moderate drinking can be harmful to those individuals who possess genetic or other biological factors that predispose them to specific organ pathologies. Illicit and prescription drugs rarely cause the kind of organ damage seen with extensive alcohol abuse.

Biomedical Consequences of Substance Abuse

Alcohol is the most physically damaging drug of all the commonly used substances. Chronic alcoholism can adversely affect all the organs of the body. Adverse effects to the gastrointestinal tract can begin immediately following ingestion of alcohol and extend to the liver as well as other organs following absorption. The liver is particularly susceptible to alcohol-associated injury, because it is the site where most of the metabolism of alcohol occurs. Until the liver has broken down ingested ethanol, alcohol is present in the bloodstream and can affect the function of the brain, heart, muscles, and gonads. Not only is ethanol toxic per se, but its breakdown may produce toxic metabolites such as acetaldehyde and acetate, which are also damaging to the body.

Alcohol abuse interacts with the physiological and metabolic processes of digestion, which contribute to nutritional deficiencies and associated diseases. Anemia, convulsions, small-bowel dysfunction, and Wernicke-Korsakoff syndrome are some of the disorders associated with alcohol-derived nutritional deficiencies. Excessive consumption has been associated with impotency, amenorrhea, infertility, and chemical diabetes. Alcohol consumption alters numerous functions of the endocrine system (Eckardt et al, 1981; Lieber, 1979).

Alcohol abuse has also been found to be damaging to the unborn child. Fetal Alcohol Syndrome (FAS), which has been identified among children of alcoholic women, is characterized by central nervous system (CNS) dysfunction, growth deficiency, a specific cluster of facial abnormalities, and other abnormalities, particularly skeletal, urogenital, and cardiac (Clarren & Smith, 1978). Research is currently under way to determine the effects of moderate maternal drinking and paternal drinking on the developing fetus (Anderson, 1982; Burns et al, 1984).

Volatile substances (glue sniffing), large doses of codeine, propoxyphene (Darvon), methaqualone, amphetamine, ritalin, as well as alcohol have been associated with a number of adverse effects on the cardiovascular system. These include alcoholic cardiomyopathy, low mean cardiac output, depressed myocardial contractility, and cardiac arrhythmias. Significant increases in blood pressure have also been associated with heavy drinking and amphetamine use (Jones-Witters & Witters, 1983).

Adverse effects associated with illegal substances such as cocaine, heroin, or marijuana are due to variability in dose, lack of hygienic administration, and a variety of adulterous compounds used to dilute the drugs. Respiratory depression and subsequent respiratory failure due to overdose of depressant-type drugs are common among illegal substance users. Pulmonary complications include pneumonia, abscess, infarction, and tuberculosis. These problems occur because of the poor nutritional status of addicts, inhaling the substances into the lung, and the respiratory depressant effects of many substances. Skin abscesses, cellulitis, and thrombophlebitis are the most frequent complications among heroin or "T's and Blues" (Talwin and Pyrabenzamine) addicts who inject the substances subcutaneously. Septicemia and acute and subacute bacterial endocarditis with involvement on either side of the heart are also seen among these addicts. Viral hepatitis transmitted by communal use of contaminated needles is a frequent complication in intravenous drug use. This condition is serious and can be fatal. Among pregnant addicts there is a high incidence of toxemia and of prematurity in the infants (National Institute on Drug Abuse, 1979). Impaired judgment, memory, and motivation are common with marijuana users. Medical consequences of substance abuse are frequently seen by nurses, but there are also other consequences to the individual, the family, and the community that may not be obvious to the nurse.

Social Problems

An association between drug use and depression in both men and women is described throughout the literature. The relationship between substance abuse and depression is complex and not easily assessed in the addicted client, but it is important for community health nurses to know that the addicted client and his or her family may be suffering from depression. Combinations of alcohol with other drugs often have greater lethal potential than either substance alone. Alcohol and other substances alter mood, judgment, and self-control. It has been shown that in the family constellation of manic-depressive disease there are more alcoholics than expected in the general population. Affective disorder is seen significantly more often in the female relatives of alcoholics than would be expected by chance alone (Winokur & Clayton, 1967). Suicide actions are likely to be more damaging with people under the influence of mood-altering substances. The risk of suicide is thirty times greater among substance abusers compared to the general population (Finkle, McCloskey, & Goodman, 1979; Beck, Weissman, & Kovacs, 1976).

Uninvolved members of the community may suffer from the consequences of substance abuse as well. It is estimated that 35 to 64 percent of all fatal automobile accidents involve a drinking driver. Moreover, the economic costs of alcoholism and alcohol misuse in terms of lost production, health care expenditures, motor vehicle accidents, fire losses, violent crimes, and social responses have been estimated to cost $58 billion a year (Department of Health and Human Services, 1982). In addition to these alcohol statistics, studies have shown that a majority of heroin users engage in criminal behaviors involving selling drugs, prostitution, burglaries, shoplifting, and stealing cars in order to obtain drugs to support their habit (Inciard, 1981).

Theories of Etiology

While there are many theories of etiology regarding substance abuse, no one theory completely explains the phenomenon. There are multiple patterns of substance use and abuse, and some explanations are more appropriate for certain types than others. Some of the current theories are disease model, genetic model, learning and developmental model.

Disease Model

Prior to the 1960s, scientific clinical studies of alcohol and drug problems were rare. The ideas that developed during that period were based on the experience of persons who had alcohol problems and the clinical experiences of those who dealt with these patients. The traditional ideas emerging from this period are still popular today and are embodied in the work of Alcoholics Anonymous and E.M. Jellinek (1946).

Alcoholics Anonymous, or AA, was founded in 1935. The ideas of this organization are simple but congruent with medical science prevailing at the time of its inception. People with alcohol problems are seen as victims of both physical and psychological aberrations. Those people predisposed to alcohol problems are said, after considerable drinking experience, to develop an allergy to alcohol. The allergy refers specifically to physical dependence. The allergy is described as "craving." This "craving" does not connote a desire for a first drink but rather a need to continue drinking once it has started. The natural history of alcoholism is described as "progressive" (Anonymous, 1976).

Jellinek (1946) gave scientific status to the ideas of AA. He did not speculate much about individual differences that might lead to alcoholism. However, he did postulate a psychological component to explain why some individuals develop alcohol problems and why, having experienced adverse consequences of drinking, they nevertheless drink again. For these individuals, he postulated that drinking had become a compulsion as an effective means to cope with emotional stress. With repeated drinking experience, however, the development of tolerance required these persons to drink increasing quantities to achieve the desired effect. In a clear analogy to the AA position, Jellinek (1952) also theorized that the physiology of some persons changes after a great amount of drinking. He introduced the term "loss of control" to char-

acterize the state of physical dependence in that the addicted drinker could not simultaneously stop drinking and avoid withdrawal symptoms. Jellinek proposed that alcoholics suffer from a disease. He contended that once such persons have begun to drink and become physically dependent on alcohol, they depart from normal health and need medical treatment. Acceptance of the disease concept is responsible for helping health professionals to see alcoholism as a treatable illness rather than a problem or moral weakness (Keller, 1976).

Genetic Model

Substance addiction seems to run in families. Observations of this phenomenon date back to the eighteenth century (Miller, Nirenberg, & McClure, 1984). Although the reasons for this occurrence are not clear, the possible hereditary basis of alcohol problems has been examined from three main perspectives: twin studies, adoption and half-sibling studies, and genetic marker studies. Adoption studies have been the most successful in demonstrating that alcoholism is genetically linked and in some cases and that susceptibility for males, in particular, increases with the number of alcoholic relatives, the severity of the alcohol problems in relatives, and the degree of genetic closeness of the relatives (Goodwin, 1979).

Another promising area of research pointing to a genetic factor involved in alcoholism is the presence of atypical alcohol metabolizing enzymes in the liver of certain ethnic groups (Ijiri, 1974). Schuckit (1981) has also found that male offspring of alcoholics have significantly higher levels of acetaldehyde than normal. EEG (Electroencephalogram) studies have also indicated changes that are specific to alcohol-addicted people, and many studies have been conducted on the C57BL strain of mice, which are higher consumers of alcohol than other strains (Murray & Gurling, 1980). While research indicates that there is biochemical uniqueness in some alcoholics and their offspring, there are no definitive answers about the genetic etiology of alcohol problems. Much research still needs to be done in this area. Not all children from alcoholic families grow up to be alcoholics themselves or even abstainers, and clearly not all substance-dependent people have a family history of substance abuse. Thus, other factors beyond heredity must be involved in the development of a substance abuse problem.

Learning and Developmental Model

Substance use is a learned behavior—learning how to take a substance, learning to recognize the effects of a substance, and learning to define these effects as pleasurable. For the most part, such learning occurs in a social context (Harford, 1984).

Peer Influence In American society, peer influences are much more powerful after puberty than are home and family values. When breaking away from family, the adolescent seeks other sources of support—usually from age-mates—to supply dependency needs, to provide reassurances, and to bolster self-esteem. The passport entry into the peer support group is adoption of the group's mores in dress, recreation, likes and dislikes, and values and beliefs. Thus, if alcohol, cigarettes, marijuana, or other drugs are what the group is "doing," then the newcomer will seek acceptance by doing the same. Substance usage is further rationalized by the knowledge that it is commonplace in the adult world, with little or no deleterious effects for the majority of adults (Jessor & Jessor, 1977; Kandel, 1975).

Sexual anxiety is another feature of the adolescent condition that demands relief. Sexual anxiety appears in many guises: concern about one's physical attractiveness; fear that heterosexual performance failure signifies homosexuality; belief that an insufficient sexual interest is indicative of "abnormality" or guilt over homosexual or heterosexual interests. Mood-altering substances work in two opposite ways to affect this complex array of related anxieties. The immediate effect of relief of inhibition and loss of self-consciousness facilitates social interaction, sexual approach, and performance. Loss of inhibition also dilutes homosexual anxiety, enabling a degree of experimentation whereby the young person can either confirm or disprove a homosexual orientation. Mood-altering substances, on the other hand, can also lead to impotence and diminished sex drive.

Role Modeling Other social reinforcements may come from the model of use and misuse set by older adolescents, young adults, parents, teachers, and even community health nurses, who may see substance use as a usual, essentially harmless, temporary phase of growing up. Parental factors that may play a role in substance abuse include lack of supervision, emotional or physical unavailability, and parental abuse of alcohol, illicit drugs, or prescription drugs.

Drug abuse appears initially to be an adolescent phenomenon. It is tied to the normal but often difficult process of growing up, experimenting with new behaviors, becoming self-assertive, developing close (usually heterosexual) relationships with people outside the family, and leaving home. Kandel (1975) proposes that there are three stages in adolescent drug use and that each has different concomitants. The first is the use of legal drugs, such as alcohol, and is mainly a social phenomenon. The second involves use of marijuana and is also primarily peer influenced. The third stage, frequent use of other illegal drugs, is predominantly a family phenomenon.

Family Dynamics It is useful to view any family in terms of its place in the family developmental life cycle. Most families go through a number of stages as they progress through life, such as birth of the first child, child attending school, children leaving home, and death of a parent or spouse (see Chapters 2 and 16). Most normal families are able to master these crises points without severe problems. Symptomatic families are not able to adjust to the change. They become "stuck" in a particular stage and are unable to progress beyond it (Haley, 1976). Substance-abusing families are often families who are developmentally "stuck."

Research (Coleman & Stanton, 1978) indicates that a high proportion of families with a drug abuse problem have experienced traumatic, untimely, or unexpected loss of a family member. This has led to the hypothesis that the high rate of death, suicide, and self-destruction among addicts is actually a family phenomenon in which the addict's role is to die or to come close to death as part of the family's attempt to work through the trauma and loss. Alexander and Dibb (1975) and Vaillant (1966) have reported a high rate of addiction for offspring of people who have immigrated either from another country or from a different section of the United States. What appears to happen is that many immigrant parents tend to depend on their children for emotional and other support, clinging to them and becoming terrified when the offspring become adolescents and start to separate (Coleman & Stanton, 1978).

Fear of separation is a significant problem for most families with an addicted member. The importance of the developmental stage of adolescence in the abuse of substances becomes more apparent when the family system is considered. The prototypic drug-abusing family is described in most of the family therapy literature as one in which one parent is intensely involved with the abuser, while the other parent is more punitive, distant, and/or absent. Usually the overinvolved, indulgent, over-protective parent is of the opposite sex, although the same sex parent may assume this role in some middle-class families. Sometimes this overinvolvement reaches the point of incest. Further, the drug-abusing offspring may serve a function for the parents, often as a channel for their communication or as a distraction from their own dissatisfying relationship. Consequently, the onset of adolescence, with its threat of the launching phase can bring on parental panic. The family then becomes stuck at this developmental stage, and a chronic, repetitive process sets in, centered on the individuation, growing up, and leaving of the substance-abusing family member (Stanton, Todd, & Associates, 1982).

Understanding the family dynamics underlying substance-abusing behavior is important because it helps community health nurses to understand the phenomenon as a treatable medical problem. Belief that substance addiction is a sin or a sign of little will power interferes with professional nursing intervention.

The earlier a problem of substance abuse can be identified, the better it is for the family, the substance-abusing individual, and society. Biomedical consequences are usually reversible with early intervention, and the family unit remains intact.

Diagnosis and Early Identification

Diagnostic Criteria

The American Psychiatric Association classifies the pathological use of substance as substance abuse and substance dependence. The diagnosis of substance abuse has three criteria: (1) pattern of pathological use; (2) impairment of social or occupational functioning; and (3) duration of at least one month. Pathological use involves intoxication throughout the day, inability to cut down or stop use, repeated efforts to control use through periods of temporary abstinence or restriction of use to certain times of the day, continuous use despite serious physical problems, the need for daily use in order to function, and episodes of a complication due to substance intoxication (alcoholic blackouts or narcotic overdose). Impairment in functioning is manifested in disturbed family or social relationships, legal difficulties, or problems on the job or in school (American Psychiatric Association, 1980).

Substance dependence is a more severe form of abuse and requires tolerance and/or withdrawal to

Table 26-1   Signs of Substance Abuse

Substance	Physical Signs	Behavioral Signs
Alcohol	An illness under treatment that does not respond as expected	Preoccupation with alcohol
	Burns on hand, chest, and forearms from careless smoking while drinking	"Doctor shopping" for sedative prescriptions
	Periorbital edema due to fluid retention	Coming to scheduled appointment with alcohol on breath
	Flushed face due to vasodilation	Frequent Monday morning absences
	Appearing older than stated age	Lowered performance on job or at school
		Poor self-image
		Dropping out of nondrinking relationships
		Giving up old hobbies or interests
		Employment choices that facilitate drinking
		Mood swings
Depressants	May seem intoxicated, but no alcohol odor on breath	Staggering or stumbling movements
		Falling asleep in class (even if interested in subject) or at work
Hallucinogen	Often appears to be daydreaming or in a trancelike state	May touch objects and examine everyday things carefully for long periods
		Body image and sense may be distorted, causing the person to panic
Marijuana	Odor of burned marijuana on clothes	
	Whites of eyes may appear irritated	
Narcotics	May have raw, red nostrils if sniffing; needle tracks if "shooting up"	Lethargic, drowsy behavior when high; purposive when obtaining money or locating source for drug
		Needs money to support habit, more so than other drugs
Phencyclidine (PCP)	Dazed, blank-stare expression, side-to-side eye movements	Poor physical coordination as if drunk, but no odor of alcohol
	Sweating, flushed skin, and excess salivation	

(continued)

Table 26-1   *(continued)*

Substance	Physical Signs	Behavioral Signs
Stimulants	Pupils may be dilated	Excessive activity, irritability, nervousness, and aggression
	Mouth and nose dry; bad breath; user licks lips frequently	Goes long periods without eating or sleeping
	May have needle marks if "shooting up"	
	Weight loss	
Volatile substances	Odor of substance on clothes and breath	
	Runny nose	
	Irritation and ulcerations around mouth	
	Watery eyes	
	Poor muscular coordination; drowsiness	

SOURCES:
Jones-Witters P, Witters W: *Drugs and Society: A Biological Perspective.* Monterey, Calif.: Wadsworth Health Sciences, 1983.

Williams E B: Assessment and identification of the problem. In: *The Community Health Nurse and Alcohol Related Problems.* Rockville, MD: NIAAA, 1978.

be present. Tolerance is the condition in which an increased amount of drug is necessary to produce the same effect or in which less effect is produced by the same dose of drug. Withdrawal is defined as the physiologic disturbances occurring after sudden cessation of large amounts of addictive substances that have been used for a long period of time. Depending on what substances are involved, withdrawal can include the following symptoms: nausea and vomiting, tinnitus, visual disturbances, pruritis, paresthesia, muscle pain, sleep disturbances, hallucination, agitation, tremor, sweats, depression, clouding of the sensorium, gait disturbance, and nystagmus.

Community health nurses may be very frustrated or puzzled by the client who is unable to cut down or stop taking substances when serious social or physical consequences are obvious. This inappropriate use of substances is called loss of control and is a key symptom of the addicted person. If the individual were able to control or stop the use of

these substances, there would be no need for treatment centers or self-help groups. Often a substance-abusing person will come to the attention of professionals, including the community health nurse, because of cardiac arrhythmias, hypertension, diabetes control, gastritis, constipation, pancreatitis, or other problems that are actually secondary to substance abuse. Figure 26-1 shows common clinical disorders associated with substance abuse.

Nursing Assessment

During assessment of a new client, nurses need to be aware of signs of substance abuse. Table 26-1 lists certain physical and behavioral clues indicative of substance abuse.

If nurses suspect substance abuse or addiction, further investigation is required as to the nature and extent of the patient's alcohol or drug involve-

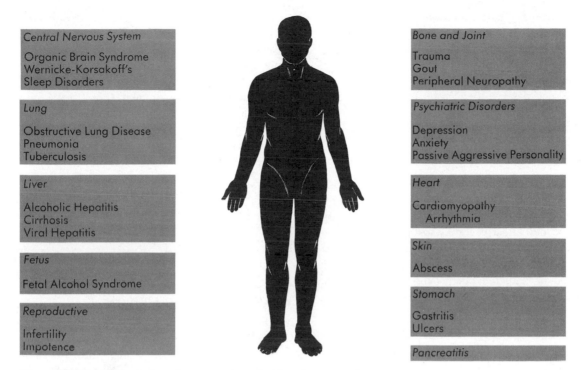

Figure 26-1 Clinical disorders associated with substance abuse.

ment. How has personal, social, physical, and mental functioning been affected? Are other serious mental or physical problems involved? What is the client's treatment history? How do the client and the family perceive the problem?

Community Health Nurse's Role

Attitude of the Nurse

Community health nurses are ideal persons to make early identification of the substance-abusing or substance-addicted person. They are usually the only health professionals who see people in the community. They can identify clients in need of help, refer them to appropriate treatment, and participate in follow-up care after treatments.

Often a substance-addicted person will come to the attention of the nurse because of problems that are actually secondary to substance abuse (see Figure 26-1). Treatment of these problems without attention to the primary cause leads to frustration and negative attitudes toward the addicted client.

Counterproductive Beliefs Studies of the attitudes of professional caretakers, including nurses, reveal that the following beliefs are especially counterproductive for success in nurse-client relationships (Kendal, 1978):

- Substance addiction is a self-inflicted disease.
- Substance addiction is hopeless.

- Recovering from addiction is a matter of will power.
- Drinking is sinful. All people should be abstinent.
- Addicts are simply people who won't accept life's responsibilities.
- Addicts deserve their problems.
- The capacity to hold your liquor is the test of a man.
- Women drive men to drink.

Nurses need to be aware of their own attitudes and to be capable of seeing the addicted client as an ill person who is capable of recovery. Nurses will be most effective if they are open-minded, positive, patient, realistic, empathic, and compassionate. Moralistic or negative attitudes are quickly sensed by addicted clients and will impede the development of trust so necessary between nurse and client.

Nurse–Patient Relationship The nurse-patient relationship provides unique opportunities to:

- Confront the patient in a nonjudgmental, serious manner about the consequences of his or her substance use
- Elicit the help of family in all efforts to confront and motivate patient to treatment
- Acquaint the patient with progressive nature of substance abuse
- Encourage the patient to enter treatment
- Discuss treatment options and inform the patient of available treatment resources in the community
- Acquaint the patient with telephone numbers of self-help groups such as AA, Alateen, Al-Anon, Narcotics Anonymous, and Women for Sobriety

Referral to Treatment

The first step in treating an addicted person is to assist him or her through detoxification. Attempting any counseling intervention with an intoxicated person is fruitless. Developing a treatment plan for detoxification requires nurses to take a careful history of substance use. The following information should be obtained: length of recent substance use; approximate quantity of alcohol and drugs consumed per day; time of last drink intake; nature of past withdrawal symptoms; presence of other chronic disease or acute conditions; and sources of assessment from significant others or previous hospital records. More critical withdrawal—seizures or delirium tremens—can be avoided with anticipatory nursing observations and interventions. Pulse, BP, and observation of disorientation provide most accurate clues to impending withdrawal problems. Any severe change in these parameters should alert the nurse to have the client transported to an emergency room.

Working Through Denial

Community health nurses cannot expect an addicted person to have immediate insight into how substances are affecting his or her life. Denial is the primary defense mechanism employed by the addicted person and by the significant others. Every effort is put forth by the client and the family members to protect themselves from the truth and the negative image of the addict label. The function of denial is to maintain the addiction. In denial, the person denies reality and blames external factors for the problems actually precipitated by the substance. By continuing to alter the meaning of the behavior, the substance-dependent person can continue to deny the relationship between substance use and its consequences. Denial can take many forms: minimizing the seriousness of the problem, attributing the drug use to factors no longer present, or blaming others.

The strength of the denial system is directly related to the duration of the substance problem. Thus those persons in the beginning stages of addiction are usually more open and capable of seeing the impact of substance use on their lives than those clients with long, involved addiction problems. Chronically addicted people can be reached only after prolonged confrontation in a drug-free environment.

Breaking through denial involves the establishment of trust and the use of confrontation and support. Intervening in the denial process may require the help of significant others or the environment of a therapeutic group. The purpose of breaking down the denial is to assist the patient to see the reality and consequences of his or her substance use. To achieve this end, some emotional pain will be encountered. The patient may respond to confrontation with anger or tears, which may make the nurse very uncomfortable. Nonetheless, confronting a client can be learned like any other nursing skill.

Working with the Family

Substance abuse by a parent is a stressful event that disturbs the family homeostasis. Family members can no longer expect the affected parent to behave in a predictable manner or to meet the demands of his or her role. Other members are forced to take on the responsibilities and roles of the substance-abusing parent. The family becomes capable of only responding to crises and incapable of maintaining a routine for meals, bed time, and other normal activities. For example, in a family where the mother is addicted and is incapable of preparing meals on time or caring for small children, older children may be forced to take on the roles of meal provider and nurturer of the young before they are developmentally ready. These children may or may not come to the attention of the community health nurse depending on how the child responds to the situation at home.

According to Booz, Allen, and Hamilton (1974), three major types of adaptation have been noted among children of substance abusers: flight, fight, and super good. Flight, or escape, is the most common way a child copes with a substance-abusing parent. Young children may hide under the bed, and older children may stay away from home as much as possible. Other children may escape emotionally and withdraw into themselves or block out all of the painful past. Fight, which is characterized by rebellion, physical and verbal aggression, and

acting out in socially unacceptable ways, are other methods of adapting. These children often get into trouble with the police. "Super good" children are those who never do anything wrong. They are excellent students and obedient to authority figures. Super good children usually do for others rather than themselves. These children often end up as professional care-givers such as social workers and nurses. Although adaptations of the super good child may seem desirable to teachers and parents, these children should not be overlooked. Children who adapt by achievement and caretaking for others frequently have problems as adults with relationships, depression, and substance abuse.

The nurse can be helpful to children with substance-abusing parents by providing a sympathetic ear. Referral to an Alateen group would be very appropriate for teenage children. The school nurse can also visit the home and refer the mother and/or family members to the appropriate services.

Jackson (1954) described seven stages of adaptation of the family crises of alcoholism. These stages can also be seen in families confronting other kinds of substance abuse.

1. Attempts to deny the problem. The family minimizes the seriousness of the drinking episodes and avoids problems related to alcohol.
2. Attempts to eliminate the problem. Family becomes socially isolated in order to decrease the visibility of the addicted person. Tension increases and relationships deteriorate.
3. Disorganization. Family experiences inept communication, role organization, and inconsistency.
4. Attempts to reorganize in spite of problem. Spouse takes over control of family with increased self-confidence. Alcoholic spouse is ignored and treated like a child.
5. Efforts to escape problem. Spouse may separate. Children may escape into achievement, daydreaming, or peer activities.
6. Reorganization. Spouse and children reorganize without the alcoholic person.
7. Recovery and reorganization of the whole family or reuniting if sobriety is achieved. Adaptation to life without alcohol.

Case Example 26-1: Family Dynamics in Substance Addiction

Mrs. B, mother of three children ages seven, ten, and eleven, is addicted to alcohol and Valium. Her husband attributes her behavior to depression and the strain of the children. Mr. B. rationalizes that alcohol helps Mrs. B. to relax. He buys alcohol for his wife so that she won't go out to buy it herself and drive while under the influence. He tells the children that their mother is sick and needs their help. Jennifer, the oldest child, often takes over the parenting role when her mother cannot function. She prepares meals for the younger children, does grocery shopping, and helps her mother to bed when she passes out. Jennifer gets excellent grades in school and is considered a model student by her teachers. Tom, the second oldest child, has become active in many school sports and is often absent from the home because of practices and games. Timothy, the seven-year-old, has many school problems. He finds it difficult to sit still and has a learning problem. Timothy is often the subject of case conferences at the school where Nancy N. is the school nurse. Concern about Timothy and failure of Mrs. B. to attend parent conferences has led Nancy N. to make a home visit where she is able to assess substance addiction as the problem and make appropriate referrals to treatment for the family and Mrs. B.

Father denies problem.

Daughter adapts to parental addiction by taking on parental roles and excelling in school.

Older son adapts by escaping into sports.

Youngest son may be suffering from minor manifestations of Fetal Alcohol Syndrome.

Nurse assesses problem and makes appropriate referral.

Families experience many problems when addiction is present. It is important that community health nurses remember the children, the parents, and the spouses when making referrals (see Case Example 26-1).

Treatment of Substance Abuse

Treatment Programs

There are many forms of treatment currently available depending on the condition and the financial resources of the client. Also the nature of the substance used must be taken into consideration.

Appropriate candidates for outpatient treatment are in stable physiological condition, have low potential for severe withdrawal symptoms, have no history of prescription or street drugs, possess a stable social support system, and are motivated to stop drinking or using drugs. Appropriate candi-

dates for inpatient treatment are: persons drinking large quantities of alcohol for long periods of time (1 pint of hard liquor per day for ten days or more or the equivalent in beer or wine); persons who have been drinking heavily while ingesting prescription or street drugs; persons using large quantities of street drugs or prescription drugs; and persons with a history of serious withdrawal reaction (seizures, hallucinations, delirium tremens, psychosis).

The major goal of treatment has been abstinence—based on the assumption that the disease cannot be cured but its course can be arrested by total abstinence from mood-altering substances. This concept is a basic tenet in Alcoholics Anonymous and dominates current treatment practices of most agencies.

General Hospital More hospitals have been admitting substance-abusing patients in the last decade, and guidelines for treating addicted clients have been established by the American Hospital Association. Earlier hospital policies excluding addicts were based on the traditional belief that they caused trouble and did not pay their bills. Even so, many addicts were admitted to acute care hospitals in the past, although treatment was usually focused on the biomedical consequences of the illness, not on substance abuse as a primary diagnosis.

The basic elements of hospital-based programs for addicted clients still include detoxification, physical rehabilitation, education about substance abuse, counseling, group therapy, and Alcoholics Anonymous sessions. However, a variety of new therapies have been tried during the last decade. Family therapy is one of these. It has been used successfully with both alcohol and drug abusers.

Family Therapy Family therapy is based on a systems theory approach. It emphasizes interactional exchange among family members with interdependence on each other. All members of the family unit are seen as contributing to how family members relate to each other and how the symptoms of substance abuse erupts. The substance abuser or addict is seen as the signaler of distress within the family system. The family unit, rather than the individual substance abuser, is seen as troubled. Therapy is focused on the entire family, rather than on the symptomatic member.

Behavioral Therapy Behavioral therapy has also been used in various programs throughout the United States. These therapies are based on the belief that drinking is a learned behavior involving social situations and customs, emotional and cognitive experiences, personal expectations, and reinforcing conditions. Some of the techniques used in behavioral therapy include aversion therapy, assertiveness training, and progressive relaxation. These techniques are designed to either extinguish the pleasurable response to chemicals or to teach skills that decrease the need for chemicals as a coping mechanism.

Nonmedical Detox Centers Nonmedical detox centers are in operation in some large cities. These centers provide a safe environment in which chronic users can detoxify. Although these services provide a desirable alternative to jail, they have some negative aspects. First, the nonmedical approach eliminates the opportunity for early diagnosis of medical problems. Second, the centers have often been used by substance abusers as emergency shelters rather than an opportunity to change their lifestyles. Nevertheless, there is some promise that detoxification centers can be safe and effective for the sick abuser. They also provide an entry into comprehensive treatment programs.

Therapeutic Communities The therapeutic community emerged as a treatment for drug abuse in 1958 as an option to established social institutions. Synanon, Daytop Village, Phoenix House, and Gateway House are examples of this type of treatment. The therapeutic community model includes encounter group therapy, tutorial–learning sessions, remedial and formal educational classes, residential jobs, and eventually conventional occupations. The primary staff are nondegreed professionals who are former addicts. Traditional therapeutic communities require the addict to remain in residence for at least fifteen months. The basic goal of the treatment is to effect a complete change in life-style: abstinence from drugs, elimination of antisocial behavior, development of employable skills, and self-reliance.

Treating Alcoholics and Drug Addicts Together Treating alcoholics and drug addicts in the same program has stirred both interest and controversy. In general, alcoholics tend to be older and middle class, and to have a history of relatively stable lives. Opiate addicts tend to be young and uneducated, and often have shown criminal ten-

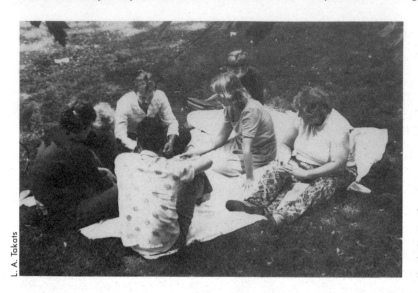

L. A. Takats

Therapeutic communities offer recovering addicts a suggested environment for systematic therapy and psychosocial rehabilitation.

dencies. Opponents of combined treatment argue that these differences militate against successful results in a program with both groups. Even the combined treatment advocates recommend caution in mixing heroin addicts with skid row and lower-class alcoholics, because experience has shown that there is considerable potential for conflict. Integrating treatment approaches that are appropriate in the same program can be difficult. For some addicts, replacing their drug with a substitute such as methadone can be a significant component of their treatment. Alcoholic treatment programs that follow the AA model are oriented toward abstinence. Although many researchers have noted the problems posed by combined treatment, little strong opposition to the general idea is evident. Pros and cons are involved in the financial and administrative aspects as well. Although combined programs may seem to be more efficient—particularly in smaller communities—categorical funding creates serious administrative problems when treatment is combined.

Pharmacological Agents Used in Treatment

Certain drugs have been used in treating substance abusers. It is important to remember that *all* of these agents must be used in conjunction with therapy; in other words, these drugs cannot stand alone in treating substance abusers.

Substitution Therapy Methadone maintenance is an approach in the treatment of opiate dependence. This mode of therapy emphasizes social and emotional functioning rather than abstinence. The treatment is based on the use of methadone, which is a chemical substitute for heroin that is long acting (twenty-four to thirty-six hours) and can be administered orally. The dose of methadone is gradually increased until reaching a stabilization level, at which point patients will be tolerant to the euphoric effects of the drug and experience no persistent craving for the opiates. Maintenance of methadone has been shown to improve the functioning of addicts in school and work and to decrease their involvement in criminal activities. Long-term methadone maintenance has been shown to be medically safe when properly administered. Methadone maintenance is controversial because it involves substitute addiction. It is aimed at reducing the consequences of the substance addiction rather than at abstinence.

Detoxification Agents Paraldehyde, chloralhydrate, barbiturates, and alcohol have been successfully used for alcohol withdrawal. Benzodiazepine tranquilizers are the most appropriately used at the present time. Methadone is the drug of choice for withdrawal from opiates, although Catapress has also been used. Haldol (haloperidol) is sometimes used for psychotic reactions or hallucinations associated with the abuse of stimulants, hallucinogens, or cannabis. Phenothiazines have been used for withdrawal but are not desirable because they tend to increase the incidence of convulsions. The trend currently is toward no drugs for detoxification if possible to avoid development of another drug dependency.

Alcohol Sensitizing Agent Disulfiram (Antabuse) is a drug that produces nausea and vomiting, tachycardia, sweating, flushing of face and neck, and dizziness when alcohol is consumed. It inactivates aldehyde dehydrogenase in the liver and produces an accumulation of unmetabolized acetaldehyde in the liver when alcohol is ingested. This type of therapy can help an alcoholic get past momentary impulses to drink. Requiring individuals addicted to both alcohol and heroin to take disulfiram in order to obtain methadone maintenance has also been useful.

Lithium Carbonate The incidence of depressive disorders correlate highly with substance abuse and addiction. Currently lithium carbonate, an antidepressant, is being investigated to determine its usefulness in addiction treatment. Since lithium is not addictive, it does not pose a threat in the development of an additional drug dependency.

Self-Help Groups

Many substance abusers have found great support and relief in joining groups of other substance abusers. Families of substance abusers can also join groups of people in similar situations. All of these groups offer a sense of belonging and of not being alone in their problem.

Alcoholics Anonymous The oldest and best known treatment of alcoholism is Alcoholics Anonymous (AA), a self-help group started in 1935. The AA program is based on twelve steps that guide the individual through the process of admitting powerlessness over alcohol, asking God (as he or she is understood) for guidance, reflecting on one's assets and shortcomings, making amends, and carrying the message of AA to other alcoholics. AA successfully provides a strong community-based social support system for abstinence. Attendance at AA meetings can be effective by itself or in conjunction with other therapies. There are no dues, and the only requirement for membership is the desire to stop drinking.

Al-Anon and Alateen Al-Anon and Alateen are self-help groups for family members of alcoholics and are based on the same twelve steps as AA. The Al-Anon and Alateen programs emphasize powerlessness over the alcoholic instead of alcohol itself. These programs help significant others to learn detachment and to work through the shame, guilt, and anger produced by involvement with a chemically dependent person. Al-Anon is for family members and significant others, while Alateen is organized for teenagers. Another group, Adult Children of Alcoholics, organized as an outgrowth of Al-Anon and Alateen, has been growing extensively.

Women for Sobriety Women for Sobriety is a recently formed organization to help women alcoholics in their recovery. The organization also has steps guiding their members through a comfortable sobriety.

Group attendance, successful role modeling, peer pressure, and helping oneself through helping others are the therapeutic factors involved in self-help groups. These groups are free of charge and are valuable sources of referral for the community health nurse. Telephone numbers for these groups are usually available in local telephone directories.

Strategies for Health Promotion

According to Miller, Nirenberg, and McClure (1984), all three levels of prevention can be effective in dealing with substance abuse and dependence.

Primary Prevention

Primary prevention attempts to prevent alcohol and drug problems before they begin. Most educational programs of this nature target junior high students. It is during this period when experimentation with substances begins (Jessor & Jessor, 1977).

Three general primary prevention approaches are currently in use: (1) educating individuals about responsible use of substances; (2) monitoring the influence of mass media on substance-taking attitudes and behaviors; and (3) setting alcohol and drug control policies that include minimum drinking age laws, pricing and taxation, situational controls, criminalization, and scheduling of drugs according to addictiveness by the federal government (Miller, Nirenberg & McClure, 1984).

According to Banonis (1978), community health nurses are in an excellent position with clients and families to implement substance-specific primary prevention strategies. All of the settings in which community health nurses work offer opportunities to introduce the subject of alcohol and drugs in day-to-day health care and teaching. When checking medication use, the nurse can teach clients about the dangers of mixing alcohol and prescribed drugs or combining prescriptions with over-the-counter preparations. Clients should also be alerted to the addictive properties of prescription drugs. Instruction on any dietary problems should always include information about alcohol use.

School nurses are in an especially strong position to encourage educational programs on substance use in health, science, or marriage and the family courses. The school nurse is also able to identify trouble signs of absenteeism or behavior associated with substance use. He or she can also act as a consultant to teachers on matters of substance abuse.

Nurses in occupational settings have a similar advantage of being able to observe illnesses or behaviors that are consequences of substance use. Those nurses working in industry can foster prevention by encouraging employers to initiate an employee assistance program (EAP). These programs have been remarkably successful in reducing the economic loss from alcohol-related problems of workers by requiring the employee to accept company-financed help (Banonis, 1978).

The nurse in a prenatal clinic or obstetrician's office has an excellent opportunity to promote prevention of the damaging effects of drugs and alcohol on the developing fetus. Mothers who are unable to abstain from alcohol or drugs during pregnancy or breast feeding should be referred to treatment for this problem. Some cities have a special clinic for such mothers. An example is the Perinatal Addiction Clinic at Northwestern Memorial Hospital in Chicago.

Secondary Prevention

Secondary prevention is aimed at people who are abusing substances and beginning to develop problems. These prevention efforts have been educational in nature and targeted toward college students, the military, and drunk drivers.

Community health nurses can carry out secondary prevention by being sensitive to the following five conditions that usually characterize special populations that are at risk for addiction problems.

1. *Family History:* Research shows that approximately 50 percent of all alcoholic men and women state either a parent, grandparent, or sibling was alcoholic (de Fuentes, 1975). Whether the phenomenon is environmentally or genetically caused is not known. Drinking problems occur less in families in which chil-

dren are introduced to drinking within the context of social occasions or meals (Banonis, 1978). In families where alcohol is prohibited for religious or disciplinary reasons, children are more predisposed to an alcohol problem should they drink. For such families, community health nurses can teach about the occurrence of alcohol problems in families and also teach some alternate methods of relaxation through exercise, meditation, or progressive relaxation.

2. *Past History:* The person who has become addicted once seems to acquire addiction to another substance relatively easily. This is probably due to physiologic alteration in the body. Nurses should be aware of this potential for cross-addiction. Any person who has been through treatment of an addiction problem should be warned about taking potentially addicting substances.

3. *Emotional Problems and Disruption in Life:* Drinking or taking drugs to relieve stress is always potentially harmful. Community health nurses can help clients under stress by encouraging them to talk out their problems and by teaching stress management techniques such as exercise, massage, and progressive relaxation. People under stress should be encouraged to reduce as much stress as they can and to be particularly good to themselves when stressful conditions are present.

4. *Minority Groups:* Membership in a minority racial or ethnic group does not by itself predispose an individual to substance abuse problems. For instance, the prevalence of alcohol and drug use is lower among blacks than in the general population. However, those blacks who use alcohol or drugs are more likely to develop a problem. American Indians and Spanish Americans also have unique problems with mood-altering substances. It should be noted that general socioeconomic conditions, particularly unemployment, contribute heavily to the stress experienced in these groups. Education and available treatment are very important. Those community health nurses who are themselves members of the minority group may work most effectively, because it is often very difficult for these clients to trust professionals outside of their group.

5. *Health Professionals:* Health professionals, particularly doctors and nurses, assume tremendous responsibility for their clients, and many experience high levels of stress and may abuse chemical substances as means of coping. In addition, compared to members of other occupational groups, they have easy access to various chemically abusing substances. Consequently, community health nurses should be sensitive to the potential for substance abuse among health professionals and be alert to make appropriate referrals for treatment whenever necessary. The unique problems of the impaired nurse are discussed in the next section.

Tertiary Prevention

Tertiary prevention refers to direct treatment of substance abusers, which usually does not involve community health nurses. Nurses can, however, play a meaningful role in helping to prevent already identified clients from relapse and further deterioration. Being alert to early signs of substance abuse and referring these clients to appropriate treatment as soon as it can be arranged are key strategies. Community health nurses should also be concerned about the issue of substance abuse among their colleagues.

The Impaired Nurse One of the reasons nurses have difficulty with caring for substance-abusing clients is that the nursing profession has been ineffectual in dealing with substance abuse among colleagues. Prevention is as important in nursing as it is in any other population. It has been estimated that there are 75,000 nurses in the United States who are addicted to mood-altering substances (Wright, 1982).

Historically, there has been very little effort on the part of nursing administrations or organizations to take responsibility for these individuals or to

Box 26-1   Educational and Support Agencies for Management of Substance Abuse

Addiction Research Foundation
33 Russell Street
Toronto, Ontario M55 251

Al-Anon Family Groups
P.O. Box 182, Dept. G
Madison Square Garden Station
New York, NY 10010
(212) 475-6110

Alcohol and Drug Problems Association
of North America (ADPA)
1101 15th Street, N.W.
Suite 204
Washington, DC 20005

Alcoholics Anonymous
P.O. Box 459
Grand Central Station
New York, NY 10017
(212) 686-1100

Distilled Spirits Council of the
United States, INC. (DISCUS)
1300 Pennsylvania Bldg.
Washington, DC 20004

National Center for Alcohol Education
1901 North Moore Street
Arlington, VA 22209

National Clearinghouse for Alcohol
Information (NCALI)
P.O. Box 2345
Rockville, MD 20852

National Institute on Drug Abuse (NIDA)
11400 Rockville Pike
Rockville, MD 20852

Pills Anonymous
P.O. Box 473
Ansonia, NY 10023

Women for Sobriety
P.O. Box 618
Quakertown, PA 18951

World Service Office of Narcotics Anonymous
P.O. Box 622
Sun Valley, CA 91352

---

provide guidance for their recovery. In many ways the denial of the nursing profession parallels the denial of the family with an addicted member. As a consequence, most nurse addicts are allowed to function marginally on night shifts and in unobtrusive jobs until termination is inevitable.

Failure to assist addicted nurses is a loss to the profession. Studies show that most of these nurses graduated in the top third of their nursing class, have achieved advanced degrees, and were highly respected for their work prior to their substance addictions (Bissell & Jones, 1981). As peers we have a responsibility to identify these nurses and assist them in receiving treatment. Some clues that may be helpful in identifying these nurses are:

1. Absenteeism
2. Tardiness or job shrinkage (doing the minimum work necessary)
3. Inability to meet schedules and deadlines
4. Illogical or sloppy charting
5. Excessive errors
6. Personality changes (irritability, withdrawal, mood swings)
7. Forgetfulness
8. Unkempt appearance (Jefferson & Ensor, 1982).

Once these nurses are identified, they should be allowed to take a leave of absence in order to obtain treatment. Termination from the job can be used as leverage to get the nurse to treatment, but firing should only be a last resort.

Appropriate treatment should be recommended and supported. Follow-up support and guidance should be provided for at least two years after treatment. The nurse should be allowed to return to the practice of nursing when abstinence is established. The care and prevention role in community health nurses should begin "at home" so to speak. If we can learn to take care of our own, we will certainly be more effective and confident in dealing with substance-abusing clients in the community. To assist community health nurses in their education and referral role, Box 26-1 provides a list of agencies that are sources for information materials, technical assistance, and funding.

Summary

Community health nurses can be critical agents of change in providing education, early assessment, referral, and prevention of substance abuse and addiction in the community. The scope of the problem in this and other countries suggests that the nurses' contribution in these areas is extremely valuable and essential. Such contributions may exceed community boundaries. For example, it is important for community health nurses to be aware and involved in all efforts to pass legislation either locally or nationally regarding substance abuse. In such efforts nurses can collaborate with some of the many political interest groups involved in the use of media or legislation for the prevention of substance abuse. For instance, it may seem logical to have an ordinance against teenage home parties that involve alcohol and drugs. However, such an ordinance would be difficult to pass if the local liquor dealers would be economically affected and would oppose such legislation. Consequently, community health nurses must view substance abuse as a problem affecting not only individuals, families, and special communities, but also society at large.

Topics for Nursing Research

• How can community health nurses identify children at risk who are from chemically dependent families?
• What are the consequences of moderate maternal drinking on the human fetus?
• How can education about mood-altering chemicals decrease the prevalence of chemical dependency?
• What are the variables that can best predict successful identification and treatment of the impaired nurse?

Study Questions

1. The most physically damaging of the following commonly abused substances is:
   a. Cocaine
   b. Alcohol
   c. Heroin
   d. Marijuana
2. Some of the negative consequences of substance abuse on society at large are:
   a. Lost production
   b. Health care expenditures
   c. Motor vehicle accidents
   d. All of the above
3. Tolerance to an abusing drug is reached when:
   a. An increased amount of the drug is necessary to produce the same effect
   b. The desired effect of the drug is reached
   c. The drug user realizes that he or she has a problem
   d. The drug user has been taking the drug for at least six months
4. A client with a previous history of drug abuse comes to the family planning clinic for contraceptives. The community health nurse observes what appear to be skin abscesses and cellulitis over the client's legs and thighs. The client denies emphatically that she has been using drugs and says she has been "off drugs for a while." Which of the following is appropriate action for the nurse to take?
   a. Recognize that the client is telling the truth and refer her to the skin clinic.
   b. Recognize that the symptoms are frequent complications of injecting substances subcutaneously and further assess the client for drug abuse.
   c. Recognize that the client is not telling the truth and refer her immediately to a drug detoxification center.
   d. None of the above.

5. Which of the following defense mechanisms are most often used by substance abusers?
   a. Reaction formation
   b. Substitution
   c. Denial
   d. Projection

References

Alexander BK, Dibb GS: Opiate addicts and their parents. *Family Process* 1975; 14: 499–514.

American Psychiatric Association: *Diagnostic and Statistical Manual of Mental Disorders*, 3rd ed. Washington, DC: Author, 1980.

Anderson RA: Possible role of paternal alcohol consumption in the etiology of fetal alcohol syndrome. In: Abel EL (editor) *Fetal Alcohol Syndrome: Animal Studies*, vol. 3. Boca Raton, Fla.: CRC Press, 1982, pp. 83–112.

Anonymous: *Alcoholics Anonymous*, 3rd ed. New York: Alcoholics Anonymous World Service, 1976.

Banonis BC: The community nurse as an agent in primary prevention. In: *The Community Health Nurse and Alcohol Related Problems*. Rockville, Md.: National Center for Alcohol Education, NIAAA, 1978.

Beck AT, Weissman A, Kovacs M: Alcoholism Hopelessness and Suicide Behavior. *J Stud Alcohol* 1976; 37: 66–77.

Bissell L, Jones RW: The alcoholic nurse. *Nurs Outlook* (February) 1981: 96–101.

Booz, Allen, and Hamilton, Inc.: *An Assessment of the Needs of and Resources for Children of Alcoholic Parents*, Final report. Rockville, Md.: National Institute on Alcohol Abuse and Alcoholism, 1974.

Burns EM et al: The effects of ethanol exposure during brain growth spurt. *Teratology*, 1984; 29: 251–258.

Clark WB, Midanik L: *Alcohol Use and Alcohol Problems among U.S. Adults: Results of the 1979 National Survey*. Rockville, Md.: NIAAA, 1980.

Clarren SK, Smith DW: The fetal alcohol syndrome. *N Engl J Med* 1978; 298: 1063–1067.

Cohen S: The effects of combined alcohol/drug abuse on human behavior. In: Gardner SE (editor), *Drug and Alcohol and Abuse: Implications for Treatment*. DHHS Publication No. (ADM) 80–958. Rockville, Md.: NIDA, 1981.

Coleman SB, Stanton MD: The role of death in the addict family. *Journal of Marriage and Family Counseling* 1978; 4: 79–91.

de Fuentes N: Houseguest. *The Alcoholism Digest* 1975; 4 (10): 6–11.

Department of Health and Human Services: *Alcohol Consumption and Related Problems*. Alcohol and health monograph no. 1, Rockville, Md.: NIAAA, 1982.

Eckardt MJ et al: Health hazards associated with alcohol consumption. *JAMA* 1981; 246: 648–666.

Finkle BS, McCloskey KL, Goodman LS: Diazepam and drug association deaths: A survey in the United States and Canada. *JAMA* 1979; 242: 429–434.

Goodwin DW: Alcoholism and heredity. *Arch Gen Psychiatry* 1979; 36: 57–61.

Haley J: *Problem-Solving Therapy*. San Francisco: Jossey-Bass, 1976.

Harford TC: Situational factors in drinking: A developmental perspective on drinking contexts. In: Miller PM, Nirenberg TD (editors), *Prevention of Alcohol Abuse*. Plenum Press, 1984.

Ijiri I: Studies on the relationship between the concentrations of blood acetaldehyde and urinary catecholamine and symptoms after drinking alcohol. *Jpn J Stud Alcohol* 1974; 9: 35–59.

Inciard JA: Crime and alternative patterns of substance abuse. In: *Drug and Alcohol Abuse: Implications for Treatment*. Treatment Research Monograph Series, NIDA. DHHS Publications No. (ADM) 80–958. Rockville, Md.: NIDA, 1981.

Jackson JK: The adjustment of the family to the crises of alcoholism. *Q J Stud Alcohol* 1954; 15: 526–586.

Jefferson LV, Ensor BE: Confronting a chemically-impaired colleague. *Am J Nurs* 1982; 82: 574–577.

Jellinek EM: Phases in the drinking history of alcoholics: Analysis of a survey conducted by *The Grapevine*, official organ of Alcoholics Anonymous. *Q J Stud Alcohol* 1946; 7: 1–88.

Jellinek EM: Phases of alcohol addiction. *Q J Stud Alcohol* 1952; 13: 673–684.

Jessor R, Jessor SL: *Problem Behavior and Psychosocial Development: A Longitudinal Study of Youth*. New York: Academic Press, 1977.

Jones-Witters P, Witters W: *Drugs and Society: A Biological Perspective*. Monterey, Calif.: Wadsworth Health Sciences, 1983.

Kandel O: Stages in adolescent involvement in drug use. *Science* 1975; 190: 912–914.

Keller M: The disease concept of alcoholism revisited. *Q J Stud Alcohol* 1976; 37: 1694–1717.

Kendal EM: Effect of attitudes on delivery of health care. In: *The Community Health Nurse and Alcohol-Related Problems*. Rockville, Md.: NIAAA, 1978.

Lieber CS: Alcohol-nutrition interactions. In: Li TK, Schenker S, Lumeng L (editors), *Alcohol and Nutrition*. NIAAA Research Monograph 2. Washington, DC: Government Printing Office, 1979.

Miller PM, Nisenkey TD, McClure G: Prevention in alcohol abuse. In: Rush B, *An Inquiry into the Effects of Ardent Spirits upon the Human Body and Mind, with an Account of the Means of Preventing and of the Rem-*

edies for Curing Them. Brookfield, Mass.: Meriam, 1814. Reprinted *Q J Stud Alcohol* 1943; 4: 324–341.

Miller PM, Nirenberg TD, McClure G: *Prevention of Alcohol Abuse.* Plenum, 1984.

Murray RM, Gurling HMD: Genetic contributions to normal and abnormal drinking. In: Sandler M (editor), *Psychopharmacology of Alcohol.* New York: Raven Press, 1980.

National Institute on Drug Abuse: *Drug Dependence in Pregnancy: Clinical Management of Mother and Child.* Services Research monograph series, DHEW Publication No. (ADM) 79–678. Rockville, Md.: NIDA, 1979.

National Institute on Drug Abuse: *National Household Survey on Drug Abuse.* Rockville, Md.: NIDA, 1982.

Schuckit MA: A prospective study of genetic markers in alcoholism. In: Hanin I, Usden E (editors), *Biological Markers in Psychiatry and Neurology.* Oxford, England: Pergamon Press, 1981.

Stanton DM, Todd TC, Associates. *The Family Therapy of Drug Abuse and Addiction.* New York: Guilford, 1982.

Vaillant GE: Parent-child cultural disparity and drug addiction. *J Nerv Ment Dis* 1966; 142: 534–539.

Williams EB: Assessment and identification of the problem. In: *The Community Health Nurse and Alcohol Related Problems.* Rockville, Md.: NIAAA, 1978.

Winokur G, Clayton P: Family history studies: II. Sex differences and alcoholism in primary affective illness *Br J Psychiatry* 1967; 133: 973–979.

Wright W: Nurses' drug problems are cloaked in denial. *The Journal* (February 1) 1982: 16.

Chapter 27

Chronic Mental Illness

Linda Chafetz

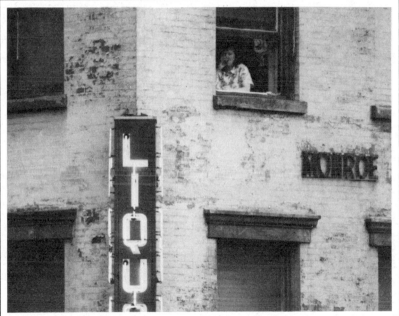

Inefficiencies in service structures and attitudes toward the mentally ill often leave individuals with long-term psychiatric disorders stranded and isolated. Community health nurses can provide a balanced, objective viewpoint in planning care for this special group.

Chapter Outline

Chapter Objectives

After completing this chapter, the reader will be able to:

- Define the chronically mentally ill in terms of criteria for psychiatric chronicity
- Identify the major mental illnesses most often associated with hospital treatment and/or disability
- Identify at least two issues in daily living confronting the chronically ill individual in a community setting
- Discuss at least two types of problems encountered by families of community-based clients
- Identify at least one form of problematic community response to the chronically mentally ill
- Discuss strategies a community health nurse might employ to assess clients with chronic psychiatric problems
- Provide at least two reasons for collaborative work with psychiatric nursing specialists and mental health consultants
- Discuss the reasons why the chronically mentally ill can benefit from advocacy efforts by community health nurses

This chapter focuses on an important and vulnerable client group in community settings: the chronically mentally ill. Long-term psychiatric disorders constitute major public health problems among adults in the United States, touching upon the lives of many individuals both directly and indirectly. However, the attitudes surrounding mental illness differ in type and intensity from those associated with other chronic health problems. Community reaction to the psychiatrically disabled frequently serves to isolate those most in need of interpersonal and material assistance. Since community living for the chronically mentally ill is a recent development, the health and social welfare systems have not always fully accommodated to their presence. Gaps and inequities in service structures may undermine the community adaptation of those with the fewest personal resources.

Although they share a set of common problems, the chronically mentally ill are nevertheless diverse—a factor that precludes generalization about their care. Long-term psychiatric disorder occurs within a series of diagnostic categories, each implying somewhat different clinical problems and treatment approaches. Within any given diagnostic grouping, individuals vary still more in terms of functional level. The term *schizophrenia*, for example, may refer to persons living independently and managing their own care. It may also apply to severely disabled individuals who require assistance in almost all facets of daily living. As in any illness situation, the person's age and developmental concerns determine his or her expectations for the future and use of services. The meaning of mental illness itself and the values attached to psychiatric treatment, symptoms, dependency, and disability are largely products of sociocultural background.

In view of this diversity, this chapter will not attempt to specify any common set of nursing interventions for the community-based mentally ill. Rather, it will begin by considering the nature and extent of serious psychiatric illness in the United States today. Next, it will review the transition from institutional to local care that has occurred over the past two decades in this country, looking at its impact on individuals, their social networks, and on communities. Using these factors as a backdrop, we may then consider the role of the community health nurse with the chronically mentally ill, and the approaches that may be used to provide individualized services consistent with clients' values, beliefs, clinical status, and treatment expectations.

Who Are the Chronically Mentally Ill?

Criteria for Psychiatric Chronicity

In the past, when criteria for chronic mental illness and institutional treatment overlapped, there was little pressure for a common definition of *psychiatric chronicity*. However, the transition to a system of community-based care has produced more discussion about the meaning of this term and the parameters of the population to which it refers. (See Box 27-1.) Persistence of symptoms, in and of itself, cannot determine chronicity, since many long-term psychiatric problems interfere minimally with social and occupational functioning. In an effort to distinguish chronic disorders from such lesser problems in living, three related criteria have been proposed: duration of hospital or residential treatment; disability; and diagnosis (Goldman, Gatozzi, & Taube, 1981; Minkoff, 1979).

The first of these, duration of institutional treatment, refers to a clear but limited part of the target population. If long-term care (of twelve months of more) in psychiatric facilities indicates chronicity,

Box 27-1   Terms Dealing with Chronic Mental Illness

Chronic mental illness: Persistent disorder involving either moderate to severe functional impairment (disability), or the occurrence of disability in the absence of treatment (continuing or intermittent). The major mental illnesses most often involve chronic disability. The population in long-term psychiatric institutions generally have chronic mental illnesses.

Community support services: Models of care that coordinate a broad range of therapeutic and social services, often using case management or resource management (by a single provider or team of providers) to coordinate care and reduce fragmentation or duplication of services.

Deinstitutionalization: Reduction in long-term hospital care for mental disorders and the expansion of community-based mental health services.

Homelessness: Absence of a stable place to live and consequent dependence on emergency type housing in shelters, use of unconventional dwelling places such as public buildings, or living in streets and parks.

Major mental illness: Schizophrenic, major affective, and chronic organic syndromes that imply pervasive and severe disturbance of the personality.

Psychosis: Psychiatric condition involving pervasive disturbance of functions and often involving reduced ability to test or perceive reality.

Transinstitutionalization: Movement of the population in long-term psychiatric hospitals to new institutional settings such as nursing homes or boarding homes with a custodial care approach and limited opportunities for community participation.

many chronic patients also reside outside these settings. The criterion of disability has more general meaning. In this sense we may consider the chronically mentally ill as those persons experiencing persistent problems that produce moderate to severe functional impairment, or that would imply such impairment in the absence of treatment.

Major Mental Illnesses

Certain diagnoses frequently imply disabling symptoms and are associated with at least occasional use of inpatient and residential care. The "major mental illnesses"—schizophrenic, recurrent affective, and progressive organic mental disorders—fall into this grouping. These involve the possibility of pervasive disturbance of the personality and "psychotic" symptoms, or disturbance reducing the individual's ability to test reality and to make safe judgments about the environment. They have traditionally been discussed in terms of "functional" (schizophrenic, affective) vs. "organic" psy-

choses—a categorization based on the assumption of physiological etiology in dementias associated with age-related and medical factors. In fact, the biochemical processes involved in all major mental illnesses have come into clearer focus during the past decade, making the functional-organic dichotomy somewhat obsolete. While these developments hold much promise for prevention and treatment in the future, they are at the level of hypotheses and do not as yet provide the means to arrest or to cure chronic disorders. For this reason, treatment of both "functional" and "organic" syndromes frequently involves symptom control and environmental support of social functioning.

Schizophrenic Disorders The schizophrenic disorders are estimated to affect between 500,000 and 900,000 persons in the United States (Goldman, Gatozzi, & Taube, 1981) and usually have their onset during the second and third decade of life. They have been attributed to psychodynamic and environmental factors (Arieti, 1974) as well as biochemical processes (Bowers, 1980).

Genetic studies show an elevated risk of illness in children and siblings of schizophrenics (Kessler, 1980). Schizophrenic illness appears to vary inversely with socioeconomic status, which has been interpreted in several ways: the impact of poverty on development and psychological status; the result of labelling of the poor as schizophrenic, and a reflection of the loss of socioeconomic status which attends chronic disability (Turner & Gartrell, 1978).

There is no one symptom, or group of problems, defining schizophrenic illnesses to the exclusion of other conditions. The acute symptoms seen in these disorders may occur in a number of other psychoses. What distinguishes schizophrenic disorders are a set of these clinical signs within a recognized pattern of prodromal, acute, and residual illness phases. The *Diagnostic and Statistical Manual (DSM III)* (American Psychiatric Association, 1980) stipulates a prodromal period of at least six months for a schizophrenic diagnosis. During this phase, changes may occur in the person's cognition, perception, mood, and functional ability. Bizarre or illogical beliefs may develop, often combined with social withdrawal and deterioration in self-care. During "active" or acute episodes, more dramatic symptoms occur: hallucinations, disorganized and incoherent speech patterns, delusions, and false ideas about self and others. Neuroleptic medications are generally employed to reduce acute symptomatology. In some cases, these may induce full remission. More often, however, the active illness phase gives way to milder "residual" symptoms (such as those in the prodromal period), which require continuing medication. Progressive functional deterioration, while by no means inevitable, constitutes a risk, particularly for clients experiencing repeated acute episodes with increasing impairment during each residual period.

Major Affective Disorders The major affective disorders follow a more variable course than schizophrenias. Some of the problems falling within this category occur as single episodes only. Even among the recurrent disorders, the possibility of a return to full premorbid function is far greater than for the schizophrenic illnesses. Affective ill-

ness, like the schizophrenic disorders, has been attributed to social, genetic, and psychological factors, as well as neurophysiological processes (Akisal & McKinney, 1973). Depression has been traditionally overrepresented among women. Bipolar affective disorder, however, appears to affect both sexes equally (American Psychiatric Association, 1980).

Major depression (single-episode or chronic) is prevalent among our general population, a fact at least partially explained by its possible occurrence at any point in the life span. It involves not only the feelings of hopelessness, helplessness, and loss observed in milder depressive reactions (including normal grief), but their persistence over time (continually, for at least several weeks, according to the DSM III), and the presence of other symptoms such as disturbances of appetite and sleep, weight changes, altered energy level, psychomotor retardation or agitation, and loss of pleasure in normally satisfying activities. Should acute psychotic symptoms emerge, they may reflect the underlying mood disorder. For example, "voices" may accuse and condemn the individual; delusions may center on guilt and unworthiness. Antidepressant agents provide a major form of treatment. The *DSM III* estimates that as many as 50 percent of persons with major depression may experience a recurrence, and that a proportion of these experience residual impairment between episodes (American Psychiatric Association, 1980). This group may be particularly at risk for development of bipolar affective disorder.

Bipolar disorder involves manic illness episodes, or alternating manic and depressive episodes. According to the *DSM III*, it occurs among 0.4 to 1.2 percent of the adult population, with onset in most cases before the age of thirty. Historically, bipolar illness has shown less association with low socioeconomic status than the schizophrenic disorders (Hollingshead & Redlich, 1958). The greater possibility of full remission between episodes may permit these individuals to maintain social resources. Also, practitioners in the United States tended for a long period to overdiagnose schizophrenic illness. In view of a new diagnostic system, the relationship between social factors and bipolar illness may be reconsidered to some extent in the future.

Like the schizophrenic disorders, bipolar illness involves a prodromal period of moderately depressed or "hypomanic" symptoms. In the latter, symptoms of inflated well-being, overactivity, irritability, and emotional lability predominate. Because of a sense of exaggerated competence and a high energy level, hypomanic persons may exhaust themselves. Mood state may seriously compromise judgment, resulting in inappropriate, intrusive, or impulsive behavior. During acute mania, frank psychotic symptoms such as hallucinations and delusions, often of a grandiose or a persecutory nature, may emerge. Gross impairment in concentration and attention, pressured and rapid speech, "flight of ideas," and extreme agitation are common. Neuroleptic medications may reduce acute symptoms; mood stabilization is more often managed through lithium. A proportion of persons diagnosed as bipolar affective disorder will experience a chronic course, with residual impairment in function and with the implied need for continuing or intermittent medication (American Psychiatric Association, 1980).

The division between major affective disorder of a recurrent nature and schizophrenic illness is not always clear-cut. Bipolar illness and severe depression may involve psychotic symptoms of a bizarre, or "mood incongruent," nature; depressive symptoms are often prominent among schizophrenics. The syndromes described here offer a sense of the types of chronic problems affecting groups, not the means to identify or diagnose individuals. When community health nurses require more detailed information relevant to their individual clients, several excellent references are available. These include the *DSM III*, as well as nursing texts on the care of the mentally ill (Burgess & Lazarre, 1981; Kalkman & Davis, 1980; Krauss & Slavinsky, 1982; Wilson & Kneisl, 1983).

Organic Mental Disorders Organic mental disorders of a chronic nature account for a substantial proportion of the institutionalized population (in mental hospitals and nursing homes), as well as a segment of the community-based group

(Schneck, Reisberg, & Ferris, 1982). They may currently affect between 600,000 and 1.25 million persons (Goldman, Gatozzi, & Taube, 1981). Chronic syndromes known as "dementias" differ from acute and more reversible organic problems (delirium), because the former do not usually involve a clouding of consciousness. Rather, their primary symptom is intellectual impairment, or loss of previously acquired cognitive abilities. When dementias arise from treatable medical causes (traumatic, metabolic, or infectious), impairment may be arrested or reversed. Dementias can occur at any age, but are most prevalent in later adulthood. This is particularly true of the primary degenerative forms (Alzheimer type diseases and multi-infarct or vascular dementia). These develop insidiously and imply at least some degree of progressive impairment. A particular variety of chronic organic disorder, called the amnestic syndrome, involves memory loss as a primary symptom. While not limited to alcoholics, it is well known in some alcohol-dependent persons with concomitant nutritional problems.

Although symptoms of disturbed cognition (impaired pervasively in progressive syndromes of the Alzheimer's type or selectively in amnestic syndrome) form the primary impairment in these disorders, personality changes, affective disturbance, and psychomotor problems are common. Indeed, when the individual is aware of increasing intellectual impairment, severe anxiety and depression may occur. This overlay of "functional" problems may prove extremely important in care of organically impaired clients.

Progressive deterioration of this type is sometimes assumed to be a "natural" risk of the aging process, despite the fact that it differs vastly from the minor problems of memory seen in normal later adulthood. Recent research efforts have treated chronic organic problems as the diseases they are, and propose hypotheses about their etiology that may someday permit their effective treatment (Schneck, Reisberg, & Ferris, 1982). The acceptance of dementia as "natural" will also sometimes lead to inadequate consideration of alternative diagnoses for older adults with cognitive dysfunction. This is a serious issue, since other syndromes (depression in particular) may be manifest as "pseudodementia," and be amenable to pharmacological therapy (Burnside, 1976; McAllister & Trevor, 1982).

Other Chronic Psychiatric Problems Additional disorders encountered among the chronically mentally ill do not necessarily imply disability and are prevalent in less severe forms among the general population. Substance abuse (a pattern of pathological use and functional impairment of at least one month's duration) and substance dependence (involving an abstinence syndrome) demonstrate a continuum of severity in terms of persistence over time, impairment of role performance, and need for mental health services. (See Chapter 26 for a detailed discussion of substance abuse.) The group at the moderate to severe end of this continuum may experience "chronic" mental illnesses, while others with similar diagnostic characteristics do not.

Severe personality disorders also affect a small but significant percentage of the chronically mentally ill. These disorders involve maladaptive and inflexible patterns of behavior causing functional impairment or distress. They represent extensions or exaggerations of what might be termed "personality styles," so that the degree to which they actually reduce functional level below socially accepted norms is variable. More severe personality disorders may be paranoid in nature. "Borderline" disorders, also potentially disabling, are characterized by strong feelings of depression and anger, unstable relationships, and impulsive behavior, which is frequently self-hurtful (Goldfinger, 1982). A potential for brief episodes of acute psychosis, a tendency to abuse drugs and alcohol, and a "lack of fit" with traditional services for long-term patients place these clients in special jeopardy (Schwartz & Goldfinger, 1981).

Chronic Mental Illness in Community Settings

Using the joint criteria of duration, disability, and diagnosis, observers have estimated that the chronically mentally ill number between 1.7 and 2.5 million individuals (Goldman, Gatozzi, & Taube, 1981). This large group is expected to increase in response to demographic trends. Young adults between eighteen and thirty-four, the age group at risk for onset of schizophrenic and bipolar disorders, now account for one third of our general population, so that the numbers of the chronic mentally ill may increase (Bachrach, 1982; Kramer, 1977; Segal & Baumohl, 1980). The general aging of our population also increases the risk of chronic organic mental disorders associated with later life, medical morbidity, and substance abuse (Lipowski, 1978).

Not all of this population resides in community settings. A sizable group continues to use long-term or institutional care. Among these are approximately 150,000 individuals in residence in state and county hospitals because of severe disabilities or special care needs, and some 750,000 persons with psychiatric disorders (primary or secondary) who reside in nursing home settings (Goldman, Gatozzi, & Taube, 1981). This leaves a community-based population of between 800,000 and 1.5 million. It is difficult to estimate the size of the group who receive community health nursing services. Whatever their numbers, their current living situations must be understood as a function of the deinstitutionalization policy that has characterized American psychiatry for the past twenty years.

The Deinstitutionalization Process

Deinstitutionalization refers to more than the effort to remove the mentally ill from long-term hospitals. From its inception, the policy of deinstitutionalization had other goals, including the development of a range of local services for the mentally ill and promotion of their human rights through appropriate care in the least restrictive environment possible (Bachrach, 1978; Scheper-Hughes, 1981). To examine deinstitutionalization in a chronological sense, we might best consider it as a treatment reform effort, implemented through advances in biological psychiatry and shaped through legislation.

The Psychiatric Institution and the Movement for Its Reform

Prior to the nineteenth century, the mentally ill, like the poor or the disabled in general, depended upon the generosity of families and local communities. If their poverty or deviant behavior exceeded the limits of these small social groups, they were subject to movement to almshouses, prisons, and the like. The moral treatment movement of the early 1800s considered psychiatric disorder as a form of disease, exacerbated by environmental factors, and therefore treatable in curative social settings located far from towns and villages. Patients in early, rural mental hospitals were socially similar to staff, who participated in the life of the institution. Preliminary results were enthusiastic, providing support for establishment of more hospitals.

By 1860, all but five of the thirty-three states had public mental hospitals, and "treatment of the insane became virtually synonymous with residence in an asylum" (Davis, n.d., p. 9). Reformers, the best known being Dorothea Dix, urged expansion of the state mental hospital system to accommodate the new population of psychiatric patients produced by the joint forces of immigration and industrialization. However, the enlightened treatment philosophy that characterized the early asylum began to give way to a model of custodial care. A number of factors have been cited to explain this, including increasing social distance between staff and patients (who became increasingly poor and foreign born), overcrowding of poorly funded facilities, and disappointment at the failure of moral treatment to achieve its initial promise of therapeutic success (Caplan, 1969; Davis, n.d.).

By the twentieth century, problems of funding and staffing undermined the quality of care in even the best of the state hospitals. In the worst, as described in critical reports of the postwar period (Deutsch, 1948), patients were subject to coercive and dehumanizing conditions. Research in institutional settings suggested that some of the behaviors associated with long-term psychiatric illness (apathy, inertia, withdrawal, and deterioration of social skills) might represent responses to the public hospital environment (Belknap, 1956; Chafetz, Goldman, & Taube, 1983; Goffman, 1961; Gruenberg, 1967).

In 1961 the Joint Commission on Mental Health and Illness published its report, *Action for Mental Health,* calling for the reform of the institutional system (Joint Commission, 1961). It advised use of smaller, more treatment-oriented psychiatric hospitals for the most severely ill, and community placement for others. If deinstitutionalization was an idea whose time had come, it was in part because of the introduction of neuroleptic medications, which provided the means to move the chronically mentally ill to the community.

Neuroleptic Medications

The first neuroleptic medication employed widely in the United States was chlorpromozine, or "Thorazine." Known as "major tranquilizers," thorazine and other such agents that followed did not in fact merely tranquilize or sedate. They also acted selectively upon psychotic symptomatology, reducing the thought disorder, hallucinations, and delusions seen in serious mental illness, as well as relieving agitation and distress. Neuroleptics do not "cure" chronic mental illness, nor are they without risk. However, such symptomatic treatment did permit discharge of long-term patients. It also shortened the duration of treatment for newer admissions, and promoted diversion of the mentally ill in the community to nonhospital sites of care whenever possible. In 1955, public hospital census began to decline from its high of 558,922 residents, falling to approximately 137,810 by 1980 (Goldman, Adams, & Taube, 1983).

Community Mental Health Legislation

If pharmacological treatment provided the basis for hospital reform, legislative efforts determined the shape of evolving community services. However, the transition to local care involved great variations between regions. To accurately understand the system's evolution in any one area, the community health nurse should study the impact of local statutes carefully. A number of events also had a national impact (Chafetz, Goldman, & Taube, 1983).

The Community Mental Health Centers Act The Community Mental Health Act of 1963 provided for the establishment of a network of federally assisted mental health centers and mandated a standard range of services (including inpatient care, crisis services, ambulatory treatment, daycare and partial hospitalization, community education, and consultation) for residents of each defined catchment area. These centers provided a model for community services structures. Since mental health plans in various states mandated similar resources, local systems began to develop.

Entitlement Programs to Support Community Living In 1965, Medicaid and Medicare benefits were introduced as a means of supporting health care for the indigent and the elderly. These programs spurred the development of local services, since they permitted fee-for-service reimbursement and transferred part of the cost of care to the federal government. For example, the elderly could now be transferred from long-term psychiatric institutions (state supported) to privately operated extended and intermediate care facilities.

Patients' Rights Statutes In 1963, Aid to the Totally Disabled (ATD) was extended to the mentally ill. In 1975, the Supplemental Security Income replaced ATD funding. This provided financial support without the label of disability. Supplemental Security Income offers the means to purchase essential services such as housing, meals, and clothing once furnished by institutions.

Patients' rights legislation in many states limited the criteria for involuntary treatment. While they were by no means uniform, criteria often stipulated dangerousness (to self or others) or grave impairment (inability to secure food, clothing, and shelter because of mental illness) as exclusive grounds for involuntary care (Slaby, Lieb, & Tancredi, 1981). These regulations served to reduce inappropriate hospitalization and to limit the duration of inpatient care.

The mandate to establish a community-based system has in some ways been accomplished. The resident census of state and county facilities has been reduced by approximately 75 percent. Extra-hospital services accounted for 73 percent of all psychiatric patient care episodes by 1975 (Goldman, Adams, & Taube, 1983). The chronically mentally ill no longer face the inevitability of institutional care, and the isolation and loss of personal autonomy that this often implied. However, full social integration has not always replaced hospital residency. New difficulties have emerged for the chronically mentally ill during the transition to community-based care.

The Impact of Deinstitutionalization

When dealing with the impact of deinstitutionalization, community health nurses interact with individuals, families, and communities; therefore, they need to understand the effects on all three groups.

Impact on Individuals with Chronic Mental Disorders

The impact of deinstitutionalization on individuals has been as diverse as the chronically mentally ill themselves. Initially, this process affected the former residents of long-term facilities whose community relationships had long been disrupted. Increasingly, deinstitutionalization also affects younger adults with little experience of long-term care (twelve months or more). In both groups, many individuals have successfully adapted to community living and have relatively little visibility in public services. If this discussion focuses on a more visible and service dependent group, it is because they concern community health nurses more directly and experience the most problems in community living.

The Risk of Readmission to Acute Care   The need for periodic hospital care constitutes one of the newer problems of the chronically mentally ill. As state mental hospitals reported a decline in long-term population, they noted rising rates of admissions for short-term care (under ninety days), including many readmissions. Inpatient psychiatric services in the community also expanded their volume of services to short-term patients. It now appears that for many clients, brief hospitalization has replaced long-term institutionalization. According to one review, 25 to 50 percent of hospitalized patients are readmitted each year, with 60 to 70 percent rehospitalized at the five- or ten-year follow-up (Anthony, Cohen, & Vitalo, 1978).

This pattern of service use is sometimes called a "revolving door syndrome." The negative tone of this phrase reflects the disappointment of early advocates for community care who assumed that any hospitalization is undesirable, and who hoped to prevent readmission through rehabilitation (Arnoff, 1975; Bachrach, 1978). Although selected community programs have decreased readmission rates, the notion that good programs always reduce hospitalizations has not been fully supported in the literature (Test & Stein, 1978). Certainly some individuals return to acute care because of ineffective treatment. For example, severely disabled patients who are discharged prematurely or without attention to follow-up are destined to return to hospital settings. However, many clients better served by community programs nevertheless require episodic inpatient care to reduce acute exacerbation of symptoms and to resolve crises.

Whatever its cause, rehospitalization tends to disrupt whatever stable living situation the individual has been able to establish. Since development of residential, social, and occupational supports represents a major personal accomplishment to many of the psychiatrically disabled, the loss, threatened or real, of such supports may be overwhelming. The client may feel like the mythical Sisyphus, who pushed a boulder to the top of a hill forever, only to watch it roll back.

Even where the social situation is stable, rehospitalization threatens self-esteem. It may represent a form of failure—to maintain independence, to control behavior, or to exercise mastery and competence in daily life. These feelings are compounded when family and mental health workers share a view of acute illness as "treatment failure." Individuals sometimes report a sense of embarrassment or shame in reestablishing contact with family and friends or aftercare services. When hospitalization occurs on an involuntary basis, it reinforces the sense of loss of personal autonomy and promotes a view of mental health providers as agents of social control. While frequent admissions, and particularly involuntary treatment, do not occur among all of the target population, they represent potential problems to a larger group, so that concerns about recurrence of illness influence daily living.

The Burden of Medication Regimens After resolution of an acute care episode, individuals deal with psychotropic medications (principally neuroleptics, antidepressants, and lithium preparations), which substitute pharmacological controls of symptoms for the institutional restraints practiced in the past. This represents both an advance in care and a new order of burden for the individual, who must integrate a therapeutic regimen into everyday life. The burden is most severe when medication is administered with a long-term maintenance model. Although persons with chronic disorders may sometimes be treated without psychoactive medication, and while even among the schizophrenic subgroup, drug-free trials may be advisable for specific clients (Herz, Herman, & Simon, 1982), a substantial segment of the target population uses medications on a more or less ongoing basis. For those diagnosed as schizophrenic, medication noncompliance appears to constitute a major predictor of hospital readmission (Davis et al, 1980). Long-term use of psychoactive medications creates a number of subsidiary physical, social, and psychological problems for the individual.

A diabetic-insulin analogy is frequently invoked to discuss medication maintenance for schizophrenia and major affective illnesses. In fact, to the extent that it suggests a form of simple replacement therapy, this comparison is severely flawed. It is true that antipsychotics, antidepressants, and lithium effect specific target symptoms. However, these agents do not provide a "missing" substance that eliminates all symptoms of major mental illnesses for every person. Residual problems may persist after treatment of acute illness, and secondary effects are common, ranging from mild and transitory discomfort to severe and potentially irreversible problems such as the tardive dyskensia. Medications influence individuals differently in terms of therapeutic effects, side effects, and dosage necessary to produce both. Since the reason why one agent to produce both. Since the reason why one agent

or dosage will best suit a particular client remains obscure, medications are sometimes administered on a trial-and-error basis until a regimen that balances benefit with risk for the individual can be established.

These physical discomforts constitute only part of a constellation of problems associated with secondary medication effects. Constraints to daily living may prove more annoying in the long run and ultimately pose more of a threat to compliance. Changes in motor behavior and energy level may influence occupational and social role performance. Altered sexual function affects family and other intimate relationships. Medication interactions limit the person's ability to use other prescribed drugs and to engage in social drinking. Finally, medications exert an impact on personal identity. Intended to promote normal living and social integration of the mentally ill, they sometimes produce visible symptoms such as a shuffling gait or muscular rigidity, which identify the user as a psychiatric patient. Estroff develops this issue in depth in her study of the community based mentally ill, *Making It Crazy* (1981). She states: "In understanding medication as a permanent aspect of clients' lives, it is foolish not to consider at what price clinical improvement and community tenure is maintained" (p. 95).

Occupational and Economic Problems Financial dependence also poses an enduring issue in the lives of some individual clients. The community mental health movement placed a strong emphasis on vocational rehabilitation programs to enhance community adaptation and to promote autonomy. The more successful model programs for the chronically mentally ill often incorporated innovative vocational components, such as graduated levels of responsibility within the program itself, or within sheltered occupational settings, as a prelude to competitive employment (Beard, 1978; Fairweather et al, 1969; Test & Stein, 1978).

However, despite this emphasis, competitive employment is not always possible. A review of the literature on rehabilitation outcome finds 10 to 30 percent of expatients in full-time employment

(Anthony, Cohen, & Vitalo, 1978). Another study of 1,471 chronically disabled adults notes that while 25.9 percent of the sample were employed, only 41.8 percent of those were holding jobs on the "open market," with others in sheltered workshops, transitional employment programs, unpaid training programs, or volunteer positions (Tessler et al, 1982). If individual disability plays a major role here, this situation is also a function of general unemployment and competition with "well" groups for paid positions. In times of economic hardship, even nondemanding jobs may be taken by skilled workers, pushing the more disabled population to the fringes of the labor market.

Work is so strongly associated with social value in our society that financial dependence may seriously erode self-concept. Sheltered workshops, transitional programs, and volunteer jobs may provide the means to mitigate these effects by offering social interaction and meaningful activities. However, these may also be experienced as poor substitutes and as symbols of chronicity and disability (Estroff, 1981). Sheets, Prevost, and Reihman (1982) point out that younger adults, in what they call a "high functioning–high aspiration group," may not wish to be associated with older chronic or deteriorated patients encountered in some community programs (p. 201). It may be especially difficult for such individuals to find transitional occupational settings appropriate to their skills and self-image.

Income maintenance programs (including disability benefits and public assistance payments) provide economic support for a large number of persons with chronic psychiatric disabilities. Often, this means life on a fixed and low income. In one study, where more than half of the subjects received assistance, the median income was estimated to be $325.07 per month (Tessler et al, 1982). Many income and entitlement programs, Supplemental Security Income among them, include provisions for part-time employment and retention of benefits during rehabilitation and gradual entry into the employment market. However, disability benefits may also promote a "psychiatric sick role" over time

and reduce motivation for financial independence (Lamb & Ragowski, 1978).

Limited Options for Housing Given the problem of finances, it is not altogether surprising to note that residential possibilities for this population are sometimes limited. Many, perhaps more than 25 percent, live with families (Minkoff, 1979; Tessler et al, 1982) and are less subject to problems of affordable housing than others. Where living at home is not advisable or available, some form of group living may provide similar social connectedness, and reduce individual expenses. These arrangements may be seen on a continuum from those promoting autonomy, such as subsidized cooperative apartments, to more structured forms of residential aftercare (Apostoles, Depp, & Scarpelli, 1980; Campanelli, Lieberman, & Trujillo, 1983).

In an ideal sense, this continuum of residential options should permit placements on the basis of individual needs and preferences. Unfortunately, the ideal placement may not exist for every person. Options such as subsidized apartments are not as yet widespread. Active treatment programs, such as halfway houses, frequently focus on progressive independence and do not absorb a large population on a long-term basis. Proprietary boarding homes, adult homes, and similar facilities have thus absorbed a disproportionate number of the community-based group, perhaps 400,000 nationally (Goldman, Gatozzi, & Taube, 1981). While many of these offer excellent support services, some that are more custodial in focus appear to perpetuate dependent patterns of behavior seen in institutions (Reynolds & Faberow, 1977). Poor general living conditions have been reported in a segment of these facilities as well (Turner & TenHoor, 1978). Such environments can induce a sense of hopelessness and a fear of progressive chronicity among residents.

Those individuals who prefer to live independently may have trouble finding decent low cost housing. In this sense the chronically mentally ill share the same problem as other disabled or disadvantaged groups. In the absence of personal

Case Example 27-1: Mr. Thompson

Mr. Thompson, a single, thirty-four-year-old, white male, called the police today, asking to be taken from his boarding home to the psychiatric hospital. He complained of hearing "voices."

Mr. Thompson is the only child of elderly parents who live in a retirement community. He experienced his first psychiatric hospitalization at the age of nineteen and terminated his college studies at that time. He has been diagnosed as having a schizophrenic illness since age twenty. For several years after his initial illness, Mr. Thompson worked sporadically as a dishwasher. However, he found his medications were too sedating for this job. Efforts to terminate medication led to relapse and loss of employment. For the past seven years, he has lived on a disability income, most of which is used to pay his room and board. Mr. Thompson describes his residence as safe and comfortable, but he expresses boredom with daily routine (which appears limited to meals and television) and is fearful of becoming a "basket case" like several fellow residents with severely disturbed behavior.

Economic and occupational problems are ongoing concerns.

Medications affect physical and psychological well-being.
Housing options may be limited.

The current emergence of acute symptoms (auditory hallucinations) is very troubling to Mr. Thompson, who has not been hospitalized for three years, and who fears "going through all this again and starting over." He admits to stopping medications one month ago and to recent heavy drinking "so I can sleep," but he cannot offer a clear reason for this change in behavior. Upon questioning, however, he reveals increasing feelings of despondency and loneliness over the past weeks, particularly when watching television. He states, "I remember when I watched the hostages coming back to America. They were hugging people, and I'd get this feeling. I don't know, maybe you'd call it remorse." He also describes his sense of dependence upon his parents, "They're old and I'm supposed to be helping them, but I'm the one who needs help. When I called today, they said, 'Call the police.' "

The risk of readmission can lead to fear or hopelessness.

Medication noncompliance must be considered in the context of the individual's life.

Depression and anger are common concerns.

resources (economic resources and/or family assistance), they frequently reside in urban hotels and other single-unit housing available to the elderly, the disabled, and the single poor (Ekert, 1981; Mealey, 1981; New York State Dept. of Social Services, 1980). The substandard nature of a large amount of single-unit housing in our cities has become a concern of mental health and community agencies. The national report on the chronically mentally ill, looking at the quality of residential placements and the restricted number of adequate individual rentals, identifies housing as a major issue at this time (Talbott, 1981).

Reactions to Problems in Community Living
Problems of housing—like medication issues, repeated hospital admissions, and financial problems—confront only a segment of the community-based population on a day-to-day basis but represent risks to others. Where these problems in community living are felt most intensely, depression and anger are common clinical issues that cross diagnostic categories. Some individuals express these feelings in clear and straightforward terms. In other cases problematic behaviors may sometimes represent attempts to resist, avoid, or protest conditions of daily life (see Case Example 27-1). Self-

medication via alcohol or substance abuse, poor follow-up with referrals, and impulsive "acting out" sometimes express frustration with the system of care and rejection of what appear to be uncaring and unresponsive services. Movement from city to city may be used as a coping strategy to avoid surroundings that promote depression and loss of hope.

The degree to which individuals avoid some pitfalls attending deinstitutionalization is variable. Good outcomes, with adequate quality of life, depend to some extent on clinical status (functional level, response to and tolerance of medication). However, social factors also influence living situation. Problems in community living may be mediated in both direct and subtle ways by the presence of a family group or other network of supportive relationships. The transition to community-based care has exerted an impact, not only on the mentally ill themselves, but on these social groups who serve as crucial determinants of community adaptation.

Impact on Families of the Chronically Mentally Ill

The chronically mentally ill, like any socially vulnerable group, may be protected and assisted by a network of supportive relationships extending practical and interpersonal resources. In a general sense, family connectedness appears to be positively associated with good psychiatric outcome. This relationship is seen consistently in studies of marital status and schizophrenic prognosis (Turner & Gartrell, 1978), and is supported by the growing body of research on social support and mental illness (Greenblatt, Bercerra, & Serafetinides, 1982).

However, the meanings of these associations are open to several interpretations. Such good outcomes may reflect the individual client's ability to maintain relationships. Or, more helpful families may also establish the most enduring ties. Some evidence exists that contact with "high stress" families promotes less favorable outcomes (Falloon et al, 1982), and that certain communication styles perpetuate dysfunction. It appears that family

involvement is highly individual in its style and effects. Although a large body of literature exists on families and mental illness, it does not stipulate the "best" approach for any given unit.

Family Response to Psychiatric Disorder   As used here, the term *family* refers to a wide network of kin relationships that vary in terms of size, geographical proximity, economic resources, and attitudes about mental illness. Although less than one half of the chronically mentally ill actually remain at home, the family, whatever its structure and size, generally responds in some way to the phenomenon of chronic psychiatric disorder. Identification of mental illness creates a crisis situation in the family system, and like any crisis, evokes coping behaviors that lead to some new form of stability or crisis resolution (Glick & Kessler, 1980). Prior to deinstitutionalization, family members might cope with long-term placement itself. Currently, they have a wider range of options, but also a larger burden of choice. Given the long-term nature of the illness, decision making may recur at many points in time.

New Issues for Families   Among the new issues facing families of the mentally ill is the persistence of anger and resentment. When onset of a chronic psychiatric disorder is insidious, many forms of behavioral disturbance precede acute decompensation and "naming" of the illness. Social withdrawal or suspicion may serve to undermine existing relationships. Impulsive, intrusive, or angry behavior can create a reservoir of resentment in those closest to the client. Feelings of animosity, disappointment, or distrust may be difficult to resolve and may decrease motivation to assist the client at a further point in time.

This burden of ambivalent feelings is compounded by knowledge of psychological theories that attribute psychosis to family dynamics and child-rearing practices. These ideas have been popularized to a great extent, not only through psychological publications for general audiences, but also through films and television, so that few families do not show some degree of concern about their possible impact on the client's illness. In some cases, mental illness represents stigma to the group, in the sense of making a psychological defect public. Under these conditions biological explanations of psychiatric disorder may be seized upon with relief. Since they downplay the "psychology of blame" and relieve family members' guilt, they are important to self-help and family support groups.

Where institutionalization took control from clients and families, they may now choose between a variety of public and private agencies for help. However, this plurality of services may not assure families of the precise information they desire. Families may request instructions on how to "cure" the client, or may wish to negate one diagnosis by finding a second opinion. To resolve these problems, they may engage in "doctor shopping" behavior, going from one service to another. These difficulties are complicated by very real questions of reliability of psychiatric diagnoses and prognoses. Early diagnoses are often tentative, and even an established diagnosis does not predict individual functional status or outcome. Conflicting opinions from multiple sources can lead to frustration, and to a sense that there is nowhere to turn for clear guidance.

Conflict also arises when family members request psychiatric intervention to control distressed or disturbing behavior. In light of patients' rights legislation, psychiatric clinicians cannot impose treatment of worrisome but nondangerous behavior. Families may interpret this as abandonment of responsibility for the seriously ill. One father telephoned a hospital to express his dismay about his adult son's decision to leave inpatient care some time before his planned discharge date. His father reported finding him in a disheveled and helpless state "standing by the phone booth where he called us, . . . he didn't even have any shoes on. . . . How could they let him go like that?"

The strain imposed on families by acute illness is sometimes more easily accepted than a long-term burden of economic support. One article notes that while the schizophrenic clients rated fear of relapse and rehospitalization as major concerns, with financial strain following, their parents focused first on "fewer jobs, dependence on others, and financial strain" (Schultz et al, 1982, p. 508). Where the client's disability appears most obvious, the economic burden may produce the least conflict. For example, families may accept the need to support a confused and helpless person. However, more functional and organized persons may be perceived by their families as unwilling rather than unable to manage money. This type of situation is likely to produce discord. The family's desire to help sometimes competes with the need to extricate themselves from the client's financial life, particularly where independence and autonomy are clinical goals.

Assumption of a therapeutic or care-giving function also taxes the social system. Medication maintenance provides a common example. While it is highly desirable that individuals take responsiblity for their own regimens, family involvement tends to influence compliance. Greenberg and Underwood (1980) point out that families may be uncertain about the utility of medications, and must be assisted to supervise and support the regimen, rather than to undermine it because of their fears of "pill pushing."

Families sometimes act as intermediaries between the client and the health care system in general. Because they see the client in a day-to-day living situation, they are frequently in the best position to identify needs, psychiatric and other, requiring professional attention. They help to locate services, to alert staff to important changes in behavior, and to attend to general health problems. Many clients should ideally be able to manage their own care. However, given the limitations of some services, and the schism between medical and psychiatric agencies, some form of intermediary may be necessary to shore up the cracks in the system.

In the case of repetitive acute episodes, family burdens may be extreme. Although this applies to only a small subset of the chronic mentally ill, it is costly in emotional terms. In essence, the client and family adapt to a state of chronic crisis, which undermines hope for any form of stability in the future. The story of Sylvia Frumkin, a pseudonym for a severely disturbed young woman with a "revolving door" illness pattern, is described by Sheehan in *Is There No Place on Earth for Me?* (1982). The Frumkin family experiences their daughter's rehospitalizations as a form of respite from the stress caused by her illness. As Sylvia's mother says, having a daughter back in a state hospital was like a "vacation" (p. 119).

Factors Influencing Degree of Family Support   The type and quality of symptoms tolerable within the family may prove critical in decisions to maintain the individual at home. These, in turn, are determined by the family's social and cultural values, and their beliefs about mental illness. To be sure, certain problematic behaviors are likely to tax the limits of most families. Withdrawal, for example, is sometimes better tolerated than substance abuse, suicidal actions, or aggressive behavior. "Peculiar" qualities that have low visibility, such as strange but private ideas, may be easier to deal with than bizarre appearance and statements.

However, the family's internal resources also play a role in the decision to remain involved in the client's care. Economic resources enable the family to purchase services for the client or for themselves. In a study of maternal caretaking, for example, Archbold (1982) distinguished between those daughters who gave direct care to their mothers, and those who could afford to manage such care through purchase of services. The latter group made a more positive psychological and physical adjustment to the burden of care overall. Where families can provide themselves with housekeeping services, legal advice, and a host of other requirements to meet their own needs, they may be more available to help over a long period. On the other hand, where family burden must be assumed directly, it may prove exhausting to the system.

Families of the mentally ill, like most of the general population, cope with multiple responsibilities, including care of young children and aging family members with other medical disabilities. The question of home placement becomes complex when the varied needs of several dependent persons must be considered. Spouses and partners of the chronically mentally ill may themselves have psychiatric problems. This provides mutual acceptance and support, but it also means that client and partner may share similar economic and social problems. In this sense, they may be unable to extend the material resources available through more traditional families.

In addition, the resources within the family change over time. The family, including the chronically ill member, experience life changes related to their own growth and development, socioeconomic factors, and evolving health status. Solutions to the problem of a psychiatric illness within the family are thus not static but constantly renegotiated in response to shifts in needs and resources.

In this respect, families may negotiate solutions that represent "the best for the most," balancing the needs of one member against the available resources existing within the group and the competing requirements of other members. Often this means that if living at home is not the best option, the family continues to extend some form of interpersonal support and/or crisis assistance. Good community services play a crucial role in this regard: day treatment programs to support home placements; respite or hostel services to relieve the burden of continuing responsibility; residential resources near to the family that allow the client autonomy and privacy but promote family contacts. In the absence of such "support to the supporters," families may be unable to negotiate a solution beneficial to all members. Some may fall into an "all or nothing pattern" in which cycles of overinvolvement, detrimental to the client's independence, alternate with rejection.

Non-kin Networks of the Mentally Ill   For a sizable number of the community-based mentally ill, family networks are functionally nonexistent. Like most Americans, the psychiatrically ill and their families are mobile, with geographic separation affecting type and amount of contacts. Middle-aged and elderly clients may have no living relatives to assist them. People with long institutional histories frequently have no kin networks to return to because of long separations. A proportion of the chronically mentally ill choose to sever contacts with relatives, particularly where prior patterns of interaction have been conflictual and disruptive. Finally, certain subgroups of clients have a need for distance and protection from interpersonal closeness, and opt for what may appear to be isolated living circumstances in the interests of their own well-being.

The nonkin networks developed by the individual may bolster family support or replace it. They include "planned" social networks in treatment settings, as well as naturally developing networks in neighborhoods, apartments and hotels, church groups, and recreational programs. These do not necessarily operate in the same manner as family groups, particularly if most members share similar problems in living. Cohen and Sokolovsky (1978), for example, identify smaller, less reciprocal networks among more disabled schizophrenics in hotels. Estroff (1981) discusses a "culture of schizophrenia" among clients, which limits social contacts to "insiders" (fellow patients and mental health staff). This situation restricts the amount and type of interaction.

Friendship networks, not unlike families, can be considered in light of their own internal resources. In order to provide long-term support, both groups require an identification of their own limits and the backup of appropriate community services. Thus, the situation of the chronically mentally ill must be considered within the wider context of the community.

Community Responses to the Chronically Mentally Ill

The Development of Local Systems of Care As a result of the deinstitutionalization process and the movement of the mentally ill to community settings, a network of local psychiatric services has evolved in most parts of the United States. These offer a range of treatment options not widely available some twenty years ago, including crisis services, outpatient clinics, residential treatment centers, rehabilitation programs, day treatment centers, and home visiting and outreach teams. This means varied forms of care to a broad population including, but not limited to, those with chronic disorders. Because of the wide clientele they serve, community agencies reduce some of the stigma once associated with psychiatric treatment. Use of mental health services does not necessarily connote disability, as did state mental hospitals. It does not automatically imply poverty, since community agencies treat individuals from varied social backgrounds (Frank, Eisenthal, & Lazarre, 1978). Psychiatric services have become an integral component of community health systems. They constitute sites of training and employment for a new generation of psychiatric practitioners, who have never experienced work in the "total institution," and whose attitudes have been molded in less restrictive surroundings.

The Problem of Social Integration Despite this proliferation of services, community response to the chronically mentally ill has not always proceeded as planned. By the mid-1970s, the situation of the more severely disabled was the subject of serious concern. A recurring issue was the failure of communities to fully integrate this group (Bachrach, 1978; Reich, 1973). One manifestation of this problem was the placement of many individuals in twenty-four-hour settings, which seemed to isolate them as effectively as the psychiatric institution. Sometimes called "transinstitutionalization," this process applies to the situation of elderly patients moved from mental hospitals to nursing homes. It also refers to conditions in some boarding facilities. Acknowledging the care and concern provided in many of these settings, a number have been described as new "backwards" (Chase, 1973; Kirk & Thierren, 1975; Lamb & Goertzel, 1971).

The mentally ill frequently cluster in specific neighborhoods as well. Boarding homes themselves may be concentrated in districts where opportunities to interact with the general community are rare (Chase, 1973). Central commercial areas and urban hotel districts house also many of the chronically mentally ill. Because of the "skid row" character of some such neighborhoods, the mentally ill within them have been called a "ghetto" population (Aviram & Segal, 1973; Bassuk & Gerson, 1978). In fact, these districts offer advantages, among them access to inexpensive rentals, a tolerant social atmosphere, and proximity to social service agencies. However, these are sometimes obtained at the cost of poor general living conditions, high incidence of substance abuse, high crime rates, and victimization of the disabled.

To some extent this isolation of the chronically ill reflected a poorly defined notion of "community," which became confused with the administrative entity of the catchment district. For example, former state hospital residents were often discharged, not to their neighborhoods of origin, but to those catchment areas providing placements. Frequently they had no preexisting social ties to facilitate their integration (Kirk & Thierren, 1975). Since hospital discharges sometimes proceeded more rapidly than development of aftercare services, other clients pursued a course of least resistance in moving to those urban areas that have historically housed disadvantaged or deviant populations. These explanations suggest a kind of passive failure on the part of communities—failure to anticipate the full range of needs of expatients and to keep pace with rates of hospital releases. However, transinstitutional placements and "skid row" living conditions affect younger adults as well, many of whom have never experienced long-term hospitalization. To understand the continuing isolation of subgroups of the mentally ill, more active resistance to their social integration must be considered.

In a widely cited article published in 1973, Aviram and Segal argued that communities had developed new strategies to "exclude" the mentally ill, in lieu of institutionalization. For example, they mentioned zoning statutes that restrict the neighborhoods where residential facilities may be located. A study in a Boston suburb similarly describes vigorous opposition to psychiatric facilities. Here deinstitutionalization, like school busing, was seen as a threat to local control and autonomy (Scheper-Hughes, 1981). "Exclusion" of the men-

tally ill has not been inevitable. A California survey indicates that specific types of neighborhoods, particularly those characterized by political liberalism and social nonconformity, promote greater social participation. However, the authors of this study contend that these areas cannot absorb large numbers of the disabled (Segal, Baumohl, & Moyles, 1980).

Community response to chronic mental illness also involves control of disturbed or disturbing behavior. Rising arrest rates in some regions suggest that the criminal justice system sometimes serves this function. Arrest affects a minority of the mentally ill, however, and this group may not be representative of the chronic population in general (Steadman, 1981). Some sources link criminalization to inability of conventional mental health services to deal with "difficult" clients. Those individuals who fit poorly into existing ambulatory and residential programs may risk arrest because of inappropriate or dangerous behavior (Whitmer, 1980).

Individuals at Risk for Poor Social Integration The more negative forms of social reaction to the mentally ill do not affect all of the target population. It is difficult to reconcile the extreme problems in community living of some individuals with the successful community adaptation of others. Individual characteristics such as personality style and preference no doubt play a role in some cases. As Estroff (1981) reminds us, we do the chronically mentally ill a disservice if we consider them as passive victims of social processes. However, the risk of problems such as isolating residential placements, movement to "skid row," or arrest appears to particularly affect the more disadvantaged and disabled. Those with the fewest family supports and economic resources depend most directly on services from communities. If they additionally lack social skills, they may encounter the most difficulty in obtaining services and be most subject to social rejection.

There is some evidence that the more successful model programs for the chronically mentally ill have limited contact with the most disturbed and disadvantaged subgroups, treating more functional and socially connected individuals (Lamb, 1981). This means allocation of resources to those most capable and willing to use them, which is in itself a sensible idea. However, it implies a severe level of clinical and social problems in the group excluded from experimental care. For the community health nurse, this means that a major role consists of linking severely ill and disadvantaged clients to agencies providing both treatment and general support services such as financial assistance, housing, and general medical care.

Homelessness and the Chronically Mentally Ill The presence of the mentally ill among the urban homeless provides an example of extreme social isolation and disadvantage. Homelessness refers to the absence of a stable place to live, with movement to public shelters, unauthorized dwelling places, or the streets. In 1981, an estimated 36,000 persons required shelter in New York City alone, with figures in excess of 200,000 cited nationally (Baxter & Hopper, 1981). While not all of this population suffers from psychiatric disorder, the chronically mentally ill account for a significant segment (Baxter & Hopper, 1981; Farr, 1982). This has been linked to their difficulty in competing for low cost housing and their inability to obtain basic welfare services. Since inexpensive rentals such as hotel rooms are diminishing in some areas, and since the mentally ill may be seen as undesirable tenants (especially where appearance and behavior are bizarre), they may be the first to lose housing and the last to mobilize resources to regain it (Baxter & Hopper, 1981; Larew, 1980; Shapiro, 1972).

The magnitude of this problem can be seen in a survey conducted in a Northern California crisis clinic (Chafetz & Goldfinger, 1984). This unit has responsibility for emergency treatment of residents in a central urban area. It was designed to respond to acute psychiatric problems, with referral of more long-term social difficulties to other ambulatory clinics. This structure works best for those clients with families or friends to return to, and with a place to stay until the acute problem is resolved.

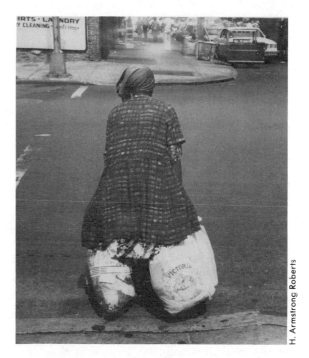

Some portion of the chronically mentally ill become "street people." Their homelessness can exacerbate crises and reduce personal resources. It also reminds community mental health professionals to focus services on basic needs and resources, not just treatment of a disorder.

However, for a disturbingly large segment of the clientele, the chief complaint includes the phrase "I have nowhere to live."

In order to explore this problem, the author reviewed the records of 440 cases for information on residence. Where the client could not provide a local address, the case was considered to be homeless. The group without a local address included both long-term "street people" and transients temporarily without housing. By this criterion, the homeless mentally ill accounted for 27.3 percent of all cases. In other words, approximately a quarter of the clients in this setting reported no stable place of residence at the time of emergency care.

This homeless group was compared to other cases (those with a local residence) to determine any significant differences between groups in clinical or demographic terms. Results showed that the homeless were essentially comparable to other cases. They were young—26 percent under twenty-five years of age, and an additional 44 percent between twenty-five and thirty-four. Most of the homeless, like others, were unmarried (93.6 percent), although 30 percent reported former marriages hence loss of prior relationships. White males predominated, but nonwhites (23 percent) and women (26.7 percent) were present as well. Not surprisingly, a larger number of those without housing reported no source of income, and few claimed to have any recent occupational activities.

The homeless clients shared the same diagnostic profile as others, with psychotic illnesses accounting for the highest proportion of cases (50 percent of the homeless, 44 percent of others). These were followed by nonpsychotic problems (28 percent and 36 percent) and substance-related pathology (13.4 percent and 9 percent). These diagnoses may be unreliable in any long-term sense, since they were made during the course of a brief clinical contact. However, they probably identify the crisis problem itself with reasonable accuracy. In this sense, there is no set of clinical characteristics that seems to distinguish them. Like others, they are heterogeneous. This impression is supported by ratings of functional level made for each case using the Global Assessment Scale (Endicott et al, 1976). Mean scores for both groups were almost identical (37.2 vs. 38.8) on this 100-point scale. Low ratings were a function of psychotic diagnosis, with no effects determined by residential status alone.

Implications for Service Planning The profile emerging here is one of youth, financial need, and absence of family and occupational supports. Like recent reports on the younger adult chronic population, it reminds us that even recently diagnosed individuals who have never been institutionalized may be at risk for extreme social isolation and disadvantage (Bachrach, 1982; Segal & Baumohl, 1980). Data of this kind do not explain individual reasons for homelessness, the critical life events

or individual problems that may lead to residential loss. However, this survey suggests that whatever these processes, they affect a sizable and varied group. It appears that these clients are making their presence felt in a mental health system that did not anticipate them and that believed that communities would be able to meet their housing needs. From a community health perspective, it shows that planning for the chronically mentally ill must focus on basic services and resources, not only on treatment of disorder.

Community Support Services A community support model of treatment has been widely recommended as the means to improve community resources for the mentally ill, and to correct the lack of fit between their needs and existing services (Turner & TenHoor, 1978). Community health nurses will probably work in conjunction with many such programs in the future. The case management or resource management concept, which is central to this model, generally involves coordination of a broad range of rehabilitative and supportive services through intervention of a single provider or team of providers. Psychiatric services (individual or group treatment, medication, etc.) are complemented by assistance in the area of housing, finances, social services, and general health care. Services may be offered directly by the case manager, or indirectly, such as through purchase of services and referrals, but the responsibility of the mental health agency is clear. Periodic assessment and planning provide the means to continually realign client needs and community resources, adapting to changes in both. Advocacy activities by case management agencies seek to maintain appropriate resources in communities and increase the accessibility for the chronically mentally ill.

While these programs do not offer a blanket "cure" for all problems of community living (Lamb, 1981; Talbott, 1981), they incorporate elements from some of the more successful experimental programs for the chronically mentally ill (Turner & TenHoor, 1978). Placing the mental health system in an important position between clients and community reduces the friction between both groups that has sometimes attended deinstitutionalization. In this sense community support type programs have potential for decreasing negative reaction to mental illness and for improving social integration of persons with psychiatric disabilities.

Implications and Strategies for Community Health Nurses

Community health nurses encounter the chronically mentally ill in a number of settings. Some of these are psychiatrically defined, as when community health nursing services are integrated into a mental health system. More frequently, however, nurses practice in settings associated with their broader health maintenance functions: home care and visiting nurse services, and services for special target groups such as the elderly, or ambulatory medical care units. These nonpsychiatric roles carry advantages, among them less identification with a social control function than that of psychiatric providers. Working in the client's natural environment (home or neighborhood), community health nurses have a good understanding of the social context of care and the environmental stressors confronting the client. They develop direct contacts with the people forming the client's social network, as well as relationships with mental health providers. This allows them to serve as a natural intermediary between the client and the larger systems of social and mental health services.

Nursing Assessment of Community-Based Mentally Ill Clients

In order to assume these functions, community health nurses require not only an understanding of common issues for the community-based population, but a method to identify their specific impact on individuals, and determine their role with any given client. Certain major problems may confront the chronically mentally ill at any point in time:

acceptance of and management of both chronic disorder and constraints to daily living, coping with stigma and social isolation, negotiating assistance from family, and developing adequate social and economic resources for daily living. However, the need for care varies in terms of individual clinical status, socioeconomic resources, attitudes and beliefs about mental illness, and concerns about the future.

In assessment community health nurses must apply some structure or method that considers both the multiple risks to well-being among the chronically mentally ill, and the ways in which these affect the individual client. The benefit of a systematic approach to assessment is two-fold: (1) it allows nurses to decide where the client requires an intermediary, to identify legitimate areas of intervention, and to clarify their own role and objectives in multiproblem situations; and (2) it also permits evaluation of work with the individual and assessment of change over time. Perhaps the most helpful approaches to assessment are those that consider three major types of information: the client's specific psychiatric problem (usually described by the referral agency), the client's functional status, and the existing supports that may be mobilized within the client's environment.

Strengths and Problems An assessment of functional status (strengths and deficits) should proceed with the question "To what extent can this person perform independently in expected social roles?" This is a deceptively simple beginning, since it begs the questions of role expectations. The client's *self*-expectations are primary, as are behaviors and social skills anticipated by the social network. These may be, in large part, a reflection of sociocultural factors. Within a group where mental illness means stigma, "visible" deficits in function may be the unacceptable, while other problems that remain "inside the family" are well tolerated. For instance, an inability to manage finances might not violate group expectations, while problems in grooming would. Age-related factors are of enormous importance in terms of functional expectations. Younger clients, grappling with developmental questions of relationships and work, may find deficits in these areas troubling. Middle-aged residents of aftercare facilities may have different ideas about their own expected functioning. Community health nurses may require multiple contacts with a client to determine what constitutes expected social performance, not in terms of their own perceptions of independence, but in terms of client-based criteria.

One of the more useful ways to organize impressions about an individual's functional capacity is evaluation of "self-care." Underwood (1978) has developed a psychiatric nursing assessment tool based on Orem's self-care model. It suggests evaluation of function in four areas: (1) air, food, and fluid; (2) elimination and personal hygiene; (3) activity and rest; and (4) solitude and social interaction. These categories permit assessment of areas where profound deficits may be observed (problems of malnutrition, difficulties in shopping, or inability to manage bathing and grooming) as well as the more complex functions such as self-regulation of activity or development of social skills and relationships. This allows application of the self-care assessment to a wide variety of persons among the chronically mentally ill, and permits evaluation of changes in need or level of dysfunction for the individual. Evaluation of type and severity of disturbance in each area leads to formulation of realistic objectives regarding resources to supplement the individual for a given period of time.

A comfortable way to assess these areas of function is to ask about a typical day. Clients with limited problems can use a question like this to discuss their needs and their feelings about daily living freely. Where communication is more difficult, particularly with profoundly impaired clients, nurses may have to adapt their own interactional style to the individual, and to use (where appropriate) alternative sources of information, such as family members. The goal remains the same—to explore daily routine. What times does the client arise? What meals were eaten? What activities took place? Who came to visit? An analysis of this kind of factual data will lead to a sense of both problems in self-care and the subjective meaning of these problems to the client.

From Problem Identification to Intervention
Where individual problems are identified, another series of questions should be asked: Is anyone currently helping? How well? At what cost? The gap between performance and expectations does not necessarily imply a need for professional intervention. For example, a woman incapable of the full responsibilities of child care may live within a social group that provides for this function, allowing her partial forms of participation. A hotel resident who cannot use coin machines to wash his clothing may be supported by staff who attend to this.

Where problems seem to be adequately resolved within the client's environment, nursing care needs may be minimal, even for the severely ill. However, if needs are not addressed, or if the social burden threatens the client's living situation, some form of assistance is probably indicated. Nursing intervention may also be required where a too-helpful network does not allow enough autonomy.

Community health nurses have a unique contribution to make because they see clients in familiar surroundings where their abilities and resources become evident. A common example is the elderly client who may appear more impaired in a formal psychiatric interview than is actually the case. The same individual, seen at home, may safely attend to household chores, make coffee, and visit with the neighbors, showing considerable functional ability. In the same sense, persons described by hospital staff as withdrawn and seclusive may be far more socially skilled on their "home ground."

The natural environment additionally allows community health nurses to make a realistic appraisal of the burden of the client's illness on others. Psychiatric personnel may assume that the more independently the client and his or her network function, the better. However, signs of impending problems related to caretaking and support may signal a legitimate need for services. Early identification and problem solving may prevent a crisis and withdrawal of support.

Supporting the Supporters

In light of the heightened vulnerability of the mentally ill without interpersonal and social resources, maintaining the client's family or social network becomes an important nursing function. Families may, first, appreciate a confidential and accepting situation to express their feelings. They may have many questions as well: How do we manage medications? How much help is too much? What does the diagnosis mean, and how will it affect the future? Does our behavior contribute to this disorder? What are the chances of other persons in the family producing offspring with the same problem, or what are the chances of our developing the same illness as we age?

Supportive listening may be all that is necessary to allow families to problem-solve and explore their own feelings. If specific problems are identified, practical forms of assistance may be suggested to alleviate stress. Some of these involve referrals to mental health services (i.e., day treatment center and family therapy services). Others may supplement household resources: homemakers, home visiting services, and legal or economic aid. Referrals to the growing network of self-help and family support groups may be of significant long-term value. These offer helpful information and alleviate the isolation sometimes associated with management of mental illness. Local mental health associations may be of assistance to community health nurses in locating support groups for families coping with similar disorders or similar types of problems.

The decision to place the client in a residential or hospital setting may be especially charged with emotion. As in any situation where changes in health status create a crisis situation, community health nurses can offer a safe relationship for expression, problem solving, and planning. Greenberg and Underwood (1980) suggest that a "here and now" attitude that focuses on realistic issues and that downplays guilt will be most effective (p. 252).

For a considerable number of the chronically mentally ill without family supports, community health nurses serve to maintain a different kind of interpersonal environment. Nontraditional supports may be found in neighborhoods, hotels, apartments. Liaison work with shopkeepers, staff in places of residence, churches, and other community contacts may enable the natural network to function better, or to accommodate to crises. For example, home visits to a hotel resident may alleviate strain on staff and promote residential stability. Neighborhood merchants distressed by peculiar or bizarre dress may respond well to explanations about illness. Work by community health nurses in the urban districts where the mentally ill are concentrated demonstrates the considerable support they can provide to individuals and to the social network (Mealey, 1981; Sweeney et al, 1982).

Planning for Crises

Even under the best of circumstances, acute psychiatric problems may periodically disrupt the client's living situation. To help both client and family or friends, community health nurses should be aware of signs of potential crises, and the types of events that may precipitate them. For the chronically mentally ill, as for all of us, stressful life changes and significant losses (real or threatened) may undermine function. Such precipitating events do not necessarily precede acute decompensations, which may occur regardless of environmental factors. However, the impact of stressful life events should not be overlooked because of the individual's diagnosis or chronicity. Identification of stressors can be used to promote early intervention and to reduce disruption of the client's social situation.

The client's decision to discontinue psychotropic medication is frequently a key event signaling relapse. On one level this reflects a relationship between medication effect and symptomatology. However, it is important to ask why the client chose to stop medications at a particular time. This decision can be due to a personal crisis, the beginning of prodromal symptoms, a desire to try drug-free living, a concern about secondary effects, or other factors grounded in the individual meaning of medications. Exploration of the issues involved may help to avoid relapse and rehospitalization.

Planning for crises involves identification of appropriate backup services that can intervene if necessary to resolve acute psychiatric problems. By locating these resources before a crisis situation occurs, client and family will be better able to manage their own fears about the possibility of acute illness. These include twenty-four-hour crisis units, respite or hostel care, outreach teams, and telephone crisis lines, which may be available in the client's area. These resources may be needed, not only in the case of individual illness, but when the family or social system is strained by other factors and is temporarily unable to provide support. Nurses perform a very important function in helping the client and family or friends to identify the specific services available to them, and the manner in which they may be contacted. A telephone list of such resources prepared before a crisis can lead to smooth management of acute problems. (See Case Example 27-2 and Chapter 16 for further discussion of crisis intervention.)

Working with Psychiatric Nurse Specialists and Mental Health Consultants

To assess, plan, and deal with crises, community health nurses may require their own base of support. They may feel ill at ease about their lack of knowledge of specific psychiatric issues, and question their own competence to deal with the chronically mentally ill. This is unfortunate, since it promotes a withdrawal from the psychiatrically impaired, reinforcing the current schism between mental health and general health care services. In fact, community health nurses have made substantial contributions to the care of this population (Pasamanick, Scarpitti, & Dinitz, 1967). However, in order to define their roles and function effectively, they may require consultants. Community health nursing agencies may themselves provide these services. Community mental health agencies and local nursing organizations can generally provide or suggest psychiatric consultants as well.

The kinds of questions that may require special expertise include the signs of acute crises, the meanings of specific diagnoses and symptoms, the signs of potentially dangerous behavior, the management of problems regarding medications, and legal aspects of psychiatric care. Clinical issues are so varied, and their resolution so individual, that an ongoing relationship with an expert consultant is more valuable than a "crash course" in psychiatric care. Community health nurses may also require support and guidance in establishing contact with disturbed or distressing clients and their social networks. Here the consultant can offer guidance concerning the process of care, and can offer suggestions for dealing with issues such as disturbed communication, suspicion, and withdrawal. Like mental health workers in other settings, community health nurses may benefit from an objective outsider with special skills and knowledge who helps to analyze interactions with client and others, and to identify the nurse's own impact on these relationships.

Special Issues in Working with Mental Health Systems

Legal and Ethical Issues   Legal and ethical questions sometimes develop in the care of the psychiatrically disabled (Slaby, Lieb, & Tancredi, 1981). One of these, perhaps the major one, is confidentiality. While all client records are considered private, psychiatric records are generally subject to even stricter controls. Community health nurses should inform themselves as to procedures

Case Example 27-2: The Kelly Family

The Kelly family is well known to the community health nurse who visited them last year during Mr. Kelly's recovery from surgery. They request a home visit to discuss their need for a vacation and the problem of their daughter, Sarah, age forty-two. Sarah has a history of recurrent depressions and is unable to work. Her parents encourage her to attend a day treatment program and monitor her medications. The Kellys are dismayed at Sarah's anxiety about their absence and her fears that "their plane will crash."

Talking with Sarah, the nurse finds that she competently manages her own meals and shopping, that she can use familiar bus routes to go to day treatment, and that she apparently enjoys her group activities there. However, Sarah expresses fears of being alone in the house, a feeling that "I will lose it and have to go to the hospital," and obsessive concerns about her parents "dying and never coming back." The nurse obtains Sarah's permission to consult with her therapist about her fears and to explore options for help during the vacation. She develops a series of alternative community services that may be used during the Kellys' vacation (including short-term residential care, home visiting services, and day treatment on a daily basis) to present to the family. She also helps Sarah formulate a list of people to call in case of a crisis and alerts local emergency services to the situation. She also refers the Kellys to a family support group, which may help in the future to discuss member problems.

Community health nurses encounter the chronically mentally ill in a variety of nonpsychiatric roles.

Community health nurses assess the client in the natural environment.

Family burden may signal a need for services.

A review of daily activities will help to identify strengths and deficits.

Stressful life events may undermine function.

Specific problems may require consultation with psychiatric specialists.

Community services may support or give respite to the supporters.

Planning for crises may be helpful to client and family. Support groups reduce isolation and share information.

---

in their region. They also should inform themselves of the legal basis for privileged communication in their state (including whether or not nursing records are subject to subpoena) and what criteria may be used to justify involuntary detainment procedures or judgments of incompetence to manage daily affairs.

Nurses should be aware of types of information that *must* be communicated to outside sources. Behavior indicating suicidal risk or imminent harm to others falls into this category. So may disorganized or disturbed behavior that seriously compromises the client's ability to clothe, feed, and shelter himself or herself. An initial contract with the client should include an agreement that while communication is confidential, the nurse cannot withhold any information that would jeopardize the person's safety or the safety of others. In those rare situations involving clear and imminent dangerousness, the course of action may involve calling the police. Local mental health systems sometimes provide mobile forms of psychiatric emergency care as well (i.e., outreach teams). Community health nurses may want to determine both the extent of local resources and the procedures for their use.

Calling for help in a clear-cut emergency may be less disturbing than deciding whether or not a true emergency exists. The latter situation is also far more likely to occur in the course of community health nursing practice. Remarks about suicide or harm to others do not necessarily mean dangerousness in the clinical or legal sense. To make correct clinical judgments, and to deal with their own values and ethical questions, nurses may require their own backup services. For this reason, the benefits from a collaborative and supportive relationship with members of the mental health system are invaluable.

Dealing with Territoriality Negotiating such a relationship with psychiatric professionals may be complicated by another issue—territoriality. Mental health workers sometimes have only a vague idea of the nature of community health nursing practice. They may require explanations as to how community health nurses define their role, particularly the difference between family nursing and family therapy. Psychiatric providers are sometimes protective of their functions. They may require assurance that community health nurses support the client and the interpersonal environment to maximize adaptation, and that they will not compete with their specialized skills of therapy. They may also require assurance that the kinds of observations made in the client's home or neighborhood do not undermine their practice, but rather add a new source of information. Once these questions are worked out, mental health providers and community nursing agencies may negotiate ways to complement each other and to work toward better patient care, without fears of encroachment on professional territory.

Dealing with "Burn Out" among Mental Health Providers Another general issue that may surface in working with the mental health system is fatalism among psychiatric staff, who withdraw from a "difficult-to-treat" or "unmotivated" patient. Particularly among clients who have failed to comply with referrals, or who show high rates of relapse, psychiatric staff may express feelings of "burn out" and disinvestment. When attempting to reestablish the client's links with the system, nurses may encounter behaviors reminiscent of the "all or nothing" responses of families. In fact, for the more isolated and service-dependent of the chronically mentally ill, mental health systems sometimes function in something of a surrogate family role, offering ongoing interpersonal contact and crisis assistance. Problems arise when failure to improve, or to comply with treatment are interpreted as indications that prior efforts were wasted. Under these conditions, mental health providers may require support themselves.

A common pitfall in these situations involves side-taking, with the assumption that the client is fully responsible for the problem or the inverse idea, that the mental health worker is unfeeling. A more balanced approach, based on reestablishing communication and defusing anger may help to link the client with psychiatric care. In some cases, by their own supportive actions on behalf of the client and the social network, community health nurses may help to diminish excessive dependency on the mental health system and encourage more appropriate use of resources.

The Community Health Nurse as Client Advocate

Assessment of individual functional status, mobilization of environmental resources, and assistance to the client's support system all constitute forms of direct nursing care in the community. However, some of the fundamental problems affecting the chronically mentally ill cannot be resolved within the individual environment or social network. Social isolation, economic difficulties, and problems of access to comprehensive support services require action at another level. Community health nurses can also serve as advocates for this underserved and vulnerable client population.

Settings for Advocacy

Advocacy may involve work with voluntary groups such as mental health associations, self-help and family groups, patients' rights advocates, and neighborhood organizations seeking to maintain and extend resources for the mentally ill. Community health nurses can also serve as advocates for the chronically mentally ill in their roles within social and medical agencies. They function in this manner when they build better links between psychiatric and other community services, when they promote conservation of welfare and social service programs for the psychiatrically disabled, and when they support public education efforts that widen the base of support for this population and that reduce their isolation.

Issues in Actions on Behalf of the Mentally Ill

Advocacy efforts on behalf of the chronically mentally ill may involve more controversy and resistance than similar actions for other groups at risk. Since mental disorder does not produce a visible handicap, it often elicits less understanding and sympathy than other chronic health problems. The more disadvantaged and isolated clients may even

be "blamed" for their poverty. The failure of some mental health programs to meet the needs of the most seriously ill may be interpreted, not as an indication for better support services, but as a justification for restricting therapeutic resources. Baxter and Hopper (1981) advise us that advocacy for the mentally ill must be "double-edged and consciously so," focusing on both treatment and the subsistence services fundamental to community adaptation.

The Special Contribution of Community Health Nursing

While the brunt of responsibility for clients may fall upon the psychiatric sector itself, community health nurses have a special role to play. Psychiatric professionals and consumers may be seen as promoting their own interests, or as expressing the inherent biases of those heavily invested in community mental health systems. Community health nurses bring a balanced and objective point of view to planning because of their general health promotion role. They have traditionally concerned themselves with the environmental determinants of health and their effects on target groups at risk. Such a perspective may help to correct some of the problems in community care to date, and to create a service system more responsive to the needs of the chronically mentally ill, their social networks, and their neighborhoods.

Summary

The chronically mentally ill constitute a population of concern to health professionals and society in general. Although a heterogeneous group, members of this population share the commonalities of previous hospitalization, the experience of persistent psychiatric symptoms and some level of functional impairment related to psychiatric symptoms. This group is of concern to community health nurses because of their numbers in communities. As a result of the deinstitutionalization policies of the 1960s and 1970s, many chronically ill clients received community care, rather than long-term institutional treatment. Their successful mainte-nance in the community has been complicated by such problems as lack of employment, limited options for housing, inadequate family and social support, medication maintenance, and frequent psychiatric rehospitalizations. Roles community health nurses can play to help improve the health and well-being of this population include nursing assessment of their health status, problems, and needs; strengthening of their family and other social support networks (supporting the supporters); planning for crisis intervention; and working with colleagues such as psychiatric mental health nurses or other mental health consultants whenever nec-essary. Given the nature of this population and their unique needs, community health nurses also have an important role as advocates and to link individuals to appropriate community services.

Topics for Nursing Research

• How many of the chronically mentally ill are seen by community health nurses, and what are their most frequent needs?
• What is the effect of community health nurs-ing services on client satisfaction and compli-ance with medication regimes?
• In what ways can community health nurses support nonkin networks of the chronically mentally ill?

Study Questions

1. Certain major mental illnesses frequently imply either hospital treatment or disability. These include which of the following?
   a. Progressive organic disorders
   b. Schizophrenic and recurrent affective illnesses
   c. Phobias
   d. a & b
2. Individuals with serious psychiatric disorders generally resided in state mental hospitals until

recently. Which of the following factors changed that situation?
   a. Prevention and the drop in incidence of serious disorders
   b. A movement for hospital reform supported by legislative changes and introduction of new medications
   c. Diversion of the chronically mentally ill to veterans hospitals
   d. Enthusiasm of communities about integra-tion of the chronically mentally ill
3. A host of new problems confront families of the community-based client. A way to approach families should include:
   a. Assurance that residing at home is always better than a residential placement
   b. An explanation of the ways that family interaction contribute to the client's illness
   c. An assessment of the strengths and prob-lems of the particular family, and the resources it uses
   d. An explanation that all mental illness is curable
4. Psychiatric nursing specialists can help the community health nurse with which of the fol-lowing issues:
   a. Understanding the meaning of specific diagnoses
   b. Exploring feelings about the client and family, as well as the nurse's own impact on the recipients of services
   c. Understanding medication-related prob-lems
   d. All of the above
5. Many of the community-based mentally ill have little or no family contacts. The community health nurse can help these individuals by:
   a. Locating their families and convincing them to take care of the client
   b. Supporting nonkin networks in neighbor-hoods and places of residence
   c. Urging the client to contact his or her own family
   d. Reporting this to the health department
6. Self-help and family support groups are important because:
   a. They offer both practical information and a sense of support with difficult problems
   b. They replace coercive treatment facilities and provide home care

c. They help families to realize that the client's problems may be their fault

d. They offer alternative therapies for chronic mental illnesses

7. The position of the chronically mentally ill individual is different than that of other persons with long-term health problems. This is due to which of the following:

   a. Poor understanding of psychiatric disorder among the general public and a tendency to hold the person responsible for his or her illness

   b. The fact that most of the chronically mentally ill are dangerous

   c. The problems within the developing mental health service structure

   d. a & c

References

Akisical HS, McKinney WT: Depressive disorders: Toward a unified hypothesis. *Science* 1973; 182: 20–29.

American Psychiatric Association: *Diagnostic and Statistical Manual of Mental Disorders* 3rd ed. Washington, DC: Author, 1980.

Anthony WA, Cohen MR, Vitalo R: The measurement of rehabilitation outcome. *Schizophr Bull* 1978; 4 (3): 365–383.

Apostoles FE, Depp FC, Scarpelli AE: *A Cooperative Community Residence within the Aftercare System: A Feasibility Study* (unpublished report). Washington DC: Elizabeth's Hospital, 1980.

Archbold P: An analysis of parentcaring by women. *Home Health Care Services Quarterly* 1982; 3: 5–26.

Arieti S: An overview of schizophrenia from a predominantly psychological approach. *Am J Psychiatry* 1974; 131: 241–249.

Arnoff RN: Social consequences of a policy toward mental illness. *Science* 1975; 88: 1278–1281.

Aviram U, Segal SP: Exclusion of the mentally ill. *Arch Gen Psychiatry* 1973; 29: 126–131.

Bachrach LL: A conceptual approach to deinstitutionalization. *Hosp Community Psychiatry* 1978; 29 (9): 126–131.

Bachrach LL: Young adult chronic patients: An analytical review of the literature. *Hosp Community Psychiatry* 1982; 33 (3): 189–197.

Bassuk EL, Gerson S: Deinstitutionalization and mental health services. *Sci Am* (February) 1978; 46–53.

Baxter E, Hopper K: *Private Lives/Public Spaces: Homeless Adults in the Streets of New York City*. New York: Community Service Society, 1981.

Belknap E: *Human Problems of a State Mental Hospital*. New York: McGraw-Hill, 1956.

Beard JH: The rehabilitation services of fountain house. In: Stein L, Test MA (editors), *Alternatives to the Mental Hospital*. New York: Plenum Publishers, 1978.

Bowers MB: Biochemical processes in schizophrenia: An update. *Schizophr Bull* 1980; 6 (3): 393–403.

Burgess AW, Lazarre A: *Psychiatric Nursing in the Hospital and the Community*, 3rd ed. Englewood Cliffs, N.J.: Prentice-Hall, 1981.

Burnside IM: *Nursing and the Aged*. New York: McGraw-Hill, 1976, pp. 148–163.

Campanelli PC, Lieberman HJ, Trujillo M: Creating residential alternatives for the chronically mentally ill. *Hosp Community Psychiatry* 1983; 34 (2): 166–167.

Caplan RB: *Psychiatry and Community in Nineteenth-Century America*. New York: Basic Book, 1969.

Chafetz L, Goldfinger SM: Residential instability in a psychiatric emergency setting. *Psychiatric Quarterly* 1984; 56 (1): 20–34.

Chafetz LC, Goldman HH, Taube CA: Deinstitutionalization in the United States. *International Journal of Mental Health* 1983; 11 (4): 48–63.

Chase J: Where have all the patients gone? *Human Behavior* (October) 1973: 14–21.

Cohen CI, Sokolovsky J: Schizophrenia and social networks; Ex-patients in the inner city. *Schizophr Bull* 1978; 4 (4): 546–560.

Davis AJ: *Moral Treatments in 19th Century American Psychiatry: Roots, Rise, Decline, and Effects* (unpublished manuscript). San Francisco, Calif.: University of California, n.d.

Davis JM et al: Important issues in the drug treatment of schizophrenia. *Schizophr Bull* 1980; 6 (1): 71–87.

Deutsch A: *The Shame of the States*. New York: Harcourt, Brace, 1948.

Ekert K: *The Hidden Elderly*. San Diego: Campanile Press, 1981.

Endicott J et al: The global assessment scale. *Arch Gen Psychiatry* 1976; 33: 766–771.

Estroff SE: *Making it Crazy: An Ethnography of Psychiatric Clients in an American Community*. Berkeley and Los Angeles: University of California Press, 1981.

Fairweather GW et al: *Community Life for the Mentally Ill*. Chicago: Aldine Publishing Co., 1969.

Falloon IRH et al: Family management in the prevention of exacerbations of schizophrenia. *N Engl J Med* 1982; 306 (24): 1437–1440.

Faris REL, Dunham HW: *Mental Disorders in Urban Areas*. Chicago: University of Chicago Press, 1939.

Farr RK: *Skid Row Project, Los Angeles County Department of Public Health* (unpublished report). January 1982.

Frank MS, Eisenthal S, Lazarre A: Are there social class differences in patients' treatment conceptions? *Arch Gen Psychiatry* 1978; 35: 61–69.

Glick ID, Kessler DR: *Marital and Family Therapy,* 2nd ed. New York: Grune and Stratton, 1980.

Goffman E: *Asylums.* New York: Doubleday, 1961.

Goldfinger SM: The client with a borderline condition. In: Gorton J, Partridge R (editors), *The Practice and Management of Psychiatric Emergencies.* New York: Mosby, 1982.

Goldman HH, Adams NH, Taube, CA: Deinstitutionalization: The data demythologized. *Hosp Community Psychiatry* 1983; 34 (2): 129–134.

Goldman HH, Gatozzi AA, Taube CA: Defining and counting the mentally ill. *Hosp Community Psychiatry* 1981; 32 (1) 21–27.

Greenberg S, Underwood PR: The family model and psychiatric nursing. In: Glick I, Kessler D (editors), *Marital and Family Therapy.* New York: Grune and Stratton, 1980.

Greenblatt M, Bercerra RM, Serafetinides EA: Social networks and mental health: An overview. *Am J Psychiatry* 1982; 139 (8): 977–984.

Gruenberg EM: The social breakdown syndrome: Some origins. *Am J Psychiatry* 1967; 123 (12): 1481–1498.

Herz MI, Herman VS, Simon JC: Intermittent medication for stable schizophrenic out patient: An alternative to medication maintenance. *Am J Psychiatry* 1982; 139 (7): 918–922.

Hollingshead AB, Redlich FC: *Social Class and Mental Illness.* New York: Wiley, 1958.

Joint Commission on Mental Illness and Health: *Action for Mental Health.* New York: Basic Books, 1961.

Kalkman ME, Davis AJ: *New Dimensions in Mental Health: Psychiatric Nursing,* 5th ed. New York: McGraw-Hill, 1980.

Kessler S: The genetics of schizophrenia: A review. *Schizophr Bull* 1980; 6 (3): 404–416.

Kirk SA, Thierren ME: Community mental health myths and the fate of former hospitalized patients. *Psychiatry* 1975; 38: 209–217.

Kramer M: *Psychiatric Services and the Changing Institutional Scene, 1950–1975.* Rockville, Md.: National Institute of Mental Health, 1977.

Krauss JB, Slavinsky AT: *The Chronically Ill Psychiatric Patient and the Community.* Boston: Blackwell Scientific Publications, 1982.

Lamb HR: What did we really expect from deinstitutionalization? *Hosp Community Psychiatry* 1981; 32 (2): 105–109.

Lamb HR, Ragowski AS: Supplemental security income and the sick role. *Am J Psychiatry* 1978; 135 (10): 1221–1224.

Lamb HR, Goertzel V: Discharged mental patients: Are they really in the community? *Arch Gen Psychiatry* 1971; 24: 29–34.

Larew BI: Strange strangers: Serving transients. *Social Casework* (February) 1980; 61: 107–113.

Lipowski ZJ: Organic brain syndromes: A reformulation. *Compr Psychiatry* 1978; 19 (4), 309–322.

McAllister TW, Trevor RPP: Severe depressive pseudodementia with and without dementia. *Am J Psychiatry* 1982; 139 (5): 626–629.

Mealey A: Provision of a multi-range program for clients in a downtown hotel by baccalaureate nursing students. *J Psychosoc Nurs Ment Health Serv* 1981; 19: 11–16.

Minkoff K: A map of chronic mental patients. In: Talbott JA (editor), *The Chronic Mental Patient.* Washington, DC: American Psychiatric Association, 1979.

New York State Dept. of Social Services: *Survey of the needs and problems of single room occupancy hotel residents on the upper west side of Manhattan.* New York: State Department of Social Services, 1980.

Pasamanick B, Scarpitti FR, Dinitz S: *Schizophrenics in the Community: An Experimental Study in the Prevention of Hospitalization.* New York: Appleton-Century-Crofts, 1967.

Reich R: Care of the chronically mentally ill: A national disgrace. *Am J Psychiatry* 1973; 130: 911–912.

Reynolds DK, Faberow NL: *Endangered Hope: Experiences in Psychiatric Aftercare Facilities.* Berkeley and Los Angeles: University of California Press, 1977.

Scheper-Hughes N: Dilemmas in deinstitutionalization: A view from inner city Boston. *Journal of Operational Psychiatry* 1981; 12 (2): 90–99.

Schulz PM et al: Patient and family attitudes about schizophrenia: Implications for genetic counseling. *Schizophr Bull* 1982; 9 (4): 504–513.

Schneck MK, Reisberg B, Ferris SH: An overview of current concepts of Alzheimer's disease. *Am J Psychiatry* 1982; 139 (2): 165–173.

Schwartz SR, Goldfinger SM: The new chronic patient: Clinical characteristics of an emerging subgroup. *Hosp Community Psychiatry* 1981; 32 (7): 470–474.

Segal SP, Baumohl J: Engaging the disengaged: Proposals on madness and vagrancy. *Social Work* 1980; 25: 358–365.

Segal SP, Baumohl J, Moyles EW: Neighborhood types and community reaction to the mentally ill. *J Health Soc Behav* 1980; 21 (4): 345–359.

Shapiro J: *Communities of the Alone.* New York: Association Press, 1972.

Sheehan S: *Is There No Place on Earth for Me?* Boston: Houghton Mifflin, 1982.

Sheets JL, Prevost JA, Reihman J: Young adult chronic patients: Three hypothesized subgroups. *Hosp Community Psychiatry* 1982; 33 (3): 197–203.

Slaby AE, Lieb J, Tancredi LR: *Handbook of Psychiatric Emergencies.* New York: Medical Examination Publishing Co., 1981.

Steadman HJ: Critically reassessing accuracy of public

perceptions of the dangerousness of the mentally ill. *J Health Soc Behav* 1981; 22 (3): 310–316.

Sweeney D et al: Mapping urban hotels: Life space of the chronic mental patient. *J Psychosoc Nurs Ment Health Serv* 1982; 20: 9–14.

Talbott JA: The national plan for the chronically mentally ill: A programmatic analysis. *Hosp Community Psychiatry* 1981; 32 (10): 699–703.

Tessler RC et al: The chronically mentally ill in community support systems. *Hosp Community Psychiatry* 1982; 33 (3): 208–211.

Test LI, Stein MA: Community treatment of the chronic patient: research overview. *Schizophr Bull* 1978; 4 (3): 350–364.

Turner RJ, Gartrell JW: Social factors in psychiatric outcome: toward the resolution of interpretive controversies. *Am Sociol Rev* 1978; 43: 368–382.

Turner JC, TenHoor WJ: The NIMH community support program: Pilot approach to a needed social reform. *Schizophr Bull* 1978; 4 (3): 319–342.

Underwood P: *Nursing Care as a Determinant in the Development of Self Care Behavior by Hospitalized Adult Schizophrenics* (dissertation). San Francisco, Calif.: Department of Mental Health and Community Nursing, University of California, 1978.

Whitmer G: From hospitals to jails: The fate of California's deinstitutionalized mentally ill. *Am J Orthopsychiatry* 1980; 50: 65–75.

Wilson H, Kneisl CR: *Psychiatric Nursing,* (2nd ed.) Menlo Park, Calif.: Addison-Wesley, 1983.

Chapter 28

Family Violence

Rose Odum

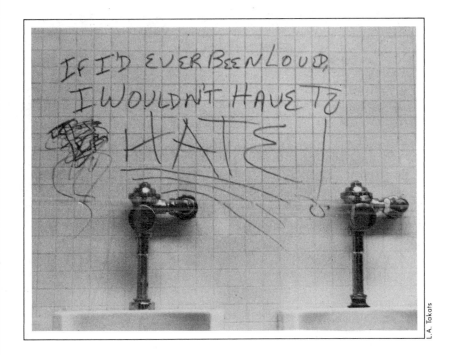

Research shows that the majority of abusive and aggressive behaviors are learned—often in the context of violent families.

Chapter Outline

Chapter Objectives

After completing this chapter, the reader will be able to:

- Identify types of violence and recognize signs of potential violence
- List and describe the various factors associated with domestic violence and abuse including societal factors, intrafamilial factors, perpetrator factors, and victim factors
- Discuss the responsibilities and opportunities of nurses in various clinical settings to prevent and to intervene in situations of potential and actual domestic violence and abuse
- Discuss the role of community health nurses in social, political and community organizations in the construction of primary and secondary prevention programs for domestic violence and abuse
- List issues related to the evaluation of health care today for families with problems of domestic violence and abuse
- Describe the nurse's legal role in the reporting of child abuse to child protective service officials

We should not . . . direct attention from the real sources of man's aggression and destructiveness, namely, the many false and contradictory values by which, in an over-crowded, highly competitive, threatening world, he so disoperatively attempts to live. It is not man's nature, but his nurture, in such a world, that requires our attention.

Montagu, 1968

This chapter concerns the nature and extent of violence and abuse directed toward members of families. Basic concepts and factors thought to be associated with domestic violence and abusive situations will be defined and described as they are used in this work and in much of the associated literature. Legal issues are well covered in Chapter 24 of this text. The related interface of legal, family, and nursing concerns will be discussed here. The final segment of this chapter addresses nursing practice from the perspectives of primary, secondary, and tertiary prevention activity by community health nurses.

Families, Society, and Violence

Within the last half of this century, the nature and function of the "family" in America have been changing, making it more difficult to generalize approaches to nursing care for each familial unit (see Chapter 17). For example, the proportion of children being born to unmarried women has increased from 5 to 18 percent in the last two decades; the number of unmarried couples has tripled in the past ten years; about 50 percent of married women with children under six years of age are employed in the paid work force; nearly half of all children will live in one-parent households before the age of eighteen, and, finally, the proportion of adults living alone has tripled in the last thirty years (*The Stanford Observer*, 1983). Scanzoni (1983) refers to "family-like" structures rather than "family" because there are so many variations on the theme of how persons dwell together in this country. There are more "blended" families than ever before—families that include children from one or more prior marriages. There are greater numbers of senior citizens, and more of these are living at home independently or have sought new partners in marriage or in "living together" arrangements. Households with same-sexed partners are more frequently reported, and America continues to broaden its multiethnic representation (Naisbitt, 1982). Never before in history have there been so many women in graduate schools or working in such traditionally male professions as medicine, engineering, and law. The extent to which men have altered their professional or domestic roles to accommodate the changing roles of women is debatable (Condran & Bode, 1982; Eisenstein, 1982).

These and other shifts from traditional familial structures to the more "progressive" forms complicate efforts to define family for purposes of health-related research and clinical planning (Scanzoni, 1983). Perhaps the most accurate definition of family would be that supplied by the respondent to research questionnaires or clinical interviews. That is, one's family is defined as the member(s) define it.

However, any discussion of family violence and abuse cannot proceed without at least a minimum understanding of what is meant by family. In Chapter 2, Knafl identified commitment to one another as an important criterion for defining family. For the purposes of this chapter, family will be defined as a primary social group made up of individuals who are interdependent in socioeconomic needs, who claim emotional, psychological, and affective ties among themselves, and who may be related by blood or by legal proceedings such as marriage or adoption. Further, this group is characterized by patterns of interaction and communication, which develop over time and which reflect the values and beliefs of other social institutions of the broader community.

Definition of Violence and Abuse

Family violence and abuse are terms that have only recently begun to appear frequently in popular media, clinical journals, and textbooks. Certainly there is no one common definition of family violence and abuse that is well grounded in research. While a fair amount of data have been gathered regarding child abuse and neglect, less is reported about battered women in the home or the abuse of the elderly person at home. Like most health problems, battering, abuse, and neglect are to some extent value judgments. For some individuals, corporal punishment of family members for disciplinary or any purpose is undesirable whether or not physical injury results. For others, it is the duty of parents to deliver "necessary" spankings. Scholars in both religion and law identify traditions upholding a man's right to discipline his wife and children (Humphreys, 1984; Waterman & Young, 1982).

For purposes of this chapter, *family violence and abuse* is defined as those behaviors of family members that are intended to result in the physical or psychological trauma or pain of another member, or in that member's failure in normal growth and development. Violence is a deliberate, aggressive act or set of acts; abuse may be passive, as in acts of omission leading to failure-to-thrive (Gelles, 1979; Kempe & Helfer, 1980). Violence may occur between parent and child (even when the child is adult and the parent is elderly); between spouses or adults living together as a couple; between siblings; and/or between child and adult caretaker in the home other than the biological parent, such as boyfriend, stepfather, stepmother, or uncle. Violence and abuse are not mutually exclusive for any given family or victim; both can, and do, happen together.

The forms that family violence and abuse may take include physical violence, psychological abuse,

material or environmental abuse, and sexual abuse. Precise research-based clinical definitions have not been developed; however, some of the more commonly reported behaviors and consequences can be enumerated. Physical abuse or violence includes bodily injuries, deprivations, and living conditions that do not support physical and mental development. In the case of child physical abuse, medical diagnostic guidelines have been put forth by radiologists and pediatricians (Schmitt, 1979). Some nonaccidental injuries and failure-to-thrive cases are more easily identified than others. Among children, burns, bruises, and fractures can be fairly easily ruled out as being nonaccidental given a reasonable history of the injury provided, the age and abilities of the child, the medical diagnostic findings, such as X-ray, and developmental parameters that are fairly standardized for a given population. In part, the advancement of criteria for differential diagnosis of accidental and nonaccidental injury and failure-to-thrive among children reflects the increased responsibility felt by clinicians who are compelled by law to report child abuse to the state departments of child protective services. Similar laws for detection of such trauma among battered women or the elderly have yet to be put forth.

Violence is one form of abuse. Explosive aggression is the form most commonly associated with violence. The word *violence*, however, might also be applied by some to the shocking sight of an extremely emaciated seven-month-old girl among thriving brothers in a relatively stable, if not wealthy, family, where extensive examination revealed no organic causes other than food deprivation. The clinical observer can also feel a sense of violence when visiting an abused wife who lives daily under the intimidating, towering dominance of her husband. The atmosphere of fear, entrapment, and agitated depression would support this sense.

Violence, then, is one form of abuse that may be physical, psychological, material, or environmental (Foley, 1983). The underlying factor in violence is that it threatens life and creates disabling fear in the victim in domestic settings. This is most true when the setting is socially isolated from the rest of the immediate community.

Violent behavior has roots that are neurophysiologic, psychologic, and sociologic. The physiologic basis for behavior has not been fully described by research. While structures in the central nervous system and certain hormonal levels, such as testosterone, have been associated with episodes and patterns of violent behavior, the empirical research establishing cause and effect is weak. Aggressive behavior expressed by a subject who is artificially stimulated, as by electrical stimulation of the brain, must still be evaluated on the basis of the immediate situation and how it is interpreted by the subject and by his or her previous learning with that and similar situations (Bandura, 1973; Laborit, 1978). The behavior is stimulus-bound and regulated by cognitive processes, experience, and expectations. Similarly, when individuals ingest alcohol, the response of violence will vary among them. Some people will become violent at times when drinking, others will not. It is more clear that alcohol leads to changes in intellectual operations and mood; it is not yet established that these alterations will necessarily lead to violent behavior (Graham, 1980).

The relationship of learning to violence seems to be somewhat clearer. The person who is more likely to become violent is that person whose past experiences or learning, and whose assessment of the immediate situation, combine to produce a violent response or behavioral expression of violence. While social learning theorists point out that violence and violent behaviors are learned through modeling, imitation, and reward or reinforcement for such performance, not all individuals who have learned violent behaviors (and who demonstrate skill in these) will necessarily repeat the behavior in future situations. Police officers and returning war veterans may be cases in point. However, when there are social sanctions and rewards for violent behavior, when the motivations for the behavior are thought to be "valid," and when certain emotional needs are gratified in the behavior, then violence is more likely to occur. For instance, when aggressive and violent behavior results in a felt increase in self-esteem, then violence is more likely to result. Finally, social psychologists and anthropologists have pointed out that some societies have been virtually free of injurious aggression or violence, thus negating the theories that such behavior is inevitable in genetic predisposition or necessary to the survival of the species (Campbell & Humphreys, 1984).

Further, certain subcultures are thought to be at greater risk for violence; some cultures, such as those that value "machismo," routinely devalue women, physically punish children, and maintain the social sanction of the right of men to be dominant. Some sociologists have postulated that dominance-subordination relationships, such as in male dominance over women and children, are common in established and "organized" society. If this is true, perhaps the progressive social changes of the women's movement, having upset this "balance," are contributing to the increase in violence against women and children that we are witnessing in today's society (Easton, 1975; Resick, 1983).

Causes of violence are thus multifactorial, making it difficult for researchers in any discipline to demonstrate direct and simplistic cause-and-effect relationships. Most theorists agree, however, that social learning by the perpetrator, victim, and family is involved in the production of violence. Additional factors include the social sanction of violence as a means of conflict resolution and approval of rigid roles of dominance-subordination among members of social groups, including families.

Nurses and other clinicians will be able to exercise primary prevention principles only to the extent that the complex causes of violence are understood. Interventions on broader social, political, and health care levels are necessary if abuse resulting from violence is to be reduced in American society and in the world.

Sexual Abuse and Incest

Sexual abuse in the home has not been differentiated significantly from other forms of physical and psychological abuse. The two problems (physical and sexual abuse) frequently coexist, and sexual victimization and physical abuse are often manifestations of similar home situations (Schmitt, 1979). Definitions of sexual abuse of children rest on the assumption that children and minors cannot be said to give "consent" to sexual involvement. This assumption underscores the intellectual immaturity of the child and his or her emotional and economic dependency on the adult caretaker (Burgess, 1984; Herman, 1981).

Sexually abused children may show up in emergency rooms, clinics, or physicians' offices with bruises, cuts, burns, and lacerations on and around the genital areas (Schmitt, 1979). In some instances, parents with a misguided sense of disciplinary practice abuse children in sexual areas as a punishment for the child's masturbation, sexual explorations, or bedwetting. Interestingly, these parents recall having received very similar punishments as children.

Psychological sexual abuse is more difficult to document. In this instance, the adult intimidates, teases, and exploits the child around inappropriate sexual themes; forcing or seducing children into pornographic activities is an example that popular media has reported increasingly in recent years.

Finally, incest as a form of child sexual abuse has become a major source of official reports to child protective services (Herman, 1981). More and more adult women from various socioeconomic levels are reporting histories of having been victimized and molested by fathers and older brothers. The problem of incest is becoming increasingly common (Anderson, 1983; Carson & Finkelhor, 1982). Estimates place the rate of incest to daughters at between 20 and 30 percent of all adult women (Burgess et al, 1978). Incest has been defined as "any physical contact between parent and child that had to be kept secret," including seductive behaviors such as exhibitionism and peeping as well as the outright demand for intercourse (Burgess et al, 1978).

Incestuous fathers are described as domineering, patriarchal personalities who have low or marginal self-esteem, who have had poor relationships with women, and who are typically socially isolated and socially unskilled (Authier, 1983; Selby, et al, 1979). Indeed families where incest has been routinized, whether overtly avowed or not, are socially isolated as a group. Some clinicians report that daughters are unaware that the incestuous activity

is unusual until conversation with adolescent peers reveals it to be so. That these girls later come to suffer guilt and a range of psychiatric and interpersonal problems has been well reported (Greenberg, 1979; Sgroi, 1982).

Following Freud, modern psychiatry has, to a large extent, kept the problem of sexual abuse hidden or at least has denied its significance in clinical reports (Herman, 1982; Hogan, 1980). Many observers believe that it has been the women's movement and the sexual revolution that have brought the "closeted" problem of domestic incest and sexual abuse into public awareness; now women and children have the much needed support to have the courage to report such cases and seek legal and clinical assistance in dealing with the problems. Men, too, are finding support in these movements as they are enabled to develop less "macho" roles, learn broader social skills in relating to women and children, and experience related gratifications in flexible parenting and marital roles.

Spousal rape studies suggest that between 14 and 37 percent of married or cohabiting women experienced forced sex with their mates (Brownmiller, 1975; Walker, 1979). There seems to be an implicit assumption that when a woman marries she relinquishes her right to refuse sexual intercourse or activity (Finkelhor & Yllo, 1978). For women who are economically dependent on spouses, who have no job or career skills, and who have dependent children, the choice seems limited.

Although sexual abuse may be perpetrated by wives, mothers, and sisters, the existing data suggest that these situations are minimal by comparison to the adult male perpetrator. Certainly, much research is needed to get a clearer picture of domestic sexual abuse carried out by female perpetrators.

Patriarchy and Family Violence

In recent years much has been written about sexism in American and other cultures (Easton, 1975; Lewis, 1979; Martin, 1976). *Sexism* is the process of assigning societal and familial roles on the basis of beliefs, values, and myths that hold that one sex can more properly or successfully fulfill the role than can the other (Driefus, 1977; Nelson & Taylor, 1981). In the family system, marital or conjugal responsibilities, rights, privileges, and power have traditionally been allocated a priority on such gender-linked principles; the predominant system has been patriarchy. In that system, the male, husband, father, and sometimes older brother, controlled the decision making and held primary economic and political power in the family (Brownmiller, 1975; Eisenstein, 1982; Hare-Mustin, 1978; Schaef, 1982). Locating primary power with the family's males naturally placed the family's females in a dependent position.

Kalmuss and Strauss (1982) conducted a national survey of 2,143 adult men and women to explore relationships between women's marital dependency and wife abuse. Both psychological and economic dependency were positively related to abuse, with more serious abuse occurring around economic dependency. This becomes an important consideration for both research and planning interventions into the problems of wife abuse since it is well established that women, on the average, tend to earn about half as much as male counterparts. At the same time, it has become commonplace for the typical middle- and lower-class family to need both spouses' employment to maintain an adequate and stable family economy. Increasingly, working wives in traditional patriarchal families become targets of their spouse's frustration; their employment, though necessary, is a source of embarrassment and threat to the husband's economic role or self-esteem. Similarly, when husbands lose their jobs, they too become subject to the emotional problems associated with economic dependency and become more vulnerable to angry outbursts. An increase in child abuse has been associated with unemployment of husbands and economic hardships (Light, 1973)

Logically, the contemporary American family must consider alternatives to traditional patriarchy as a family system life-style (Scanzoni, 1983) and has begun to do so. More egalitarian family patterns can help to avoid the violent consequences of failing to adapt to the increasing stresses of modern society.

The Women's Movement

Perhaps one of the most significant social shifts in America during the decades of the 1960s and 1970s was the women's movement. The failure of the Equal Rights Amendment in no way reflects a "return" to traditional role performance. Indeed the traditional distribution of labor and power in the family was never much changed (Condran & Bode, 1982); working women just must work twice as hard. Naisbitt (1982) highlighted the directions for women of the future in his report of a national study, entitled "The Nation's Families, 1960–1990," conducted by the Joint Center for Urban Studies of MIT and Harvard. For instance, "Husband-wife households with only one working spouse will account for only 14% of all households as compared with 43% in 1960. Wives will contribute about 40% of family income compared to about 25% now" (p. 233). Naisbitt further points out that women are experiencing an "option explosion" in both work and career. "More women are working and many more are going to college. Today there are more women in college and graduate school than men" (p. 235). More women are preparing for professions and to acquire blue collar money-making skills as well.

Clearly, the nature of the family is changing. The question now is, to what extent will individual families and other social institutions define this change as hardship and regression as opposed to opportunities for growth and development of *all* family members. "Whether the sex-segregated labor market will accommodate the growing economic needs and personal aspirations of working women is still being questioned, even though 50% of women of working age are gainfully employed. Women continue to earn about fifty cents of every dollar earned by men including college-educated women" (Nash, 1981).

Depending on how families interact with social, political, economic, and religious institutions, roles for members will be traditional and fixed, or futuristic and flexible. There is increasing evidence that victims of family violence are those members with the least economic and social power. Victims are women, children, and the elderly. While occasional abuse of male heads of households does occur, the reported incidence remains relatively small (Gelles, 1979). Women who do use violence most frequently are retaliating for abuse initiated by their spouses. Most murders committed by wives occur after years or months of battering and abuse.

Much more sociological investigation is needed to identify how limit-setting practices are initiated and sustained. However, children with nonaccidental burns, wives with repeated cuts and bruises,

and elderly parents with unexplained fractures are examples of the point of departure from limit-setting to abuse. As more women need and want to work outside the home and to experience economic and social equality, and as social legislation affording improved rights and protection for children are established, the incidence of violence resulting in injury to the dependent or helpless family member may diminish. At the same time, a man who holds rigidly to values of male dominance may be caught between the psychologic needs of a "macho" head-of-household role and pragmatic needs imposed by economic austerity and may certainly be vulnerable to violent expressions toward his family.

Family Dynamics

Balance of Power and Division of Labor

Since the 1950s development of the view of family as a system, researchers have taken an increased interest in the system's power distribution and division of labor. For a variety of reasons, the traditional family system is not working as well as it was assumed to work in America around the turn of the century; this is reflected in rates of divorce, runaways, violence, and selection of alternative life-styles (see Box 28-1). An examination of power and the division of labor within an individual family can shed light on that family's potential for violence. Available research indicates that men still do not fully share the responsibilities of household labor (Condran & Bode, 1982). While this may be changing, much additional research and accommodation are essential if progress is to be maintained. After his extensive review of domestic violence and its causes, Gelles (1979) concludes:

The sexist character of society must change. An underlying cause of family violence is the fact that the family

is perhaps the only social group where jobs, tasks and responsibilities are assigned on the basis of gender and age, rather than interest or ability. . . . An elimination of the concept of "women's work"; elimination of the taken-for-granted view that the husband is and must be the head of the family; and an elimination of sex-typed family roles are prerequisites to the reduction of family violence (p. 19).

Rigid Role Prescriptions

An open, flexible family system may reduce the potential for violence among family members. Such a system would recognize each individual's need to change, grow, and be unique, and would not maintain a facade of harmony and sameness by denying familial conflict. The open family system can acknowledge and properly identify its internal problems, and it can seek help from external individuals and systems whenever necessary (Farrar, 1982).

An oppressively traditional, or closed, family system would allow for none of this flexibility. Individual family members would be tightly locked into

Box 28-1   Families at Risk for Violence

The following characteristics can typify families at risk for violent and dysfunctional crisis resolution and can also make them unlikely to seek counseling or other health care:

- Poor self-esteem
- Resistance to external environment and lack of spontaneity in social or interpersonal activities
- Belief in strict disciplinary habits and corporal punishment

- Excessively high expectations of family members, often beyond the individual's development or innate capacity
- Rigid role prescriptions and patriarchal family structure
- Denial of any internal problems
- Lack of necessary and sufficient social supports

---

rigid roles. Leadership would be autocratic and inflexible (Cromwell & Olson, 1975). Members would not share in the rights or responsibilities for decision making. Problems would not be acknowledged, or they would be defined by the autocratic leader according to his values and beliefs.

By definition, closed family systems do not often open themselves to change, alternative ways of living together, or different patterns of communication. When the usual patterns are those of violence and abuse, the victims have little hope for rescue. Probably the most dramatic example of how the closed family system victimizes its members is the problem of incest. Judith Herman's recent book, *Father-Daughter Incest* (1982), makes it abundantly clear that this problem is very contemporary, as most family therapists and clinicians are aware, and that the closed nature of that family system virtually precludes intervention from outside. Similarly, families who abuse children and wives are more often shut off, without belief that things can or even should be different in family life, or that any real help is available (Gelles, 1979; Odum, 1981; Pagelow, 1981).

Social Isolation and Lack of Gratification

Apparently the rigid and closed family system is subject to social isolation. Family members are expected to meet each other's basic psychosocial needs without outside help. Children are expected to gratify parental needs for love and esteem, and parents are expected to fulfill children's developmental needs, such as socialization.

Spouses are not expected to have significant or abiding interpersonal involvement with others outside the marriage. Obviously there is enormous pressure in this rigid crucible of family life; when children fail to gratify parents, they are more at risk for abuse (Justice & Justice, 1976; Kempe & Helfer, 1980). Wives who complain that their daily life is dull and ungratifying are perceived as threatening and unfaithful by patriarchal, unreasonable husbands, and subsequent abuse occurs (Roy, 1977). Farrar (1982, p. 173) has sorted out the following characteristics of rigid and closed family systems:

- Control is by authoritarian leadership.
- Discipline is autocratic and overly strict.
- Negotiations are limited.
- Roles are rigid and stereotyped.
- There are many explicit rules that are strictly enforced.
- Feedback loops are primarily negative with few positive loops.
- Stability is maintained by tradition.
- Exploration of alternatives is closed.
- A strong religious or ethical value is used as a rationale for avoiding conflict.
- There is resistance to and denial of change.
- Poor adaptability encourages family stasis, limiting growth and autonomy.

Those characteristics are certainly applicable to abusive families. The clinical problems presented by the rigid family to clinicians are enormous because such systems avoid change and external influence. The broader society functions to facilitate the traditional, patriarchal balance of power in families. The clinician faces not only the resistance of the family system, but of many shapers of social policy at large. This has recently become an issue among family therapists who realize the vast influence of societal norms used by therapists which support patriarchal balance of power (Taggart, 1985).

Intergenerational Transmission of Violence

Social learning theorists and family therapists alike postulate that children will grow up to emulate many of their parents' behaviors and attitudes. The extent to which this is actually universal has yet to be established with controlled and replicable research. However, those reporting on the cyclical nature of child abuse point out that parents who abuse their children were themselves, in the majority of cases, abused as children (Gelles, 1981; Milner & Wimberley, 1979; Roy & Earp, 1980). Of course, what is considered abusive in one generation—child labor, for instance—may not have been considered abusive in previous generations.

Historically, it has been not only legally but socially acceptable to abuse one's wife physically (Martin, 1976). Men were expected to discipline their wives and children, and parents who neglected corporal punishment of children were held to be irresponsible—hence, the traditional maxim, "Spare the rod and spoil the child." While research has not fully explained the relationship of the parenting of a child and that child's subsequent abusive or violent behavior in adulthood, there seems to be some connection that perpetuates the cycle of family violence. It may be, then, that by helping an individual victim, community health nurses can disrupt the cycle of violence for an entire family.

Victims of Family Violence

Victims of family violence include women, the elderly, and children. Although much more has been written about abused and neglected children than other groups, this does not mean that the problems of spouse and elderly abuse are less important than those of child abuse. Indeed, a recent report on the abused elderly concludes that older victims are as frequently abused as the children in our society (Crouse et al, 1981).

Child Abuse and Neglect

In 1974, the National Center of Child Abuse and Neglect was formed by the federal government to develop programs and projects for research, prevention, and treatment of child abuse. A model law for reporting of child abuse was derived from that center and provided impetus for similar laws now active in all fifty states. Kempe and Helfer (1976) reported that in 1975 at least 550,000 cases of suspected child abuse and neglect were reported in the United States. The number today is estimated to be closer to two million (Erickson, McElroy, & Colucci, 1984).

In the last decade, much work has been done to develop causal or explanatory models of abuse (Caulfield, Disbrow, & Smith, 1977; Garbarino, 1977; Kempe & Helfer, 1980). Two perspectives emerge from this body of work: an ecological perspective, which looks at the environment surrounding the child and family, and an intrafamilial focus on the individual family itself.

The ecological, or social-psychological, perspective views child abuse and neglect as a failure of society to adequately protect and nurture its children. Maldistribution of jobs, lack of resources for education and training, underdeveloped social support systems, and inferior legal rights for women, children, and minorities are seen as the true precursors to abusive practices. Preventive measures thus include improved health and social policies for the care of *all* children, not only the abused.

If we take the dynamics of the individual family as the focus of study, child abuse is related to parental psychopathology and familial transmission of abusive parenting patterns (Justice & Justice, 1976; Logenberry, Nilsson, & Lundetin, 1979). This perspective incorporates the medical and disease models of abuse, both of which may be more effective for intervention after the fact than for primary prevention. Some theorists attempt to combine both the social-psychological and the intrafamilial models, and see the various factors of abuse on a continuum from environmental conditions to individual details of family function.

Research on Child Abuse Prediction and Identification   Although research in the area of child abuse is fraught with a range of methodological problems (Gelles, 1981), a review of current efforts to examine different pieces of the overall etiological puzzle does reflect commonality in ideas, formulations, and data about the nature of the problem. Conceivably, these generalizations could lead to integrated productive approaches to prevention and intervention.

Information found to be helpful in identifying high-risk mothers during prenatal labor, delivery, and postpartum periods included:

1. Maternal (and paternal) passivity or hostility with the infant
2. Expressed disappointment over some physical characteristics of the child
3. No eye contact with the baby
4. Nonsupportive spouse interaction
5. Parents' expectations of baby beyond the child's developmental capacity
6. Mother sees child as too demanding or repulsive

7. Negative reactions to baby by other family members
8. Mother receives little or no support from husband or family
    (Caufield, Disbrow, & Smith, 1977; Helfor, Schneider, & Hoffmeister, 1978)

Among other similarities, abusive parents are frequently abused as children, are low in empathy, have few close friends and are socially isolated, show role reversal with children, have strict disciplinary practices with corporal punishment, and have excessively high expectations of their offspring (Bavolek, 1978; Gray & Kaplan, 1980). Additionally, abusive parents or caretakers have shown poor self-esteem, limited interpersonal skills, and inability to cope with crisis situations (Helfer, Schnieder, & Hoffmeister, 1978; Parke & Collmer, 1975).

Problems abound in the effort to research child abuse and neglect, as well as other areas of family violence. It has been very difficult to establish control or comparison groups. Most studies are retrospective or after the fact investigations, and samples are usually small. Theoretical models are generally simplistic, single-variable types of explanations of abuse. The private, sensitive nature of violence in families complicates finding willing, voluntary subjects for research, and many "false positives" are identified. Consequently, evaluative studies of interventions have little scientific merit. Caution should be applied to any effort to diagnose abuse or neglect and violence. Thorough data gathering and assessment are essential to the derivation of accurate clinical inference (Berger, 1983).

Multidisciplinary and Interdisciplinary Screening Teams   Precisely because of the rudimentary state of knowledge and research about abuse and violence, a screening team is more effective than the individual diagnostician. The team should include experts from medicine, nursing, psychology, sociology or social work, and, whenever possible, home care workers. Ideally, at least one of these individuals will have specific training in family therapy. The team members offer mutual support and share responsibilities. Expertise in child abuse is limited, since there is so little research-based information available. Therefore, no single team member can make all the decisions and judgments for the group. Leadership will be assumed by the worker who is best informed about the particular and unique family under discussion and who knows what research and intervention efforts have been reported in the literature. (See Chapter 12 for a further discussion of group leadership.) It is important that team members are comfortable with each other so that they, in turn, can be supportive to reporting staff or to families seeking help. By its very nature, working with child abuse or neglect "burns out" staff and leads to mutual withdrawal and resistance between family, clients, and workers. Indeed the resistance behaviors of families can affect the decisions about distribution of services to families (Odum, 1981). It is not a good idea for one worker who has an interest or inclination to handle all the abuse cases. Cases should be spread evenly among staff so that no one worker is allowed to burn out and in turn withdraw support from families. However, once a positive therapeutic alliance is established by one worker with a family, everything possible should be done to protect that relationship. Having a different worker to see a family every week will only serve to increase the distrust and resistance in that family.

Abuse in Homes, Hospitals, and Community Agencies One can observe child abuse or neglect in any place where children are found. Community health nurses making home visits to a diabetic family member, for instance, may also observe abusive behavior or potential. Nurses in hospital emergency rooms or even pediatric waiting rooms will see parent-child interactions that lack empathy or tenderness and that include battering behaviors. Taking a routine family history in the perinatal period should contain assessment for abusive potential. It is both the prerogative and the responsibility of nurses to observe for abusive behaviors in any work setting. Substantial observation should be shared verbally with supervisory personnel and

carefully documented in the client's record when possible. (See Case Example 28-1.)

Spouse Abuse

Women as Victims While reports of husband abuse by wives do occur, they are much less frequent and less severe on the average than wife abuse by male partners (Carson & Finkelhor, 1982, p. 10; Gelles, 1979; Roy, 1977). Because men are typically stronger than women, have greater individual and economic freedom, and in most states enjoy laws and attitudes that discourage outside intervention into domestic assault or rape, the problem of battered and assaulted women is clearly the more pressing social and health care problem (Gaquin, 1978). It is also interesting to note that battered women have been found to be three times more likely to be pregnant than nonbattered women seen in emergency rooms (Carson & Finkelhor, 1982).

Gelles (1979) estimated that "no fewer than two million women are victims of severe physical violence each year" (p. 92). Actual numbers are difficult to establish because of the reticence of women to identify injuries as abuse, physicians' reluctance to diagnose the etiology of these women's trauma, and the closed nature of the families in conflict (Hornung, McCullough, & Sugimoto, 1983). However, public health and other officials have clearly recognized the problem of wife abuse as a serious national concern (Finkelhor & Yllo, 1978; Gaquin, 1978; Gelles, 1979; Schechter, 1982).

Societal and Historical Sanctions of Wife Abuse It is difficult to bring claims of spouse abuse forward and to have them effectively litigated. Marital rape or sexual assault of wives is difficult to establish and successfully prosecute (Geis, 1983). The ambiguity of laws dealing with spouse abuse has negative effects on the problem, such as the failure of women to seek medical, social, or legal intervention; prejudicial attitudes among law enforcement officials who blame victims rather than

Case Example 28-1: Childhood Sexual Abuse

Jane is a seven-year-old blond, blue-eyed child in the first grade. She is shy and withdrawn and seems to have problems keeping her attention span at an appropriate level.

Behavior problems at school are often signs of child abuse and sexual abuse at home.

On this morning Jane makes an unusual number of requests to go to the bathroom. The teacher decides to spend time talking with Jane over the lunch hour. Jane begins to cry and is unable to speak clearly, as if about to become hysterical.

Children may "act out" their fear and stress of sexual abuse through some part of the body associated with sexuality.

Over the next several days the teacher talks with the school nurse about Jane's behavior. With the aid of anatomically correct hand puppets and drawings, the nurse is able to learn that Jane is being sexually molested at home by her father.

Play therapy and the use of dolls are very effective in helping children express problems with abusive parents.

After talking with the school administration, it is decided to try to contact the mother for a conference. During the conference with the mother (the father is unable to get away from work to attend), the mother becomes very angry and denies that any such behavior on the part of the father could ever occur. She praises her husband for his warm generosity with the daughter and for his devotion to her. She later takes her daughter out of the classroom and enrolls her in a private school.

Families with incest may develop a "conspiracy of ignorance" about the sexual acting out.

The teacher and the nurse complete a written report of suspected sexual abuse by the father (incest). However, since there is very little confirming evidence and a complete denial by the mother, no intervention is made.

Even though no action is taken, this state may have a central registry of confirmed cases. Should another report be filed about this family, the case for intervention would become much stronger.

---

the abusers; and the reluctance of the courts to intervene. Marital sexual assault will likely continue to be a seriously underreported problem until state and federal laws clearly acknowledge and prohibit such actions (Campbell & Humphreys, 1984; Roundsaville, 1978; Stank, Filcroft, & Frazier, 1979).

Learned Helplessness and Victimization Basically, learned helplessness is a concept derived from social learning theory (Walker, 1979). Over time the abused develops beliefs, expectations, and responses that help to establish the notion that she

deserves the abuse, that she has no power to interfere with the abuse, and that the abuse is a naturally occurring fact of life (see Case Example 28-2). She gradually learns to settle down into a routine or cycle of abuse, often coupled with depression and/or substance abuse. Feeble efforts to control the abuser might include such coping mechanisms as deliberately irritating him and thus feeling "in charge" of when the abuse will occur.

These women feel that all control for what happens to them in life lies outside of the self, and the self can only just respond to the will of the external powers. Closely aligned with the concept of learned helplessness is victimization. Attitudes in society toward the victim of abuse or crime, in the home or on the streets, have been in themselves abuse (Williams, 1983). The victim is sometimes blamed for being passive, weak, unthinking, and sinful, and for bringing the assault on herself. Sex-role stereotyping in the society can reinforce this sense of victimization. As Williams sums it up: "The male role, as defined by this culture, usually shows a mixture of aggression and macho. . . . Women are socialized to accept the passive role and to expect victimization" (p. 43).

Psychoanalytic theory was also a source of support for the victimization of women by teaching that women are innately masochistic. Psychiatrists, consciously or not, subscribed to ideas of female inferiority and immaturity, a position that was not exposed and questioned until very recently (Sturdivant, 1980).

Diligent and carefully designed research into the sources of destructive myths about women's needs, wants, and abilities is essential to the healthful development of women and families. Accordingly, sound social and clinical programs for helping women to unlearn the patterns of beliefs and behaviors that lead to ongoing victimization and helplessness need vigorous development and evaluation. Community health nurses, as clinicians, researchers, husbands or wives, and fathers or mothers, can contribute enormously to this growth through their questioning, role-modeling, and educating at work and at home. Such contributions begin, however, with the individual nurse's willingness to raise questions about traditional roles for women in a rapidly changing society.

Elderly Abuse in the Home

"Grannybashing," a term new to the last decade, has found growing recognition here and abroad (Select Committee, 1980; Walshe-Brennan, 1977). However, unlike child abuse, the physical and psychological maltreatment of older persons in their families has received very little clinical and research attention. Few statistics are available, but what

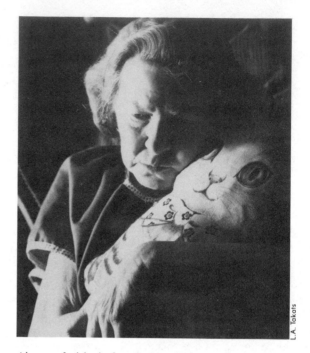

Abuse of elderly family members is a phenomenon receiving increasing attention from health professionals. Abuse can be physical, psychologic, or material and can result in injury or mental and affective changes such as disorientation and paranoid ideation.

information does exist suggests that older victims are white and have at least one chronic illness, and that abuse may be of multiple types. Physical disability is frequently observed (Block & Sinnott, 1979; Lau & Kosberg, 1979). Beck and Ferguson (1981) have made initial efforts to classify types of abuse, including physical abuse, psychological abuse, and material abuse. Physical abuse involves both battering and neglect and improper administration of drugs and medication. Psychological abuse is represented in verbal condescension, devaluing attitudes, and caretaker's failure to be empathetic or sensitive to the losses and grief of aging. Material abuse includes the theft or misuse of the older person's monetary or other possessions and resources. Hickey and Douglas (1981a) did not include material abuse per se; they did explore sexual abuse or molestation.

Case Example 28-2: Spouse Abuse

Tom and Mary arrive at the emergency room together looking nervous and upset. Tom states that Mary, his wife, had fallen down the stairs to the basement. Mary neither confirms nor denies that this occurred. She sits quietly, eyes downcast.

The history of the trauma given by couples involved in abuse are often not congruent with the affect of the persons reporting.

Mary has one blackened eye, bruises on both forearms, bruises around her breasts, and bruises on upper ribs on front and back. She reports that she is three months pregnant.

It is not unusual for batterers to strike victims on parts of the body usually covered by clothing.

Tom provides some social history. They do not have health insurance since he lost his job some months ago in the steel mills. They have two children, ages two and three years.

Economic stress of unemployment and the related loss of self-esteem are associated with domestic violence.

The physician applies emergency treatment for Mary's injuries and suggests she see an OB/Gyn physician regarding her pregnancy at her earliest convenience.

Many health care providers choose not to identify injuries as domestic violence, for fear of "meddling" in nonmedical concerns.

Then the physician discharges the couple.

Two months later the same physician treats Mary for her miscarriage. Mary now reports that her husband has been abusive to her and that he had kicked her in the abdomen. However, she refuses to press charges against Tom because she has nowhere else to go and she does not want to leave her small children. Besides, she says, Tom is very sorry and vows never to hit her again.

Failure to intervene in domestic violence can, and often does, lead to death and disability.

Mental and affective changes, such as confusional states, depression, disorientation, irritability, and paranoid ideation may be the effects of neglect and poor nutrition, hydration, and inadequate exercise. Bruises and fractures from falling because physical assistance was not provided during ambulation may also be classified as abuse. Unnecessary roughness during physical assistance or care may result in dislocations of joints and fractures. Obviously, health care workers, social workers, police officers, and others can best assess the health and welfare of older citizens in their homes if the potential for abuse is made a routine part of their evaluation.

The current literature on the causes of elder abuse in the home clusters around several themes and issues. These include the development of violence-prone personalities across several generations of a family; victimization of the weak or helpless; inadequate social policies and laws to protect the elderly; unresolved parent-child-parent conflict and life cycle role-reversals; social isolation of elder persons and/or family; stress on the homemaker-caretaker (usually an adult female); and situational/developmental crises (Champlin, 1982; Crouse et al, 1981; Hickey & Douglas, 1981b).

In many cases, the victim lives in the home of the abuser, suggesting that the added burden on the abuser's family increases the likelihood of impulsive acting out. Steuer and Austin (1980) associated abuse with alcohol use, continued unresolved conflict between elderly parent and child, the abuser's own childhood history of abuse, and inadequate social supports with coexisting increased economic and psychological dependency needs.

Case finding and detection are further complicated by the frequent denial by victims and family that abuse occurs, and by the prevailing attitude that what goes on inside a family dwelling is its own business. Violence may be a family's technique for dealing with conflicts. However, it is not the family's prerogative and should not preclude intervention (Block & Sinnott, 1979; Rathbone-McCuan, 1980).

Problems of the caretaker, typically a middle-aged daughter or daughter-in-law, include many stresses and few gratifications. She finds herself with teenaged children needing support for their own socialization. She may be experiencing midlife crisis—feeling that life has passed her by, that old age is just around the corner, and that she is losing attractiveness and value on the job market. These are frequent sources of depression and irritability. When the health care and emotional or economic needs of grandparents are imposed onto this already large pile of demands, they can tip the scales of self-control, and abuse may result.

Of course, old age brings with it the increased risk of mental health problems; forgetfulness, confabulation, paranoid ideas, and general senility are common examples. The caretaker-spouse, child, or wife may also have mental health problems that aggravate existing tension or interfere with his or her ability to give necessary and sufficient care to the elderly parent. The health care worker in the clinic or at home should carefully observe the psychosocial makeup of caretakers for evidence of existing mental illness. Appropriate psychiatric-mental health consultation is very helpful in these assessments and interventions. The already burdened caretaker is at greater risk of becoming an abuser when these problems receive little or no professional attention or intervention.

Those who plan services for the elderly, including prevention and intervention with abuse in home settings, need to appreciate the limitations of the family as care-giver. Today's family is less likely to be stationary and stable. Both parents are working outside the home and may be compelled to move job locations. Also, many elderly are now migrating to the warm weather states, often without familial support. It may be helpful, in the long run, to follow interstate and interagency referrals and planning for such basic moves. The U.S. Census Bureau, for instance, has planned changes in classification of data on the older citizen. The plan is to break down age into smaller categories and to cross-reference these with many socioeconomic and demographic variables. Such data might be useful in research that seeks to predict who will most likely be abused and under what circumstances. Does abuse occur more often in mobile families? Is abuse more likely in those areas of migration of the elderly? How do these conditions of smaller and more transitory families, often with both spouses working, and the aging migration to warm climates reflect cultural changes in felt values of concern and responsibility for the elderly family member (Long & Brady, 1983)?

Community health nurses and other professionals working with the elderly in their homes need to be mindful that their services might well serve the elderly in much the same way as did the "extended family" in earlier days. Without the available middle-aged female care-giver, other older children, or extended family members, the older person may no longer be able to count on total or sometimes even partial care from the family. The risks may even increase with the person's age. A recent study of twenty-two abused elderly in a major community program for the homebound elderly revealed that the abused older person is older than his or her nonabused counterpart; the abused experience feelings of helplessness, depression, and isolation. Also, there was frequent mention of histories of conflict with the now adult children caretakers (Vandenbos & Buchanan, 1983).

Nurses and agencies who expect that families

Case Example 28-3: Domestic Abuse

Dr. Smith, a nurse consultant in Psychiatric-Mental Health Consultation for a Community Health Service to the Homebound Elderly arrives at the agency's office for routine consultation with the staff nurses and social workers. Nancy, a social worker, and Barb, a community health nurse, begin to discuss Mr. Pasatori, a seventy-eight-year-old Italian patient. He has medical diagnoses including diabetes, COPD, and depression.

During their last visit, the nurse and social worker noticed that Mr. Pasatori had multiple bruises on both forearms. His skin turgor was very poor beyond his normal appearance. He complained of stiffness in his neck and shoulders, and he seemed listless and withdrawn.

Many abused elderly have several medical problems, are depressed, and are slightly older than non-abused elderly.

Bruises suggest that he has been forcibly held and/or shaken. Correspondingly, his uncommonly sad affect increases the nurse's concern about abuse.

Mrs. Pasatori, the patient's wife of fifty-five years, and an adult daughter were present for the visit. Their faces were tired and sullen. When the nurse asked about their care of Mr. Pasatori, they mumbled one-word answers, frequently finding reasons to leave the room.

Frequently, middle-aged adult daughters are stressed by two sets of burdens: caring for their parents and caring for their own families.

The adult daughter lives next door; she is married and has three high school aged children. Her husband is employed as a janitor at the local Catholic church where they attend services. Mr. and Mrs. Pasatori also have two adult sons who live out of state and who rarely visit. They are said to hate their father for past abuses and rigid punishment in discipline.

Dr. Smith, the consultant, encourages close, ongoing evaluation of nutrition and hydration, but also encourages the nurse to spend more time sitting with the daughter. Dr. Smith also emphasizes the importance of supporting the caretaker and recommends that Nancy begin to identify appropriate resources, such as homemaker assistance. Finally, Dr. Smith mentions the possible need for referral to family counseling.

When there is a history of intergenerational conflict, abuse may result.

---

can provide all health care for the elderly will be disillusioned and less effective than those who approach families as "temporary extended family members." Continuity and integration of caregivers' activities and interagency cooperation among health and social workers are essential. While patient and family education is very important, it is not enough. Real help in the form of homemakers, meals on wheels, financial planning, and family therapy or counseling is necessary (see Case Example 28-3). See Chapter 23 for a more detailed discussion of health services for the older adult.

Legal Aspects

Perhaps chief among the legal concerns of clinicians in their work with violent families is that of confidentiality. Generally speaking, communication and recording about work with families are protected when the nurse is working with an agency, hospital, or physician who assumes responsibility for treatment with the patient and family. Many health care agencies and hospitals employ attorneys who offer counsel to nurses and others who become involved in legal proceedings for whatever reasons in the course of their practice (Munro, 1984). Nurses should be aware of laws that detail rights and responsibilities in their jurisdiction of practice. Independent nurse practitioners with graduate preparation may need to seek private counsel on the legal aspects of working with family violence.

With regard to child abuse and neglect, all states have passed mandatory reporting laws that require that health and social welfare workers, among others, report actual or potential abuse (Humphreys, 1984). Community health nurses often visit families with such problems over many months and have opportunities to observe reportable abuse or potential abuse. This situation can pose conflict for nurses who wish to comply with the law, but who also seek to shelter the working rapport and trust they have managed to establish with the family. In most cases, it is preferable to be honest with the family that a report is being contemplated or prepared. A candid, clear, nonvalue-laden rationale should be presented with the specific dangers to health and development carefully spelled out. The nurse can ask family members to help develop the statement of concerns. In some situations the nurse can talk with the abusive parent or spouse and help them initiate a phone call to the appropriate official.

There are no specific protective services for reporting abuse to wives or the elderly, although many states are working on the development of policies. Nurses will need to seek additional supervisory and peer support in encouraging legal action, criminal or civil, to those victims. It would be very worthwhile to make visits to battered women's shelters such as those described recently (McEvay & Brookings, 1982). If the community does not have such shelters, nurses may wish to organize to develop a shelter. It would also be instructive to visit public court hearings on spouse abuse cases and to discuss the problems of litigation with attorneys who are active in these cases.

Most state nurses' associations have sister organizations or political arms such as SNAPI, State Nurses Active in Politics in Illinois. This organization supports lobbying activities that put forth such legislation as the Domestic Violence Act and Elder Abuse Act (HB2376 and HB2339, respectively). Professional nursing organizations can also foster legislation that will further protect nurses involved in legal proceedings. Such organizations benefit greatly from the participation of all professional nurses.

Strategies for Community Health Nursing Intervention

Primary Prevention: A Predictive Model of Abuse

Primary prevention of family violence can occur only to the extent that the problem can be predicted. Primary prevention strategies are therefore limited by the absence of predictive clinical tools and by the continuing tendency, at both individual and societal levels, to deny that the problems of family violence exist. Because of their excellent opportunities to reach out to victims in the home environment, community health nurses can, however, begin to make a difference.

Family violence research has thus far not been able to provide clinicians with the ability to predict potential or actual situations of abuse. Despite this uncertainty, the community health nurse can find conceptual frameworks and working models in the literature to guide clinical assessments. Figure 28-1 represents an effort to identify, from research and from the existing literature, the basic factors most likely to predict abusive situations. In this model the family is viewed as an open and interactionist system. Also implicit in the model are the forces of formal and informal social institutions, psychodynamic factors of family members,

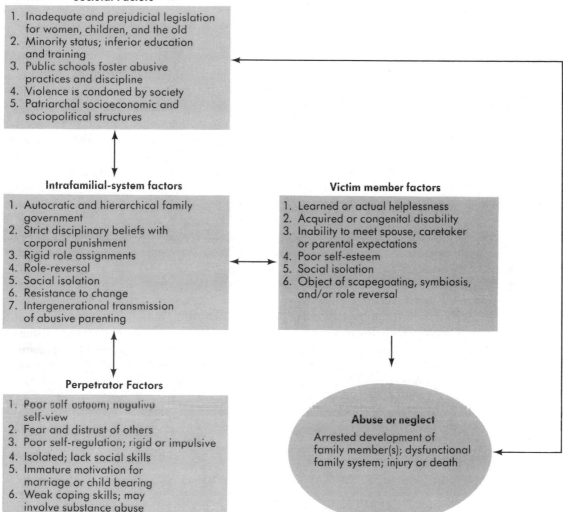

Figure 28-1 Family violence model: Domestic abuse of children, women, and the elderly. (Instrumentation for validating the most critical factors is being developed. Presentations of the model have included MNRS Minneapolis, April 1984; UCLA, School of Nursing, July 1984; and the National Behavior Medicine Conference, St. Paul, University of Minnesota, Fall 1983.)

changes in family systems over time, and the family's interaction with society.

Often community health nurses visit families in their homes over prolonged periods of time. Having this opportunity, nurses can observe the extent to which the family fits the model, whether or not actual injury has occurred. It is unlikely that every family will reflect every factor mentioned, since each family is unique. However, the family who does present many of these characteristics may become vulnerable to violent expression. While much additional research is needed in the development of predictive accuracy, especially well-controlled longitudinal studies, the practicing community health nurse can begin to sharpen observational skills on the basis of what is currently known about abusive families.

Nurses are more likely to observe and document potential for abuse in communities where economic and social support for prevention of abusive families is available. Such supports should include nonsexist family life educational programs in elementary schools, daycare centers for children, improved vocational and career opportunities for women, assertiveness and sensitivity training groups for couples, and provision of homemaker and home health aides.

Secondary Prevention

As a group, community health nurses have been leaders in the detection and care of abused and neglected children (Odum, 1981). Initially, this activity was retrospective—that is, involvement was initiated after the fact of abuse. Crisis intervention became a common mode of helping individuals and families after a violent episode. Well-developed communication skills are another important secondary prevention strategy for family violence.

Crisis Intervention   It is difficult, at best, to relate crisis theory to family violence. Crises, by definition, represent responses of a system in equilibrium to change or to threat of change. Previously existing coping strategies and the associated behaviors do not meet the demands of stressors or stressor events that threaten the system's homeostasis (Hall & Weaver, 1974; Rapoport, 1965).

If violence, such as battering behavior, is an *established strategy* for conflict resolution in an ongoing family system (indeed, across several generations of a family system), then assault is not a response to crises; it is a way of life. If it has been a family's practice to painfully wound a child as regular disciplinary behavior, or to resolve marital power struggles with spouse abuse, then change

that threatens that established practice may bring about crisis, such as when a child refuses to gratify an abusive parent, or a wife rebels. The crisis may then be expressed in the occurrence of unexpected or accidental death of the family victim; in dissolution of the family as a unit (the placement of a child in foster care by the courts); or in a grandparent's confiding to an outsider about abuse sustained in the home, rather than keeping quiet.

In other families, abuse or violence may be expressed in isolated and unpatterned behavior stimulated by situational or maturational crisis. For instance, stressors predisposing abuse to the elderly may include such factors as the caretaker's midlife phase with concurrent demands of both younger and older family members, her mandatory employment outside home, and unwanted change in body or self-image.

Whether the family crisis is reflected in new violent behavior or family dissolution—such as placement of a child in foster care, divorce, or nursing home placement for the previously home-bound elderly—the system is reacting to change. Families whose members are able to apply conscious problem-solving (including a clear perception of what has been happening in the system), who can delineate mutual goals to achieve a nonviolent resolution, and who have objective, informed, and compassionate outside support can overcome the crisis. The cycle of violence can be prevented or broken at this time of disequilibrium because the family will be more conscious of its problems and more receptive to intervention and support than at a time of equilibrium. Supporting the family's positive problem-solving efforts and mutual interaction is, therefore, one of the community health nurse's key secondary prevention strategies. Such support can result in the family's experience of developmental growth and higher order of satisfaction.

Community health nurses interact with families in their homes for longer periods of time than do more episodic care-givers. These nurses have vested interests in health promotion as well as in secondary prevention; their ability to anticipate both maturational and situational crises over time can provide opportunities to identify stressors that may precipitate or exaggerate violent coping behaviors.

Maturational crises occur at many points in the family life cycle. These points include marriage, childbirth, adolescence, midlife adjustments, old age and retirement, and death. Through anticipatory guidance, nurses can help family members recognize the stressfulness of these periods and identify the family's internal and external coping resources.

Community health nurses who are consistent in visiting, who make telephone and other contacts readily available, and who act as advocates and coordinators of care may be able to develop basic trust and permeate the otherwise closed family boundary.

Communication   Communication is the essential skill for effective nursing care with abusive families, but it is difficult for even the most advanced practitioner to master. The unique aspects of therapeutic interviewing with abusive families include:

1. Communication is directed to the family as a unit, not as a one-to-one approach.
2. More time and consistency are required than for most other types of family health problems.
3. The interviewer must have a capacity for empathy, warmth, genuineness and at the same time demonstrate assertiveness and leadership abilities.

Therapeutic communication begins with the goal of establishing at least minimal rapport with the family, especially its dominant member when that member is available. This rapport includes promoting the family's sense of trust and dependency. Dependency is not an end goal, but rather it is an attempt to have the parents experience something they have never experienced before—basic trust and fulfilled positive regard. Eventually, the family is able to extend this trust to others, becoming less isolated. Kempe and Helfer (1980) have referred to this increased ability to reach out as the establishment of "lifelines." Often these lifelines take

the form of telephone lines. The nurse who begins to receive phone calls from the abusive family has achieved progress, even when the call seems superficial or trivial. Small problems in the lives of these often desperate families can represent crisis-proportion stressors. Family members often do not have the necessary self-esteem and self-regulation to deal with "small" problems. It is important to reinforce this new reaching-out behavior by communicating openly and listening sensitively.

Including husbands in the interviewing process can be problematic, but it is essential to try. These efforts, couched in nonthreatening, positive language, may include leaving notes of invitation to join in discussions with the visiting nurse. Timing the visits very early in the day, after the husband has returned home from work, or on lunch hours is often successful, as is making appointments. Providing for the husband's inclusion can help to reduce his suspiciousness of what may be said "behind his back." It also provides an opportunity for the nurse to role-model an assertive but sensitive and caring posture with husbands who need the macho shroud and/or who tend to carry out violence when the macho image is threatened.

Active listening is effective in interviewing the family. Not only the members' words, but the non-verbal patterns of interaction should be observed and at some point shared with the family. For instance, are there threatening postures or gestures that intimidate responsiveness or communication among members?

In the initial phase of communication, it is especially important to maintain a nonjudgmental attitude and minimal advice-giving. This is most difficult when one observes harsh behavior between spouses or with children or the elderly. Unless immediate danger exists to the victimized person, however, criticism or condemnation must be avoided. Instead, the nurse may be able to divert attention and eventually come back to suggest alternative approaches to child discipline or spouse interaction. Typically, these families are not ready or prepared to listen to advice or to learn. Developing trust and rapport will lay the groundwork for later health teaching, counseling, and referral.

After the family has learned to trust the nurse, additional workers and supports can be introduced. If the nurse is not equipped to function as a family counselor or therapist, it is appropriate to introduce other qualified workers as the middle or working phase of nursing care begins to unfold. The nurse's role can shift toward that of advocate or coordinator of needed services. The family should not be allowed to feel however, that the nurse is preparing to withdraw from the family. The extension of the family's trust from the nurse to other practitioners can be tenuous at best, and premature termination at this point can usher in the family's retreat into its shell of social isolation and resistance.

As the nurse begins to observe patterns of interaction in the family, he or she can ask members to identify which of these are mutually supportive and which are prone to lead to violent conflict and abuse. For instance, a guilt-ridden middle-aged caretaker of an infirm elderly parent may assume sole responsibility for the latter all day, unable to set limits. Then in the night, when demands continue, the accumulated frustration may lead to abuse. The nurse can trace such patterns in spouse and child abuse as well.

Probably the most unique contribution community health nurses make to helping families avoid violence is the enhanced self-esteem of the members as individuals and as a group. It has been consistently suggested in the literature, that individuals who batter or abuse others have very low self-esteem. People who feel good about themselves are less inclined to use violence. Increased self-esteem can also assist the victim's perspective and problem-solving ability. A wife and mother who makes positive self-references and who attends better to grooming, diet, and dress may also begin to question the inevitability of her role as helpless victim.

Similarly, reduced social isolation as a goal of therapeutic communication can be observed. Willingness to have homemaker or home health aide assistance in the home, to visit clinics and counselors, to attend social support groups, or simply to visit neighbors are valid indicators of therapeutic gains.

Of course, reduction of violent behavior and increased capacity for verbal expression of both emotional and cognitive perceptions can be assessed in evaluation of progress. Probably many of these homes, with years of history of violence or abuse, will not become gardens of sweetness and light. The terminating phase of community health nursing therapy can begin when the home has been "safe" for all its members for several months.

Terminating with abusive families is a gradual and planned process that may take weeks. Much depends on the availability of community services and the capacity of the family to establish lifelines with these services. In some cases, community health nurses may want to maintain informal contact with the family indefinitely. One nurse known to the author continues to exchange "Mother's Day" cards with an ex-child-abusing mother years after the therapeutic alliance officially ended. Both reportedly derive much gratification from this limited, but powerful, communication.

Initiating effective referrals to other community services during and while terminating nursing care with abusive families is very helpful in achieving and maintaining therapeutic goals. Unfortunately, such services are often too limited or lacking totally (Martin, 1976). A dependent and battered wife's cooperation may be impossible to enlist when there are no supportive community resources, such as shelters, vocational training centers, daycare centers, and various psychological and legal counseling services. Communities who fail to provide such services cannot expect community health nursing intervention to have much effect on problems of family violence. Indeed, no single service, whether medical, social, or psychological, can have lasting impact standing alone. A consortium of services sharing a philosophy of intervention is the only hopeful approach to decreasing abuse in the home and its sequelae of social and cultural violence (Braen & Warner, 1983; Steele, 1980).

Tertiary Prevention

Institutional care of victims of family violence is, in many cases, the only alternative. Foster home placement of abused children, nursing home placement of the abused elderly, and imprisonment of severe abuse perpetrators have become familiar solutions.

Total care of children and old people in the home with the primary burden on the wife-homemaker is not realistic in contemporary society. The increasing necessity of two-income family economy, the rising number of aged in the population and inadequate access to birth control and planned parenthood among very young and poor women present unreasonable expectations to today's small, transient, nuclear families. Until the larger society assumes greater responsibility for child care, care of the elderly, and promotion of egalitarian family life styles, the family will continue to have major internal conflicts.

Enormous emotional and psychological pain is experienced by many families as they realize they cannot take care of their own in the home. The pain may take the form of social shame, intrapsychic guilt, depression, and anxiety. Families who are already violence-prone in their coping efforts will likely experience increased violence.

Community health nurses are commonly involved with families facing such dilemmas. In these situations, it is important for the nurse to remain nonjudgmental about the family's "failure" and to assume objective, problem-solving postures in helping the family assess and plan for the necessary placement of a member. In this process, the nurse will want to address the following questions:

- What kind of care does the member need—medical, nursing, psychological, socialization programs, or specialized housing?
- Have all existing resources (homemakers and health aides, daycare programs, meals-on-wheels, financial aid, family therapy, shelters, legal counsel, and intervention by the courts) been exhausted in helping the family manage at home?
- What does the family really want to do; is conflict with the victim insurmountable or too entrenched to be reduced? Has the family had sufficient opportunity to express frustration, anger,

and aggression without recrimination for having such feelings?
- Can the family deal with the preceding questions? If so, what do they expect the nurse to contribute toward the answers? If the family asks the nurse to decide for them about placement, nurses can make clear that this is not appropriate. To promote the family's sense of participation in their own care the nurse shares the results of assessments concerning perceived strengths and weaknesses in the family, available resources, and the success of past coping efforts. Such objective feedback from an outside observer greatly facilitates the family problem-solving activity.

Of course, the ideal solution is to help the family remain intact. While placement of a member may ease immediate crisis situations, the resulting family fracture can have years of detrimental social and psychological effects. Such effects include shame, guilt, and perceived social alienation. Few communities have developed the kinds of multiservice and coordinated programs needed to effectively intervene in family violence (Erickson, McElroy, & Colucci, 1984). Robbins outlines the types of needed services, including emergency medical care, shelters, vocational and career training, ambulatory clinics, nurse practitioners, child development centers, and advocacy and counseling services (Robbins, 1983).

Increasingly, community health nurses are realizing that effective nursing care is possible only when that care is orchestrated among an array of community health and social services. In the case of family violence, this is especially true. However, what is important is not just the existence of such services, but their strong commitment to the rights of women, children, and the elderly. Further, society must recognize that the "sanctity" of the home loses its meaning and privileges when members of the family are routinely battered, abused, and neglected. To the extent that patriarchal and macho roles contribute to the violence, communities will need to provide counseling services, sensitivity training, nonsexist couple and family therapy, and legal interventions to facilitate the perpetrator's rehabilitation.

In any case, the "conspiracy of ignorance" that for so long has clouded the extent of domestic violence in this country is over; the movement toward a more egalitarian society and family life-style has clearly begun, with increased effort to provide for the rights of women, children, and the old.

Community health nursing's contribution to this important movement goes beyond the purely clinical role. It has been estimated that one in every forty-four women voters is a nurse. Collectively,

this amounts to significant political power to invest on behalf of battered women, abused children, and victimized elderly citizens. Elected officials who note the trend toward a more representative democracy in this pluralistic country would be wise to seek the counsel of nursing in making decisions about health care dollar allocations, policy-making, and legislation that will determine the fate of victims of family violence. Ultimately, it is the courage and persistence of the individual practicing nurse that will bring this attention to nursing.

Summary

Domestic violence in this country is prevalent, acceptable, and largely unresponsive to traditional controls and interventions. Neither criminal nor civil laws are sufficiently enforced and in some areas are nonexistent. While the identification and reporting of abusive situations have increased, corrective activities are sporadic, poorly funded, and uncoordinated.

The need for broadly based and progressive social legislation to prevent victimization is eminent. Similarly, health care institutions need to develop systems for evaluation of need for social supports and referral and networking mechanisms.

Informed community health nurses can make significant contributions to solving problems of family violence when they are open to detection of the problem; are willing to get and stay involved; possess a personal capacity for assertiveness and can act as advocate for victims; keep informed of what services exist in the community and act politically to expand and coordinate those services; choose to work for agencies or hospitals who maintain nonsexist, egalitarian, and caring attitudes for victims.

Nurses prepared at the master's and doctoral level can provide private or independent counseling services for victims. These may range in focus from

couple and family therapy to rape counseling or group therapies for parents concerned about child abuse. Independent nurse practitioners may also function as consultants to community agencies. Among these are homebound elderly programs, visiting nurse associations, and schools.

Topics for Nursing Research

- What are the major characteristics of abusive families? How are abusive families different from families who do not abuse members?
- How should abuse be defined for research purposes? Should the definition include psychological and sexual abuse as well as physical battering and neglect?
- What intervention programs involving nursing exist and what is the best way to measure their effectiveness?
- What is the difference between a psychological model of domestic violence and abuse and a sociocultural model of domestic violence and abuse? Which type of model is best suited for nursing research?

Study Questions

1. Primary prevention of nonaccidental injury and failure-to-thrive in families involves the ability to predict or identify a potential for violence or abuse. Which of the following sets of factors is most indicative of such potential based on the model presented in this chapter? (Choose one.)
   a. Psychosocial history of abuse or neglect in the family; social isolation; societal sanctions for violence as means of conflict resolution; dependency and learned helplessness among victims; and patriarchal family structure
   b. Symptoms of psychosis or paranoia; frequent use of marijuana; social deviancy in dress and mannerisms
   c. Poverty; lack of motivation to find employment or keep a job; lack of religious training; and shiftless character
   d. Working mothers neglect their children; health care officials and law officers are overly eager to pry into the domestic affairs of families; and society encourages domestic conflict by providing shelters for women and daycare facilities for children

2. If a family *habitually* uses violence to resolve conflict and to maintain its equilibrium, what kinds of events might stimulate or lead to crises, such as the loss of a member or the breakup of the family through divorce or placement? (Choose one.)
   a. An increase in victim's helplessness and dependency
   b. A member's disclosure of abuse and active seeking of help
   c. Increased power or autonomy of the victim
   d. b and c

3. In a family that has *not* used violence, but which has relied on rigid patriarchal structure and social isolation to maintain its equilibrium, what kinds of circumstances might prompt their use of violence and abuse? (Choose one or more.)
   a. Birth of a child or pregnancy
   b. Loss of a job for the "head" of household
   c. Major physical illness of a member, especially a parent
   d. Conflict between a parent and an emerging adolescent's autonomy

4. Incest is described as:
   a. An avowed relationship between a parent and child or siblings involving sexual behavior
   b. Coerced sexual performance by a child on demand of a parent or older or more powerful sibling or relative
   c. Any verbal or physical sexual behavior between a minor and an adult in a familial unit, which must be kept *secret*
   d. b and c

5. On the level of secondary prevention of family violence and abuse, the role of the nurse includes:
   a. Active participation in the community to promote daycare centers, shelters for battered women, consciousness-raising groups for men in relations with women and children, and educational programs to educate children about appropriate refusals to adult overtures for physical contact
   b. Working with other members of the health care professions to be willing to identify violence and abuse injuries and to get involved in the treatment and referral processes
   c. Working with the state nurses associations to promote legislation that would support legal interventions into domestic violence and abuse, such as mandatory reporting of child abuse, agencies to investigate domestic abuse of the elderly, and the renaming of rape as "criminal sexual assault"
   d. All of the above

References

Anderson K: Cover story. *Time*, September 5, 1983.

Authier K: Incest and sexual violence. In: Hansen J (editor), *Sexual Issues in Family Therapy*. Germantown, Md.: Aspen Systems Corporation, 1983.

Bandura A: *Aggression: A Social Learning Analysis*. Englewood Cliffs, N.J.: Prentice-Hall, 1973.

Barnhill L, Hansen J: *Clinical Approaches to Family Violence*. Germantown, Md.: Aspen Systems Corporation, 1982.

Bavolek S: *Primary Prevention of Child Abuse and Neglect: Identification of High Risk Adolescents Prior to Parenthood* (doctoral dissertation). University of Utah, 1978.

Beck CM, Ferguson D: Aged abuse. *Journal of Gerontological Nursing* 1981; 7 (6): 333–336.

Berger AM: The child abusing family: Methodological issues and parent-related characteristics of abusing families. In: Olson D, Miller C (editors), *Family Studies Review Yearbook.* Beverly Hills, Calif.: Sage Publications, 1983.

Block M, Sinnott J (editors): *The Battered Elder Syndrome: An Exploratory Study.* College Park, Md.: University of Maryland, 1979.

Braen G, Warner C (editors): *Management of the Physically and Emotionally Abused.* New York: Appleton-Century-Crofts, 1983.

Brownmiller S: *Against Our Will: Men, Women, and Rape.* New York: Simon and Schuster, 1975.

Burgess A: Intra-familial sexual abuse. In: Campbell J, Humphrey J (editors), *Nursing Care of Victims of Family Violence.* Englewood Cliffs, N.J.: Reston Publishing Company, 1984.

Burgess A et al.: *Sexual Abuse of Children and Adolescents.* Lexington, Mass.: Heath, 1978.

Campbell J, Humphreys J (editors): *Nursing Care of Victims of Family Violence.* Englewood Cliffs, N.J.: Reston Publishing Company, 1984.

Carson B, Finkelhor D: The scope of contemporary social and domestic violence. In: Barnhill L, Hansen J (editors), *Clinical Approaches to Family Violence.* Germantown, Md.: Aspen Systems Publications, 1982.

Caufield C, Disbrow M, Smith M: Determining indicators of potential for child abuse and neglect: Analytical problems in methodological research. *Commun Nurs Res* 1977; 12: 141–163.

Champlin L: The battered elderly. *Geriatrics* 1982; 37 (7): 121.

Condran J, Bode J: Rashomon, working wives, and family division of labor: Middletown, 1980. *Journal of Marriage and the Family* 1982; 44 (2): 421–426.

Cromwell R, Olson D (editors): *Power in Families.* New York: Wiley, 1975.

Crouse J et al: *Abuse and Neglect of the Elderly in Illinois.* Springfield, Ill.: Sagamon State University, 1981.

Dobash RE, Dobash RP: *Violence Against Wives: A Case of the Patriarchy.* New York: Free Press, 1979.

Driefus C (editor): *Seizing Our Bodies.* New York: Vintage Books, 1977.

Easton B: Feminism and the contemporary family. In: Scott N, Pleak E (editors), *A Heritage of Her Own.* New York: Simon and Schuster, 1975.

Edwards J, Kluck P: Patriarchy: the last universal. *Journal of Family Issues* 1980; 1 (3): 333.

Eisenstein Z: The sexual politics of the new right: Understanding the crisis of liberalism. *Signs* 1982; 7 (3): 567–584.

Erickson E, McElroy A, Colluci N: *Child Abuse and Neglect,* Holmes Beach, Fla.: Learning Publications, 1984.

Farrar F: Family rigidity. In: Clements I, Buchanan D (editors), *Family Therapy.* New York: Wiley, 1982.

Finkelhor D, Yllo K: Rape in marriage. In: Finkelhor D et al (editors), *The Dark Side of Families.* Beverly Hills, Calif.: Sage Publications, 1983.

Fitzpatrick J et al: *Nursing Models and their Psychiatric-Mental Health Applications.* Bowie, Md.: Robert Brady Company, 1982.

Foley T: Nursing intervention in family abuse and violence. In: Stuart G W, Sundeen S (editors), *Principles and Practice of Psychiatric Nursing.* St. Louis, Mo.: Mosby, 1983.

Gaquin D: *Spouse Abuse: Data from the National Crime Survey.* Washington, DC: Visage Press, 1978.

Garbarino J: The human ecology of child maltreatment: A conceptual model for research. *Journal of Marriage and the Family* 1977; 39: 721–735.

Geis G: Interaction with the legal system. In: Braen G, Warner C (editors), *Management of the Physically and Emotionally Abused.* New York: Appleton-Century-Crofts, 1983.

Gelles R: *Family Violence.* Beverly Hills, Calif.: Sage Publications, 1979.

Gelles R: Violence in the family: A review of research in the seventies. In: Olson D, Miller B (editors), *Family Studies Yearbook Vol. 1.* Beverly Hills, Calif.: Sage Publications, 1981.

Germain C: Sheltering abused women: A nursing perspective. *J Psychosoc Nurs* 1984; 22 (9): 24.

Gettys C, Humphreys W (editors): *Understanding the Family: Stress and Changes in American Family Life.* New York: Appleton-Century-Crofts, 1981.

Gil D: Violence against children. *Journal of Marriage and the Family* 1971; 32 (17): 637–648.

Graham K: Theories of intoxicated aggression. *Canadian Journal of Behavioral Science* (April) 1980; 12: 141–158.

Gray J, Kaplan B: The lay visitor program: An eighteen month experience. In: Kempe CH, Helfer R (editors), *The Battered Child.* University of Chicago Press, 1980.

Greenberg N: The epidemiology of childhood sexual abuse. *Pediatr Ann* 1979; 8 (5).

Hall J, Weaver R: *Nursing of Families in Crises.* Philadelphia: Lippincott, 1974.

Hare-Mustin R: A feminist approach to family therapy. *Family Process* 1978; 17: 181.

Helfer R, Schneider C, Hoffmeister J: *Report on the Research Using the Michigan Screening Profile of Parenting.* East Lansing, Mich.: Michigan State University, 1978.

Herman J: *Father Daughter Incest.* Cambridge, Mass.: Harvard University Press, 1981.

Hickey T, Douglas R: Mistreatment of the elderly in the domestic setting: An exploratory study. *Am J Public Health* 1981a; 71 (5): 171.

Hickey T, Douglas R: Neglect and abuse of elder family

members: Professionals' perspectives and care experiences. *Gerontologist* 1981b; 21 (2): 171.

Hogan R: *Human Sexuality.* New York: Appleton-Century-Crofts, 1980.

Hornung B, McCullough R, Sugimoto T: Status relationships in marriage: Risk factors in spouse abuse. In: Olson D, Miller B (editors), *Family Studies Yearbook,* vol. 1. Beverly Hills, Calif.: Sage Publications, 1983.

Humphreys W: The nurse and the legal system: Dealing with abused women. In: Campbell J, Humphreys J (editors), *Nursing Care of Victims of Family Violence.* Englewood Cliffs, N.J.: Reston Publishing Company, 1984.

Justice B, Justice R: *The Abusing Family.* New York: Human Sciences Press, 1976.

Kalmuss D, Strauss M: Wives' marital dependency and wife abuse. *Journal of Marriage and the Family* (May) 1982: 277.

Kempe CH, Helfer R: *The Battered Child.* University of Chicago Press, 1980.

Kempe CH, Helfer R (editors): *Child Abuse and Neglect: The Family and the Community.* Cambridge, Mass.: Ballinger, 1979.

King, I: *Toward a Theory for Nursing.* New York: Wiley, 1971.

Laborit H: The biological and sociological mechanisms of aggression. *International Social Science Journal* 1978; 30: 728–749.

Lau E, Kosberg J: Abuse of the elderly by informal care providers. *Aging* (September) 1979: 10–15.

Laws J: A feminist review of marital adjustment literature and the Rape of the Locke. *Journal of Marriage and the Family* (August) 1971; 483–485.

Levant R: Sociological and clinical models of the family: An attempt to identify paradigms. *American Journal of Family Therapy* 1980; 8 (4).

Light R: Abused and neglected children in America: A study of alternative policies. *Harvard Educational Review* 1973; 43: 198–240.

Logenberry D, Nilsson K, Lundetin C: Life style patterns in families with neglected children. *Child Abuse and Neglect* 1979; 3 (2).

Long A, Brody E: Characteristics of middle-aged daughters and help to their mothers. *Journal of Marriage and the Family* 1983; 45 (1): 193–202.

Martin D: *Battered Wives.* San Francisco: Glide Publications, 1976.

McEvoy A, Brookings J: *Helping Battered Women.* Holmes Beach, Fla.: Learning Publications, 1982.

Milner J, Wimberley RL: An inventory for the identification of child abusers. *J Clin Psychol* 1979; 35 (1).

Montagu MFA: *Man and Aggression.* New York: Oxford University Press, 1968; 16.

Munro J: The nurse and the legal system. In: Campbell J, Humphreys J (editors), *Nursing Care of Victims of Family Violence.* Englewood Cliffs, N.J.: Reston Publishing Company, 1974.

Naisbitt J: *Megatrends.* New York: Warner Books, 1982.

Nash J: Book review. *Signs* 1981; 7 (2): 492.

Nelson M, Taylor P: Power relationships in marriage: The fine print in the oral tradition. In: Getty C, Humphreys W (editors), *Understanding the Family: Stress and Change in American Family Life.* New York: Appleton-Century-Crofts, 1981.

Odum R: Retrospective analysis of relationships between developmental and health parameters of abused children and parental responses to helping-persons (unpublished dissertation). Chicago: Rush University, Ill., 1981.

Pagelow M: *Woman Battering: Victims and their Experiences.* Beverly Hills, Calif.: Sage Publications, 1981.

Parke J, Collmer CW: Child abuse: An interdisciplinary analysis. In: Heatherington E (editor), *Child Development Research.* University of Chicago Press, 1975.

Rapoport L: The state of crisis: Some theoretical considerations. In: Parad J (editor), *Crisis Intervention.* New York: Family Service Association of America, 1965.

Rathbone-McCuan E: Elderly victims of family violence and neglect. *Journal of Contemporary Social Work* (May) 1980; 296.

Resick P: Sex role stereotypes and violence against women. In: Rothblum E, Frank V (editors), *The Stereotyping of Women: Its Effects on Mental Health.* New York: Springer Publishing Company, 1983.

Robbins J: Community planning. In: Braen G, Warner C (editors), *Management of the Physically and Emotionally Abused.* New York: Appleton-Century-Crofts, 1983.

Roundsaville B: Battered wives: Barriers to identification and treatment. *Am J Orthopsychiatry* 1978; 46 (3).

Roy M: *Battered Women.* New York: Van Nostrand, 1977.

Rory M, Earp J: Child maltreatment: An analysis of familial and institutional predictors. *Journal of Family Issues* 1980; 3 (3): 339.

Scanzoni J: *Shaping Tomorrow's Family: Theory and Policy for the 21st Century.* Beverly Hills, Calif.: Sage Publications, 1983.

Schaef AW: *Women's Reality.* Englewood Cliffs, N.J.: Reston Publishing Co., 1982.

Schechter S: *Women and Male Violence.* Boston: South End Press, 1982.

Schmitt B: *Child Abuse and Neglect: The Visual Diagnosis of Non-accidental Trauma and Failure-To-Thrive.* Denver: University of Colorado Medical Center, 1979.

Selby J, et al: Families of incest: A collation of clinical impressions. Department of Psychology, University of North Carolina, 1979.

Select Committee on Aging: *Elder Abuse: The Hidden Problem.* Committee Publication 96–200, 1980.

Sgroi S: *Handbook of Clinical Intervention in Child Abuse.* Lexington, Mass.: Lexington Books, 1982, 9–36.

Stanford Observer, October, 1983.

Stank E, Filcroft A, Frazier W: Medicine and patriarchal violence: The social construction of a private event. *International Journal of Health Services* 1979; 8.

Steele B: Psychodynamic factors in child abuse. In: Kempe C H, Helfer R (editors), *The Battered Child.* University of Chicago Press, 1980.

Steuer J, Austin E: Family abuse of the elderly. *Journal of the American Gerontological Society* 1980; 28 (8): 372–377.

Sturdivant S: *Therapy with Women,* vol. 2. New York: Springer Publishing Company, 1980.

Taggart M: The feminist critique in Epistemological Perspective: Questions of context in family therapy. *Journal of Marital & Family Therapy* 1985; 11 (2): 113–126.

Vandenbos G, Buchanan J: Research on aging and national policy: A communication with Robert Butler. *American Psychologist* 1983; 38 (3): 300–307.

Walker L: *The Battered Woman.* Harper and Row, 1979.

Walshe-Brennan K: Grannybashing. *Nursing Mirror* 1977; 145: 32–34.

Waterman J, Young J: Educational approaches to management and prevention of family violence. In: Braen R, Warner C (editors), *Management of the Physically and Emotionally Abused.* New York: Appleton-Century-Crofts, 1983.

Whall A: Congruence between existing theories of family functioning and nursing theories. *Adv Nurs Sci* 1980; 3 (1): 66.

Williams LM: Changing attitudes toward victims of violence. In: Braen R, Warner C (editors), *Management of the Physically and Emotionally Abused.* New York: Appleton-Century-Crofts, 1983.

Chapter 29

Health Policies:
Managing Change in Community Health Nursing

Helen K. Grace

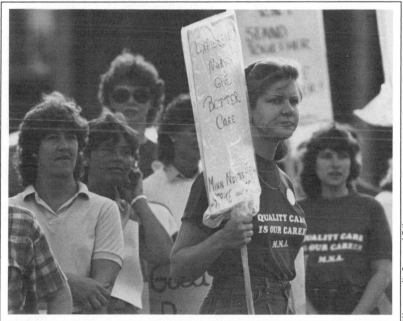

Minneapolis Star and Tribune

Nurses' increasing professionalism and activism will pave more powerful avenues for their influence on the formation of health policies.

Chapter Objectives

After completing this chapter, the reader will be able to:

- Discuss the relationship between health care issues and health policy formation
- Give examples of health policies that affect community health nursing practice
- Describe the role of the federal government and other institutions in health policymaking
- Outline challenges community health nurses may face in the future, and discuss strategies they may employ to assist them to meet these strategies

Community health nursing has undergone many changes during its history and must survive many current and future changes to remain a viable speciality. Heinrich (1983) compares the changes community health nursing has experienced to a pendulum swinging between sets of opposites: "community focus versus individual and family focus; health education versus treatment of illness; generalization versus specialization; apprenticeship versus higher education; hospital care versus home care; nursing integrated with welfare services versus separate, generally available public health services" (pp. 317–318).

These contrasting influences on community health nurses date back to the nineteenth century when William Rathborn, with support from Florence Nightingale, established district nursing in England (Heinrich, 1983; Monteiro, 1985). The motivation to establish district nursing to provide health care to the sick poor was fueled by some of the same issues facing health care providers today:

- The need to provide health care to the poor and indigent
- Unavailability of hospital beds
- High cost of hospital beds
- Suitability of the home environment to provide cost-effective care
- Need to incorporate family members in the care of sick members
- Preference of some people to be cared for in their homes

- Advantages of caring for some people (the chronically ill and terminally ill and those who are confined) in their homes rather than in the hospital

In addition to these issues, another integral aspect of district nursing still relevant for health providers in the community is the orientation toward, and emphasis on "health nursing" (health promotion and wellness) as opposed to "sick nursing" (disease prevention and cure) (Heinrich, 1983; Monteiro, 1985).

The health issues that community health nurses face now are a reflection of the dominant health policies at this moment in history. Also, they affect not only community health nursing but all nursing specialties and the health care system in general.

Since the post–World War II period, health policies have reflected the predominant focus on hospital-based, acute care services for the treatment of disease. Beginning in the late 1970s, and accelerating into the 1980s, health policies were confronted with new influences such as increased public concern over the costs of health care, alternatives to institutionalization, home health care, and a growing interest in health promotion and disease prevention. This chapter will trace the social, economic, and political issues that are reflected in changing health care policies and the implications that can be drawn for family-centered community nursing.

Historical Perspective

The Post–World War II Years

Prior to World War II, most medical care was provided in the home; hospitals were primarily used for the treatment of those who had no families to care for them. The physician made home calls to oversee treatment of the ill, and private duty nurses provided nursing care for those patients requiring specialized care over and above that which the family could provide. Nurses were educated within hospitals, and students, as part of their training, provided most of the nursing services to hospitalized patients. However, once training was completed, most nurses practiced in the home setting. Only a few registered nurses remained in hospitals as administrators and teachers. The bulk of nurses in practice served to supplement the family's efforts in caring for the sick within the home. Nurses carefully followed physicians' directives, but their social contract was with the family, who paid directly for the services rendered. Within this structure, nurses had a great deal of autonomy and were responsible for their own practice.

World War II totally transformed this system of medical care for the ill. First, nurses were enlisted into the army for the care of the sick. This served to deplete the numbers of nurses available to provide home-based nursing care services. Second, while student nurses continued to provide the bulk of nursing services to hospitalized patients as part of their training, upon completion of their training large numbers of them went into the armed services. A policy that gave significant support for this trend was the establishment of the Nurse Cadet Corps; under auspices of this program a large number of nurses had their education financed in exchange for serving a term of duty in military service.

The role of nurses in the war effort was markedly different from that of the family-based nurse of the past. While at the front line, nurses had wide-ranging responsibilities for care of the wounded soldier. When wounded soldiers were removed from the front-line emergency treatment centers, they were taken to the equivalent of the modern acute treatment hospital. Here, in an institutional setting, nurses became directly involved in patient care and in the accompanying management of other health-related personnel, such as aides and orderlies. With the high numbers of wounded soldiers and the limited numbers of doctors, physicians were primarily involved in treatment of injuries in the acute stage, while nurses were responsible for ongoing nursing care and rehabilitation. Thus, the circumstances of war gave nurses continued autonomy and independence in their practice, but the setting had moved from the home to the hospital. Meanwhile, reliance on sophisticated technology and a controlled setting for the treatment of disease began to increase.

When the war ended, the hospital became the commonly accepted locus of care. Hospitals were rapidly built, fueled by support from the federal government. As every community saw its own hospital as an essential part of the community, the need for nurses and nursing personnel to staff hospitals accelerated. Prior to the war the family had been the major care-giver for the ill. Removal of the patient from the family, however, necessitated that services previously provided by the family now be the responsibility of the hospital. The need for nursing personnel to staff hospitals was enormous.

It had been anticipated that nurses engaged in the war effort would return to staff the burgeoning hospitals, but this did not happen. Nurses went in one of two directions. First, the enactment of the GI bill provided support for nurses to enroll in educational programs to earn academic degrees, both at the baccalaureate and graduate levels. A large number of nurses availed themselves of this opportunity. Another large group pursued the post–World War II American dream: marriage and family. This latter group of nurses largely retired from nursing, except for those who worked part-time to supplement the family income.

In the meantime the proliferation of hospitals, fueled by public policy, resulted in an acute shortage of nurses. A new field of hospital administration was also emerging. The lay hospital administrator replaced the physician, or in some instances the nurse, as the chief manager of the hospital. Hospital administrators viewed nurses as blue-collar workers. In contrast, nursing was moving toward a greater degree of professionalization.

The trend toward professionalization was most profoundly reflected in nursing education. Nurses who had moved into programs of higher education became nurse educators. Many of these educators, concerned about the limited background provided nurses in nurse training programs, sought to upgrade nursing education, and concluded that the only way to accomplish this was to move nurse training out of hospital-based programs and into universities. Shifting baccalaureate and graduate level nursing education away from the hospital setting thus created what has been called the "education-practice gap." Education in the university became increasingly theoretical with limited amounts of clinical practice.

Although university programs drew increasing enrollments, these lengthened programs did not have the capacity to prepare the numbers of nurses needed to staff hospitals. The baccalaureate-prepared nurse added to the number of categories of nursing personnel that emerged to meet the need created in the burgeoning hospital field. The nurse's aide, the licensed practical nurse, and the registered nurse prepared out of the hospital-based diploma schools formed the backbone of nursing care delivery in the late 1940s and 1950s. In the 1960s, the two-year associate degree nurse emerged as yet another category of nurse. The interest in producing adequate numbers of nurses grew out of the prevailing concerns for staffing the acute care hospital. During this period, interest and concern for family-centered community nursing was minimal at best, with only a limited amount of content included in baccalaureate nursing educational programs. Nevertheless, throughout the history of public health nursing, nursing leaders, including Florence Nightingale, had emphasized the need for special training for nurses who work in the community and in families' homes. Following World War I, the Committee for the Study of Nursing Education, funded by the Rockefeller Foundation, specifically recommended postgraduate training in public health for nurses working in that area (Heinrich, 1983).

The 1960s and 1970s

As nursing began to be recognized as a national priority, the federal government established the Nursing Division within the United States Public Health Service. The importance of nursing as a national resource was reflected in public policy establishing support for advanced nursing education. In the meantime, hospitals were becoming increasingly labor-intensive and medicine more highly specialized. With federal support for nursing education, graduate programs followed the model of clinical specialization. While early graduate programs prepared administrators and teachers, the vogue of clinical specialization increased the numbers of graduate students seeking specialized preparation within medical-surgical nursing, obstetrics, pediatrics, and psychiatric/mental-health nursing. In community health, nurse practitioner programs were begun to prepare baccalaureate-level nurses for advanced specialty roles in family adult and school health.

In 1965 the first nurse practitioner program was initiated in Colorado (Ford, 1982). The program began as a demonstration project in which nurses were prepared as pediatric nurse practitioners to provide comprehensive care to well children. Preparation in other specialty areas such as adult and family followed (Ford, 1982).

In the practitioner model the nurse became skilled in assessing physical problems and the management of patients with a wide range of chronic conditions. Here also the model was that of increased specialization and a focus on the individual and the family rather than on a broader perspective— that is, the community as client. This emphasis in practitioner programs led to conflict among some groups over what constitutes the proper focus for nurses prepared to work in communities (Anderson, 1983). Nurse practitioner programs were perceived as deviating from the traditional roles and functions of public health nursing—that is, away from the population-based nursing of aggregates and whole communities, and toward the care of individuals in the community setting. As discussed in Chapter 1, the question of what constitutes the proper focus of community versus public health nursing is still an issue debated among leaders in the field. Consequently, although many graduate programs had a community health component, this field became somewhat fragmented between those who viewed community health in a traditional framework and those advocating preparation as nurse practitioners caring for individuals and families as well as communities.

Nursing education reflected the prevailing focus on preparing nurses for the high technology, specialized hospital of the 1960s. While a limited number of nurse practitioners were prepared, nurses generally practiced in the hospitals.

The ethos of the 1960s, characterized by its emphasis on the unlimited resources and the brave new frontier of outer space, served to influence public policy in an expansionist direction. In all aspects of life the federal government was becoming increasingly involved. This was certainly evident in the health field. Describing the history of the National Institutes of Health, Young notes: "In the 1960s many lay people and experts with personal experience with specific diseases gave testimony to Congress (parents whose children had died of cancer, individuals suffering from multiple sclerosis, kidney failure, epilepsy, cancer, heart disease, etc.). . . . This period of medical research has been nicknamed 'The Disease of the Month Club' " (Larson, 1984, p. 354).

Increasingly, the government was getting centrally involved in public policymaking that directly influenced the shape and direction of medical care delivery for the decades ahead. The orientation was toward the "conquering of disease" as epitomized by President Nixon's 1971 State of the Union speech declaring "war on cancer" (Larson, 1984, p. 354).

Since the late 1960s and early 1970s the federal government has played a major role in determining health policies that affect nursing, including community health nursing. The federal government had paid for the health care of many of the nation's poor and elderly. It has financed health and health-related research, education of health professionals, and the construction and renovation of health facilities. The federal government's commitment and involvement in health care is evidenced by its ever-expanding budget for health expenditures (Aiken, 1982). Because of its involvement, the federal government has had a major stake in the formation of health policies designed to improve the public's health. In addition, health providers increasingly look to the government for solutions to problems affecting not only health services but also the daily working conditions of health providers (Aiken, 1982).

Health policy formation is a process that includes the way issues are raised on the public agenda and how laws are passed committing resources to programs that affect people. An example of a health policy having significant impact on the health sector including nurses is the Health Planning and Resources Act of 1974. The goal of this policy was the improvement of health care for all people. It was designed to decrease cost of care, to increase quality of care, and to increase access of care to the medically underserved (Sovie, 1978). Strategies to accomplish these goals were created through health planning structures such as Certificate of Need bodies and Health Systems Agencies (Diers, 1985). Community health nursing was able to meet the challenges of this policy by supplying primary care nurse practitioners to establish clinical practices to meet the needs of the medically underserved. However, this led to quests for changes in the legislative bodies to allow such nurses autonomy and reimbursement to do their jobs effectively. In addition to their clinical roles, some nurses were also available to serve on health planning boards and to participate in the health care decision-making process.

During this period, however, nursing was relatively inactive in the public policy field. Federal funding for nursing was a reflection of the public concerns for an adequate supply of prepared nurses, for specialty preparation to meet the need for clinical specialists to staff the high technology hospital, and for specialized approaches to increasing numbers of unrepresented groups in the nursing field. A concern for health care for rural, underserved populations resulted in federal funding for nurse practitioners. Ironically, this funding initiative served to stimulate a number of public policy debates, particularly at the state level. On the one hand, the federal government was providing support for training programs preparing nurse practitioners, while on the other hand, these practitioners, once in practice settings were constrained from providing care to underserved populations because of state licensure restrictions and lack of reimbursement mechanisms. As a result of the increase in numbers of nurse practitioners in the field, a number of state boards of nursing opened the state licensure acts to change the language to cover expanded roles for nursing. This resulted in heated battles between nursing and medicine.

The hospital as the focal point for care was reinforced by health insurance coverage that became a part of worker benefit packages. Under this arrangement, the individual patient rarely felt the impact of the increasing cost of care; payment was handled under insurance coverage that was paid for by the employer. With the development of Medicare and Medicaid in the mid-1960s, the federal government became the payer for medical care services for the elderly and for the indigent. While the entrance of the federal government into the Medicare-Medicaid field was initially resisted by medicine, very quickly the government was integrated into the field as a primary bill-payer for both hospitals and physicians.

The rush toward an ever-expanding "health care industry" continued. Within the triumvirate of hospitals, physicians, and third-party payers, the reimbursement system revolved around payment for the treatment of disease, usually within institutional settings such as hospitals and nursing homes. Reimbursement for home health care, on the other hand, was at best minimal. Fees for services delivered were largely to physicians, although dental services in some instances were reimbursable from third-party payers. Within this structure there was little opportunity for nurses to function independently of either hospitals or physicians. The cost of nursing services in hospital settings was subsumed as part of the room charges for patients.

In conclusion, despite the nurse-practitioner movement, the medical community increasingly focussed on specialization and sophisticated treatment of diseases. Care of the ill was carried out almost totally in hospital settings. Nurses who worked in the community were either employees of private practice physicians, or worked for public health departments or visiting nursing services on a salaried basis. Although nurses had little autonomy, they were the invisible "glue" that kept the health system functioning.

Nursing in the 1980s: Health Care Policy Issues

The 1980s have ushered in a new era of cost consciousness in the health care field. Among the indicators that the current system must be altered are the threatened insolvency of the Medicare-Medicaid trust funds, the possible bankruptcy of the Social Security system, a growing awareness in the business community that the costs of the health care component of their worker benefit packages are exorbitantly high, and an increasing percentage of the gross national product going toward support of health care services. These concerns, coupled with the rising numbers of elderly in society and the cost of care for this population, have made issues of cost control a matter of top concern in the public policy domain. As a reflection of these concerns, currently one of the most important policy issues is related to reimbursement and controlling costs.

Prospective Payment and Diagnostic Related Groups   Changes in the system of reimbursement for care from retrospective to prospective payment through diagnostic related groups (DRGs) are influencing the total pattern of health care delivery within this country. By paying hospitals a set fee for the care of patients within DRGs the federal government is no longer paying for the actual costs of care that, prior to this time, had been charged as part of the patient's bill. This is reducing the number of patients being admitted to hospitals for care and decreasing the length of stay for patients that are hospitalized. The result of this shift is that increased numbers of ill patients are being maintained in the community without admittance to the hospital, and those being discharged are in need of follow-up nursing care that normally would have been provided within hospitals.

This change in reimbursement, while highly controversial, is creating an entirely new climate in the health field. As hospitals struggle to survive in a new competitive environment, many are becoming part of multihospital networks, where the emphasis is on hospitals as a business enterprise. As this business emphasis builds, the first priority becomes profit, and patient care is given secondary focus. Given these shifting priorities, it is anticipated that many hospitals will not survive, and that the total number of hospital beds will ultimately be reduced.

The Family and the Community: Settings for Service Delivery Within this changing climate, family-centered community health care is once more coming into the foreground. Recognizing that a large percentage of the costs of health care is associated with institutional overhead, policymakers are once more looking on the family and the community as essential adjuncts to the health care delivery process. Indicators of this trend include development of hospice care for the terminally ill, daycare programs for the elderly, alternative birthing centers for delivery of infants, and outpatient surgical centers. A growing public awareness of the need for health promotion and individual involvement in maintenance of personal health are reflections of an underlying changing value system.

These changes within the health care system, and their inherent conflicts, offer enormous opportunities for nurses but also pose serious challenges. Within the health care delivery system of the future, nursing could become the predominant profession; alternatively, new categories of health care workers could be prepared to take over functions that traditionally have belonged to nursing. For example, in the health promotion field a whole new profession of health promoters could well develop that would capitalize on the newfound interest in maintenance of a healthy life-style. Alternative birthing centers, while developed by nurse midwives, have rapidly been added as adjuncts to hospitals that recognize an interest in a family-centered approach to birthing. There is the potential for a proliferation of new health care workers who are extensions of physicians and hospitals. If nursing is to assume the leadership role it is capable of, it must first take responsibility for charting its course and promote family-centered community health nursing as the wave of the future.

The Challenge of the Future

The models for family-centered community health nursing are embedded in our past. Nurses have always practiced in the community and have provided services within the home, even while the emphasis was on acute care hospitals. With this as a background, nurses have the opportunity to become the architects of the health care system of the future, bringing together their knowledge of the community with that of the acute care setting. But if nursing is to play this role, nurses must help to shape public policy. Several of the factors that will contribute to the ability of community health nurses to shape public policy in the health arena are discussed in this section.

Social and Political Awareness

Nursing's success in shaping public policy will depend on an understanding of social, political, and economic forces. Nursing has traditionally been in a dependent position, controlled by physicians, on the one hand, and more recently by hospital administrators, on the other. A first step in overcoming this constraint is to recognize the web of social forces that has served to surround nursing and to develop a systematic approach to surmount these forces.

The recently completed study of the National Commission on Nursing (National Commission, 1983) and the Institute of Medicine study (Institute, 1983) point to the potential role that nursing has in shaping the health care system of the future. If the nursing profession can reach internal agreement over educational preparation and credentialing, it can speak with a unified voice about its participation in the health care delivery system of the future.

Speaking with a unified voice, nurses can clearly state that "nursing is an independent profession that has a set of activities, theories, and practices that have intellectual and clinical autonomy; and that its authority in institutions does not match its responsibility and accountability" (Diers, 1985, p. 55). Knowing this, nurses must then take the initiative to compile data to specify what nursing is, what it costs, and ultimately what is needed to gain control over nursing practice and reimbursement of nursing services.

Nurses should actively participate in making policies (rather than implementing policies already made by others) and engage in political action necessary to get policies implemented. It is important for nurses to know what health care agendas are current, how to fit into them, and how to formulate health policies beneficial to nurses within these agendas.

While the role of the federal government in policy decisions that affect health and consequently nursing is certainly crucial, nurses need to realize that health policies are also made at state and local levels and within the private foundations. Community health nurses have opportunities to work with people at all levels in the community and with different communities. They have the responsibility to participate in political decisions that affect clients' health and to work for the improvement of health and well-being of the clients in the communities in which nurses live and work (Archer, 1983).

Recognizing and Using Power

Nurses need to recognize the immense power that they have, and also to see that their destiny in large measure is in their own hands. Nurses are more effective in using power when they work together—cooperating and collaborating with their colleagues both within and across specialty areas—rather than working alone. Nurses can realize tremendous power in collective action to achieve mutual goals (Boyle, 1984), both in the practice setting and in the political arena. Acting as a single force rather than as dissenting factions, nurses can find solutions to their common problems.

As a predominantly female profession, nursing has not always acknowledged nor consciously used its power. However, as a professional group, nurses need power in order to control their profession and deliver nursing services on their own terms. They need power to:

- Help shape health policy
- Alter the disproportionate leverage of physicians
- Provide competent, humanistic, and affordable care to people
- Ensure that nursing is an attractive career option for bright women and men (Ferguson, 1985, p. 90)

Community health nurses can use power effectively and constructively when they care for individuals, families and communities; when they collaborate and form partnerships with other nurses, other health professionals, consumers, and community leaders; and when they engage in political action to bring about quality health care.

Overcoming Economic Constraints

Nurses need to overcome the economic constraints that have served to limit their practice. Current public policy in the health field is based on a pro-competition argument. Fagin has summarized the essential components of pro-competition proposals as including (1) consumer choice from a variety of health care plans, (2) provision of subsidy to the individual by the government and insurers so that individuals may use this subsidy to purchase health services of their own choosing, (3) tax rebates for choosing least costly health plans, and (4) competition between physicians and other providers to offer a range of health services (Fagin, 1982). In these proposals the role of the consumer in the purchase of health services and the role of other health providers are minimally discussed. Fagin further notes, "Physician services are at the core of all pro-competition proposals. This is to be expected since physicians are the dominant providers, control their own and others' practice, serve as gatekeepers to the system, and drive the vast majority of health care costs" (Fagin, 1982 p. 57). Although physicians currently serve as gatekeepers for the system, overwhelming evidence is mounting regarding both the quality of care provided by nurses and its cost effectiveness. The pro-competition climate of today provides the opportunity for nursing to legitimize its role within the health care system. If community health nurses are to profit from future opportunities, they must devise ways to market their services and manage their financial affairs, including their own budgets.

Marketing Community Health Nursing Services With origins in the church and the military, nursing has traditionally been unconcerned with economics, and has been considered woman's work done out of dedication, not for profit (Camunas, 1986). Community health nursing in particular has always been concerned with providing nursing care to those who need such care. Much of that care has been provided through municipalities or tax-supported programs. Consequently community health nurses did not have to "sell" their services to consumers. This may well be changing. In the midst of rising health care costs, an oversupply of highly trained physicians, underpayment for health promotion and wellness care (the major emphasis of community health nursing), a health care system that places high value

on sophisticated high technology, and a generally better informed consumer, community health nurses will find it increasingly necessary to determine the kind of health care the public needs and will use, as well as the best ways to deliver such services to them. In essence, as nurses we must devise ways to "sell" or market our services not only to meet the public's need but also to ensure our own survival.

Marketing is an exchange process. Applying the concept to public health nursing, Archer (1983) defines it as "a systematic approach to planning and evaluating a public health nursing organization's exchange relationships with its target aggregates" (p. 305). Thus marketing is more than advertising to increase sales. Its goal is to fulfill the needs and wants of the consumer (Camunas, 1986). Community health nurses can develop marketing skills enabling them to provide cost-effective care. Marketing strategies involve several steps that can be summarized as follows (Camunas, 1986):

1. *Identify markets*—target aggregates or specific geographic areas or population segments; specify health needs of each segment and identify goals, strategies, and tactics to meet needs
2. *Gather detailed information about the market*—assessment of segments; qualitative and quantitative methods may be used
3. *Develop marketing strategies and tactics*—planning requires clear statement of goals and objectives as well as limitations
4. *Define product*—nursing services need to be clarified for consumers so that they can know what to expect
5. *Promote product*—communication between providers and the market to meet the market's need for the product and to enable providers to accomplish their goal
6. *Determine place of practice and price for service*—may be influenced by competition analysis and existence of other organizations providing similar services.
7. *Evaluate steps of the marketing strategy*
8. *Promote services*—through media, word of mouth, written materials, and marketing consultants

Other marketing strategies community health nurses may consider are summarized by Archer (1983, pp. 308–309). They include:

- Client involvement—clearly and behaviorally defined goals and objectives based on and congruent with client priorities
- Additional services built on those the target aggregate originally wanted
- Accessibility to clients
- Systematic outreach and follow-up
- Short waiting times
- Convenient hours of service
- Employment of members of target aggregates
- Few restrictive eligibility categories—programs responsive to community needs are more easily sold to community residents

These strategies can increase the appeal of nursing services delivered to the community, and thus make it easier for community health nurses to reach the market for their services.

Managing Finances and Budgets

As the health care climate becomes more competitive with respect to price and cost of services, health professionals including nurses will be required to "cost out," or itemize, their services. As an example, in 1983 Maine enacted a bill requiring that nursing costs be identified on patients' bills as separate from other hospital costs (Booth, 1985). This trend can be expected to continue, and in the near future community health nurses may also be required to cost out their services.

The costs and benefits of health promotion services such as health education and counseling will need to be specified. The institution of DRGs is expected to result in greater numbers of sicker patients being discharged to their homes and families. This will require that community health nurses determine how the management and care of these patients in their homes will be reimbursed. While community health nurses in the past have been primarily concerned with the quality of their services as opposed to the cost, they must now be equally concerned with both. They must seek out and compile the data that will keep them informed about cost and payment for their services. They must also seek out alternative and innovative ways of payment for services provided to those who cannot afford it. It is vital that community health nurses carefully monitor their financial expenditures and do ongoing cost-accounting of their services. One way to accomplish this goal is for nursing managers to have control over their budgets.

Budgeting is a planning tool that enables managers to control and influence behaviors and outcomes as well as achieve their organizational goals. Community health nurses long have worked within budget constraints, but most have not had the knowledge or the political skills to influence and control the budget's development (Ruth & Mahr, 1984). Budgeting in organizations, whether they are public, nonprofit, or proprietary, involves a set of activities that occurs throughout the year and involves several phases: (a) preparation; (b) submission for approval; (c) approval by governing bodies; (d) implementation or execution; and (e) evaluation and audit (Lee & Johnson, 1977; Ruth & Mahr, 1984). Understanding and participating in the budget process may require time and persistence, but such involvement will enable community health nurses to improve their services and the overall management of their health care agencies (Ruth & Mahr, 1984).

Taking Political and Legislative Actions

The significant role that the government plays in health policymaking includes influencing reimbursement systems; financing health research and programs, thus determining what health care problems will be researched and/or implemented; determining who will receive what kind of care; and what health care agendas will determine future goals and objectives. Government also influences health care agencies and health professions, including the legal definitions of specialized professionals such as nurses. Because the role of the government is so pervasive, nurses must devise ways to influence the government at local, state, and federal levels.

Currently the American Medical Association and the American Hospital Association constitute two of the most effective lobbying groups in Washington. If the health care delivery system and the nurse's role within it is to change, these powerful lobbying groups must be counterbalanced. Nurses constitute the largest professional group in all of the health care arena; mobilization of this powerful group is the challenge confronting us. The effectiveness of nurses in the political arena is hampered by a number of factors. First, the way in which nurses view themselves has already been pointed out as a handicap. Coming from a traditional female perspective, nurses tend to view their dependent position in health care delivery as their proper place as women. Second, because of the ways in which the profession has been controlled in the economic realm, nurses do not have a clear image of their economic worth in the delivery of health care. With this deflated sense of self-worth, it is difficult to envision how the system might be changed.

There are, however, several opportunities for individual nurses to actively participate in the political and legislative process in order to effect positive changes in the profession itself, in nursing practice, and in the improvement of care to clients. Such opportunities or activities are as follows:

- Political action
  Learn political and legislative process—Local political representatives are often good sources to learn from
  Communicate with legislators—monitor their performance on health issues; know their record
  Participate in the election process—run for office; manage political campaigns; support candidates
  Join political action committees
- Legislative Action
  Serve as experts on selected, relevant health issues

Inform legislators—provide health information that can be drafted into health bills
  Prepare and give testimonies
  Serve as expert witness at health-related hearings
  Write letters to support or oppose legislation as appropriate
- Lobbying
  Be well informed about issues
  Advocate for desired changes such as policies and laws favorable to nursing
- Involvement in Professional Organizations
  Know issues relevant to the organization
  Assume active role in organization's committees
  Support N-CAP
- Community Participation
  Assume community leadership positions
  Become involved in community coalition groups with similar interests
  Be visible in community
  Establish meaningful partnerships with community leaders and consumers

The community is a natural power base for community health nurses. Political involvement should begin in, and in partnership with, the community. Families in the community with whom nurses work can be nursing's strongest allies. Together they can pressure political representatives to work for high-quality family-centered health care in the community. Provision of such care may require innovative programs and approaches.

Exploring Innovative Programs and Approaches

In addition to providing nursing services in traditional settings such as local health departments and county and state facilities, community health nurses can explore alternative practice settings such as health maintenance organizations (HMOs), preferred provider organizations (PPOs), community health nursing centers, and individual or nurse-partnership kinds of entrepreneurships. Community health nurses can also seek special (private or governmental) funding to launch family-centered programs such as demonstration projects for special population groups such as single-parent and dual-career families, gay families, the chronically ill, the elderly, and pregnant adolescents. Health services delivery sites can be expanded to include facilities such as churches, YMCAs, and other community centers. Community health nurses can capitalize on the trend toward wellness and fitness among

consumers, and collaborate with them to establish and maintain family-oriented health centers. Such centers would have wellness and holistic care as their focus and would emphasize client participation. The nurse works with the consumer as coparticipant or as partner (Bakken, 1983) committed to the goal of improving the health and welfare of the whole community.

Summary

Nurses and consumers working together can build a case for changes in the reimbursement system and for improvement of the health and welfare of individuals and families in the community. Nursing is often referred to as the sleeping giant whose power would be overwhelming if awakened. One out of every forty-nine voters in the United States is a nurse. Their sheer numbers give nurses the ability to change the system, particularly if they take their case to the health care consumer in such a way that the consumer can understand the role that nurses seek to play. Traditionally, nurses have taken care of the poor, minorities, and the aged, groups with little political power. Demonstration of improved health care delivery, communicated clearly by nurses and addressing consumer concerns, is a powerful political device.

Concerns over monopoly and restraint of trade are political indicators that the time might be ripe for nurses to carefully organize and orchestrate their approach to changing the system. Consumers' discontent with the experiences they encounter indicates a readiness for change and an acceptance of nurses as care-providers far beyond what nurses envision for themselves.

While some may argue that the goals described here constitute only a self-serving political cause to advance nursing, we would respond that it is only as nursing's role in health care delivery is expanded that the system can change so that the

care delivered can more effectively meet the health care needs of the people served.

Nurses have the capability of changing the system; to do so, they must recognize their power and join with the consumer in the political process of public health policy change.

References

Aiken L: The impact of federal health policy on nurses. In: *Nursing in the 1980's.* Aiken L H, Gortner S (editors), *Nursing in the 1980's.* Philadelphia: Lippincott, 1982.

Anderson E: Community focus in public health nursing: Whose responsibility? *Nurs Outlook* 1983; 31 (1): 44–48.

Archer S: Marketing public health nursing services. *Nurs Outlook* 1983; 31 (6): 312–316.

Ashley J: This I believe about power in nursing. *Nurs Outlook* 1973; 21 (10): 46.

Bakken K: Integrated health care: The whole person in community. *Nursing Economics* (November–December) 1983; 1: 178–180.

Booth R: Financing mechanisms for health care: Impact on nursing services. *Journal of Professional Nursing* 1985; 1 (1): 34–40.

Boyle K: Power in nursing: A collaborative approach. *Nurs Outlook* 1984; 32 (3): 164–167.

Camunas C: Marketing as a nursing skill. In: Mason D, Talbott S (editors), *Political Action Handbook for Nurses.* Menlo Park, Calif.: Addison-Wesley, 1986.

Diers D: Policy and politics. In: Mason D, Talbott S (editors), *Political Action Handbook for Nurses*. Menlo Park, Calif.: Addison-Wesley, 1986.

Fagin CM: Nursing as an alternative to high cost care. *Am J Nurs* (January) 1982; 82 (1): 56–60.

Ford L: Nurse practitioners: History of a new idea and predictions for the future. In: Aiken L H, Gortner S (editors), *Nursing in the 1980's*. Philadelphia: Lippincott, 1982.

Ferguson V: Powers in nursing. In: Mason D, Talbott S (editors), *Political Action Handbook for Nurses*. Menlo Park, Calif.: Addison-Wesley, 1986.

Heinrich J: Historical perspectives on public health nursing. *Nurs Outlook* 1983; 31 (6): 317–320.

Institute of Medicine: *Nursing and Nursing Education: Public Policies and Private Actions*. Washington, DC: National Academy Press, 1983.

Larson E: Health policy and NIH: Implications for nursing. *Nursing Research* 1984; 33 (6): 352–356.

Lee D and Johnson RW: Public budgeting systems 2nd ed. Baltimore, Md., University Park Press, 1977.

Monteiro L: Florence Nightingale on public health nursing. *American Journal of Public Health* 1985; 75 (2): 181–185.

National Commission on Nursing: *Summary Report and Recommendations*, 1983.

Ruth MV and Mahr CA: Budgeting in community health agencies. *Nursing Economics*. 1984; 2: 47–50.

Sovie M: Nursing: A future to shape. In: Chaska N (editor), *The Nursing Profession*. New York: McGraw-Hill, 1978.

Appendices

Appendix 1

Family Assessment Tool

Assessment of _____ Family

Child of Concern _____ Birthdate _____

Address _____ Telephone _____

Purpose of Assessment _____

Report Submitted by _____ Date _____

Observations

I. Description of Home and Environment
II. Significant Socio-Cultural Influences
III. Interaction of Family Members

Area of Inquiry

I. **Family's Perception**

  *A. "What does the family see as a problem?"
  *B. "What has the family already tried?"
      "What does the family think might be a
      solution?"
  *C. "If special education is considered, how does
      the family feel about it?"
  *D. "Describe your child in a few sentences."
  *E. "What goals does the family have for the
      child?"

II. **Health Interview**

  A. Growth and Development
     Antenatal: Age and health of mother during
pregnancy, other pregnancies, AP care and
experiences, weight gain, drug ingestion,
illnesses, blood type, length of gestation.

Natal: Length of labor, anesthesia, type of
delivery, condition of baby at birth (cry,
color, O_2, incubator), birth weight.

Postnatal: Problems in nursery, feeding or
sleeping problems, excessive weight loss.

Development: Rolled over, sat alone, walked,
talked (meaningful words, 2 word sentences), feeding history, teeth eruption, urine
and bowel control, establishment of hand
preference, development compared to siblings and parents, school experiences,
developmental testing, developmental tasks.

Disturbances: Speech delays or irregulari-
ties, lethargy, attention disorders, hearing
and vision difficulties, clumsiness of motor
tasks, enuresis, encopresis, pica, thumb
sucking, failure to grow or unusual growth,
antisocial behavior.

Learning Patterns: Self-reliance, self-control, approach tendency, learning style.

B. Health History
Childhood diseases, illnesses, accidents, seizures, hospitalizations, ear infections, medications, allergies, immunizations. Last P.E. date? Where? By whom?

C. Present Status
Eating, sleeping, elimination, interests, peer relationships, exercise/play, method of discipline, sexuality.

D. Review of Systems
Skin, Eye, Ear, Nose, Throat, Cardio-Respiratory, Gastro-Intestinal, Genito-Urinary, Musculo-Skeletal, Neurological.

III. **Family History**

A. Family Composition: age, sex, present status of siblings, age of parents, extended family.
B. Health Status of Family Members.
C. Educational and work experiences of parents.
*D. "How do all family members get along together?"
"What activities do they share?"

Items with asterisk [*] are subjective questions that require nurse to elicit expectations, understanding of problem, general feelings and values that family has about child of concern.

Closing Discussion with the Family

I. Review goals with family
A. Define the problems.
B. Discuss information to be shared with school staff.

C. Emphasize family sharing in decision making process.

II. Arrange for follow-up contacts.

Nursing Summary

I. Assessment
A. Interpret data and summarize impression.
B. List and prioritize problems.
C. List family's strengths and weaknesses.

II. Plan
A. Meet with staffing team and family to review information.
  1. Identify problem areas.
  2. Identify family, school, and community resources.
  3. Discuss alternative solutions.
B. Identify a solution if possible.
  1. Designate team members to be involved with the family.
  2. Involve family
C. Develop an individualized Educational Program (IEP) with a health component.
D. Determine evaluation criteria and procedure (when, by whom, how, and where).

III. Implement Health Component of Individualized Educational Program.

IV. Evaluation — Determine success of plan based on criteria established in II. D.

SOURCE:
Holt S, Robinson T: The school nurse's assessment tool. *Am J Nurs* (May) 1979; 950–953.

© 1978 Sandra J. Holt and Thelma M. Robinson
1979 Revised.

Appendix 2

The Consumers' Health Survey

(A Survey of Health and Health Care Needs Conducted by Suburban Cook County—Dupage County Health Systems Agency, Inc. 1010 Lake Street, Oak Park, Illinois, 1977. Reprinted with permission.)

These questions are excerpted from *The Consumers' Health Survey*, which begins with questions concerning basic demographic information, such as name, familial relationships, gender, race, education, and occupation. The survey is intended to be filled out by one family member but answered for *each* household member. The form allows for responses for up to eight persons. The survey consists of two parts: Part A concerning individual information and Part B concerning household information.

Part A: Individual Information

II. Medical Care—Individual Family Members

1. During the past year, what was the total number of times this person went to a doctor for medical care?
2. How long has it been since this person visited a doctor about his/her health?
3. How long has it been since this person had a complete physical check-up or examination?

III. Dental

1. About how long has it been since this person last visited a dentist?
2. If this person visited a dentist during the past year, was any of the following work done? (Please indicate number(s).)
   1. Cleaning
   2. Fluoride treatment
   3. Exam or X-ray
   4. Fillings or repair
   5. Extraction or surgery
   6. Gum treatment
   7. Straightening (orthodontia)
   8. Dentures (false teeth or bridgework)
   9. Other (specify) _____
   10. Did not visit the dentist during the past year.

IV. Lifestyle

1. How many drinks of alcoholic beverages (wine, beer, or liquor) does this person have during a usual week?
2. Does this person use any form of tobacco?
3. If this person smokes cigarettes, on the average, about how many cigarettes does he/she smoke per day?

V. Health—Individual Conditions

Did this person have any of the following conditions in the past year? (Please indicate number(s) for each.)

1. Allergies
2. Anemia or "low blood"
3. Appendicitis
4. Arthritis or rheumatism
5. Asthma
6. Bladder or urinary problems
7. Bronchitis or frequent coughing
8. Cancer
9. Chicken pox
10. Dental problems
11. Diabetes
12. Emphysema
13. Epilepsy
14. Frequent attacks of sinus trouble
15. Frequent colds
16. Frequent constipation
17. Frequent diarrhea
18. Frequent ear infections
19. Frequent gallbladder or liver trouble
20. Frequent headaches
21. Frequent nausea, vomiting
22. Frequent nervous troubles
23. Frequent skin troubles
24. German measles (Rubella, 3 day)
25. Hardening of the arteries
26. Heart trouble
27. Hemorrhoids or piles
28. Hepatitis (yellow jaundice)
29. Hernia or rupture
30. High blood pressure (hypertension)
31. Kidney stones or chronic kidney trouble
32. Measles (8 day or red)
33. Menstrual troubles
34. Mononucleosis (kissing disease, mono)
35. Mumps
36. Overweight
37. Palsy
38. Pneumonia
39. Pregnancy
40. Prostate trouble
41. Senility (poor orientation as to time, place, people)
42. Shortness of breath
43. Shingles
44. Sleeping difficulty (insomnia)
45. Strep throat or sore throats
46. Stomach ulcer
47. Stroke or effects of stroke
48. Swelling of legs or other swelling
49. Thyroid trouble or goiter
50. Trouble with varicose veins
51. Tumor, cyst or growth
52. Vaginal infection

VI. Hospital Use

1. During the past 12 months, has this person received care in a *hospital emergency room?*
2. If 1 is yes, how many times in the past 12 months was the *emergency room* used for each of the following reasons:

1. An emergency
2. A "non-emergency" service
3. During the past 12 months, has this person received *hospital outpatient care?*
4. If 3 is yes, how many times in the past 12 months did this person receive *hospital outpatient care?*
5. If 3 is yes, at which *hospital(s)* was care received? Please give name and city.)
6. Was this person an *overnight* patient in a hospital at any time in the past 12 months?

If no, skip remainder of section for this person. Go to section VII.

7. How many times in the past 12 months was this person admitted to the hospital and stayed overnight? (Indicate number of admissions.)
8. How many nights was this person in the hospital in the past 12 months?
9. For which of the following reasons did this person enter the hospital during the past 12 months? (Please indicate number(s).)
   1. Sickness or illness
   2. Accident or injury
   3. Childbirth or related
   4. Operation (surgery)
   5. Medical tests
   6. Other (specify) _____
10. To which hospital(s) was this person admitted in the past 12 months? (Please give name and city.)

VII. Senses—Hearing, Vision and Speech for Adults 18+ Only

1. Does this person presently receive any help from specially trained people in any of these areas: (Indicate number for each.)
   1. Hearing
   2. Speech
   3. Sight
   4. No
2. Does this person need help from specially trained people, but is not receiving help in any of these areas: (Indicate number for each.)
   1. Hearing
   2. Speech
   3. Sight
   4. No
3. If this person needs help from specially trained people

but is not receiving help in any of these areas (hearing, speech, sight), which of the following is the major reason help is not being received? (Please indicate number.)

1. Problem not serious enough
2. Could not afford
3. Not sure where to seek
4. No transportation
5. Afraid to seek care
6. Have been refused services (specify where)

   _____

7. Other (please specify) _____

   _____

VIII. Mobility (all ages)

1. Does this person have any trouble getting around freely?

   If no, skip remainder of section for this person. Go to section IX.

2. Which of these statements fits this person best in terms of health and ability to get around?
   1. Must stay in bed all or most of the time.
   2. Must stay in the house all or most of the time.
   3. Needs the help of another person to get around.
   4. Needs the help of a special aid such as a wheelchair or walker to get around.
   5. Does not need the help of another person or a special aid but has trouble getting around outside of the hosue.
3. If this person has a problem getting around, about how long has this person had the problem?
4. If this person has trouble getting around, has this person seen a doctor in the past year about his/her condition?
5. If this person has trouble getting around, what is the specific condition which causes this problem?
   1. Missing or deformed fingers, hand, arm, toes, etc.
   2. Palsy or paralysis of any kind
   3. Arthritis or other stiffness
   4. Accident or injury
   5. Calcium deposits or cartilage problems
   6. Old age or sickness
   7. Other (specify) _____
6. Is this person presently helped at home on a continuing basis?

IX. Long Term Care and the Elderly for Adults 65 + Only

1. Has it ever been suggested that this person be placed in a nursing or convalescent home?
2. If 1 is yes, for what reasons might this person not be placed in a nursing or convalescent home?
   1. Person will not consent to such care.
   2. Person will consent to such care, but his/her spouse or other family relation does not wish to place him/her in such care.
   3. Person is unable to afford such care.
   4. Person's family is unable to afford such care.
   5. This care is not available in the area.
   6. Other (specify) _____
3. If 1 is yes, do you anticipate this person will require nursing or convalescent facility care in the next: (Indicate number.)
   1. 1–6 months   4. 3–5 years
   2. 7–12 months   5. Never
   3. 1–3 years   6. Don't know

X. Health Activities for Adults 18 + Only

1. Is this person limited for health reasons in the kind or amount of work or other activities that he/she can do?
2. During the past two weeks, how many days did his/her own illness keep this person from his/her job, school, housework, or other normal daily activities.
3. If retired, did poor health cause this person to retire earlier than he/she wished?

Health Activities for Children 6–17 Only

4. Has health affected this child's school attendance to a point where school performance has been affected?
5. During the past two weeks, how many days did illness or injury keep this person from going to school?
6. Is this child limited in the kind or amount of play or recreation because of health?
7. Does this child need special help or school resources

for any of the following reasons: (Indicate number(s) for each.)

1. Hearing
2. Sight
3. Speech
4. Orthopedic handicap (braces, special shoes, etc.)
5. Gifted
6. Learning disability
7. Mentally retarded
8. Emotionally disturbed
9. Other (specify) _____
   _____
10. No

8. If 7 is yes, does this child presently attend special classes for any of the following: (Indicate number(s).)

1. Hearing
2. Sight
3. Speech
4. Orthopedic handicap (braces, special shoes, etc.)
5. Gifted
6. Learning disability
7. Mentally retarded
8. Emotionally disturbed
9. Other (specify) _____
   _____
10. No

XI. Accidents and Injuries (all ages)

1. Has this person had an accident or injury requiring treatment during the past 12 months?

If no, skip remainder of section for this person. Go to part B.

2. How many separate accidents or injuries requiring treatment has this person had in the past 12 months?

3. Where did the latest accident or injury occur?

1. Inside home
2. At home but outside
3. Friend's home
4. Store
5. Farm
6. Industrial place
7. School
8. Place of recreation and sports, except school
9. Motor vehicle
10. Other (specify) _____
    _____

Part B: Household Information

I. Environmental Health

1. Are your living quarters in:
   1. _____ A one family home?
   2. _____ A building for 2–6 families?
   3. _____ A building for more than 6 families?
   4. _____ A mobile home or trailer?

2. How many rooms do you have in your living quarters not counting bathrooms, porches, balconies, hallways, or utility rooms?
   _____ Number of rooms

3. Check if any of the following conditions exist in any part of your living quarters:
   1. _____ Water leaks through walls, floors, windows, doors, or ceilings.
   2. _____ Water collects on walls, floors, windows, doors, or ceilings.
   3. _____ Basement floods (storm water).
   4. _____ Plumbing leaks.
   5. _____ Sewage back-up into basement.
   6. _____ A room which has no window which opens and no other ventilation.
   7. _____ Holes and/or cracked or falling plaster in walls, ceilings, or floors.
   8. _____ Peeling paint inside of house.
   9. _____ Steps or porches poorly constructed or not maintained.
   10. _____ None

4. Which of the following statements best describes the heating in your living quarters:
   1. _____ Always enough heat in all rooms
   2. _____ Usually enough heat in all rooms
   3. _____ Seldom enough heat in all rooms
   4. _____ Too much heat
   5. _____ No heat

5. Is there any room which has no electricity?
   1. _____ Yes   2. _____ No

6. Do your kitchen and bathroom sinks provide hot and cold running water?
   1. _____ Yes   2. _____ No

7. Do your kitchen and bathroom sinks empty into:
   1. _____ Public sewer system
   2. _____ Septic tank
   3. _____ Neither
   4. _____ Don't know

If you have a septic tank, does it do any of the following:

8. _____ Smell badly; Odor
9. _____ Pools on top of ground
10. _____ Drain into a ditch
11. _____ Drain into a stream
12. _____ None of the above
13. Does the cooking stove in your living unit use:
   1. _____ Gas or electricity
   2. _____ Wood
   3. _____ Coal
   4. _____ Oil
   5. _____ No working stove
   6. _____ Don't know
14. Is there an operating refrigerator in your living unit?
   1. _____ Yes   2. _____ No
15. Is there a working flush toilet inside your living unit?
   1. _____ Yes   2. _____ No
16. Within the last year, have you seen any of the following things in or around your living quarters? (Check each that you have seen.)
   1. _____ Rats
   2. _____ Roaches
   3. _____ Stagnant water
   4. _____ Piles of paper stored for more than one week
   5. _____ Junk automobiles
   6. _____ Weeds to the extent they cause a nuisance
   7. _____ Unlighted halls or stairways
   8. _____ Cracking or peeling paint on outside of home
   9. _____ None of these
17. Do you share the kitchen or bathroom with another household?
   1. _____ Yes   2. _____ No
18. Where do you usually dispose of your garbage and trash?
   1. _____ City or county pickup
   2. _____ Private pickup
   3. _____ Private dump
   4. _____ Public dump
   5. _____ Dump on own property
   6. _____ Other (specify) _____

II. Public and Social Services

In the following list of health and public services, check each that your household is *not* satisfied with:

1. _____ Garbage and trash collection
2. _____ Housing code inspection
3. _____ Rodent and pest control
4. _____ Dog control
5. _____ Street cleaning
6. _____ Ambulance service
7. _____ Public health dept.
8. _____ Blood banks
9. _____ Mental health services
10. _____ School health programs
11. _____ Satisfied with all
12. _____ Other (please specify)

_____

_____

Check each of the following conditions that you consider serious in the entire community. Also check those that you consider serious in your neighborhood or immediate area.

	(1) Community	(2) Neighborhood	
13.	_____	_____	Need for housing
14.	_____	_____	Health care
15.	_____	_____	Drinking water quality
16.	_____	_____	Noise
17.	_____	_____	Drug addiction
18.	_____	_____	Air pollution
19.	_____	_____	Lack of public transportation
20.	_____	_____	Need for drug stores
21.	_____	_____	Need for a hospital
22.	_____	_____	Need for a doctor
23.	_____	_____	Other (specify)

_____

_____

Please check the *one* service you feel is the most important to provide or increase in your community (*check only one*).

24. _____ Places where people with problems can go to stay and work on their problems (mental hospitals, homes for delinquents).
25. _____ Educational events to help people learn ways to deal with their problems (seminars to help parents raise their children).
26. _____ Vocational and social rehabilitation day pro-

grams where people can receive specialized help and continue living at their homes (vocational training, special education services).

27. ____ Groups of people meeting on mutual concerns (senior citizens, Alcoholics Anomymous).

28. ____ Counselors or therapists to help people with their specific problems (outpatient mental health clinic, family service agency).

29. ____ Round-the-clock emergency service for mental health problems (psychiatric emergency room).

Check any of the following social and health services someone in your household presently needs and would probably use.

30. ____ Alcoholism help
31. ____ Child day care
32. ____ Dental services and education
33. ____ Drug abuse help
34. ____ Expectant parent classes
35. ____ Family planning and birth control
36. ____ Home inspection
37. ____ Immunizations (shots)
38. ____ Coronary care services
39. ____ Nutrition program
40. ____ Mental health and psychiatric services
41. ____ Pre and post birth home visits by nurses
42. ____ Rat/insect control
43. ____ Services for retarded
44. ____ V.D. clinic and education
45. ____ Visiting nurses
46. ____ Well-baby child care
47. ____ Poison control services
48. ____ First-aid training
49. ____ Home nursing
50. ____ Rescue squad
51. ____ Other (please specify) _____

_____

52. Which of these health professional people would you rather talk to about an emotional problem? (*check only one*)

1. ____ Psychiatrist   4. ____ Nurse
2. ____ Psychologist   5. ____ Physician
3. ____ Social worker   6. ____ None of
                              the above

III. Household Information

1. How much income was received by all members in this household in 1976 before taxes, including earn-

ings (wages, salary, commissions, bonuses, tips), social security, retirement pensions, interest and dividends?

1. ____ $0–2,520
2. ____ $2,521–3,999
3. ____ $4,000–6,999
4. ____ $7,000–9,999
5. ____ $10,000–12,999
6. ____ $13,000–15,999
7. ____ $16,000–19,999
8. ____ $20,000–24,999
9. ____ $25,000–34,999
10. ____ $35,000–49,999
11. ____ $50,000 +

Or household monthly income before taxes $ ____

2. Did any household member receive assistance payments in the past 12 months?

1. ____ No
2. ____ Don't know
3. ____ Aid for dependent children (ADC or AFDC-U)
4. ____ Old age assistance (SSI)
5. ____ General assistance or township general assistance
6. ____ Aid to the blind (SSI)
7. ____ Aid to the disabled (SSI)
8. ____ Food stamps
9. ____ Don't know type of aid

IV. Household Medical Care

Please fill in the following information about the doctor or clinic that your household uses for the kinds of medical care indicated. Use the spaces at the right for your answers.

1. Type of Practice (enter number)
   1. Private doctor
   2. Doctor clinic
   3. Private chiropractor
   4. Chiropractic clinic
   5. Christian science practitioner
   6. Company or industrial clinic
   7. Health department clinic
   8. Hospital emergency room or outpatient clinic
   9. Osteopath
   10. Other (please specify)

   _____

2. Location or Place (address, city).

3. Total number of office visits in the past 12 months for all household members. (Specify number of visits for each doctor.)

	Family General Care	Obstetric Gynecology (Female)	Pediatric (Children)	Special Condition (Specify)	Special Condition (Specify)
1.					
2.					
3.					

4. Does your household have a doctor you consider to be your family doctor?
   1. ____ Yes (skip to question 17)
   2. ____ No (continue to next question)

The following are reasons why some households have no regular doctor or clinic. Please check the major reason why your household has no regular doctor or clinic (*check one only*).

5. ____ Have recently moved here and have not yet sought medical care.
6. ____ Have never needed medical care.
7. ____ Just never have gotten around to trying to find a doctor.
8. ____ Get medical care at many different places— no regular place.
9. ____ Use nonprescription drugs for medical care.
10. ____ Do not know how to find a doctor.
11. ____ Have tried to find a doctor but was refused care.
12. ____ Do not wish to see doctors.
13. ____ Doctor recently retired.
14. ____ Cost of care.
15. ____ Disliked service received previously.
16. ____ Other (please specify) _____
17. In general, would you say that you are very satisfied, satisfied, dissatisfied, or very dissatisfied with the medical care you and your family get?
    1. ____ Very satisfied
    2. ____ Satisfied
    3. ____ Dissatisfied
    4. ____ Very dissatisfied

Has anyone in your household been refused medical care by a doctor in the past year?

18. ____ No
19. ____ Don't know
20. ____ Yes. . .
    21. How many times? _____
    22. Where? _____
    23. Why were you refused? _____

V. Medical Care— Doctor Use

The following are reasons why some people do not go to the doctor. Please check each reason which explains why members of your household did not go to the doctor if they should have.

1. ____ Did not realize that the problem was serious at the time.
2. ____ Expense of seeing doctor, medicine.
3. ____ Don't want charity.
4. ____ Just never have gotten around to trying to find a doctor.
5. ____ Don't like long waits.
6. ____ Don't like being in waiting room with others.
7. ____ They don't take a very long time with you anyway.
8. ____ Afraid of doctors, shots, etc.

9. ____ Can't understand their explanations.
10. ____ They don't explain much to me.
11. ____ Don't see the same doctor all the time.
12. ____ Previous bad experience in family.
13. ____ Doctors are busy and I hate to bother them.
14. ____ Afraid of being refused service by a doctor.
15. ____ Don't know how to find a doctor or medical help.
16. ____ No transportation to get to doctor.
17. ____ Too expensive to get to doctor.
18. ____ Was turned away due to full practice.
19. ____ No one to care for children.
20. ____ Too sick to travel.
21. ____ Unable to get there at time service is offered.
22. ____ Distance to doctor.
23. ____ Other (please specify) _____
24. Has your household changed doctors in the past 12 months? That is, have they stopped going to one doctor in favor of going to another doctor for the same kind of care?
    1. ____ Yes
    2. ____ No (*skip to question 40*)
    3. ____ Don't know (*skip to question 40*)

The following are reasons why some people change doctors. Please check each reason for the change of doctors in your household.

25. ____ Household moved during past year.
26. ____ Moved office away or too far away to travel to.
27. ____ Died or stopped practicing.
28. ____ Would not make house calls willingly for a serious problem.
29. ____ Treatment given did not seem to be effective.
30. ____ Disliked personality of doctor.
31. ____ Poor communication (difficult to contact or language barrier)
32. ____ Did not seem to keep up with medical progress.
33. ____ Charged too much.
34. ____ Prescribed too many expensive drugs.
35. ____ Seemed uninterested in helping me.
36. ____ Disliked doctor's assistants or nurses.
37. ____ Doctor reduced number of patients in his practice.
38. ____ Other family member wanted to change doctors.
39. ____ Other (please specify) _____
40. Has your household called anyone besides a doctor in the past year for medical advice?
    1. ____ No
    2. ____ Don't know

____ Yes, was this:
    3. ____ Health department
    4. ____ Visiting nurse
    5. ____ Druggist
    6. ____ Medical society
    7. ____ Library
    8. ____ Hospital
    9. ____ Faith healer
    10. ____ Friend
    11. ____ Other (specify) _____

41. Everyone has some idea on what the "best" or ideal medical care should be. Please compare the care you have now or have received in the recent past to *what you think is the ideal care* (*check one*).
    1. ____ My current care is the ideal care.
    2. ____ My curent care is almost the ideal care.
    3. ____ Some parts of my current care are ideal or almost ideal but others are not.
    4. ____ Not much of my current care is close to my ideal.
    5. ____ Almost none of my current care is close to my ideal.

VI. Household Medical Care

1. Has anyone in your household been refused service at a hospital in the past year?
    1. ____ No
    2. ____ Don't know
    3. ____ Yes—At which hospital(s)? (Please give name and city.)

       _____

       Why did you seek care? _____

       _____

       Why were you refused? _____

       _____

2. In the past year did any household member use an emergency rescue squad and/or ambulance?
    1. ____ No
    2. ____ Don't know
    3. ____ Yes—Number of times _____

3. In the past year has any household member used a hospital emergency room or outpatient clinic rather than contacting a doctor?
    1. ____ No
    2. ____ Don't know
    3. ____ Yes—Number of times _____

VII. Medical Care—Last Visit

Please answer only for yourself if you have seen a doctor in the past year. Questions refer to only your last visit.

1. What was the main reason that you went to the doctor on your last visit?
    1. _____ Illness
    2. _____ Accident or injury
    3. _____ Chronic condition
    4. _____ Needed shots
    5. _____ Voluntary check-up
    6. _____ Pregnancy or birth control
    7. _____ Check-up needed for work, school, insurance, camp, marriage, or military
    8. _____ Medical tests
    9. _____ Surgery or surgical follow-up
    10. _____ Psychiatric care
    11. _____ Other (please specify) _____
    _____

2. How long ago was this visit?
    _____ Days   _____ Weeks   _____ Months
3. After you decided that you needed this last visit to the doctor, how much time was it from when you called for the appointment until you were actually able to see the doctor?
    1. _____ Standing appointment
    2. _____ Under 1 day
    3. _____ 1 day
    4. _____ 2–6 days
    5. _____ 1–2 weeks
    6. _____ 3–4 weeks
    7. _____ More than 4 weeks
    8. _____ Dropped in—no appointment
    9. _____ Don't remember
4. Did the doctor ask you non-medical questions, such as about possible home, social, or mental problems?
    1. _____ Yes
    2. _____ No
    3. _____ Don't remember
5. Did the doctor explain your illness or problem so that you were satisfied that you understood it?
    1. _____ Yes
    2. _____ No
    3. _____ Don't remember
6. Did the doctor or nurse provide adequate instruction for future care of your illness or problem and medicine to be taken?
    1. _____ Yes
    2. _____ No

3. _____ Don't remember
4. _____ Does not apply

Questions 7 and 8 for *women only*

7. On the average, how frequently do you receive a Pap smear from your doctor? (*check one*)
    1. _____ Every six months
    2. _____ Once a year
    3. _____ Every two years
    4. _____ Less often than every two years
    5. _____ Never
    6. _____ Don't know
8. How often do you do a breast self-examination (for cancer detection)? (*check one*)
    1. _____ At least once a month
    2. _____ Several times a year
    3. _____ Never
    4. _____ Not familiar with self-examination
    5. _____ Don't know

VIII. Household Dental Care

If your household has a regular or usual source of dental care, please answer questions 1–8. If your household has no regular or usual source of dental care, please answer questions 5–20.

Please fill in the following information about the dentist or clinic that your household uses for the kinds of dental care indicated. Use the spaces at the right for your answers.

1. Type of Practice (Please enter number.)
    1. Private dentist
    2. Dental clinic
    3. Company or industrial clinic
    4. Health department clinic
2. Location or place (address, city)
3. Do you visit a dentist regularly?
    _____ Yes   _____ No
4. In general, would you say that you are very satisfied, satisfied, dissatisfied, or very dissatisfied with the dental care you and your family get?
    1. _____ Very satisfied
    2. _____ Satisfied
    3. _____ Dissatisfied
    4. _____ Very dissatisfied
5. Has anyone in your household been refused dental care by a dentist in the past year?
    _____ Yes
    _____ No
    _____ Don't know

If yes:
6. How many times? ____
7. Where? ____
8. Why were you refused? _____
_____

The following are reasons why some households have no regular dentist or clinic. Please check the major reason why your household uses no regular dentist or clinic (*check one only*).

9. ____ Have recently moved here and have not yet sought dental care.
10. ____ Have never needed dental care.
11. ____ Just never have gotten around to trying to find a dentist.
12. ____ Get dental care at many different places—no regular place.
13. ____ Have no teeth or false teeth—do not need a dentist.
14. ____ Do not know how to find a dentist.
15. ____ Have tried to find a dentist but was refused care.
16. ____ Afraid of dentist.
17. ____ Dentist recently retired.
18. ____ Cost of care.
19. ____ Disliked service received previously.
20. ____ Other (please specify) _____
_____

(*Note: The remainder of the survey contains specific questions that address household medical costs and health insurance.*)

Appendix 3

A Typology of Nursing Problems in Family Nursing Practice

First-Level Assessment

I. Presence of health threats, health deficits, and foreseeable crisis or stress points in the family.

    A. Health Threats—conditions that are conducive to disease, accident, or failure to realize one's health potential. Examples of these are the following:

        1. family history of hereditary disease—e.g., diabetes

        2. threat of cross infection from a communicable disease case

        3. family size beyond what family resources can adequately provide

        4. accident hazards—e.g., broken stairs, pointed sharp objects, poisons, and medicines improperly kept, fire hazards, fall hazards

        5. nutritional
       a. inadequate food intake both in quantity and quality
       b. excessive intake of certain nutrients
       c. faulty eating habits

        6. stress-provoking factors—e.g.,
       a. strained marital relationship
       b. strained parent-sibling relationship
       c. immature parents
       d. interpersonal conflicts between family members

        7. poor environmental sanitation
       a. inadequate living space
       b. inadequate personal belongings/utensils
       c. lack of food storage facilities
       d. polluted water supply
       e. presence of breeding places of insects and rodents
       f. improper refuse disposal
       g. unsanitary waste disposal
       h. improper drainage system
       i. poor lighting and ventilation
       j. noise pollution
       k. air pollution
       l. unsanitary food handling and preparation

        8. personal habits/practices—e.g.,
       a. excessive drinking of alcohol
       b. excessive smoking
       c. walking barefooted
       d. eating raw meat/fish
       e. poor personal hygiene
       f. self-medication

        9. inherent personality characteristics—e.g., short temper

      10. health history which may precipitate/induce the occurrence of a health problem, e.g., previous history of difficult labor

      11. inappropriate role assumption—e.g., child assuming mother's role; father not assuming his role

      12. inadequate immunization status, especially of children

      13. family disunity—e.g.,
       a. self-oriented behavior

      b. unresolved conflicts of member(s)
      c. intolerable disagreements

B. Health Deficits—instances of failure in health maintenance. These include:
1. illness states, regardless of whether they are diagnosed or undiagnosed
2. failure to thrive/develop according to normal rate

C. Stress Points/Foreseeable Crisis Situations—anticipated periods of unusual demand on the individual or family in terms of adjustment/family resources. Examples of these include:
1. marriage
2. pregnancy, labor, puerperium
3. parenthood
4. additional member of a family—e.g., newborn, lodger
5. abortion
6. entrance at school
7. adolescence
8. loss of job
9. death of a member
10. resettlement in a new community
11. illegitimacy

Second-Level Assessment

II. Inability to recognize the presence of a problem due to:

A. Ignorance of facts

B. Fear of consequences of diagnosis of problem
1. social—stigma, loss of respect of peer/significant others
2. economic—cost
3. physical/psychological

C. Attitude/philosophy in life

III. Inability to make decisions with respect to taking appropriate health action due to:

A. Failure to comprehend the nature, magnitude/scope of the problem

B. Low salience of the problem

C. Feeling of confusion and resignation brought about by failure to break down problems into manageable units of attack

D. Lack of knowledge/insight as to alternative courses of action open to them

E. Inability to decide which action to take from among a list of alternatives

F. Conflicting opinions among family members regarding action to take

G. Ignorance of community resources for care

H. Fear of consequences of action
1. social
2. economic
3. physical/psychological

I. Negative attitude towards the health problem—A negative attitude is one that interferes with rational decision making

J. Inaccessibility of appropriate resources of care
1. physical—location
2. cost

K. Lack of trust/confidence in health personnel/agency

L. Misconceptions of erroneous information about proposed course(s) of action.

IV. Inability to provide nursing care to the sick, disabled, or dependent member of the family due to:

A. Ignorance of the facts about the disease/health condition (nature, severity, complications, prognosis, and management); child development and child care

B. Ignorance of the nature and extent of the nursing care needed

C. Lack of the necessary facilities (equipment and supplies) for care

D. Lack of knowledge and skill in carrying out the necessary treatment/procedure/care

E. Inadequate family resources for care
1. responsible family member
2. financial
3. physical resources—e.g., isolation room

F. Negative attitude towards the sick/disabled or dependent member of the family

G. Presence of personal/psychological conflicts

H. Attitude/philosophy in life

I. Self-oriented behavior of family members

V. Inability to provide a home environment which is conducive to health maintenance and personal development due to:

A. Inadequate family resources
1. financial
2. responsible/competent family members
3. physical—e.g., lack of space to construct facility

B. Failure to see benefits (especially long-term ones) of investments in home environment improvement

C. Ignorance of importance of hygiene and sanitation

D. Presence of personal/psychological conflicts, e.g.,
  1. identity crisis/role confusion
  2. jealousy/rivalry
  3. guilt feelings

E. Ignorance of preventive measures

F. Attitude/philosophy in life

G. Family disunity, e.g.,
  1. self-oriented behavior of members
  2. intolerable disagreements
  3. lack of support to member in crisis

VI. Failure to utilize community resources for health care due to:

A. Ignorance or lack of awareness of community resources for health care

B. Failure to perceive the benefits of health care/ services

C. Lack of trust/confidence in agency/personnel

D. Previous unpleasant experience with health worker

E. Fear of consequences of action (preventive, diagnostic, therapeutic, rehabilitative)
  1. physical/psychological
  2. financial
  3. social—e.g., loss of esteem of peer/significant others

F. Unavailability of required care/service

G. Inaccessibility of required care/service
  1. cost
  2. physical—location

H. Lack of or inadequate family resources
  1. manpower—e.g., baby sitter
  2. financial—e.g., cost of medicine prescribed

I. Feeling of alienation to/lack of support from the community, e.g., mental illness

J. Attitude/philosophy in life

SOURCE:
Bailon SG, Maglaya AS: *Family Health Nursing—The Process.* Quezon City: SG Bailon and AS Maglaya, University of the Philippines College of Nursing, 1978: pp. 37–41. Reprinted with permission.

Appendix 4

Michigan Alcoholism Screening Test (MAST) (Revised 11/14/77)

Melvin L. Selzer, M.D., Professor of Psychiatry, University of Michigan

Points			Yes	No
	0.	Do you enjoy a drink now and then?	____	____
(2)	*1.	Do you feel you are a normal drinker? (By normal we mean you drink less than or as much as most other people.)	____	____
(2)	2.	Have you ever awakened the morning after some drinking the night before and found that you could not remember a part of the evening?	____	____
(1)	3.	Does your wife, husband, a parent, or other near relative ever worry or complain about your drinking?	____	____
(2)	*4.	Can you stop drinking without a struggle after one or two drinks?	____	____
(1)	5.	Do you ever feel guilty about your drinking?	____	____
(2)	*6.	Do friends or relatives think you are a normal drinker?	____	____
(2)	*7.	Are you able to stop drinking when you want to?	____	____
(5)	8.	Have you ever attended a meeting of Alcoholics Anonymous (AA)?	____	____
(1)	9.	Have you gotten into physical fights when drinking?	____	____
(2)	10.	Has your drinking ever created problems between you and your wife, husband, a parent, or other near relative?	____	____
(2)	11.	Has your wife, husband, or other family members ever gone to anyone for help about your drinking?	____	____
(2)	12.	Have you ever lost friends because of your drinking?	____	____
(2)	13.	Have you ever gotten into trouble at work because of drinking?	____	____
(2)	14.	Have you ever lost a job because of drinking?	____	____
(2)	15.	Have you ever neglected your obligations, your family, or your work for two or more days in a row because you were drinking?	____	____
(1)	16.	Do you drink before noon fairly often?	____	____
(2)	17.	Have you ever been told you have liver trouble? Cirrhosis?	____	____
(2)	**18.	After heavy drinking have you ever had delirium tremens (D.T.s) or severe shaking, or heard voices or seen things that really weren't there?	____	____
(5)	19.	Have you ever gone to anyone for help about your drinking?	____	____

(5)	20.	Have you ever been in a hospital because of drinking?
(2)	21.	Have you ever been a patient in a psychiatric hospital or on a psychiatric ward of a general hospital where drinking was part of the problem that resulted in hospitalization?
(2)	22.	Have you ever been seen at a psychiatric or mental health clinic or gone to any doctor, social worker, or clergyman for help with any emotional problem, where drinking was part of the problem?
(2)	•••23.	Have you ever been arrested for drunk driving, driving while intoxicated, or driving under the influence of alcoholic beverages?
		(If YES, how many times? _____)
(2)	•••24.	Have you ever been arrested, or taken into custody, even for a few hours, because of other drunk behavior?
		(If, YES, how many times? _____)

* Alcoholic response is negative.

** 5 points for delirium tremens

*** 2 points for *each* arrest

Scoring System:

In general five points or more would place the subject in an "alcoholic" category. Four points would suggest alcoholism, three points or less would indicate the subject was not alcoholic. Programs using the above scoring system find it very sensitive at the five point level, and there is a tendency to find more people alcoholic than anticipated. However, it is a *screening* test only and should be sensitive. In other words, it gives useful evidence of suspected problems but is not considered adequate for positive diagnosis of alcoholism.

SOURCE:
Selzer, M.L., The Michigan Alcoholism Screening Test (MAST): The quest for a new diagnostic instrument. *American Journal of Psychiatry*, 127: 1653–1658, 1971. Copyright 1971, the American Psychiatric Association. Reprinted by permission.

Appendix 5

Study Questions Answer Key

Chapter 1

1. c, *pp. 5–7*
2. b, *p. 12*
3. c, *p. 8*
4. d, *p. 18*

Chapter 2

1. a, *pp. 44–47*
2. c, *pp. 40–43*
3. b, *pp. 37–39*
4. b, *p. 36*
5. a, *pp. 34, 36, 51*

Chapter 3

1. a, *p. 57*
2. d, *pp. 61–62*
3. c, *pp. 61–62*
4. d, *p. 60*

Chapter 4

1. c, *pp. 78–82*
2. c, *p. 76*
3. a, *p. 83*
4. a, *pp. 78–79*

Chapter 5

1. b, *pp. 99–100, 102–103*
2. c, *pp. 100, 104*
3. b, *p. 103*
4. a, *p. 118*
5. a, *pp. 103, 123*
6. a, *pp. 103, 106*

Chapter 6

1. a, *pp. 136–137*
2. b, *p. 146*
3. c, *pp. 137–138*

4. b, *pp. 139–140*
5. d, *pp. 135–138*

Chapter 7

1. a, *p. 157*
2. b, *pp. 162–166*
3. d, *p. 167*
4. d, *pp. 168–169*
5. d, *p. 172*

Chapter 8

1. d, *p. 185*
2. b, *pp. 185–186*
3. a, *p. 187*
4. c, *pp. 195–196*

Chapter 9

1. b, *pp. 217–219*
2. b, *p. 212*
3. d, *p. 211*

Chapter 10

1. c, *pp. 229–230*
2. c, *pp. 232–234*
3. c, *p. 236*
4. d, *pp. 242–243*

Chapter 11

1. b, *p. 249*
2. c, *pp. 255–258*
3. e, *pp. 255–258*
4. b, *pp. 251–253*

Chapter 12

1. b, *p. 268*
2. d, *p. 278*
3. c, *p. 275*

4. c, *p. 283*
5. a, *p. 282*
6. c, *pp. 291–292*

Chapter 13

1. d, *pp. 298, 314–315*
2. c, *p. 302*
3. c, *p. 313*
4. b, *pp. 316–320*
5. d, *p. 323*
6. c, *pp. 310, 324*
7. a, *pp. 309, 323*
8. d, *p. 326*
9. b, *p. 329*
10. a, *pp. 325–326*

Chapter 14

1. d, *p. 337*
2. d, *pp. 343–344*
3. d, *pp. 338–339*
4. d, *p. 344*
5. d, *pp. 346–347*

Chapter 15

1. a, b, and d, *pp. 357, 358*
2. b and d, *pp. 357, 358*
3. b, *pp. 362, 363*
4. c and d, *p. 362*
5. b, *p. 368*
6. d, *p. 369*

Chapter 16

1. a, *p. 378*
2. b, *p. 385*
3. d, *pp. 378–379*
4. d, *pp. 380–381*
5. b, *p. 400*

Chapter 17

1. b, *p. 409*
2. a, *p. 410*
3. d, *p. 410*
4. c, *pp. 414–415*
5. d, *p. 418*
6. a, *p. 422*

Chapter 18

1. b, *pp. 433–435*
2. d, *pp. 435–436*
3. d, *pp. 437–439*
4. c, *pp. 438–441*
5. c, *p. 447*

Chapter 19

1. b, *p. 465*
2. d, *pp. 467–468*
3. a, *pp. 479–480*
4. c, *p. 469*
5. b, *pp. 483–484*
6. b, *pp. 477, 479*
7. d, *pp. 475–476*

Chapter 20

1. b, *p. 489*
2. b, *pp. 493–496*
3. a, *pp. 490–492*
4. d, *pp. 493–496*
5. c, *pp. 497–498*

Chapter 21

1. c, *pp. 517–520*
2. d, *pp. 520–527*
3. c, *pp. 536–541*
4. d, *pp. 537–538*

Chapter 22

1. a, *pp. 547–548*
2. c, *p. 559*
3. b, *pp. 559–560*
4. d, *pp.. 563–570*
5. b, *p. 547*
6. d, *pp. 560–562*

Chapter 23

1. a, *pp. 579, 580*
2. b, *p. 583*
3. d, *p. 585*
4. a, *pp. 580–582*
5. f, *pp. 588–590*
6. a, *pp. 597–598*

Chapter 24

1. d, *pp. 621–622*
2. b, *pp. 616–618*
3. c, *pp. 624–625*
4. d, *pp. 631–632*
5. d, *pp. 614–616*

Chapter 25

1. b, *pp. 637–638*
2. d, *p. 642*
3. a, *p. 643*
4. d, *pp. 646–647*
5. d, *pp. 651–653*

Chapter 26

1. b, *p. 672*
2. d, *p. 673*
3. a, *pp. 676–678*
4. b, *pp. 678–679*
5. c, *p. 680*

Chapter 27

1. d, *p. 696*
2. b, *pp. 700–701*
3. c, *pp. 706–708*
4. d, *p. 716*
5. b, *pp. 708–709, 715*
6. a, *p. 715*
7. d, *pp. 718–719*

Chapter 28

1. a, *pp. 742–744*
2. d, *pp. 744–745*
3. a, b, c, and d, *pp. 730–731*
4. d, *pp. 729–730*
5. d, *pp. 744–747*

Index

1930 Estelle Massey and Mable Staupers, two outstanding Black nursing leaders, were invited by the NOPHN to join committees, marking the first time Black nurses participated in organizational work of NOPHN.

1930–31 White House Conferences findings on child heath motivated the school nursing section of NOPHN, under the leadership of Leah Blaisdell and Lulu Dilworth, to revise "Functions and Qualifications of School Nurses." School nursing gained in importance as a result.

1933 The Federal Emergency Relief Administration permitted states to use federal money for nursing care of the sick at home.

1934 Pearl McIver became the first public health nurse employed by the United States Public Health Service (USPHS) to provide consultation to state health departments.

1935 The Social Security Act, of which Title VI was particularly important for public health nursing, was passed.

Tax-supported official agencies began to assume responsibilities that, previous to 1935, were the prerogative of voluntary agencies—mostly visiting nurse associations. Following the passage of the Social Security Act some bedside nursing, maternal and child health, and crippled children's services came under the aegis of official health agencies.

The Social Security Act stimulated state health departments to develop their programs. The need for public health nurse consultants resulted in the assignment of Pearl McIver to the "States Relations Division" of the Public Health Service. McIver's task was to assist states to improve their public health nursing services. Public health nursing consultation to state health departments began.

1942 The American Association of Industrial Nurses was founded. It developed independently of NOPHN.

1945 Haven Emerson's "Local Health Units for the Nation" was published. Standards were set for local health departments—among them that in a generalized public health nursing program the ratio of public health nurses to population should be 1:5000. That ratio excluded bedside nursing; the ratio for bedside nursing was 1:2500.

1946 Margaret Arnstein, USPHS, headed a project to provide an accounting plan for determining public health nursing costs. A cost manual resulted from the study, and it was used by many public health nursing agencies. This provided a plan for the establishment of payment schedules.

1946 The National Mental Health Act was passed. It assisted states in establishing community mental health centers, and it provided money for the education of nurses in psychiatric nursing.

1946 Hill-Burton Hospital Construction and Survey Act. The passage of this act allocated funds to build public health and hospital facilities.

1949 Lucille Petry was appointed Assistant Surgeon General in the Public Health Service, the first woman and the first nurse to receive such an appointment.

1951 Ruth Freeman was the first nurse to be appointed to the executive board of APHA.

1952 The study of the structure of the nursing organization begun in 1946 led to the establishment of two nursing organizations: American Nurses' Association (ANA) and National League for Nursing (NLN). NOPHN was dissolved and interests and resources merged with NLN. This was a landmark not only for nursing but for public health